# FRAGILE X SYNDROME

# Fragile X Syndrome

## Diagnosis, Treatment, and Research

### Third Edition

EDITED BY

## Randi Jenssen Hagerman, M.D.

Tsakopoulos-Vismara Chair in Pediatrics
and Medical Director of the M.I.N.D. Institute
University of California, Davis

AND

## Paul J. Hagerman, M.D., Ph.D.

Professor of Biological Chemistry
University of California, Davis

THE JOHNS HOPKINS UNIVERSITY PRESS

Baltimore and London

© 1991, 1996, 2002 The Johns Hopkins University Press
All rights reserved. First edition 1991
Third edition 2002
Printed in the United States of America on acid-free paper
2  4  6  8  9  7  5  3  1

The Johns Hopkins University Press
2715 North Charles Street
Baltimore, Maryland 21218-4363
www.press.jhu.edu

Library of Congress Cataloging-in-Publication Data
Fragile X syndrome : diagnosis, treatment, and research / edited by
Randi Jenssen Hagerman and Paul J. Hagerman. — 3rd ed.
p.    cm.
Includes bibliographical references and index.
ISBN 0-8018-6843-2 (hbk. : alk. paper)—ISBN 0-8018-6844-0 (pbk. : alk. paper)
1. Fragile X syndrome.   I. Hagerman, Randi Jenssen, 1949–   .
II. Hagerman, Paul J.

RJ506.F73F74   2002
616.85′884—dc21          2001050347

A catalog record for this book is available from the British Library.

*To our parents, who have given us life and guidance;*
*to our daughters, Karin and Hillary, who give us joy;*
*to the families touched by fragile X, who give our work meaning*

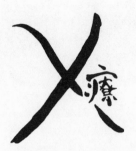

# CONTENTS

# CONTRIBUTORS

Andrea Beckel-Mitchener, Ph.D., Beckman Institute, University of Illinois, Urbana, Illinois

Loisa Bennetto, Ph.D., University of Rochester, New York

Marcia L. Braden, Ph.D., Colorado School for Psychology, Colorado Springs, Colorado

W. Ted Brown, M.D., Ph.D., Department of Human Genetics, Institute for Basic Research in Developmental Disabilities, Staten Island, New York

Franci Crepeau-Hobson, Child Development Unit, Children's Hospital, Denver, Colorado

Amy Cronister, M.S., Genzyme Genetics, Phoenix, Arizona

Jennifer L. Hills Epstein, Psy.D., Child Development Unit, Children's Hospital, Denver, Colorado

Roberto Galvez, Beckman Institute, University of Illinois, Urbana, Illinois

Louise W. Gane, M.S., M.I.N.D. Institute, University of California at Davis, Davis, California

Kristen Gray, M.A., E.C.E., Assistive Technology for All, Denver, Colorado

William Greenough, Ph.D., Beckman Institute, University of Illinois, Urbana, Illinois

Andrew Halpern, M.D., Child Development Unit, Children's Hospital, Denver, Colorado

Susan Harris, M.I.N.D. Institute, University of California at Davis, Sacramento, California

Andre T. Hoogeveen, Ph.D., Department of Clinical Genetics, Erasmus University Medical School, Rotterdam, The Netherlands

Scott Irwin, M.D., Beckman Institute, University of Illinois, Urbana, Illinois

Lisa Nobel, M.S., Assistive Technology Center, Children's Hospital, Denver, Colorado

Rebecca O'Connor, M.A., Children's Hospital, Denver, Colorado

Ben A. Oostra, Ph.D., Department of Clinical Genetics, Erasmus University Medical School, Rotterdam, The Netherlands

Bruce F. Pennington, Ph.D., Department of Psychology, University of Denver, Denver, Colorado

Karen Riley, Ph.D., University of Denver, Denver, Colorado

Sarah Scharfenaker, M.A., C.C.C., M.I.N.D. Institute, University of California at Davis, Sacramento, California

Stephanie Sherman, Ph.D., Department of Human Genetics, Emory University School of Medicine, Atlanta, Georgia

William E. Sobesky, Ph.D., Department of Psychiatry, University of Colorado Health Sciences Center, Denver, Colorado

Tracy Stackhouse, O.T.R., M.I.N.D. Institute, University of California at Davis, Sacramento, California

Ivan Jeanne Weiler, Ph.D., Beckman Institute, University of Illinois, Urbana, Illinois

# PREFACE TO THE THIRD EDITION

Since the publication of the second edition of *Fragile X Syndrome* in 1996, substantial advances in our understanding of the disorder have made a third edition essential. These advances include new knowledge of the mechanisms involved in gene expression and of the neurobiology of fragile X and new treatment programs for children, including academic interventions. All of the chapters have been substantially rewritten; there are new chapters on the neurobiology of fragile X syndrome (by Bill Greenough and colleagues), academic interventions (by Marcia Braden), and gene expression (by Paul Hagerman), which encompasses possible molecular interventions. Because our knowledge regarding cytogenetics has not changed substantially, this chapter was not included in the present edition to make room for new chapters and information.

The editorship represents a husband-and-wife collaboration that helps wed molecular and clinical correlations. We have moved to the University of California at Davis since the publication of the previous edition. Randi is now the Tsakopoulos-Vismara Chair in Pediatrics and the medical director of the M.I.N.D. Institute, and Paul is a professor of biological chemistry and a M.I.N.D. Institute investigator. M.I.N.D. stands for Medical Investigation of Neurodevelopmental Disorders; the M.I.N.D. Institute represents a remarkable collaboration among clinicians, basic researchers, and parents. The institute's goal is to find better treatments and, eventually, cures for neurodevelopmental disorders, including fragile X syndrome.

This book would not have been possible without support from parents who have taught us what we know about those affected by fragile X, who have stimulated our passion for treatment and cure, and who, in many cases, have directly supported research. We are particularly thankful to the Boory, Cooper, Kraff, Fishman, Christoff, Clark, Shelton, Mitchel, Geis, Lang, and Mulvey families. The FRAXA Research Foundation, headed by Katie Clapp, has made a great difference in the field through its support of research, both nationally and internationally. The National Fragile X Foundation, with Executive Director Robert Miller, has been remarkable in its educational endeavors for both parents and professionals and its support of research through the William Rosen Fund, established by Arlene and Jeff Cohen, and the LeCover Fund, established by Deborah and Stephen LeCover.

This book represents the dedicated efforts of the authors, who reflect the breadth and depth of the fragile X field and who have spent years in the laboratory and/or working directly with those affected by fragile X syndrome and their families. Their dedication is unsurpassed. We are thankful for the wonderful support of Susan Harris and Andrew Wheeler, who helped with the production of the manuscript and subsequent editing.

The staff and professionals of the Fragile X Treatment and Research Center at the Children's Hospital in Denver have been ever supportive, even after our move to U.C. Davis. We also thank our colleagues for fruitful discussions in Denver and in Davis, including Flora Tassone, Jennifer Hills Epstein, Rebecca Wilson, Karen Riley, Kathleen McKelvie, Rebecca O'Connor, Louise Gane, Sally Rogers, Ed Goldson, Tracy Stackhouse, Sarah (Mouse) Scharfenaker, Jim Grigsby, Lucy Miller, Penny McKenzie, Ann Reynolds, Mary Murphy, Annette Taylor, Susan Harris, Lisa Nobel, Kristen Gray, Cathy Bodine, Marcia Braden, Nancy Mann, Lauren Carpenter, Elsie Vacano, Janine Mills, Robin Hansen, Cindy and Jim Mamay, Dolores Garcia, Beth Goodlin-Jones, Meredith Miller, Maureen Leehey, Tracy Kovach, David Amaral, and the Developmental Psychobiology Research Group (DPRG).

For support of our research, we are grateful to the National Institute of Child Health and Development (NICHD), the Children's Hospital Research Foundation, the FRAXA Foundation, the National Fragile X Foundation, and the M.I.N.D. Institute.

# PART I
## Diagnosis and Research

# CHAPTER 1

# The Physical and Behavioral Phenotype

Randi Jenssen Hagerman, M.D.

## The Spectrum of Involvement in Fragile X Syndrome

Over the last decade, a broader spectrum of involvement in fragile X syndrome (FXS) has been identified than that reported in the 1980s. FXS causes not only mental retardation but also, in milder forms, a variety of learning and emotional problems without significant cognitive deficits (Franke et al. 1998; Sobesky et al. 1996; Tassone et al. 2000c; Hagerman 1999a). The molecular advances over the last decade (see chaps. 2 and 12) and subsequent molecular-clinical correlations have shown that variation in the clinical phenotype is related to changes in the fragile X mental retardation 1 (*FMR1*) gene, such as lack of methylation, the presence of mosaicism, or variation in the activation ratio (the percentage of cells with the normal X as the active X) (Tassone et al. 1999b; Mazzocco et al. 1997b; Mostofsky et al. 1998; Kaufmann et al. 1999; Cohen et al. 1996; de Vries et al. 1996a, 1996b). The immunocytochemical measure of the FMR1 protein (FMRP) in blood provides a way to measure the activity of the *FMR1* gene, and FMRP levels correlate with cognitive involvement (Tassone et al. 1999b; Willemsen et al. 1997; Menon et al. 2000; Bailey et al. 2001b).

Although the most-affected individuals have a full mutation (more than 200 CGG repeats) that is fully methylated, an appreciation for background gene effects that are additive to the effects of the *FMR1* mutation is developing. Problems in the family such as hyperactivity, anxiety, or social deficits that are genetically influenced may have a further effect on the phenotype of the child with FXS. The presence of autism with FXS is associated with severe language and social deficits in addition to a lower IQ compared to that of children with FXS without autism, so children with both disorders are usually at the lowest end of

*Fragile X Syndrome: Diagnosis, Treatment, and Research,* third edition, ed. Randi Jenssen Hagerman and Paul J. Hagerman (Baltimore: Johns Hopkins University Press, 2002), © The Johns Hopkins University Press.

the spectrum of involvement in fragile X (Bailey et al. 1998, 2000, 2001a). Recent studies have shown that FMRP levels do not correlate with the presence of autism (Bailey et al. 2001a), and there may be secondary gene effects that are additive to the *FMR1* mutation that led to autism (Rogers et al. 2001).

Recent evidence also suggests that a subgroup of individuals with the premutation may have mild clinical involvement, such as prominent ears, problems with math, anxiety, attention problems, and/or executive function deficits (Riddle et al. 1998; Lachiewicz et al. 2000a; Hills et al. 2000a; Franke et al. 1998; Hagerman et al. 1996; Tassone et al. 2000c). Tassone et al. (2000a, 2000b) reported *FMR1* gene dysregulation in some individuals with the premutation, which may be the molecular underpinning of mild involvement (see chap. 12). There is also evidence of unique phenotypes in subgroups of individuals with the premutation, including premature menopause in approximately 16% of women with the premutation (Allingham-Hawkins et al. 1999). Most disturbing is the emergence of a unique neurologic phenotype in a subgroup of older men with the premutation, which may include a progressive cerebellar tremor, memory and executive function deficits, ataxia, Parkinsonian features, and generalized brain atrophy (Hagerman et al. 2001a). These symptoms may be related to background gene effects acting in concert with the dysregulation of *FMR1* that leads to elevated messenger RNA (mRNA) levels (see below and chap. 12). The prevalence of this problem in older individuals with the premutation is not presently known.

To review the history of fragile X, it is important to remember that recognition of the classic physical phenotype in males with fragile X syndrome, including large and prominent ears, a long narrow face, and macroorchidism, evolved over a decade. In the early 1970s, Gillian Turner in Australia was impressed with the lack of unusual physical features in this group of patients with X-linked mental retardation (Turner 1983). Escalante (1971), Cantú et al. (1976), and Turner et al. (1975) reported macroorchidism in males with X-linked mental retardation, and Turner et al. (1978) subsequently linked macroorchidism and the marker X or FXS chromosome. Approximately 80% of patients with FXS will have one or more of these features, but their presence varies with age (fig. 1.1). Additional features, including velvetlike skin (Turner et al. 1980), hyperextensible finger joints (Hagerman et al. 1984), a high-arched palate, flat feet, and pectus excavatum, stimulated Opitz et al. (1984) to hypothesize the existence of a connective tissue dysplasia in FXS. This hypothesis led to further investigations concerning cardiac abnormalities, and subsequently mitral valve prolapse was found in the majority of older patients with FXS (Loehr et al. 1986). A defect in connective tissue has not been proven, but light microscopic studies by Waldstein et al. (1987) demonstrated abnormal elastin fibers in the skin, aorta, and cardiac valves in males with FXS. We have yet to understand how the mutation in the *FMR1* gene causes a connective tis-

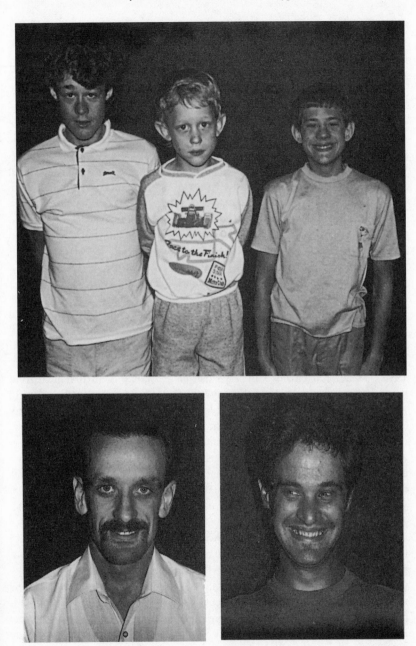

**Fig. 1.1.** Males with fragile X syndrome who show some typical facial features, such as prominent ears, prominent forehead, and/or a long narrow face.

sue problem, although it will probably involve the interaction of FMRP and mRNAs related to connective tissue structure.

The *FMR1* gene was identified and sequenced in 1991 by an international collaborative effort (Verkerk et al. 1991; Yu et al. 1991; Vincent et al. 1991; Bell et al. 1991; see chap. 2). Individuals affected by FXS were found to have an extensive trinucleotide $(CGG)_n$ sequence that was over 200 repeats in size and completely methylated such that a normal level of FMRP was not produced (Fu et al. 1991; Pieretti et al. 1991). The lack or a deficiency of FMRP causes the physical, cognitive, and behavioral features that we identify as FXS. The details of molecular studies of *FMR1* are reviewed in chapters 2 and 12, and what is known about the function of FMRP is reviewed in chapters 4 and 5. Although FMRP is thought to be an mRNA carrier protein that binds to approximately 4% of human fetal brain messages in vitro (Ashley et al. 1993), it is unclear whether the phenotype in FXS is related to the lack of carrying mRNAs from other genes or if it is simply a direct effect of the absence of FMRP in other cellular processes. What is known is that there is a spectrum of involvement in FXS, which has been better appreciated since the discovery of *FMR1*.

The spectrum of phenotypic involvement is futher expanded by females with the full mutation who also have a normal X chromosome that can produce FMRP. The degree of phenotypic involvement in females with the full mutation is most closely associated with the activation ratio (Abrams et al. 1994; Sobesky et al. 1996; Riddle et al. 1998; de Vries et al. 1996b; Mostofsky et al. 1998). Therefore, females with FXS can have a range of involvement from mental retardation and all of the physical features described below to mild learning disabilities without remarkable physical involvement. Approximately 70% of females with the full mutation will have cognitive deficits in the borderline to mentally retarded range (Rousseau et al. 1991a, 1994a; Hagerman et al. 1992; Steinbach et al. 1993; de Vries et al. 1996b; Riddle et al. 1998). However, those with a normal IQ will usually have significant learning disabilities and/or emotional difficulties (Hagerman et al. 1992; Mazzocco et al. 1993, 1997a; Abrams et al. 1994; Sobesky et al. 1994a, 1994b, 1996; Riddle et al. 1998).

The spectrum of involvement in FXS may be most easily understood by picturing a gradual decrement of FMRP production from normal levels to complete absence. In mildly affected individuals the IQ may be normal, but learning problems or emotional difficulties may be present. With lower FMRP levels more severe cognitive and physical features are present. The full FXS, including mental retardation as well as physical and behavioral features described below, is seen when there is little or no FMRP present. Chapter 6 will review the cognitive and neuropsychological deficits in FXS. This chapter will describe the physical and behavioral features of FXS and detail the molecular/clinical correlations of these features.

## Physical Phenotype

### Facial Features

The classic features of a long narrow face and prominent ears are often not present in the prepubertal child (fig. 1.2) (Chudley and Hagerman 1987; Verma and Elango 1994). However, there exists a gestalt of additional facial features that are helpful to the experienced clinician in suggesting the diagnosis of FXS. Hockey and Crowhurst (1988) attempted to characterize these features in a retrospective study of photographs from infancy in children with FXS. Common findings include puffiness around the eyes and narrow palpebral fissures, a large head relative to the body, epicanthal folds, strabismus, and hypotonia. Simko et al. (1989) found epicanthal folds in 8 of 20 boys with FXS. The broad palpebral fissures or long but narrow eye openings are a particularly helpful finding in a subgroup of young boys with FXS (fig. 1.3). Butler et al. (1988) evaluated photoanthropometric measures to demonstrate long palpebral fissures in FXS, compared to controls.

Prominent ears are common in males with FXS and are often present even in prepubertal boys. Simko et al. (1989) found long, wide, or protruding ears in 15 of 20 (75%) boys with FXS. Merenstein et al. (1996) found prominent ears in 78% of 97 prepubertal boys with the full mutation but in only 20% of 5 boys

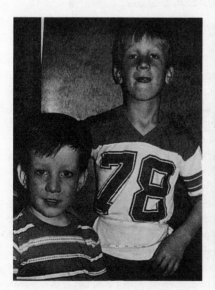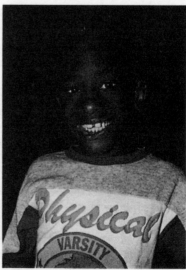

**Fig. 1.2.** Prepubertal boys with fragile X syndrome who do not have remarkably distinguishing physical features. *Source:* Hagerman (1987). Reprinted with permission.

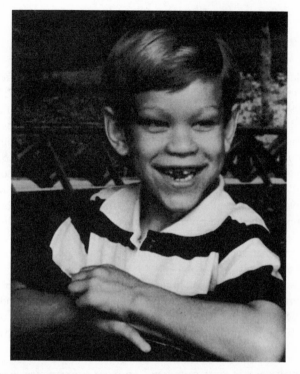

**Fig. 1.3.** Narrow palpebral fissures and puffy eyelids in a boy with fragile X syndrome.

with a partially methylated full mutation and in 86% of 29 boys with a mosaic pattern. A somewhat lower prevalence for prominent ears was seen in pubertal and postpubertal males. The ears may also be long or wide, with the occasional loss of the antihelical fold, so that the upper pinna may be cupped out (fig. 1.4). Surgical pinning of the ear is a treatment option if ear prominence is dramatic and psychologically stressful for the child. Ear width is a more discriminating feature in identifying patients with FXS than is ear length, and it is more easily quantified than is ear prominence (Butler et al. 1991; Lisik et al. 2000). Butler and colleagues (1991a, 1991b) used a combination of discriminating anthropomorphic variables including testicular volume, ear width, bizygomatic diameter (narrower in patients with FXS than in controls), and head breadth (wider in patients with FXS than in controls) and correctly distinguished patients with FXS from retarded patients without FXS in 95% of cases.

The jaw may be prominent in men and women with FXS, but it is not usually prominent in children. Loesch et al. (1993b) showed that the jaw length increases disproportionately to an increase in body height in patients with FXS

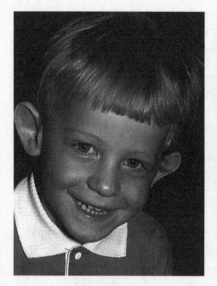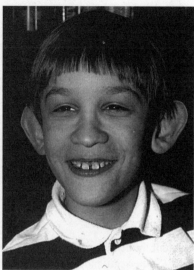

**Fig. 1.4.** Boys with fragile X syndrome who have ears that are prominent and cupped out in the upper part of the pinnae.

compared to controls. Therefore, the jaw is usually large in adulthood in patients with FXS. In addition, the face becomes long during and after puberty. A long face is clinically noticeable in 80% of adult males with the full mutation (tables 1.1 and 1.2). The cause of the long face and prominent jaw is unknown, although a mild acromegalic effect secondary to episodic growth hormone excess has not been ruled out. Growth hormone abnormalities could be related to the hypothalamic problems in FXS (discussed below). Dental maturity has also been found to be advanced in children with FXS, although it is uncertain whether this is hormonal or related to accelerated early growth in FXS described below (Kotilainen and Pirinen 1999).

A high-arched palate has been reported by several authors (Hagerman et al. 1983; Partington 1984; Sutherland and Hecht 1985). In our experience this is a common feature (tables 1.1 and 1.2), but it is hard to quantitate with measurements inside the mouth. A high palate is usually narrow and is often seen in association with dental crowding or malocclusion. Partington (1984) reported the presence of cleft palate in 5 of 61 (8%) males with FXS, and Hagerman (1987) reported a child with Pierre Robin malformation sequence including a cleft palate who was subsequently diagnosed with FXS. Four additional cases of Pierre Robin sequence in association with FXS were reported by Lachiewicz et al. (1991). This frequency of association suggests that cleft palate is not coincidental and that the connective tissue abnormalities of FXS place these patients at higher risk for the Pierre Robin sequence. Hjalgrim et al. (2000) reported histological studies in six fetuses with FXS and found delayed ossification of nasal bones, acid mucupolysaccharide malfunction in the supporting tissue, and epithelial fusion of the palatal processes persisting longer than normal. One fetus also demonstrated hand anomalies with an abnormal ossification sequence. Loesch et al. (1992) reported a family with FXS and cleft lip and palate with additional minor limb anomalies consistent with FG syndrome. A similar family with FXS and FG syndrome in several members was also reported by Piussan et al. (1996). Clearly, further research is needed for us to understand the connective tissue changes and the molecular mechanism of these changes in FXS.

## Macroorchidism

Macroorchidism (large testicles) is present in over 80% of adult males with FXS (Sutherland and Hecht 1985; Merenstein et al. 1996). However, males with FXS have been documented to be fertile and capable of reproduction (Willems et al. 1992; Rousseau et al. 1994b). Importantly, the sperm of males with the full mutation contains the premutation even though the full mutation is present in all other tissues (Reyniers et al. 1993). Malter et al. (1997) have evidence of a back mutation of a full mutation to a premutation in spermatogonia in early fetal development, such that FMRP begins to be produced in spermatogonia and subsequently in sperm. There seems to be a selection advantage for sperm with the premutation instead of the full mutation, although FMRP is not necessary for reproduction, since the knockout fragile X mouse is fertile and can reproduce (chap. 4).

Macroorchidism is seen in a much smaller percentage of prepubertal boys than postpubertal males, and a dramatic increase in the size of the testicle has been seen in boys with FXS between 8 and 10 years, presumably secondary to gonadotropin stimulation (Lachiewicz et al. 1994b). Lachiewicz and Dawson (1994b) found macroorchidism of ≥4.0 ml in only 1 of 27 boys with FXS between 2 and 7 years. Tables 1.1 and 1.2 show a higher frequency of macroorchidism, since they included measurements of 3-ml volume or larger in the prepubertal children. Lachiewicz's study demonstrated that occasionally 3 ml in volume occurs in prepubertal patients in the general population. Butler et al. (1992) documented a cross-sectional growth curve for testicular volume changes in over 185 males with FXS compared to normals (fig. 1.5). The majority of adult males with FXS have a testicular volume of 40 to 60 ml (fig. 1.6).

Macroorchidism is usually measured with an orchidometer, a series of ellipsoid shapes of a known volume that are compared directly with the testicle. The Prader orchidometer (figs. 1.6 and 1.7) includes shapes with volumes of 2–

**Table 1.1**
**Proportions of Prepubertal Boys and Girls with Features**

| | Males with Full Mutation | | | |
|---|---|---|---|---|
| Physical Feature | Fully Methylated (n = 103) | <50% Methylated (n = 10) | Male Mosaic (n = 30) | Females with Full Mutation (n = 40) |
| Long face | 50% | 20% | 47% | 48% |
| Prominent ears | 69% | 50% | 70% | 68% |
| High-arched palate | 62% | 40% | 57% | 53% |
| Hyperextensible finger joints | 72% | 70% | 77% | 60% |
| Double-jointed thumbs | 55% | 50% | 30% | 38% |
| Single palmar crease | 22% | 10% | 17% | 15% |
| Hand calluses | 13% | 0% | 13% | 0% |
| Flat feet | 72% | 80% | 83% | 60% |
| Heart murmur or click | 1% | 0% | 0% | 0% |
| Macroorchidism[a] | 39% | 30% | 13% | — |

*Source:* Adapted and updated from Merenstein et al. 1996.
*Note:* Prepubertal = up to age 12 years 11 months.
[a]Includes testicular size of 3 ml or larger.

**Table 1.2**
**Proportions of Postpubertal Males and Females with Features**

| | Males with Full Mutation | | | |
|---|---|---|---|---|
| Physical Feature | Fully Methylated (n = 64) | <50% Methylated (n = 7) | Male Mosaic (n = 22) | Females with Full Mutation (n = 27) |
| Long face | 80% | 83% | 71% | 59% |
| Prominent ears | 66% | NA | 36% | 30% |
| High-arched palate | 63% | NA | 38% | 81% |
| Hyperextensible finger joints | 49% | 17% | 50% | 30% |
| Double-jointed thumbs | 48% | 17% | 35% | 30% |
| Single palmar crease | 22% | 0% | 48% | 11% |
| Hand calluses | 52% | 0% | 40% | 0% |
| Flat feet | 60% | 17% | 50% | 26% |
| Heart murmur or click | 29% | 33% | 9% | 19% |
| Macroorchidism[a] | 92% | 83% | 91% | — |

*Source:* Adapted and updated from Merenstein et al. 1996.
*Note:* Postpubertal = age 13 and above; NA = not available.
[a]Includes testicular size of 3 ml or larger.

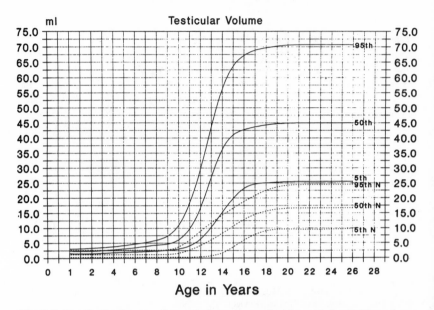

**Fig. 1.5.** Standardized curves for testicular volume of males with fragile X syndrome (*solid line*) and normal males (*broken line*). *Source:* Butler et al. (1992). Reprinted with permission.

25 ml. It can be ordered from Dr. Andrea Prader, Kinderspital Zürich, Switzerland. The Adelaide orchidometer includes volumes of up to 100 ml (Sutherland and Hecht 1985), which is useful in measuring the testicles in adults with FXS. The testicle can also be measured (in centimeters) directly with a tape or calipers, and the volume (in milliliters) can be subsequently calculated using the formula $\pi/6$ (length)(width$^2$).

Prader (1966) and Zachmann et al. (1974) found that the upper limit of the normal testicular volume was 25 ml in adult normal men. Farkas (1976) and Daniel et al. (1982), however, found larger volumes (up to 30 ml) in normal men. Therefore, significant macroorchidism is probably not present until the testicular volume is larger than 30 ml (fig. 1.6). The discrepancies in the normative data are probably accounted for by differences between international populations due to racial variation. Macroorchidism is not specific to FXS, and studies of institutionalized mentally retarded males have shown that the prevalence of macroorchidism is as high as 29%, whereas only 4–27% of men with macroorchidism have FXS (Brøndum-Nielsen et al. 1982; Primrose et al. 1986; Hagerman et al. 1988).

O'Hare et al. (1986) suggested that depletion in melatonin may be associated with macroorchidism. Both macroorchidism and precocious puberty are

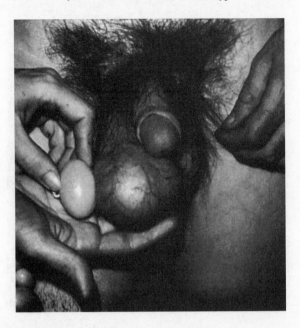

**Fig. 1.6.** Macroorchidism in an adult male with fragile X syndrome. The testicle is compared to a 25-ml volume from the Prader orchidometer. *Source:* Hagerman (1987). Reprinted with permission.

linked to destruction of the pineal gland, which produces melatonin. O'Hare et al. (1986) studied five adult males with FXS and controls and found a significant decrease of melatonin production at night during sleep. Only one patient with FXS did not have macroorchidism and did not have an enlarged penis, and this patient had the highest melatonin levels of the fragile X group. Subsequent studies, however, of saliva melatonin levels in patients with FXS demonstrated elevated melatonin levels compared to controls both during the day and at night (Gould et al. 2000). Elevated melatonin levels may be related to hypothalamic dysfunction in FXS, and elevated melatonin would be likely to inhibit the release of gonadotropins, so this is probably not the cause of macroorchidism. It is unclear how elevated melatonin levels relate to the sleep disturbances that are common in FXS (Musumeci et al. 1995; Elia et al. 2000; Hagerman 1996).

A study by Slegtenhorst-Eegdeman (1998) of the macroorchidism in the *FMR1* knockout (KO) mouse found an enhanced rate of Sertoli cell proliferation in these mice compared to controls. The Sertoli cells support the germ cells, and an enhanced number could stimulate an increase in tubule length in the testes, which has been documented in FXS (Nistal et al. 1992). The Sertoli cells are stimulated to proliferate by follicle-stimulating hormone (FSH), but serum

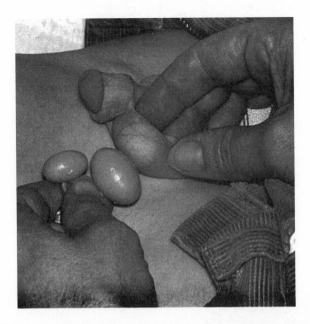

**Fig. 1.7.** Mild macroorchidism (4–5-ml volume) in a four-year-old boy with fragile X syndrome. Note comparative measurements with a Prader orchidometer.

FSH levels were not elevated in the KO mouse compared to controls. The level of FSH receptor mRNA in the testis of the KO mouse was slightly but not significantly elevated compared to controls. Perhaps the deficiency of FMRP may influence the stability of FSH receptor mRNA, and further studies are necessary (Slegtenhorst-Eegdeman et al. 1998). It is known that the germ cells are producing FMRP in normals (Bachner et al. 1993a, 1993b) and in those with FXS because there is a contraction from the full mutation to the premutation in the human fragile X male fetus (Malter et al. 1997). Therefore, it is unlikely that the germ cells are responsible for the macroorchidism, although their expression of FMRP in an environment of somatic cells that lack FMRP may be an important issue for macroorchidism (Slegtenhorst-Eegdeman et al. 1998).

Ultrastructural studies of the testicle in humans have documented an increased ground substance (Shapiro et al. 1986), interstitial fibrosis, edema (Cantú et al. 1976; Johannisson et al. 1987), and abnormal tubular morphology (Rudelli et al. 1985; Nistal et al. 1992). There is limited evidence of reduced spermatogenesis and an excessive number of malformed spermatids, which could cause decreased fertility in males with FXS (Johannisson et al. 1987). Because the sperm contain the premutation, a retarded male would pass only the premutation to all of his daughters. The male offspring would receive

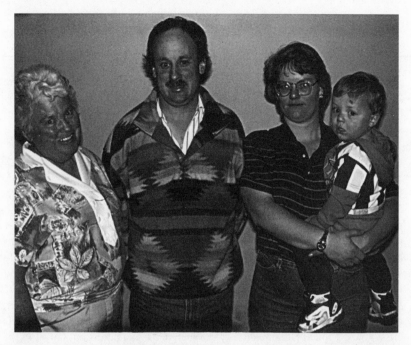

**Fig. 1.8.** An adult male with fragile X syndrome (*center*), with his mother on the left and his wife and son on the right. His mother is a premutation carrier, he is a mosaic, and his wife and son do not have the *FMR1* mutation. His son has normal development.

the Y chromosome from their father, and they would not be affected by FXS (fig. 1.8).

Two cases of testicular tumors in males with FXS have been reported, although it is unclear whether they are related to the *FMR1* gene or to macroorchidism. The first report was of a benign testicular tumor similar to a sperm granuloma in a 34-year-old man with macroorchidism (del Pozo and Millard 1983). In the second case, a classic seminoma in the left testis of a 45-year-old man was removed, but at 50 years of age the patient developed a spermatocystic seminoma in the right testis (Phelan et al. 1988).

A few other cancers have been reported in patients with FXS: a malignant ganglioma in a 17-year-old male (Rodewald et al. 1987), an adenocarcinoma of the colon in a 14-year-old boy (Phelan et al. 1988), a case of acute lymphocytic leukemia in a male (Cunningham and Dickerman 1988), myelodysplastic syndrome in a 33-year-old pregnant woman (Vorst et al. 1993), chronic lymphocytic leukemia in a 62-year-old man (Rudelli et al. 1985), an undifferentiated nasopharyngeal carcinoma in a 16-year-old boy (Ferrari et al. 2000), and a lung tumor in a 66-year-old man (de Graaff et al. 1995b). However, there is not sufficient evidence to support an increased rate of cancer associated with the *FMR1* mutation compared to the general population. The last, a lung tumor, is in a man with the full mutation; however, the lung tumor has a methylated premutation with 160 repeats. The tumor, therefore, arose from cells with the premutation, and it is postulated that all male patients with the full mutation have a low level of mosaicism, that is, a low number of cells (1%) with the premutation (de Graaff et al. 1995b).

## Physical Features in Females with FXS

Escalante (1971) was the first to report mental retardation in females in association with the marker X chromosome. His clinical descriptions included a high palate, genu valgum, and flat feet, which are similar to the connective tissue problems in males with FXS (Vianna-Morgante et al. 1982). Fryns (1986) analyzed the physical features in 135 heterozygotes. He found facial stigmata similar to those in males, including a long face, a prominent forehead, and mandibular prognathism in 28%. These findings were present in 14% of the subjects with normal intelligence and in 55% of those with mental retardation. Loesch and Hay (1988) subsequently studied 90 adult and 20 prepubertal heterozygotes. Typical facial features were seen in 37% of adults but only 14% of girls. Additionally, hypermobility of the finger joints was seen in 40% of adults and 52% of the girls. Flat feet were seen in 19% of both groups. All of the features were more prevalent in mentally impaired heterozygotes compared to normal IQ heterozygotes. Cronister et al. (1991a) compared the physical features of 105 heterozygotes to those of 90 controls but found a paucity of statistical differences, although hyperextensible MP joints and double-jointed thumbs were seen twice as frequently in impaired heterozygotes as in impaired controls. Although less pronounced, there is evidence of a connective tissue dysplasia in affected heterozygotes showing manifestations similar to those of the male. Mildly prominent ears are the most common finding in prepubertal girls with FXS compared to their normal sisters (Hagerman et al. 1992; fig. 1.9). Enlargement of the ovaries has been seen in two affected women who were evaluated by ultrasound (Turner et al. 1986) and in a young girl with FXS who presented with precocious puberty (Moore et al. 1990). Occasionally, more significant malformations, such as cleft palate, have also been reported in heterozygotes (Loesch and Hay 1988).

Physical features typical of FXS are far more common in females with the full mutation than in females with the premutation compared to controls (Hull and Hagerman 1993; Riddle et al. 1998). The earlier studies also documented this finding, but because the full mutation was not yet identified, these females were identified only as "affected" by FXS. Usually the term *affected* refers to

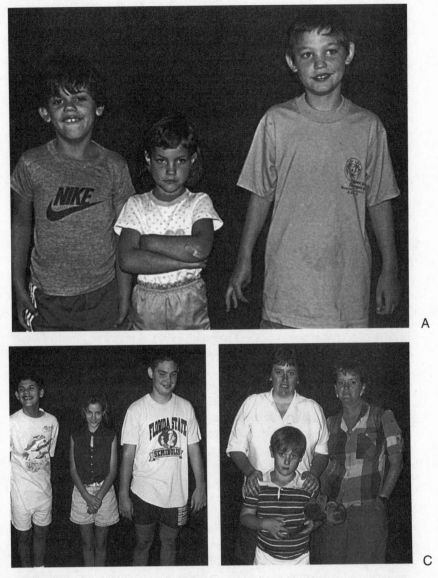

**Fig. 1.9.** *A:* Two boys and a girl with fragile X syndrome who are prepubertal. Note mildly prominent ears in the girl. *B:* The same children as in *A* who are now pubertal. The girl's face is now mildly longer, although her brothers do not have a long face. *C:* Three generations in a family: the unaffected grandmother has a premutation, her daughter has the full mutation and mild learning disabilities, and the grandson has the full mutation and mental retardation.

cognitive deficits, and approximately 70% of females with the full mutation have significant intellectual deficits, that is, an IQ in the borderline (70–84) or mentally retarded range (IQ < 70; Hagerman et al. 1992; Rousseau et al. 1994a; de Vries et al. 1996b). The majority of females with the full mutation and a normal IQ also have learning disabilities related to executive function deficits (Mazzocco et al. 1993; Sobesky et al. 1994b, 1996; Mostofsky et al. 1998) as identified by neuropsychologic testing (chap. 6). The executive function deficits may lead to attentional problems, poor topic maintenance, tangentiality in speech, and impulsive behavior. These mild deficits combined with math problems and typical physical features are helpful in clinically identifying females who may carry the full mutation but do not have mental retardation. Poor eye contact is also a helpful feature, but this problem is often present even in women with the premutation, as are prominent ears (Hull and Hagerman 1993; Riddle et al. 1998).

## Ophthalmologic Findings

Ophthalmologic problems in patients with FXS include strabismus (lazy eye), which was reported in 56% of 16 males (Schinzel and Largo 1985), in 40% of 15 patients (Storm et al. 1987), in 30% of 30 patients (Maino et al. 1991), and in 44% of 55 patients with FXS (King et al. 1995). A recent prospective study of ophthalmologic problems in 48 boys with FXS demonstrated that 25% had significant ocular findings, including 17% with refractive errors and 8% with strabismus (Hatton et al. 1998). The lower incidence of strabismus reported here suggests that previous studies had a selection bias, although even 8% is much higher than the prevalence in the general population (0.5–1%) (Hatton et al. 1998). The type of strabismus reported in all of the studies has varied, including esotropia, exotropia, and hyperdeviations (fig. 1.10). Congenital esotropia was seen in 3 of 55 patients by King et al. (1995), and a total of 5 patients with strabismus required surgery. Hatton et al. (1998) reported successful surgery in two of four patients with strabismus and FXS. Strabismus is a common problem in many developmental disorders and requires early diagnosis and treatment to avoid amblyopia (Maino et al. 1990). Flood and Sanner (1985) and Storm et al. (1987) found frequent refractive errors in patients with FXS, including both myopia and hyperopia. Hatton et al. (1998) reported that hyperopia and astigmatism composed the majority of refractive errors in their patients. Nystagmus was occasionally seen in all studies but was not coincidental with strabismus. Kranjc et al. (1998) described one 4-year-old boy with nystagmus and bilateral macular dysplasia. Although the macular dysplasia may have predisposed this patient to nystagmus, it is probable that the macular dysplasia is a coincidental finding and not part of FXS. King et al. (1995) found amblyopia in 7 patients (13%), and several patients presented with ocular prob-

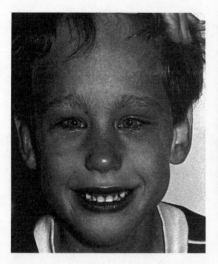 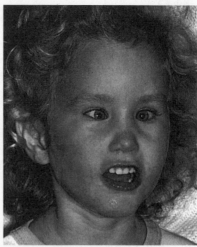

A B

**Fig. 1.10.** *A:* Mild esotropia in the left eye associated with amblyopia in a boy with fragile X syndrome. *B:* More marked esotropia in the right eye of the sister.

lems before a diagnosis of FXS was made. Therefore, ophthalmologists and optometrists should be aware of FXS, and all children with FXS should be evaluated by an ophthalmologist by 4 years of age or sooner if obvious problems are present.

Surgery and/or patching are often necessary to treat strabismus. Ptosis (lid lowering) is also occasionally seen and may require surgery for cosmetic reasons or to avoid amblyopia. Perhaps some of the ophthalmologic findings, particularly high myopia, may be related to connective tissue problems. A recent summary of medical problems, including strabismus, in males with FXS can be found in Table 1.3.

## Otitis and Sinusitis

A frequent complaint of children with FXS is recurrent otitis media (middle ear infection) in early childhood. Although this is a common disorder of all children (Teele et al. 1983), the frequency of infection is excessive in a subgroup of boys with FXS. Hagerman et al. (1987) studied 30 boys with FXS and found that 63% had recurrent otitis compared to 15% of their normal siblings and 38% of developmentally disabled children without FXS. Forty-three percent of the children with FXS required the insertion of one or more sets of polyethylene (PE) tubes in the tympanic membranes. Simko et al. (1989) also found recur-

**Table 1.3**
**Medical Problems of Males with Fragile X Syndrome**

| Problem | % of Patients with Problem |
|---|---|
| Emesis (147)[a] | 31 |
| Failure to thrive in infancy (138) | 15 |
| Strabismus (161) | 36 |
| Glasses (148) | 22 |
| Hernia (230) | 15 |
| Joint dislocation (150) | 3 |
| Orthopedic intervention (171) | 21 |
| Otitis media (291) | 85 |
| History of sinusitis (43) | 23 |
| Seizures (288) | 22 |
| History of apnea (139) | 10 |
| Diagnosis of autism in the past (211) | 20 |
| Diagnosis of ADHD (224) | 80 |
| Motor tics (188) | 19 |
| Psychotic ideation (146) | 12 |

[a]Numbers in parentheses, number of patients evaluated.

rent otitis in 45% of 20 children with FXS. A recent summary of our experience with males with FXS demonstrates that 85% have had at least one otitis infection, whereas 23% have had sinusitis (table 1.3).

Recurrent otitis media is associated with a fluctuating conductive hearing loss and subsequent language and articulation deficits (Bennett and Haggard 1999). Evidence also exists for cognitive sequelae affecting the verbal IQ and behavior problems including hyperactivity (Hagerman and Falkenstein 1987; Paradise et al. 2000; Bennett and Haggard 1999) in otherwise normal children. In the population with mental retardation, abnormal tympanograms secondary to serous otitis have also been associated with a lower IQ compared to those without ear problems (Saxon and Witriol 1976; Libb et al. 1985). Children with FXS usually have significant language and cognitive deficits that can be worsened by the sequelae of recurrent otitis. It is therefore imperative that children with FXS be vigorously monitored and treated for recurrent otitis media so that hearing is always optimal and sequelae are avoided. This often means the insertion of PE tubes when a hearing loss is documented or the use of prophylactic antibiotics to avoid otitis media when a child has a history of recurrent infections (see chap. 8).

Why children with FXS are predisposed to recurrent otitis media infections is unknown. The facial structure, including a long face and a high-arched palate, may affect the angle of the eustachian tube and prevent appropriate drainage of the middle ear. The connective tissue dysplasia and hypotonia may lead to a collapsible eustachian tube, which would also affect drainage. A transient hypogammaglobulinemia was documented in one young boy (Hagerman et al. 1987), and a second child with FXS had an immunoglobulin G (IgG) subclass 1 and 3 deficiency with recurrent otitis and sinusitis. Other cases of hypogammaglobulinemia in FXS have not been reported, so a consistent immunodeficiency is unlikely in this syndrome.

Recurrent sinusitis is not infrequent in FXS, although it is less common than recurrent otitis (table 1.3). The long and narrow face associated with FXS most likely causes problems with drainage of the sinuses. Sinus X-rays are needed to confirm the diagnosis, and treatment includes antibiotics. For recurrent problems, consultation with an ENT physician is necessary to evaluate the need for prophylactic antibiotics or surgical intervention to improve drainage.

## Orthopedic Problems

The most common musculoskeletal manifestations in FXS include flexible pes planus (flat feet), excessive joint laxity, and scoliosis (figs. 1.11 and 1.12). Davids et al. (1990) reviewed the orthopedic problems of 150 males with FXS. Fifty percent demonstrated significant pes planus, which was not associated with pain or disability but was usually associated with uneven shoe wear. Thirty-nine percent of the children with pes planus were seen by an orthopedist before the diagnosis of FXS was made, and almost all were treated with a foot orthosis or with orthopedic shoes. This usually improved the gait pattern and shoe wear. In only one case was foot surgery done, specifically an extra-articular subtalar arthrodesis.

Davids et al. (1990) also evaluated joint laxity and found that 73% of children with FXS younger than 11 years had joint laxity with hyperextensible metacarpophalangeal (MP) joints (MP extensions ≥90%), whereas 56% of those 11 to 19 years of age and 30% of those older than 20 had this finding. This suggests that the ligaments tighten with age. Tables 1.1 and 1.2 show the frequency of hyperextensible MP joints and double-jointed thumbs in the molecular subgroups in childhood and adulthood. There are no statistically significant differences in the molecular subgroups regarding these features, but the tightening of ligaments or less joint laxity is notable with age.

Theoretically, patients with FXS should be at risk for joint dislocations. Although double-jointed thumbs are common in both males and females (fig. 1.12), joint dislocations are uncommon (3%; table 1.3). We followed one patient with recurrent patellar dislocation who eventually required patellectomy (Davids et al. 1990) and a second patient with congenital hip dislocation who was treated at birth. The connective tissue dysplasia may also predispose pa-

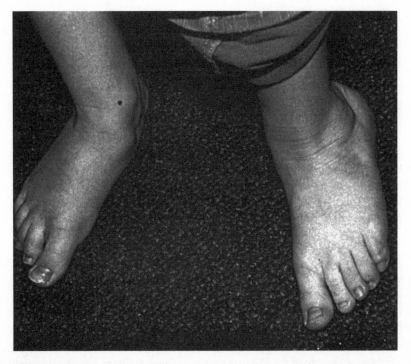

**Fig. 1.11.** Pes plenus (flat feet) with pronation (turning in of the ankle) in a boy with fragile X syndrome.

tients to positional malformations in utero. We have seen 3 cases of clubfoot deformity in 150 males with FXS (fig. 1.13).

## Skin Manifestations

The most notable feature of the skin in patients with FXS is its softness and smoothness. This is particularly noticeable on the hands. The palms may occasionally appear wrinkled, a callus is often present on the hand from hand biting, and a single palmar crease, either a simian crease or a Sydney line (fig. 1.14), is seen in 51% of males (Simpson et al. 1984). A single palmar crease was less frequent in our experience (tables 1.1 and 1.2). Striae are also common on the lateral aspects of the abdomen and sometimes on the upper aspects of the arms and legs in obese patients. This is probably related to the connective tissue abnormalities and elastin problems described below.

The microscopic correlate of smooth, soft skin was studied by Waldstein et al. (1987) in skin biopsies of five males with FXS. There was incomplete or ab-

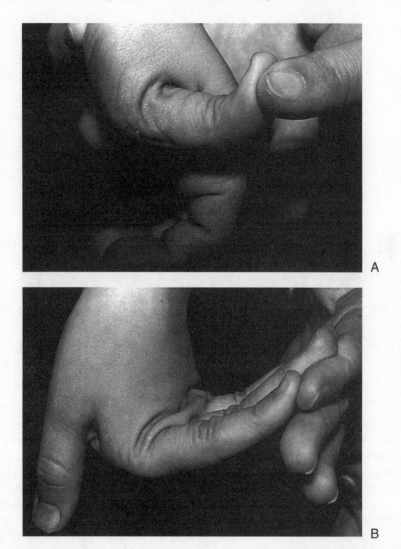

**Fig. 1.12.** *A:* Double-jointed thumb in a boy with fragile X syndrome. *B:* Hyperextensible finger joints with metacarpophalangeal extension of >90° in a boy with fragile X syndrome.

sent arborization of elastin in the papillary dermis and a decreased number of elastin fibrils in the deep dermis when compared to controls. These findings were also seen in a subsequent patient at autopsy (Waldstein and Hagerman 1988). Abnormal elastin fibrils were also present in the aorta and in cardiac

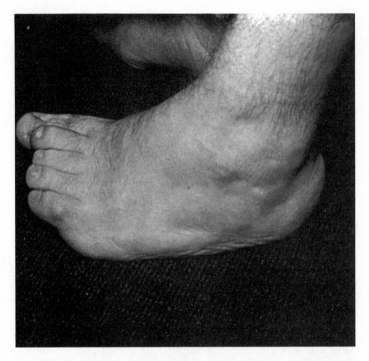

**Fig. 1.13.** Clubfoot deformity in a boy with fragile X syndrome.

valves, and there were hypoplasia of the aorta and mitral valve prolapse. It is likely that the elastin abnormality is part of the connective tissue dysplasia in FXS. Perhaps FMRP is involved in carrying or regulating mRNAs associated with elastin and/or other connective tissue components. This is an issue that requires further study, and it is to be hoped that newer techniques in the genomics or proteomics field will clarify the interaction between FMRP and connective tissue components.

The rare occurrence of cutis verticis gyrata (CVG), which is the development of furrows or folds in the skin of the scalp, giving it a convoluted appearance, has been reported in FXS. Musumeci et al. (1991a) described 2 cases and, in a survey of 20 unrelated institutionalized males with CVG, 5 were found to have FXS (Schepis et al. 1989).

## Cardiac Involvement

Concern for a possible connective tissue dysplasia in FXS led to further studies of cardiac function. Loehr et al. (1986) evaluated 40 patients, mostly adults,

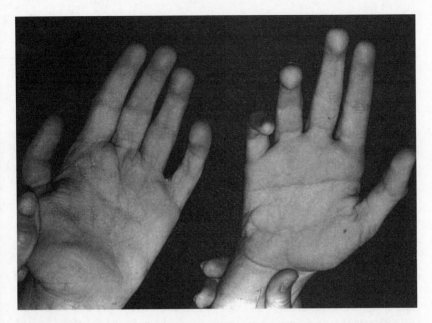

**Fig. 1.14.** The right hand demonstrates a single palmar crease in a boy with fragile X syndrome.

with FXS (including 6 females) and found mitral valve prolapse (MVP) in 55% diagnosed by echocardiographic findings in combination with clinical findings of a click or systolic murmur. A rare male demonstrated significant mitral regurgitation that required more frequent follow-up. MVP was also seen in 3 heterozygous females. Seven males (18%) also had mild dilation of the base of the aorta, but this did not seem to be progressive. These findings were corroborated by Sreeram et al. (1989), who found dilation of the aortic root in 12 of 23 (52%) and MVP in 5 of 23 (22%) men with FXS. Puzzo et al. (1990) studied 13 males and females with FXS and found not only MVP in 77% but tricuspid septal leaflet prolapse in 15% and mild pulmonary artery dilation in 23%. Crabbe et al. (1993) studied young children with FXS (16 boys and 1 girl) and found only 1 boy with auscultatory findings of MVP. None of the patients showed echographic findings of MVP, aortic root dilation, or other abnormality. Crabbe et al. suggested that these problems are less common in the young child with FXS, but rather develop in adolescence and adulthood.

If a click or murmur is present in a patient, a cardiac evaluation that includes an echocardiogram is recommended. If MVP is documented, prophylaxis for subacute bacterial endocarditis is warranted during dental procedures or operations that could contaminate the bloodstream with bacteria. MVP is usually a benign finding, although it can predispose a patient to cardiac arrhythmias. There have been no complaints of arrhythmias in affected males, although palpitations occur in 31% of normal IQ heterozygotes (Cronister et al. 1991a), and in several MVP has been diagnosed. However, MVP is also common in the general population, and we do not know whether its occurrence is increased in heterozygotes compared to controls. It is interesting that MVP is also associated with panic disorder (Hartman et al. 1982), which is a problem for some women with either the full mutation or the premutation (Franke et al. 1996, 1998; Sobesky et al. 1994b, 1996).

Males with FXS do not have a significantly shortened life-span, but cases of sudden death have been reported. One was reported in an 18-year-old with FXS (Waldstein and Hagerman 1988). This teenager presumably died from an arrhythmia precipitated by a viral myocarditis. His autopsy demonstrated a diffuse hypoplasia of the aorta and a mild postductal coarctation. This malformation had not been found previously in FXS, although I recently saw a case of a 9-year-old boy with an atretic segment of the descending aorta that had been repaired at birth. The finding of abnormal elastin fibers in the walls of the aorta and in the cardiac valves in the case reported by Waldstein and Hagerman (1988) suggests a relationship to abnormal connective tissue. A second case of sudden death occurred in a man with FXS at age 29. Death was presumably from a cardiac arrhythmia, but autopsy findings were normal except for mild MVP. DNA studies demonstrated the *FMR1* full mutation, fully methylated in all 12 tissues evaluated, including 3 areas of the brain (Tassone et al. 1999a). The patient was not taking medication, and there was no evidence of a viral infection at the time of death. In studies of young patients in the general population who experienced a sudden cardiac death, MVP is associated with approximately 5% of these deaths (Waller 1985). It is unclear in these two cases of sudden death of young males with FXS whether the MVP was related to the death. Two additional cases of sudden death were reported by Sabaratnam (2000) in older men with FXS. One patient died suddenly at 67 years of age. At autopsy, he had an abnormal dilated mitral valve with disorganization of many of the chordal tendinae and a dilated right heart. The cause of death was thought to be a combination of mitral valve incompetence, left ventricular hypertrophy, and atheromatous coronary arteries resulting in fatal ischemia or arrhythmia (Sabaratnam 2000). The second patient died suddenly at 87 years of age, but the cause of death was thought to be bronchopneumonia. At autopsy, his heart demonstrated mild concentric hypertrophy, moderate dilation of the left ventricle, and mild dilation of the left atrium with mild diffuse subendocardial fibrosis, and the mitral valve showed ballooning degeneration. The histology confirmed mucoid degeneration of the mitral leaflet. Excess acid mucopolysaccharide was present in the aorta. The role of the FMRP in the heart has not yet been clarified in normal individuals, much less the effect on cardiac function of the absence of this protein in FXS.

## Hypertension and Kidney Dysfunction

Hypertension is not uncommon in men with FXS, although its prevalence has never been studied in detail nor in comparison to other retarded males. The elevated blood pressure is often blamed on the anxiety experienced by the patient with FXS in the clinician's office during an examination. Persistent hypertension is experienced by some patients, however, and it requires a more thorough workup and subsequent antihypertensive medication. Perhaps connective tissue problems, such as abnormal elastin fibers, affect the resiliency of the vessel walls and predispose males with FXS to hypertension.

A rare patient with FXS has been noted with kidney problems, which could lead to hypertension. Three male patients in my practice have had a nephrectomy because of renal scarring and atrophy caused by dilated ureters and reflux. In addition, a female with the full mutation has also experienced significant vesicoureteral reflux without kidney damage. Perhaps the connective tissue dysplasia in FXS also influences the ureters and predisposes to reflux. A careful study of urogenital abnormalities in FXS is warranted.

Another explanation for hypertension in FXS is the excessive sympathetic response to daily stimuli in the environment in individuals affected with FXS (Miller et al. 1999). Clonidine is a medication that treats hypertension by lowering the levels of norepinephrine in the central nervous system (CNS) and peripherally, and it also decreases hyperactivity and aggression (Hagerman et al. 1995). It may, therefore, be a useful medication to treat behavior problems and hypertension at the same time (see chap. 8).

## Growth

Several authors have commented on unusual growth patterns in FXS, including increased birth weights, macrocephaly, increased or decreased height, and an acromegalic appearance in many adults (Turner et al. 1980, 1986; Fryns 1984; Meryash et al. 1984; Sutherland and Hecht 1985; Brøndum-Nielsen 1988; Borghgraef et al. 1990).

Partington (1984) evaluated 61 males with FXS and found a mean birth weight close to the fiftieth percentile and evenly spread height and weight growth percentiles. He found that 6.5% were at or below the fifth percentile for height and that no one was significantly increased over the ninety-fifth percentile. Sutherland and Hecht (1985) summarized data in several studies and found that 21 of 29 boys who were younger than 15 had growth percentiles above the fiftieth percentile and that 9 (31%) were at or above the ninety-fifth

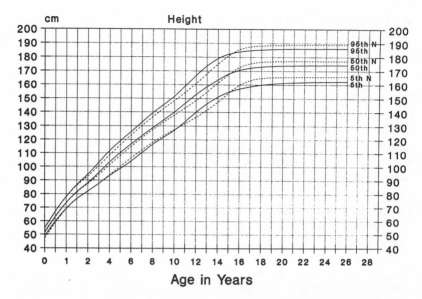

**Fig. 1.15.** Standardized curves for height of males with fragile X syndrome (*solid line*) and normal individuals (*broken line*). *Source:* Butler et al. (1992). Reprinted with permission.

percentile. The adults, on the other hand, tended to be short, with 23 of 87 (26%) measuring at or below the fifth percentile. Loesch and Hay (1988) confirmed the finding of a tendency for short stature in men with FXS and women compared to controls. In further studies Loesch et al. (1995) have demonstrated disturbed growth patterns in males and females with FXS including an increased height throughout childhood, lowered growth velocity during puberty, and a decreased height in adulthood, compared to controls. These findings are hypothesized to be secondary to hypothalamic dysfunction. Butler et al. (1992) published the growth percentiles of 185 white males with FXS between the ages of 0 and 26 years compared to previous published data of normals. Figures 1.15 to 1.18 present these data regarding height, weight, head circumference, and ear length, respectively, in patients with FXS compared to normals.

Prouty et al. (1988) reported that fetal growth, including head circumference and birth weight, were normal. They also found a mild increase in head circumference growth during childhood, which persisted into adult life. This was similar to the findings of Sutherland and Hecht (1985), who reported that the head circumference data demonstrated a mild tendency for an increased size, even in adulthood, when 70% were at or above the fiftieth percentile and 7% were above the ninety-seventh percentile. Individuals with FXS have on occa-

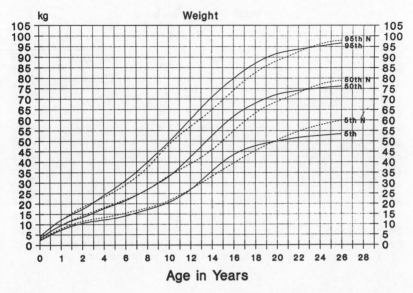

**Fig. 1.16.** Standardized curves for weight of males with fragile X syndrome (*solid line*) and normal individuals (*broken line*). *Source:* Butler et al. (1992). Reprinted with permission.

sion been misdiagnosed as having Sotos syndrome or cerebral gigantism because of the association of of developmental delay, a large head circumference, and generalized overgrowth (Fryns 1984; Beemer et al. 1986; de Vries et al. 1995). Further endocrine studies were carried out in two males with FXS and the Sotos-like phenotype. One was found to have elevated levels of insulin-like growth factor 1 (IGF-1) and insulin-like growth factor binding protein 3, although thyroid function, growth hormone (GH), luteinizing hormone (LH), FSH, and plasma testosterone levels were normal (de Vries et al. 1995). The IGFs are involved in growth processes including cartilage development and ovarian function (which is a problem in women with the premutation). IGF-1 elevations have been detected in Sotos syndrome also, and this finding is thought to be related to the overgrowth problem. Clearly, more studies are warranted in this area in FXS. Greenberg (Frank Greenberg, Houston, pers. comm., 1989) studied 15 patients with Sotos syndrome; 3 were positive for FXS on cytogenetic studies. On the other hand, a rare male with FXS will demonstrate microcephaly, although this is far less common than mild macrocephaly. Neuroanatomical studies through brain imaging techniques have demonstrated changes in brain structure, which explain the usual finding of macrocephaly in FXS as described below.

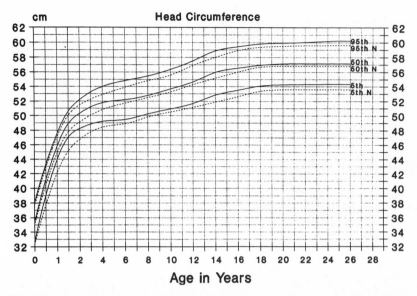

**Fig. 1.17.** Standardized curves for head circumference of males with fragile X syndrome (*solid line*) and normal individuals (*broken line*). *Source:* Butler et al. (1992). Reprinted with permission.

## Endocrine Dysfunction

The focus of early work has been on macroorchidism. In an effort to find the cause of macroorchidism, the levels of testosterone, LH, FSH, and thyroid hormone were measured and reported to be normal (Bowen et al. 1978; Cantú et al. 1978; Brøndum-Nielsen et al. 1982). However, mild elevations in gonadotropin levels (FSH and LH) were reported by Turner et al. (1975), Ruvalcaba et al. (1977), and McDermott et al. (1983). This finding is consistent with an elevated gonadotropin etiology for the macroorchidism seen in some hypothyroid patients (Castro-Magana et al. 1988). Further studies by Berkovitz et al. (1986) in males with FXS demonstrated a normal testosterone response to human chorionic gonadotropin stimulation and normal 5-alpha-reductase activity and androgen receptor binding in genital skin fibroblasts but mild elevations of androstenedione, 17-hydroxyprogesterone, and progesterone. Additional evidence for abnormal hypothalamic-pituitary function includes a blunted thyroid-stimulating hormone response to thyrotropin-releasing hormone stimulation (Wilson et al. 1988; Bregman et al. 1990) and enhanced cortisol levels in the afternoon and after stress in individuals with FXS compared to controls (Wisbeck et al. 2000). The enhanced cortisol levels are reminiscent of the enhanced melatonin levels both during the day and at night in individuals with FXS

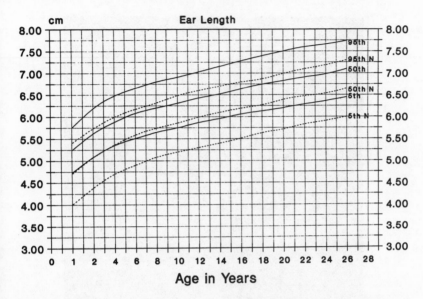

**Fig. 1.18.** Standardized curves for ear length of males with fragile X syndrome (*solid line*) and normal individuals (*broken line*). *Source:* Butler et al. (1992). Reprinted with permission.

(Gould et al. 2000). In addition, enhanced prolactin levels have been reported in FXS (Bregman et al. 1990). These enhanced levels may be secondary to a dysinhibition in the CNS, which causes a mild dysregulation of hormone release.

Clinically, Fryns et al. (1987) identified a subgroup of males with FXS with extreme obesity, short stature, stubby hands and feet, and diffuse hyperpigmentation. This phenotype is somewhat similar to that of Prader-Willi syndrome, and subsequently several additional patients with a Prader-Willi-like phenotype in FXS have been reported (de Vries et al. 1993b; Schrander-Stumpel et al. 1994). Both Prader-Willi syndrome and FXS are hypothesized to include problems with hypothalamic dysfunction, and both are associated with the absence of proteins that are involved with mRNA function. The absence of the *SNRPN* gene in Prader-Willi syndrome may affect the expression pattern of other genes, since *SNRPN* appears to have a role in mRNA splicing (Lalande 1994). Both disorders have a complex phenotype involving behavioral, cognitive, and physical problems with some important similarities that could stem from hypothalamic dysfunction and/or from diverse effects from mRNA dysfunction. A boy with FXS and a phenotype similar to that of Prader-Willi syndrome but without short stature is seen in figure 1.19. His obesity was related

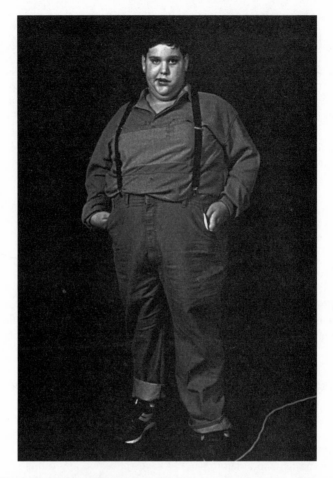

**Fig. 1.19.** Prader-Willi-like phenotype in a boy with fragile X syndrome.

to the behavioral phenotype in FXS, which includes perseverative eating, although this behavioral phenotype may certainly be influenced by hormonal problems related to hypothalamic dysfunction.

Further evidence of hypothalamic dysfunction is seen in the precocious puberty reported in an 8½-year-old girl with FXS (Butler and Najjar 1988), a 2-year and 8-month-old girl with FXS (Moore et al. 1990), and a 7-year 7-month-old girl with FXS (Kowalczyk et al. 1996). All three of these patients demonstrated advanced bone age, a mature response to gonadotropin-releasing hormone stimulation, and normal brain imaging. The girl reported by Kowalczyk et al. (1996) responded well to Lupron intramuscular (IM) monthly injections for almost two years, and menarche occurred six months after the Lupron was discontinued. Further support for hypothalamic dysfunction as a cause of the FXS phenotype comes from the report by Fryns et al. (1986) of three males without FXS but with acquired lesions of the CNS, including one with a hypothalamic tumor. All three patients had macroorchidism and facial features typical of FXS.

Premature ovarian failure (POF) is usually defined by menopause before 40 years, and it has been a consistent finding in approximately 16–24% of women with the premutation (Cronister et al. 1991a; Schwartz et al. 1994; Partington et al. 1996; Vianna-Morgante et al. 1996; Giovannucci Uzielli et al. 1999). An international study assessed 760 women in FXS families and found that 16% of those with the premutation had POF compared to none of the women with full mutation and 0.4% of normal controls (Allingham-Hawkins et al. 1999). A recent report by Hundscheid et al. (2000) found POF primarily in women who inherited the premutation from their fathers. They studied Dutch families and, among 82 women with a paternally inherited premutation, 28% had POF, whereas only 3.7% of 27 women with a maternally inherited premutation had POF. Subsequent studies, however, by Murray et al. (2000b) and Vianna-Morgante and Costa (2000) did not support a paternal-parent-of-origin effect on POF. Sherman (2000) suggested that international differences in the data sets may be related to reduced reproductive fitness in mother-daughter pairs with POF compared to father-daughter pairs, particularly in countries where women tend to reproduce at a later age (see chap. 3).

When women in the general population with POF are screened for the *FMR1* mutation, there is a significant positive yield, particularly if there is a familial pattern of POF (Conway et al. 1995, 1998; Murray et al. 1998). Giovannucci Uzielli et al. (1999) screened 108 subjects with POF and without a family history of fragile X or mental retardation, and 6.5% had the premutation. This is significantly higher than the typical 1% yield of POF in the general population and 70-fold higher than the background prevalence of the premutation in the Italian population (Giovannucci Uzielli et al. 1999). Similar results (6% positive) were reported by Marozzi et al. (2000) in screening 106 women with POF. There is ample justification now to support the screening of women with POF for the fragile X premutation (Hagerman et al. 1998; Finucane 1996). In addition, there is also evidence that screening the general female population antenatally or preconceptionally is also productive. Pesso et al. (2000) screened 9,459 women in Israel between 19 and 44 years of age with no known history of fragile X, and 134 carriers were detected, which is a frequency of 1 in 70. See chapter 3 for further discussion.

Turner et al. (1994) found that the dizygous twinning rate was three times the normal rate in women with the premutation and suggested that twinning could deplete the ovary more rapidly, leading to premature menopause. Vianna-

Morgante (1999) supported this hypothesis in her report that women with the premutation and POF had an enhanced twinning rate (10%) compared with the rate of normal relatives (1.1%) and women with the premutation but without POF (3.2%). She hypothesized that increased levels of FSH previously reported in women with the premutation could lead to enhanced twinning and to POF. Enhanced FSH levels would reflect hypothalamic dysfunction leading to over-stimulation of the ovaries. Studies by Braat et al. (1999) support this hypothesis. He studied nine women with the premutation who were younger than 40. Two of the nine had FSH elevation, and two had high progesterone levels. One had an anovulatory cycle, and two had a shortened follicular phase. Only one patient had a normal cycle. Black et al. (1995) also found ovarian dysfunction in preimplantation studies in women with the premutation. Eight of nine carriers had a poor response to hormonal ovarian stimulation, and four of the carriers had perimenopausal elevations of FSH. Murray and colleagues studied 116 women with the premutation and did not find enhanced twinning compared to controls but did find elevation of FSH in those with the premutation (Murray et al. 1999, 2000a) and a significant shift in menopause age for the entire premutation group compared to controls in the family. The age of menopause did not correlate with CGG repeat number or with activation ratio (Murray et al. 2000a). Whether this is a primary hypothalamic overstimulation problem or an intrinsic ovarian problem awaits further research. It is also known that the region Xq26-Xq28 is an important region for the maintenance of ovarian function and that women with deletions in this region have premature menopause (Tharapel et al. 1993). Perhaps other genes in this region may be interacting with the molecular dysfunction associated with the premutation, such as elevated mRNA levels, which are also seen in females with the premutation (Tassone et al. 2000a) (see chap. 12).

## Neurologic Features

Young boys with FXS are often described as hypotonic with poor motor tone (Hagerman et al. 1983; Wisniewski et al. 1991). The hypotonia seems to be a general effect of the CNS dysfunction in FXS, and the consequences may be significant. Fryns suggested that the facial features in FXS, particularly a long narrow face and joint laxity, may be a consequence of hypotonia and be unrelated to connective tissue abnormalities (Brown et al. 1991). Hypotonia, however, has also been reported in other known connective tissue disorders and was present to a severe degree in all children with Ehlers-Danlos type VI with lysyl hydroxylase deficiency reported by Wenstrup et al. (1989). Hypotonia may affect joint stability, fine and gross motor coordination, and sensory integration. These problems should be treated with early occupational therapy. Intervention techniques are described in chapter 10.

Wisniewski et al. (1989, 1991) described a lack of focal or hard neurologic findings in FXS. The most common findings on examination were soft neurologic signs indicative of motor incoordination. A rare patient, however, has cerebral palsy involving unilateral spasticity or spastic diplegia, which may be secondary to birth asphyxia (Dunn et al. 1963) in some cases, although in others there is no such history (Gillberg 1983; Fryns 1984). These findings may simply be coincidentally associated with FXS. Finnelli et al. (1985) described hyperreflexia in FXS, but this is not a consistent finding. Clonus is more common in adult patients as compared to children with FXS and may be present as the patient ages because of the neuroanatomic changes that occur over time, as described below. The palmomental reflex is often positive in men with FXS, suggesting frontal lobe dysfunction. This reflex is elicited by scraping the thumb across the palm of the patient; the patient's chin will twitch if the sign is positive (Musumeci, pers. comm., 1990).

Fryns et al. (1988) also reported an unexpectedly high incidence of sudden infant death (SIDS) in babies with FXS. Seventeen deaths before the age of 18 months occurred in 219 male offspring (8%) and 6 of 169 female offspring (4%) of obligate carrier women. The authors attributed this finding to CNS disturbances in affected offspring, although hypotonia leading to an obstructed airway, seizures, or MVP and arrhythmias may have been contributing features.

Sleep apnea has also been reported by Tirosh and Borochowitz (1992) in four patients with FXS. Two of the patients improved after a tonsillectomy and adenoidectomy, but two other patients required the use of CPAP (continuous positive airway pressure) by nasal canula for alleviation of symptoms. A careful history for snoring and obstructive symptoms should be carried out on all children with FXS, and parents should be advised to have infants sleep in the supine position to decrease the chance of SIDS. For infants considered high risk for apnea, a sleep monitor can be used.

## Neurologic Problems in Premutation Carriers

In this section, we will focus on older men with the premutation (fig. 1.20*A–C*) because we are seeing an emerging neurologic phenotype in a subgroup of these males. At the time of this writing, nine grandfathers with the premutation have developed a progressive cerebellar or intention tremor in their 50s or 60s, and the first five patients were reported by Hagerman et al. (2001a). These men all had normal previous cognitive abilities, and in fact three of them have Ph.D.s or equivalent levels of education. One case was identified after death, and he had a progressive tremor in addition to gradual dementia, which finally led to a bedridden state before death at age 69 (Hagerman et al. 2001a). All of the patients have had a progressive intention tremor that usually interferes initially with writing but subsequently may interfere with eating, drinking, dressing, and

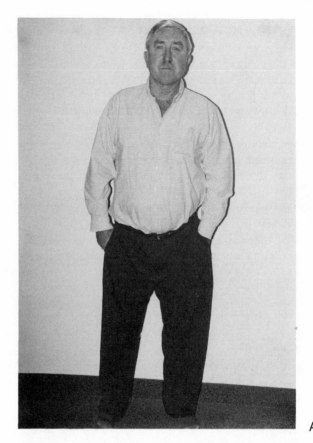

A

**Fig. 1.20.** *A:* A grandfather of a child with FXS. This man carries the premutation and does not have physical features of FXS, but he has a progressive cerebellar tremor, which began in his fifties. *B* and *C:* Magnetic resonance imaging (MRI) study of a 70-year-old grandfather with the premutation who has experienced a progressive cerebellar tremor, frequent falling, and memory problems. The MRI shows global atrophy. Note dilation of the ventricles.

eventually gait, with frequent falling. Ataxia and decreased sensation in the lower extremities have also been seen in the majority of patients. Some of these individuals have been diagnosed with atypical Parkinson disease because features of Parkinsonism, such as masked facies, resting tremor, or increased tone, have been present. All of the cases seen thus far have had significant generalized brain atrophy. Carbidopa-levodopa has been helpful for two patients, and amantadine has been helpful in two patients. All of the patients have had severe

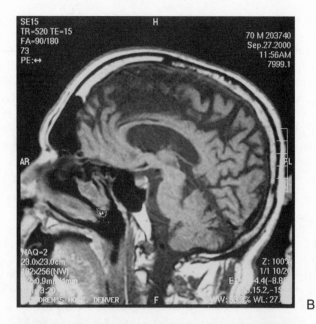

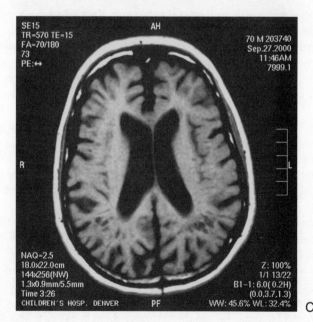

**Fig. 1.20.** *(continued)*

executive function deficits that seem to worsen over time, and two have had more global dementia.

An additional patient with this syndrome also has the survival motor neuron (SMN) mutation and has had two grandchildren who died from Werdnig-Hoffmann disease (William Landau, pers. comm., 2000). There may be background gene effects that can influence this progressive neurologic phenotype in a subgroup of older men with the premutation. All of the men have also had an elevation of mRNA levels, as described in chapter 12, and this may be related to the neurologic phenotype. Perhaps the elevated mRNA complexes with other proteins or other messages, and this leads to neuronal cell death (Tassone et al. 2000b; Hagerman et al. 2001a). An example of one of these cases is described below and was originally reported by Hagerman et al. (2001a).

## CASE HISTORY

Sid is a 70-year-old man with the fragile X premutation with 78 CGG repeats. At age 61 he developed a tremor in his right hand. He noticed the tremor when he tried to separate coffee filter papers, but it subsequently developed in the left hand and began interfering with his handwriting. Over the last three to four years, it has been noticeable intermittently at rest, but it is mainly an action tremor that worsens when he is moving his hands. He retired at age 64, although he worked part-time for two years after that time. His tremor began to interfere with his handwriting more dramatically at age 66, and at that time he also found it hard to get a key into the car door lock. More recently, he has had mild problems in spilling liquid when he tries to pour something from one container to another, and he frequently has to hold a glass with two hands. He cannot use plastic utensils because of their lack of support in association with his tremor. He may occasionally spill food from his fork when trying to get it to his mouth. He has difficulty with hygiene, such as shaving, unless he uses two hands. He also has intermittent difficulties with dressing.

Over the last four to five years, he has had occasional problems with falling. He may drift to one side in his gait, and he has had difficulties with tandem walking. He has had mild memory problems, particularly with short-term memory, but he has had no difficulty with remembering long-term events. Since his retirement, his wife says that his brain "has gotten lazier." His past medical history has included hypertension for 12 years, treated with propranolol, but his tremor has not improved on this medication.

He has never had any symptoms associated with fragile X syndrome, and his development was normal. He has worked as a professor, and at times he can be very focused on detail, even perfectionistic. He also has a history of compulsive hand washing. He was shy in childhood, but he overcame this shyness by adulthood.

Examination demonstrated normal height, weight, and head circumference, and his blood pressure was 130/80. He has a slightly long face with subtle cupping of the ear pinnae bilaterally. Lungs were clear, and the cardiac exam was normal. He had a mild scoliosis with slight elevation of the left side of his back. Genitalia were normal with a testicular volume of 15 ml bilaterally. Finger joints were not hyperextensible, and palmar creases were normal. His brother has been diagnosed with a tremor, and he has two grandchildren with FXS.

He had a marked, slow, 2 cm in amplitude and 4 Hz in frequency bilateral intention tremor that interfered with his handwriting and spiral drawing and with pouring water from one cup to another. He had mild dysmetria on finger-to-nose testing and Parkinsonian features, including moderate facial masking, mild rigidity of upper extremities, mild poverty of movement, slow foot tapping, and minimal arm swing with a mildly wide-based gait. He had difficulty with tandem walking and almost fell on examination. Deep tendon reflexes were 1+ and symmetrical in the upper extremities and at the knees but absent at the ankles, and toes were downgoing. He had decreased position sense in the right great toe and decreased vibratory sense in the distal lower extremities.

His cognitive testing on the WAIS-III showed a Verbal IQ of 117, a Performance IQ of 107, a Full-Scale IQ of 113, a Verbal Comprehension Index of 125, a Perceptual Organization Index of 123, a Working Memory Index of 104, and a Perceptual Speed Index of 88. He had very significant executive function deficits on the Wisconsin Card Sorting Test.

MRI testing demonstrated global brain atrophy involving both the cerebrum and the cerebellum (fig. 1.20).

Although this gentleman's tremor has been very slowly progressive over a nine-year period, other individuals whom we have seen have had more significant cognitive deficits and sometimes a more rapid progression of tremor. Sid's molecular testing showed only 78 CGG repeats and a normal level of FMR1 protein, specifically, 89% of his lymphocytes are positive for FMRP using the technique described in Tassone et al. (2000b). In addition, his messenger RNA level was elevated at over four times normal, and this is more thoroughly discussed in chapter 12. We do not yet know what percentage of older men with the premutation develop these symptoms and whether this neurologic problem is reflective of a second gene effect. It is also possible that environmental trauma, such as alcoholism, may further exacerbate these problems, and one of our patients, who was severely alcoholic, has more severe cognitive deficits and more rapid decline. We have not yet evaluated an older woman with the premutation and this type of tremor, so these difficulties seem to be more common in males than females. This appears to be a unique phenotype in a subgroup of those with the premutation, although those with the full mutation have not been well studied in the geriatric age group. All of the individuals whom we have studied have either normal or borderline low levels of FMRP, so we think that this phenotype is not secondary to FMRP deficiency but instead may be related to elevated mRNA levels. Examination of two brains from older grandfathers who died from this condition revealed the presence of eosinophilic intranuclear inclusions in neurons and glial cells throughout the brain, including cortex, hippocampus, substantia nigra, and cerebellum (Greco et al. 2001; Hagerman and Hagerman 2001). Further studies are needed to clarify whether these neuropathologic findings are generally present in carrier males with these neurologic symptoms, whether the elevated mRNA is related etiologically to these inclusions, and the prevalence of this neurologic condition in older carriers.

## Seizures and Electroencephalographic Findings

The most common neurologic abnormality in FXS is seizures. Sanfilippo et al. (1986) reported an electroencephalographic (EEG) pattern in three epileptic males with FXS that included medium- to high-voltage unilateral or bilateral spikes in the temporal area during sleep. Musumeci et al. (1988a) subsequently reported this finding as characteristic of FXS but not other causes of mental retardation. The temporal or central spikes were sometimes multifocal with two or more independent, occasionally alternating foci that also occurred during sleep but rarely were seen in the waking record (fig. 1.21). This pattern was present in 7 of 12 males with FXS (58%) and in 4 of 88 (4.5%) retarded males without FXS, suggesting significant specificity for FXS. The pattern was mainly present in children, and it could be identified in epileptic and nonepileptic males with FXS. Musumeci et al. (1988b) noted the similarities between this pattern and benign childhood epilepsy with centrotemporal spikes (BCECS). However, Rees et al. (1993) have shown that BCECS is not genetically linked to *FMR1* in the families they have studied.

Wisniewski et al. (1991) reported the follow-up of 14 patients with FXS with seizures. All were well controlled with anticonvulsants, usually carbamazepine (Tegretol). All of the seizures began in childhood or adolescence, they were usually infrequent, and in 10 of the 14 patients, the seizures were outgrown before adulthood. The rolandic spikes were present in 17% of 26 patients with FXS who had an EEG, and patients with these spikes included some with and some without seizures. In two patients with follow-up EEGs, the spikes disappeared at a later age, suggesting a benign, age-related effect similar to BCECS (Wisniewski et al. 1991).

The 14 patients with FXS and seizures in the study by Wisniewski et al. (1991) usually had generalized seizures. In a study by Musumeci et al. (1999) of 168 patients with FXS, 17% had seizures. Of those with seizures, 46% had generalized tonic-clonic seizures, 89% had complex partial seizures, 25% had simple partial seizures, and 7% had febrile seizures. Only 1 patient had status epilepticus, which was 3.6% of those with seizures, and this occurred when phe-

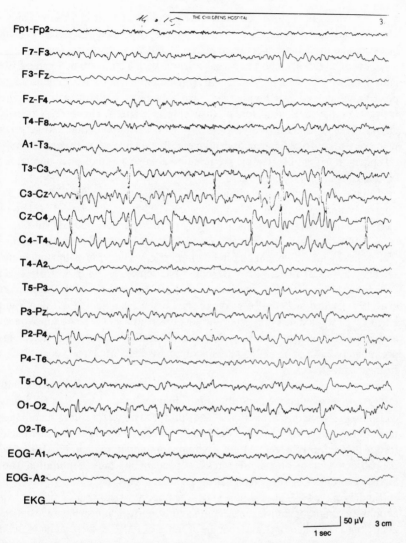

**Fig. 1.21.** Bilateral asynchronous central-temporal or rolandic spikes with extension to the occipital area on the right in a five-year-old boy with fragile X syndrome and complex partial seizures.

nobarbital and phenytoin were discontinued. Pregnancy and delivery complications were not associated with seizures, most patients were well controlled on anticonvulsants, and only 2 patients received more than one drug. Seven patients (25% of those with seizures) continued to have seizures in adulthood. An

EEG was done in 67 patients. Slow background was seen in 75% and spike wave discharges were seen in 48%, as previously described by Musumeci et al. (1988a), and these discharges were mainly in the centrotemporal regions.

Singh et al. (1999) reported partial seizures with a focal epileptogenic EEG pattern in two girls with presumably the full mutation who were cytogenetically positive and in their grandmother, who had only the premutation. Perhaps there were also other familial factors predisposing to seizures. However, Kluger et al. (1996) also found a five-year-old boy with the premutation and seizures when screening 16 patients with benign childhood epilepsy with centrotemporal spikes. It is possible that the premutation alone may predispose to seizures or at least spike wave discharges.

The prevalence of seizures in males with FXS has varied depending on the referral basis for each clinic. Musumeci et al. (1988a) found a rate of 50% (6 of 12 males studied) and a subsequent rate of 29% in 24 patients studied (Musumeci et al. 1999); however, their center specializes in epilepsy and their patient population has an ascertainment bias in favor of epilepsy. Other investigators found seizures in 4 of 27 males (15%; Brøndum-Nielsen et al. 1983), 8 of 61 (13%; Partington 1984), 4 of 20 (20%; Harvey et al. 1977), 14 of 62 (23%; Wisniewski et al. 1991), and 4 of 29 (14%; Vieregge and Froster-Iskenius 1989). Loesch and Hay (1988) studied heterozygotes and found seizures in 7.8% of adult women and 5.0% of girls. The overall prevalence of clinical seizures in males is approximately 23%, or 65 of 285 patients summarized by Musumeci et al. (1999) from several studies.

The cause of epilepsy in FXS is not known. Vieregge and Froster-Iskenius (1989) suggested that the dendritic spine abnormalities observed in FXS may cause excessive neuronal excitation and spiking. The seizures may also be related to the cerebellar vermal deficits in FXS described below. The main neurotransmitter from the cerebellum is gamma-aminobutyric acid (GABA), and the pathophysiology of some seizures is dependent on a lack of inhibition from GABA neurons (Christensen and Krogsgaard-Larsen 1984).

Studies of the FVB background knockout mice have shown a significant susceptibility to audiogenic seizures compared to normal littermates (Musumeci et al. 2000). This demonstrates that the absence of FMRP causes an increase in cortical excitability. Other evidence of cortical hyperexcitability has been reported in a patient who generated giant somatosensory evoked potentials and spikes in the EEG with finger tapping (Musumeci et al. 1994; Ferri et al. 1994) and in MEG studies described below (Rojas et al. 2001). These findings of cortical hyperexcitability may be related to enhanced dendritic connections and a deficiency of normal pruning with absence of FMRP discussed in chapter 5.

## Neuroanatomic Findings

Only a handful of postmortem neuropathologic studies have been performed on males with FXS. Dunn et al. (1963) reported findings in a 28-year-old retarded man who died from bronchopneumonia. The family was later identified as being FXS positive. This man demonstrated mildly dilated ventricles and islands of small numbers of nerve cells (heterotopia) scattered throughout the subcortical white matter. Heterotopia was also seen in an autopsy performed on a 41-year-old retarded man with FXS who died of amyotrophic lateral sclerosis (ALS) (Desai et al. 1990). This patient had significant abnormalities associated with ALS, including marked neuronal loss and degeneration of the corticospinal tracts. A small olivary heterotopic present beneath the right inferior cerebellar peduncle was unrelated to ALS. Heterotopia has been identified in many other disorders and represents arrested migration of neuronal cells (Musumeci et al. 1985). Dunn et al. (1963) also found marked siderosis of the globus pallidus and loss of myelin in the centrum semiovale and in the pyramidal tracts of the brain stem.

Rudelli et al. (1985) reported the postmortem study of a 62-year-old man with FXS and moderate retardation who died from chronic lymphocytic leukemia treated with prednisone. Malformations of the CNS were not present, but a mild degree of atrophy was seen in the frontal and parietal lobes. Rapid Golgi dendritic spine patterns were analyzed from the third and fifth layers of the cortex and the pyramidal layer. The spine morphology was abnormal, with long, thin, tortuous spines; irregular dilations were also seen in prominent terminal heads. Synaptic vesicle density was normal, but the synaptic length was reduced, with a resulting mean synaptic contact area that was 35% less than that in controls (Rudelli et al. 1985). Hinton et al. (1991) subsequently reevaluated Rudelli's case and two new cases, a 15-year-old boy and a 41-year-old man with FXS. The same abnormal dendritic morphology as described by Rudelli et al. (1985) was seen in all three males, but the neuronal density in cingulate and cortical areas was not different from controls. Jenkins et al. (1984) also saw the same dendritic spine abnormalities in a 23-week-old fetus. An additional study, reported by Fryns et al. (1988), was performed on a 3½-month-old child with FXS who died from sudden infant death. Microscopic examination showed that all organs, including the brain, were normal. Similar results were seen in two brothers with FXS who died at 48 and 73 years from natural causes (Reyniers et al. 1999). The younger brother had a mild dilation of the ventricles, but all other brain structures, including the hippocampus, were normal. The older brother had mild aging effects in the brain, but the structures were normal, including the cerebellum. In contrast, Sabaratnam (2000) studied the brains of two men who died suddenly at 67 and 87 years from cardiovascular causes, and both demonstrated abnormalities of the mitral valve, ventricular hypertrophy, and cardiomegaly. Both cases had increased brain weight and dilated lateral ventricles. Microscopic examination of the brain was done in the 87-year-old only and demonstrated focal Purkinje cell loss in the cerebellum with corresponding Bergmann gliosis, and in the hippocampus there was mild CA4 pyramidal cell loss and concomitant astrogliosis/microgliosis. A Denver case of a 29-year-old man with FXS who died suddenly also demonstrated Purkinje cell loss in the cerebellum compared to an age-matched control (Margaret Bauman, pers. comm., 1995). Most recently, Irwin et al. (2000) demonstrated an enhanced number of immature dendritic spines in three patients with FXS who are described in detail in chapter 5.

The eosinophilic intranuclear inclusions observed in two brains of older premutation carriers who had progressive intention tremor and ataxia have not been seen in patients affected by FXS. However, the two brains of the older carriers did demonstrate significant loss of Purkinje cells in the cerebellum (Greco et al. 2001), which has been seen in patients with FXS (Sabaratnam 2000).

Berry-Kravis and Huttenlocher (1992) and Berry-Kravis and Sklena (1993) reported a 50% decrease in cyclic AMP (cAMP) production in the platelets of patients with FXS, compared to normal controls and patients with autism and/ or mental retardation. Subsequent studies showed similar cAMP abnormalities in lymphoblastoid cell lines (Berry-Kravis et al. 1995), although a neurotumor line with elevated FMRP levels increased cAMP (Berry-Kravis and Ciurlionis 1998). Their data are most consistent with a depression of catalytic subunit activity, such as an abnormality within the cell membrane that influences adenylate cyclase activity. The cAMP cascade is an important second messenger system through which many neurotransmitters exert their influence to modulate synaptic functions. Interruptions or abnormalities of the cAMP cascade can produce mental deficiency, and cAMP is considered particularly important for short-term neuronal retention. Blockade of cAMP cascade pharmacologically in *Aplysia* prevents normal sensitization to sensory stimuli (Kandel and Schwartz 1982). Therefore, the cAMP abnormalities in FXS may relate to the cognitive deficits and behavioral problems, particularly the sensory disturbances, that are seen clinically.

An occasional additional abnormality may relate to factors other than FXS. One 18-year-old male with FXS followed in Denver had a history of hypoxia secondary to birth trauma and focal seizures in childhood. His MRI scan demonstrated a cystic area in the basal ganglia, most probably secondary to his birth trauma. Another Denver patient presented with growth deficiency, and MRI demonstrated an empty sella, with subsequent documentation of growth hormone deficiency. Hjalgrim et al. (2000) reported an abnormal sella turcica in two fetuses with FXS. In one fetus a notochordal tissue remnant was seen in the dorsum sellae, suggesting a delay in apotosis of ectodermally derived tissue. Wisniewski et al. (1991) described an arteriovenous malformation in the left temporal area, and Rodewald et al. (1987) reported the occurrence of a malignant ganglioma in a male with FXS.

## FMRP Studies in the CNS

Studies of FMRP expression in both animals and humans have helped to localize FMRP expression in normals (chaps. 4 and 5). Hinds et al. (1993) showed high expression of FMRP in the human brain compared to other tissues. In the adult mouse the granular layers of the hippocampus and the cerebellum had the highest expression, although moderate expression of FMRP was seen throughout the cerebral cortex, with little or no expression in white matter (Hinds et al. 1993). Khandjian et al. (1995) studied FMRP expression in mice and found significantly higher expression in young animals compared to adults. In the normal human brain, Devys et al. (1993) also found the most intense staining for FMRP in neuron-rich areas, including Purkinje cells and the granular layer of the cerebellum and neurons in the cortex. The strongest staining was in the perikaryon and the proximal part of axons and dendrites. There was very little staining of white matter. Hanzlik et al. (1993) found expression throughout fetal development. Abitbol et al. (1993) found particularly high expression in the cholinergic neurons of the nucleus basalis magnocellularis (nBM) in normal 8-, 9-, and 25-week-old human fetuses. The nBM is the major source of cholinergic innervation to the limbic area and cortex. They hypothesize that the lack of this cholinergic innervation, particularly to the limbic system, may be the reason for the overreaction of the sympathetic response to stimuli and the anxiety/mood lability problems that are common in both males and females with FXS. In addition, cholinergic dysfunction may be related to the sleep disturbances of children with FXS that are seen clinically and the physiobiological disturbances of sleep reported by Musumeci et al. (1995). Abitbol et al. (1993) also found intense staining for FMRP in the hippocampus, the thalamic and subthalamic nuclei, and the large GABAergic neurons of the nucleus reticularis thalami. For a detailed discussion of the influence of these neuroanatomic structures on behavior with special reference to fragile X, see Binstock (1995). Chapters 4 and 5 thoroughly review the recent findings of the role of FMRP in the CNS.

## Neuroimaging

Early neuroimaging studies in FXS demonstrated the nonspecific findings of ventriculomegaly in 39% of cases, suggesting mild frontal and parietal atrophy (Fryns 1984; Musumeci et al. 1991b; Wisniewski et al. 1991). Schapiro et al. (1995) demonstrated significantly larger right ventricles compared to left ventricles and significantly larger brains (12% greater intracranial volume) in 10 males with FXS compared to controls. Reiss et al. (1995a) found larger brains in females with FXS compared to controls, and both males and females with FXS had larger lateral ventricles compared to controls. Although asymmetry in the ventricular enlargement was not seen, Reiss et al. (1995a) reported a correlation between ventricular size and age and an inverse correlation between ventricular size and IQ. That is, the lower the IQ, the larger the lateral ventricles, and older individuals had larger ventricles. This later finding is reminiscent of the lateral ventricular enlargement reported in a subgroup of older men with the premutation who had brain atrophy discussed earlier (Hagerman et al. 2001a). Reiss et al. (1995) suggested that enhanced apoptosis may be occurring in some brain areas in individuals with FXS, and this may be occurring in some older men with the premutation and tremor. The finding of more rapid temporal lobe shrinkage in males with FXS compared to controls, described below, is also suggestive of apoptosis (Reiss et al. 1994).

The issue of asymmetry in ventricular dilation, specifically greater enlargement on the right compared to the left, reported by Schapiro et al. (1995), is also of interest. The neuropsychologic findings described in chapter 6 suggest that even minor deficits of FMRP affect nonverbal or perceptual performance areas initially so that the Performance IQ is most sensitive to level of FMRP or involvement from the *FMR1* mutation (de Vries et al. 1996a; Riddle et al. 1998; Tassone et al. 1999b). This suggests that the right side of the brain would be more significantly affected than the left side of the brain, leading perhaps to larger ventricles on the right. Hjalgrim et al. (1999) reported on the results of SPECT scanning in five males and one female with FXS. They found hypoperfusion of the right frontal lobe and right thalamus compared to normal controls. In addition to the right-sided hypoperfusion, there was a suggestion of basal ganglia hypoperfusion. Grigsby (pers. comm.) saw similar pockets of hypoperfusion frontally in women with FXS. In addition, Guerreiro et al. (1998) reported SPECT scan hypoperfusion of frontal areas in six patients with FXS and parietal or cerebellar hypoperfusion in two of these patients.

Right-sided abnormalities also predominate in recent volumetric MRI studies carried out in males with the premutation (Daly et al. 2000; Moore et al. 2000). Studies in ten males with the premutation found decreases in gray matter volumes in the right side of the cerebellum, middle temporal gyrus, postcentral gyrus, parahippocampal gyrus, and hippocampus compared to controls. In addition, a positron emission tomographic (PET) study of eight females with the premutation has shown relative hypometabolism of right parietal, temporal, and occipital association areas compared to controls (Murphy et al. 1999). It seems that resting brain glucose metabolism decreases with age in premutation females, and Murphy and colleagues hypothesize a premature brain aging process, in addition to differences in brain development, which is more severe for those with the full mutation than for those with the premutation, but it is still present in the latter group (Murphy et al. 1999).

Additional specific neuroanatomic differences in FXS compared to controls have been reported in several studies by Reiss et al. (1991a, 1991b, 1994, 1995a, 1995b). Both males and females with FXS have demonstrated a significantly smaller posterior cerebellar vermis compared to controls in quantitative MRI studies (Reiss et al. 1991a, 1991b; Mostofsky et al. 1998; Mazzocco et al. 1997a; Kates et al. 1997) (fig. 1.22). In addition, the volume of the right and left hippocampus was found to be larger in 15 young males and females with FXS compared to age-, gender-, and IQ-matched controls (Reiss et al. 1994). This study also revealed a volumetric decrease with age of the superior temporal gyrus, which is important in processing complex auditory stimuli and language, and a volumetric increase with age of the hippocampus. The decrease in volume of the superior temporal gyrus is worrisome because it suggests ongoing deleterious effects of the lack of FMRP during childhood and early adulthood. Although this study was cross-sectional in the evaluation of age changes, the results are supportive of findings of IQ decline in males and females with FXS (Lachiewicz et al. 1987; Wright-Talamante et al. 1996; also see chap. 6). It is also important to remember, however, that some adaptive skills, particularly self-help skills, continue to improve with age even in adulthood in FXS, in contrast to many other forms of mental retardation (Wiegers et al. 1993).

Contradictory findings to those of Reiss et al. (1994) regarding the size of the hippocampus were reported by Jakala et al. (1997). They studied males and females with the premutation and full mutation, with ten adult patients in each group. Enlargement of the hippocampus was not seen on MRI studies when the size of the hippocampus was corrected for the overall brain size, which was larger in those with the full mutation compared to those with a premutation. Perhaps the differences between studies relate to the fact that Jakala et al. (1997) studied adults, whereas Reiss et al. (1994) studied younger patients. In the Jakala et al. study, age correlated negatively with hippocampal raw volume, so older patients had smaller hippocampal volumes. However, Jakala et al. did find nonspecific changes in the hippocampal structure in >50% of those with the full mutation, including focal hyperintensities in temporal pole white matter, atypical hippocampal morphology, and enlargement of perivascular spaces.

A subsequent study by Reiss et al. (1995) found that the caudate nucleus was larger in patients with FXS compared to controls. The increased size of several brain structures in FXS may relate to abnormalities of the normal pruning process of neuronal connections, as discussed in chapter 5. Reiss et al. (1995a, 1995b) found that IQ was inversely correlated with caudate nucleus volume and that the level of *FMR1* gene inactivation also correlated with caudate nucleus volume, suggesting that these anatomic changes are related to the *FMR1* mutation. The specific neuroanatomic changes help to validate a specific neurobehavioral phenotype in FXS, which is described below.

The caudate is involved with frontal-subcortical circuits that are important

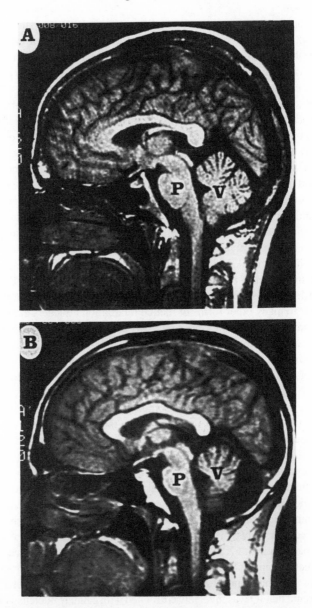

**Fig. 1.22.** *A:* An MRI scan of the brain of a normal male (midsagittal slice). *B:* An MRI scan of the brain of a male with fragile X syndrome. *P* identifies the pons. Note the decrease in size of the posterior cerebellar vermis (*V*). *Source:* Reiss et al. (1988b). Reprinted with permission.

for attention, attention shifting, executive functions, emotional lability, motor programming, and oculomotor functions, which are all problematic in FXS (Friefeld and MacGregor 1993; Mazzocco et al. 1993; Abrams and Reiss 1995; Kermadi and Boussaoud 1995). The posterior cerebellar vermis, which has been postulated to be dysfunctional in autism, is important for processing sensory stimuli and in modulation of sensory motor integration (Ornitz and Ritvo 1968; Ornitz 1989). Sensory disturbances, such as tactile defensiveness, in addition to other autistic-like features, are present in FXS and are likely related to these neuroanatomic findings. Courchesne et al. (1994) found similar size discrepancy in the posterior cerebellar vermis in individuals with autism compared to controls.

Involvement of the amygdala in FXS was first hypothesized after a study of monozygotic twin girls with the full mutation who were discordant for mental retardation (Mazzocco et al. 1995; Reiss et al. 1995). Twin A had a Full-Scale IQ of 105, and twin B had a Full-Scale IQ of 47, but both twins had similar CGG expansions, activation ratios, and neonatal course without brain trauma. Neuroimaging studies, however, showed an increased size of the amygdala in twin B (35% larger than twin A). Although their overall brain size was similar, twin A also had enlarged lateral and fourth ventricles, enlarged caudate and thalamus, and a smaller posterior cerebellar vermis than twin B (Reiss et al. 1995).

Amygdala dysfunction in fragile X has also been detected in *FMR1* knockout mouse studies. Paradee et al. (1999) demonstrated an abnormal conditioned fear response, specifically significantly less freezing behavior during contextual and cued conditions in the knockout mouse compared to controls. They hypothesize greater amygdala dysfunction than hippocampus dysfunction in knockout mice, which is supported by the lack of hippocampal long-term potentiation (LTP) abnormalities in knockout mice (Godfraind et al. 1996) (see chaps. 4 and 5). Further support for amygdala dysfunction in FXS is found in functional MRI (fMRI) studies described below.

An interesting metabolic study using positron emission tomography (PET) has been done in 10 individuals with FXS compared to controls with Down syndrome and normals (Schapiro et al. 1995). Using regional cerebral metabolic rates (rCMRglc), the investigators documented increased activity in the premotor regions, thalamus, caudate, and vermis in FXS compared to controls. In addition right/left symmetry in the rCMRglc of the parietal lobe was significantly higher in patients with FXS compared to healthy controls. Discriminate function studies that reflected rCMRglc interactions of the right ventricular and left premotor regions (frontal) distinguished patients with FXS from controls. Overall, these studies support disturbed frontal-subcortical interactions in FXS, which probably provide the basis for the behavioral dysfunction described below.

For a review of neuroanatomic studies in humans, see Kooy et al. (1999).

These authors carried out detailed MRI studies of 11 fragile X knockout mice compared to controls and found no differences in contrast to the human studies. Perhaps the changes in humans with FXS are related to higher cognitive functions that have evolved subsequent to the mouse. However, ultrastructural differences have been noted in the knockout mouse compared to controls, as discussed in chapter 5.

Recent correlations between MRI findings and cognitive/behavioral testing have given new insight into brain-behavior relationships. Mostofsky et al. (1998) used MRI to study 32 males and 37 females with FXS compared to developmentally disabled controls. The size of the posterior vermis correlated with the activation ratio and was a significant predictor of the performance on most of the cognitive measures, including Verbal IQ, Performance IQ, Full-Scale IQ, Block Design subtest, the Rey-Osterreith Complex Figure Test, and the categories achieved on the Wisconsin Card Sorting Test. This research not only confirms that the posterior cerebellar vermis is significantly affected by the *FMR1* mutation compared to controls with cognitive deficits, but also that the vermis is very important for a variety of cognitive tasks, including executive function abilities and visual spatial abilities. After removing the effect of the mean parental IQ, the size of the posterior vermis predicted up to 23% of the variance on cognitive testing in the patients with FXS (Mostofsky et al. 1998). However, there was no correlation between size of the posterior vermis and age, suggesting that atrophy was not seen (although the oldest patient was only 43 years) and that hypoplasia is the primary cause of the small size of the vermis.

In a study of 30 school-aged girls with FXS and age- and IQ-matched controls, Mazzocco et al. (1997a) found that the size of the posterior cerebellar vermis was negatively correlated with measures of stereotypic/restricted behavior, communication dysfunction, and autistic items on a neuropsychiatric developmental interview. Higher scores represent more dysfunction, and these higher scores correlated with a smaller posterior vermis size. However, measures of anxiety in these females with FXS did not correlate with IQ nor with the size of the posterior cerebellar vermis (Mazzocco et al. 1997a). These data suggest that anxiety, which is part of the behavioral phenotype of girls with FXS, may have a different neuropathologic mechanism that is unrelated to the hypoplasia of the posterior cerebellar vermis.

More recent research has involved functional MRI studies in individuals with FXS. Menon et al. (2000) studied 10 girls with FXS using a working memory task in fMRI studies. They found a significant correlation between levels of FMRP and brain activation in the right inferior frontal gyrus, the right and left middle frontal gyrus, and the right and left supramarginal gyrus, which is in the parietal cortex. Their studies suggest that reduced levels of FMRP lead to reduced transmission of neuronal signals or restriction in the neuronal network that can be recruited in response to this working memory task (Menon et al. 2000).

In a study of fMRI activation in arithmetic processing in 16 girls with FXS, Rivera et al. (2000) found decreased activation in fragile X patients compared to controls. In the most complex set of problems, the level of FMRP correlated positively with activation level in the left and right precentral gyrus, the left middle frontal gyrus, and the left supramarginal gyrus, areas known to be involved in arithmetic processing.

Regarding emotional perception, Reiss and colleagues (Reiss 2000) have studied gaze and face processing with fMRI in 16 girls with FXS. Compared to controls, girls with FXS demonstrated impaired performance in determining whether the gaze in pictures of faces was directed at them. In addition, girls with FXS showed a deficit in activation of the amygdala compared to controls. Overall, the controls showed greater activation of not only the amygdala but also the left linguinal/fusiform gyri, left cuneus, and left hippocampal/parahippocampal gyri compared to the girls with FXS (Reiss 2000). The technology of fMRI is beginning to provide new insight to our understanding of dynamic brain activity in fragile X, which will be useful in monitoring treatment effects in the near future.

## Evoked Potentials and Magnetoencephalography

A limited number of studies of evoked potentials have been done. Gillberg et al. (1986) reported that 6 of 7 autistic boys with FXS demonstrated prolonged transmission times in auditory brain stem responses (ABRs). Wisniewski et al. (1991) found prolonged latencies in waves III–V in 4 of 12 patients with FXS. Ferri et al. (1988) also found variable prolonged latencies in ABRs and slight but significantly prolonged latencies in visual pattern-evoked potentials in males with FXS. Arinami et al. (1988) confirmed the ABR findings of prolonged latencies in 12 men with FXS compared to controls. For the group data, interpeak latencies were prolonged in FXS for waves III–V but not for waves I–III, suggesting a central rather than a peripheral lesion. Individually, 5 of the 12 patients with FXS had interpeak latencies longer than 2.5 standard deviations above the control mean. Arinami et al. (1988) postulated that recurrent otitis media, which is common in FXS (Hagerman et al. 1987), may have altered the development of the brain stem portion of the auditory nervous system, as reported in patients without FXS (Folsom et al. 1983). Waves III to V represent the pathway from the superior olivary nucleus (III) to the pontine lateral lemniscus (IV) to the inferior colliculus in the midbrain (V).

Work by Miezejeski et al. (1997) demonstrated that sedation prolongs the latencies in ABRs in individuals with FXS and in those with mental retardation (MR) without FXS. They found no difference in the latencies of 13 patients with

FXS compared to normals and to those with MR. They suggest that the previous findings of Arinami and colleagues (1988) may be due to the use of sedation in some patients.

Ferri et al. (1994) studied midlatency somatosensory-evoked potentials (MLSEP) in 10 males with FXS compared to controls and demonstrated distinct cortical hyperexcitability in the supplementary motor area (SMA). One of the 10 patients with FXS demonstrated giant MLSEPs after stimulation of the right and left median nerves. In fact, just tapping the right hand induced the appearance of left parietal-evoked EEG spikes (Ferri et al. 1994). In the other patients with FXS, abnormally large N30 waves were present in the frontal region compared to controls. The SMA in the frontal region is important for motor planning, coordination, and sensory motor integration, all of which are dysfunctional in FXS (Friefeld and MacGregor 1993; chap. 10).

The use of event-related potentials (ERPs) has turned out to be a fertile area for detecting early neurocognitive processing abnormalities in infants with FXS. Hill Karrer et al. (2000b) compared infants with FXS to infants with Down syndrome and normals in a visual ERP paradigm and found very large Pb components, a positive wave in early processing that appears dramatically exaggerated, perhaps related to the deficit in dendritic pruning reported by Comery et al. (1997) and reviewed in chapter 5.

ERP methodology has also been useful in detecting more subtle neurocognitive dysfunction in normal IQ carriers of the premutation. Hill Karrer et al. (2000a) studied female carriers with a motor readiness brain potential (MRP) recording session using a paradigm involving the learning of a novel elbow movement that controlled a computerized cursor ball from a starting position to a fixed target. Carriers consistently demonstrated less neural inhibitory control from frontal recording sites in the MRP waveform compared to controls.

Another productive area of research is the use of magnetoencephalography (MEG) in the study of fragile X. Rojas et al. (2001) studied 11 adults with FXS and age-matched controls using a 37-channel MEG device. Pure tone auditory stimuli were given, and magnetic responses to approximately 100 tones were signal averaged to produce auditory evoked magnetic fields for each subject. The analysis involved calculation of the root mean square (RMS) field for all subjects, and individuals with FXS had significant increases in the RMS field across the entire waveform compared to controls. Since MEG field strength is directly proportional to the number of synchronously active cells in the cortex, these results suggest that more neurons are activated in FXS to acoustic stimuli, perhaps related to the enhanced dendritic connections in FXS (Comery et al. 1997; Weiler and Greenough 1999; chap. 5).

## Behavioral Phenotype

The behavior of males with FXS represents a phenotype that has some consistent features and may often be more helpful diagnostically than the physical phenotype. This is particularly true for young males with FXS, who usually do not demonstrate macroorchidism or a long narrow face. They typically present to their physician in early childhood because they are not speaking in sentences by two to three years of age and are temperamentally difficult children. Tantrums are frequent problems, and hyperactivity is seen in the majority. Hypotonia, irritability, and perseveration in speech and behavior are usually complicating features. Autistic-like features, such as poor eye contact, hand flapping, and hand biting, are often seen by two to five years of age. The following case history illustrates several typical features.

### CASE HISTORY

PB is a five-year-old boy who was diagnosed with the FXS after cytogenetic studies demonstrated the FXS in 29% of his lymphocytes. DNA studies showed a full mutation with 425 repeats that is fully methylated. He was born after a normal pregnancy and full-term delivery. His birth weight was 9 pounds 10 ounces, and he did well during the newborn period. In his early development, he cried frequently, nursed poorly, and had difficulty with lactose intolerance. He rolled over at 6 months, crawled at 14 months, and began walking at 17 months. He was somewhat slow in smiling and cooing, and he was unable to say several words until four years of age. He has difficulty with hand flapping and rare hand biting, but he more frequently bites his shirt. He has problems with poor eye contact, although this has improved recently. He is fascinated by glass, running water, loud noises, vacuum cleaners, and books. He is particularly interested in sharks and whales.

PB has had frequent otitis media infections, although PE tubes have not been placed. He dislikes many foods, and he reacts adversely to the texture of food, so he has failed to thrive in the past. He requires the addition of a liquid protein supplement to maintain weight and growth. He is hypotonic, and his occupational therapist in his developmental preschool program has worked on improving motor coordination and on increasing food tolerance with oral motor stimulation. He has a short attention span, particularly for preacademic work, and a high activity level related to restlessness and impulsivity. In school, he has frequently been noted to laugh abruptly or inappropriately. Perseveration and echolalia have also been problems, and he is receiving speech and language therapy. Cognitive testing at five years old using the Kaufman Assessment Battery for Children demonstrates a mental processing composite score of 60, with a significant difference between his sequential processing (56) and simultaneous processing (69) scores.

Physical examination shows that his growth is at the fiftieth percentile for height, weight, and head circumference. His face is mildly narrow with a ptosis involving the left eye and a mild strabismus. His palate is narrow. His cardiac examination is normal, and his extremities demonstrate bilateral single palmar creases and MP joint extension to 80°. Hallucal creases are seen bilaterally, and his feet are not flat. His testicles demonstrate a volume of 3–4 ml bilaterally.

## Hyperarousal and Hyperactivity

Clinically, individuals with FXS seem to be extrasensitive to sensory stimuli such that they are easily hyperaroused in situations with excess auditory, visual, or tactile stimuli. Tantrums may result from this hyperarousal, as in a supermarket or at a concert. Hyperactivity or even oppositional behavior may worsen in environments with excessive sensory stimuli. Yelling or placing demands on the child may worsen this problem (see chaps. 9 and 10 for more discussion, including intervention techniques). Cohen (1995b) postulated that arousal modulation problems characterized the behavioral phenotype in FXS and were related to problems such as poor eye contact, tactile defensiveness, anxiety, avoidant behaviors, hyperactivity, repetitive motor behaviors, aggression, and even verbal perseverations. In support of this theory, Cohen et al. (1991a) found that propranolol, a beta-blocker that reduces heart rate and blood pressure and increases relaxation, improved aggression and repetitive behavior in an adult male with FXS, perhaps related to calming down hyperarousal (see chap. 8 for more discussion). A subsequent study by Belser and Sudhalter (1995) assessed electrodermal reactivity (EDR), which is the sweat response, to direct eye contact versus lack of eye contact in two males with FXS and controls. They found enhanced EDR in the males with FXS during eye contact, and this was associated with an enhanced level of perseverative and deviant language compared to the condition of no eye contact. This preliminary study demonstrated a physiologic enhanced arousal that was linked to anxiety and tangential and perseverative language in FXS.

A subsequent study by Miller et al. (1999) included 25 individuals (19 male and 6 female) representing a broad spectrum of FXS involvement and a detailed sensory challenge protocol that assessed the EDR response to repetitive stimuli in visual, auditory, tactile, olfactory, and vestibular modalities. Compared to age-matched controls, individuals with FXS demonstrated enhanced EDR as measured by amplitude and number of peaks to all sensory modalities. The degree of EDR enhancement also correlated with the level of FMRP, which is further support that this is a fragile X–related phenomenon. In addition, the habituation to sensory stimuli was poor and significantly abnormal in those with FXS compared to controls. This work demonstrates enhanced electrodermal arousal with stimuli, which is reflective of enhanced sympathetic activity in FXS, since the sympathetic system controls the sweat response to stimuli (Miller et al. 1999). The study of EDR responses creates a quantitative physiologic measure of hyperarousal that can be applied to future measures of treatment efficacy. Hagerman et al. (2001b) used EDR measures to assess response to stimulant medications, including methylphenidate, dextroamphetamine, and Adderall in children with attention deficit hyperactivity disorder (ADHD) and FXS compared to developmentally disabled controls. The stimulants significantly decreased the enhanced EDR response in FXS compared to controls. The effect of stimulants is puzzling because they typically enhance dopamine and norepinephrine neurotransmission (Cyr and Brown 1998; Solanto 1998), which one might think would further increase EDR responses. The opposite effect seen experimentally is perhaps related to an enhancement of inhibitory pathways with stimulant treatment (Hagerman et al. 2001b) (see chap. 8).

Further support for autonomic dysregulation and hyperarousal in FXS comes from the study of heart rate variability in boys with FXS compared to age-matched normal controls (Boccia and Roberts 2000). These authors found that boys with FXS had a faster heart rate, lower parasympathetic activity, and similar sympathetic activity compared to controls. Although sympathetic activity was not enhanced, the lowered levels of parasympathetic activity represent autonomic dysfunction and another mechanism of hyperarousal.

Hyperactivity was a notable problem in early reports of males with FXS (Turner et al. 1980; Mattei et al. 1981) and was further documented in 47% of 17 boys with FXS by Finnelli et al. (1985). Largo and Schinzel (1985) reported the onset of hyperactivity by 2 years of age, whereas Fryns (1985) emphasized the disappearance of hyperactivity after puberty. Fryns et al. (1984) reported attentional problems in all 21 boys with FXS who underwent a detailed psychologic profile. Hyperactivity and attention deficits can be the presenting complaint of even high-functioning boys with FXS with a borderline or normal IQ (Hagerman et al. 1985; Hagerman et al. 1996). Hyperactivity was documented by a Conners rating score (Conners 1973; Werry et al. 1975) of 15 or higher in 73% of prepubertal boys with FXS, although all demonstrated concentration difficulties (Hagerman 1987). Bregman et al. (1988) also found attention or concentration problems in 100% of 14 males with FXS, although only 71% fulfilled criteria for attention deficit hyperactivity disorder. The residual state of ADHD was seen in a further 21%, suggesting that many of the older patients had outgrown their hyperactivity, a result similar to the report by Fryns (1985). Borghgraef et al. (1987) found ADHD in twice as many males with FXS compared to controls and found that hyperactivity improved with age, in that 80% of young boys and 54% of older school-aged boys with FXS had ADHD.

Further controlled studies of ADHD in FXS include the work of Baumgardner et al. (1995), who compared 31 boys with FXS and controls matched on age and IQ. Parent and teacher ratings demonstrated significantly higher levels of hyperactivity, stereotypic movements, and unusual speech in boys with FXS compared to controls. Overall, 73% of boys with FXS fulfilled ADHD DSM III-R criteria compared to 33% of controls. Turk (1998) compared 49 boys with FXS to 45 boys with Down syndrome and 42 boys with MR of unknown etiology on a variety of behavioral checklists, including the CBCL, for parents and teachers. Boys with FXS had significantly higher rates of inattentiveness and fidgetiness compared to controls, but hyperactivity was higher in the group with nonspecific MR by parent rating, although by teacher rating, "can't sit still, restless, or hyperactive" was a more significant problem in boys with FXS than in the other two control groups. Activity level showed a highly significant inverse correlation with developmental level in all three groups, so the youngest children were the most active.

In contrast, Kau et al. (2000) studied 41 preschool-aged boys with FXS compared to controls with developmental disability and found that the boys with FXS were not more significantly hyperactive nor inattentive than controls on a temperament scale. However, boys with FXS demonstrated more motor deficits, more positive mood, and increased initial avoidance of novel stimuli compared to controls. In another temperament study, Hatton et al. (1999) found boys with FXS to be more active but less approachable, adaptable, intense, and persistent compared to a reference sample. Although there was significant variability in the temperament profiles across the sample of 45 boys with FXS, there was no relationship between temperament scores and developmental testing. In addition, the temperament profile of individuals remained stable over the 47- to 88-month follow-up period.

A detailed neuropsychologic study of the profile of attention problems in 25 boys with FXS compared to boys with Down syndrome, boys with ADHD, and normal controls was carried out by Munir et al. (2000). Males with FXS displayed significantly worse problems on selective attention, divided attention, sustained attention, and inhibition compared to controls, but they did better on the response-organization task that required speed compared to those with Down syndrome, and their response time on the sustained attention task was comparable to that of the ADHD controls. In general, the impulsive behavior of the boys with FXS was evident on all tasks and is a consistent feature in the behavioral phenotype. In a similar study of adult males with FXS, more significant deficits were seen in a task that required attention shifting from one stimulus to another than in a task that required sustained attention compared to controls with MR (Cornish et al. 2001). This further supports the role of executive function deficits in ADHD and in FXS (discussed in detail in chap. 6).

ADHD symptoms are less frequent in girls with FXS, and approximately 35% have these difficulties (Hagerman et al. 1992; Freund et al. 1993). Further studies have not found this rate to be significantly different from age- and IQ-matched female controls (Freund et al. 1993). Girls with FXS and ADHD usually have less hyperactivity compared to boys with FXS. However, impulsivity and short attention span can be a significant problem for the girls. Significant ADHD symptoms in girls can be somewhat helpful or protective of shyness and social withdrawal, as described below (Sobesky et al. 1995, 1996). The treatment of ADHD includes a variety of interventions at home and school, in addition to medications, as described in chapters 8, 9, and 10.

## Psychiatric Comorbidity

In a study of 49 boys with FXS compared to a control group of boys with tuberous sclerosis (TS), a structured psychiatric interview in addition to cognitive testing and behavior checklists (CBCL) demonstrated a high level of psychiatric comorbidity (Backes et al. 2000). Although ADHD was high in 74%, a variety of additional problems were present, including oppositional defiant disorder in 29%, functional enuresis in 27%, functional encopresis in 20%, separation anxiety disorder in 10%, and obsessive compulsive disorder in 2%. The prevalence of ADHD was significantly different in FXS compared to TS, but the other diagnoses were not significantly different. In the FXS group, 26.5% had two psychiatric diagnoses, 8.2% had three diagnoses, and 12% had four diagnoses. The high rate of combined psychiatric problems has led to the use of more than one medication for treatment, as described in detail in chapter 8.

Results similar to those of Backes et al. (2000) were reported by von Gontard et al. (2001) in comparing the same 49 boys with FXS to 46 boys with spinal muscular atrophy and normal male controls. There was a high rate of psychiatric comorbidity, with 81.6% of the boys with FXS and only 10.9% of the boys with spinal muscular atrophy also having a psychiatric diagnosis. Families with FXS experienced a higher rate of parental stress than did families with spinal muscular atrophy, particularly if the child was disruptive.

Einfeld et al. (1999) reported on the 7-year follow-up of 46 patients with FXS now with a mean age of 22 years (SD, 5.47 years) compared to a large control group of 399 individuals with intellectual handicap on the Developmental Behavior Checklist (DBC). In the FXS group, there was a significant decline in disruptive behavior and a significant increase in antisocial behavior over the 7-year follow-up. There was no change in the items "avoid eye contact" and "shy," but these items were significantly different in FXS compared to controls even seven years before (Einfeld et al. 1994). Overall, there is a progressive and steady improvement in behavior disturbance in both those with FXS and controls between childhood and young adulthood. Perhaps the most controversial area of psychiatric comorbidity is the association of autism and FXS.

## Autism and Autistic Features

Several early reports of FXS included cases of autism in males (Turner et al. 1980; Proops and Webb 1981; Meryash et al. 1982), but Brown et al. (1982) pointed out the association between FXS and autism when 5 of 27 (18.5%) males with FXS were diagnosed with autism. Subsequently, several authors confirmed this report (Brøndum-Nielsen et al. 1983; Levitas et al. 1983; August and Lockhart 1984; Kerbeshian et al. 1984; Varley et al. 1985), which stimulated the screening of males with autism for FXS. Some smaller studies did not find FXS in the males with autism who were tested (Opitz and Sutherland 1984; Goldfine et al. 1985; Pueschel and Herman 1985), but the larger studies demonstrate a significant prevalence, with a high of 15.7% in Sweden (Blomquist et al. 1985; Fisch et al. 1988). Overall, approximately 6.5% of males with autism test positive for FXS when subjected to cytogenetic studies (reviewed in Hagerman 1991; Brown et al. 1986). A study by Li et al. (1993) used both cytogenetic and DNA studies to screen 104 autistic children (84 males and 20 females) in Taiwan. Eight (7.7%) were positive for FXS by DNA testing, but the cytogenetic expression was only 1% or 2% in 5 of the 8 positive patients. In earlier studies involving cytogenetic testing only, many laboratories may have defined expression of 2% or less as negative. The era of DNA testing has led to more accurate identification of individuals with the *FMR1* mutation and, therefore, a more accurate assessment of the prevalence of FXS in individuals with autism.

Previous research has shown that autistic-like features, such as hand flapping, hand biting, perseveration in speech, shyness, and poor eye contact are seen in the majority of individuals with FXS (Turk and Graham 1997; Hagerman et al. 1986; Hagerman 1996; Kerby and Dawson 1994; Baumgardner et al. 1995), but the majority of patients with FXS do not demonstrate the core social deficits typical of autism (see tables 1.4 and 1.5 and figs. 1.23 to 1.25). They are usually interested in social interactions, and they are usually sensitive to the facial emotional cues presented by others (Simon and Finucane 1996; Turk and Cornish 1998). The percentage of individuals with FXS who also have significant social deficits that fulfill DSM-III-R or DSM-IV criteria for autism has ranged from 15% to 28%, depending on the age of the patients (Reiss and Freund 1992; Baumgardner et al. 1995; Hagerman 1996; Cohen 1995a; Turk and Graham 1997).

Studies that directly compare patients with FXS to patients with autism have been limited but suggested more echolalia and more deviant language or inappropriate responses in autism (Paul et al. 1987; Sudhalter et al. 1990; Ferrier et al. 1991). In studies of eye gaze, children with autism tend to avoid direct eye gaze whether people are looking at them or not, whereas children with FXS are more avoidant of direct eye contact when someone looks at them, suggestive of more reactive avoidance (Cohen et al. 1989, 1991b).

**Table 1.4**
**Proportion of Prepubertal Boys and Girls with Features**

| | Males with Full Mutation | | | |
| Behavioral Feature | Fully Methylated (n = 103) | <50% Methylated (n = 10) | Male Mosaic (n = 30) | Females with Full Mutation (n = 40) |
|---|---|---|---|---|
| Hand flapping | 83% | 70% | 93% | 40% |
| Hand biting | 56% | 10% | 37% | 20% |
| Hyperactivity | 70% | 30% | 70% | 55% |
| Perseveration | 85% | 90% | 90% | 70% |
| Aggression | 42% | 10% | 33% | 28% |
| Shyness | 73% | 80% | 60% | 83% |
| Anxiety | 68% | 90% | 63% | 58% |
| Panic attacks | 25% | 30% | 27% | 25% |
| Poor eye contact | 86% | 70% | 80% | 73% |
| Violent outbursts | 14% | 0% | 17% | 3% |
| Tactile defensiveness | 81% | 60% | 80% | 68% |

*Source:* Adapted and updated from Merenstein et al. 1996.
*Note:* Prepubertal = up to age 12 years 11 months.

**Table 1.5**
**Proportion of Postpubertal Males and Females with Features**

| | Males with Full Mutation | | | |
| Behavioral Feature | Fully Methylated (n = 64) | <50% Methylated (n = 7) | Male Mosaic (n = 22) | Females with Full Mutation (n = 27) |
|---|---|---|---|---|
| Hand flapping | 81% | 17% | 68% | 26% |
| Hand biting | 64% | 17% | 50% | 22% |
| Hyperactivity | 64% | 67% | 82% | 19% |
| Perseveration | 100% | 75% | 91% | 67% |
| Aggression | 55% | 67% | 47% | 15% |
| Shyness | 61% | 100% | 100% | 96% |
| Anxiety | 79% | 100% | 91% | 81% |
| Panic attacks | 39% | 25% | 22% | 33% |
| Poor eye contact | 98% | 67% | 100% | 96% |
| Violent outbursts | 42% | 20% | 37% | 4% |
| Tactile defensiveness | 86% | 60% | 80% | 70% |

*Source:* Adapted and updated from Merenstein et al. 1996.
*Note:* Postpubertal = age 13 and above.

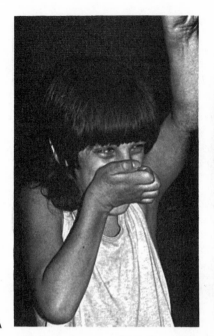
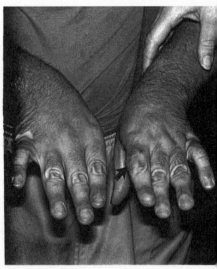

A

**Fig. 1.23.** *A:* Hand biting in a boy with fragile X syndrome. *B:* The arrow points to a hand callus that is secondary to repetitive hand biting in a man with fragile X syndrome.

Bailey et al. (1998) directly compared 57 young boys with FXS to a referral group of 391 individuals with autism on the Childhood Autism Rating Scale (CARS). They found that 25% met the CARS cutoff for autism, with a very similar profile on the CARS to children with autism. Bailey et al. also found that individuals with a lower developmental level were more likely to be diagnosed with autism. All of their nonverbal children with FXS (*n* = 7) scored in the autistic range on the CARS. In a follow-up study, Bailey et al. (2000) compared 31 children with FXS and CARS scores <30 to age-, race-, and gender-matched children with autism. Developmental testing on the Battelle Developmental Inventory showed a flat profile across five domains in FXS, whereas boys with autism had a more variable profile, but significant differences were seen only in the Personal-Social domain, with boys with autism scoring 7.8 months lower than boys with FXS. A subsequent analysis directly compared 13 boys with FXS and autism (CARS score >30), 13 boys with FXS and CARS score < 30, and 13 boys with autism. The boys with FXS and autism together scored lower than the other two groups on the Battelle, suggesting an additive effect of the two conditions with severe developmental consequences. The au-

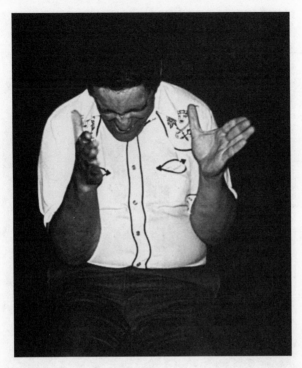

**Fig. 1.24.** An adult male with fragile X syndrome demonstrating hand flapping in addition to squinting and eye avoidance.

thors acknowledge, however, that the CARS may be more likely to indicate autistic behavior in young children with severe delays because of the delays alone (Bailey et al. 2000).

Rogers et al. (2001) studied 27 children with idiopathic autism, 24 children with fragile X syndrome, and 23 children with other developmental delays between the ages of two and four with state-of-the-art autism measures, the Autism Diagnostic Interview (ADI-R) and the Autism Diagnostic Observation Scale (ADOS-G), as well as measures of development and adaptive behavior, the Mullens and the Vineland Adaptive Behavior Scales. Unexpectedly, two distinct groups with fragile X syndrome emerged. One subgroup included 16 of the children with fragile X syndrome who did not meet criteria for the diagnosis of autism on the ADI-R, the ADOS-G, the DSM-IV, or clinician rating. Their profile on the ADOS-G, the ADI-R, and the developmental instruments was virtually identical to that of the other developmentally disabled control group. The second subgroup of fragile X children ($n = 8$) represented 33% of the total FXS group, who met all criteria for autism on all four diagnostic sys-

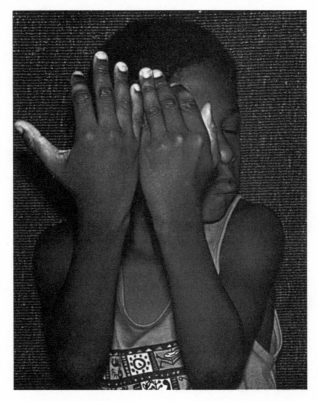

**Fig. 1.25.** A young boy with fragile X syndrome covering his eyes because of eye avoidance behavior.

tems. Their profiles on the autism instruments and on the developmental instruments were virtually identical to that of the group with idiopathic autism. This finding of two distinct fragile X syndrome subgroups makes one consider possible additional genetic influences acting synergistically, with the *FMR1* mutation leading to elevated rates of autism in FXS.

Further support for the concept of additional genetic effects leading to autism was found by Harris et al. (2000) concerning adaptive functioning and molecular relationships in individuals with FXS. They used the Vineland Adaptive Behavior Scales in 86 individuals with the full mutation or mosaic status with an age range of 1.6 to 45 years. Fourteen of these individuals were female, and 72 were male. The correlations between FMRP and various subdomains on the Vineland were significant: FMRP and Communication ($p = 0.005$), FMRP and Daily Living Skills ($p = 0.002$), FMRP and Adaptive Behavior Composite ($p = 0.002$). However, there was no correlation between FMRP and the Socialization domain on the Vineland ($p = 0.278$). The variation seen in socialization in individuals with FXS does not correlate with the variations seen in the molecular measures. This suggests that other factors, either genetic or environmental, are responsible for the variation in socialization seen within this population of individuals with fragile X.

The possibility of a second genetic hit causing autism in individuals with FXS was suggested by Feinstein and Reiss (1998) and gains further support from the FMRP studies by Bailey et al. (2001). There was no association between FMRP level and score on the CARS in 55 boys with FXS (25% of whom had a CARS score of >30). The boys with FXS and autism had lower levels of development compared to boys with FXS alone, and FMRP accounted for less variance in developmental level than did autistic behavior (Bailey et al. 2001).

Autism has also been reported in females with FXS in both mildly and severely retarded cases (Hagerman et al. 1986a; Edwards et al. 1988; Gillberg et al. 1988; Le Couteur et al. 1988; Bolton et al. 1989). Autism is not a common finding in females, but it represents the most severe end of the spectrum of social anxiety and social withdrawal, which are common in even mildly affected heterozygotes. Several studies have screened autistic females for FXS, but the numbers have been limited, with the results ranging from 0% yield (Blomquist et al. 1985; Wright et al. 1986; Matsuishi et al. 1987) to a high of 12.1% (Cohen et al. 1989a). The summation of all reports regarding the screening of autistic females for FXS yields approximately 4% positive by cytogenetic studies (Hagerman 1991). Similar results were found by Bailey et al. (1993), who screened 40 autistic females and found 5% positive for FXS. It is, therefore, recommended that all males and females with autism have DNA testing to evaluate for FXS. In addition, cytogenetic testing should be included to evaluate structural abnormalities that have been associated with autism (Mariner et al. 1986; Li et al. 1993; Cook et al. 1997; Prasad et al. 2000).

## Shyness and Social Anxiety

Shyness or social anxiety is often the presenting feature of females with FXS, particularly those with the full mutation (Hagerman et al. 1992; Sobesky et al. 1995), but it is also a common complaint of females with the premutation. Shyness is often associated with poor eye contact, which was present in 47% of females with the full mutation compared to 18% of controls, but it was also present in 36% of women with the premutation (Hull and Hagerman 1993). Although most girls with the premutation and mildly affected individuals with the full mutation outgrow shyness or social anxiety, for many females with the full mutation shyness and anxiety persist. Lachiewicz and Dawson (1994a) found that 40% of girls with FXS over nine years old had an anxiety rating (which included shy and fearful behavior) in the clinical range on the Conners Parent Questionnaire compared to none of the controls. Freund et al. (1993) carried out psychiatric evaluations on 17 females with FXS, ranging in age from 4 to 27, and found a diagnosis of avoidant personality disorder (a rather severe form of shyness) in 65% compared to 12% of IQ-matched controls. The shyness is clearly linked to anxiety, and both seem to be a core feature of FXS because they occur in individuals with the premutation who are mildly affected and in both males and females with the full mutation (Kerby and Dawson 1994, Merenstein et al. 1994, 1996; Franke et al. 1996, 1998; Hagerman et al. 1996).

To better sort out whether anxiety or depression is related to the stress of having children with FXS, Franke et al. (1998) carried out a remarkable study of psychiatric problems in women with the *FMR1* mutation. They compared 13 mothers with the full mutation, 61 mothers with the premutation, 17 women with the premutation who were siblings of the first two groups but did not have children with FXS, 18 women siblings without the *FMR1* mutation and without children, and 42 mothers without the *FMR1* mutation who had children with autism. The study used a psychiatric interview to obtain DSM IV diagnoses and to assess personality disorders, intellectual testing, and self-report questionnaires. Franke et al. found that affective disorders of all types were present in 41–56% of those with the premutation or full mutation, which was increased compared to the siblings without the mutation (11%) but similar to mothers of autistic children (38%). Anxiety disorders in general were seen in 41–46% of mothers with the full mutation or the premutation, which was significantly increased compared to those with the premutation without children (12%), siblings without the premutation (17%), and mothers of autistic children (24%). Social phobia was the most significant anxiety disorder and was significantly increased in full mutation mothers at 31% and in premutation mothers at 18% compared to mothers of autistic children at 4.8%. There was a trend for bipolar disorder to be increased in those with the *FMR1* mutation compared to controls; it was present in 15% of mothers with the full, 12% of those with the premutation either with or without children, but none of the control siblings and 5% of mothers of children with autism. Major depression was seen in 15% of mothers with a full mutation and 20% of mothers with the premutation, which was significantly different from 10% of mothers of autistic children, 0% of siblings with the premutation, and 5.6% of control siblings.

In the personality disorders area, schizotypal and schizoid personality disorder were each seen in 23% of mothers with the full mutation, which was significantly different from all other groups (Franke et al. 1998). Avoidant personality was seen in 23% of mothers with the full, 8% of mothers with the premutation, 6% of siblings with the premutation, 0% of control siblings, and only 2% of mothers of autistic children. When one combines social phobia with the personality disorder diagnoses, schizotypal personality disorder, and avoidant personality disorder, there seems to be a gene dosage effect. That is, 77% of mothers with the full, 31% of mothers with the premutation, 12% of siblings with the premutation, and 7% of mothers of autistics have one of these diagnoses. This study shows evidence of a combined effect of the *FMR1* mutation (in either the premutation or full form) and the stress of raising a developmentally disabled child on the prevalence of psychopathology in women. The IQ had no influence on the presence of a psychiatric diagnosis (Franke et al. 1998). In a previous study, however, Sobesky et al. (1996) demonstrated that the presence of executive function deficits was associated with a diagnosis of schizotypy. Therefore, the cognitive problems seem to affect some aspects of psychopathology. It is also possible for depression to influence the scoring in cognitive testing, as was demonstrated by Thompson et al. (1996).

Although most boys with FXS are shy, their level of ADHD or the severity of their mental retardation often overshadows the shyness. There is evidence in both males and females with FXS that symptoms of ADHD, particularly impulsivity, tend to counteract or improve shyness and social withdrawal (Sobesky et al. 1995; Merenstein et al. 1996). In females shyness is more of a problem clinically than in males, probably because the females have higher cognitive ability and fewer ADHD symptoms. Shyness and social anxiety also can be present with only mild to moderate deficits in FMRP. Both shyness and social anxiety are seen in high-functioning males with FXS who are producing only limited levels of FMRP (Hagerman et al. 1994; Merenstein et al. 1994; Hagerman et al. 1996; Tassone et al. 1999b).

We identified selective mutism in six girls with FXS who had had significant difficulties with shyness and social anxiety (Hagerman et al. 1999). Children with selective mutism are silent in some situations (most often in school) but are able to talk in other situations, such as the home environment. Selective mutism is related to anxiety, particularly social phobia, and the overall prevalence among 7- to 15-year-olds is approximately 1 per 500 in the general population (Kopp and Gillberg 1997). The girls with FXS and selective mutism have not had hyperactivity nor impulsivity, but anxiety has been a severe problem and they have usually responded to fluoxetine and therapy (see chap. 8). Selective mutism is uncommon in boys with FXS, perhaps because ADHD is more prevalent in boys, but it occasionally occurs, as reported by Miller et al. (2000).

Figure 1.26 demonstrates a spectrum of involvement in FXS focusing on cognitive and emotional issues and how these symptoms relate to levels of FMRP. Mild deficits of FMRP may cause only emotional problems such as shyness and social anxiety, whereas mild to moderate deficits can cause executive function deficits with mood dysregulation but perhaps without mental retardation. Moderate to severe deficits lead to mental retardation and more severe emotional and behavioral problems. From the work of Tassone et al. (1999b)

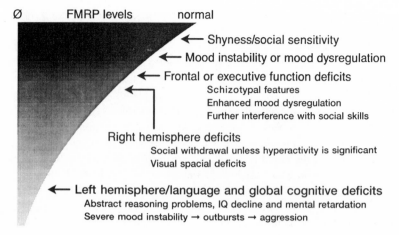

Ø          FMRP levels          normal

← Shyness/social sensitivity
← Mood instability or mood dysregulation
← Frontal or executive function deficits
　　Schizotypal features
　　Enhanced mood dysregulation
　　Further interference with social skills
Right hemisphere deficits
　　Social withdrawal unless hyperactivity is significant
　　Visual spacial deficits
← Left hemisphere/language and global cognitive deficits
　　Abstract reasoning problems, IQ decline and mental retardation
　　Severe mood instability → outbursts → aggression

**Fig. 1.26.** Hypothesized clinical/protein correlations in fragile X syndrome with an increasing deficit in FMRP production correlating with gradually more severe cognitive and behavioral involvement.

and Wright-Talamante et al. (1996), it is likely that a patient will maintain an IQ of >70 if FMRP levels are at least 50% of normal (see chaps. 4, 6, and 12).

## Stereotypies and Tics

FXS has been identified in several patients who had previously been diagnosed with Tourette syndrome. Kerbeshian et al. (1984) were the first to report this association in an 11-year-old boy, who developed both simple and complex motor tics in early childhood. Vocal tics included barking, throat clearing, and repetitive swearing or coprolalia. The boy also demonstrated compulsive mannerisms and automatic vocalizations or perseverative statements. This patient had an older brother with FXS and an atypical tic disorder. Hagerman (1987) subsequently reported a 9-year-old boy who was diagnosed with Tourette syndrome and autism before FXS was recognized. He demonstrated both simple and complex motor tics and vocal tics including coprolalia. The coprolalia was greatly exacerbated when he was placed in a self-contained setting where other children used foul language. Baumgardner et al. (1995) found a tic disorder in 22.6% of 31 boys with FXS compared to 16.7% of controls, which was an insignificant difference.

Although only an occasional patient with FXS demonstrates both motor and vocal tics that are simple and typical of Tourette syndrome patients, there exists a spectrum of Tourette syndrome–related problems in many males with FXS. Coprolalia, or repetitive bursts of swearing, is rather common in FXS in

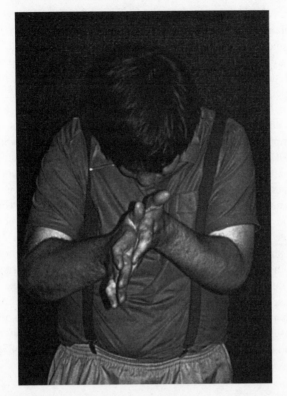

**Fig. 1.27.** A hand mannerism or stereotypy that involves rubbing the hands together is demonstrated by a man with fragile X syndrome.

our experience, particularly when individuals are exposed to foul language in their educational or social environment. There is a propensity to imitate such language, frequently manifested by a burst of pressured speech, which is perhaps a complex vocal tic. Other statements previously described as automatic verbalizations, such as "you're stupid" or "let's get out of here," are said in a perseverative, compulsive, and sometimes pressured fashion reminiscent of a complex vocal tic. These statements have also been termed *palilalia* (Newell et al. 1983) and are thought to be a language deficit, although the quality of this language seems to have some overlapping neurological features with Tourette syndrome (see chap. 6).

Complex stereotypies involving the hands and arms are also similar to complex motor tics exhibited by patients with Tourette syndrome (Fig. 1.27). Kano et al. (1988) tried to differentiate the two by pointing out that tics have a spasmodic nature, usually involving the face, and are affected by psychosocial factors, whereas stereotypies do not have these qualities. In our experience, however, complex hand stereotypies, such as hand flapping or other mannerisms (figs. 1.24 and 1.27) can dramatically increase when the patient with FXS is anxious or afraid. Burd et al. (1987) found that 12 of 59 PDD patients manifested Tourette syndrome and that tic symptoms were frequently misclassified as stereotyped movements.

Obsessive/compulsive behavior is a significant part of Tourette syndrome and is also seen in approximately 20% of first-degree relatives (Pauls et al. 1986). Compulsive or ritualistic behavior is also common in FXS, and it may respond well to fluoxetine or another seratonin agent (Hagerman et al. 1994; Hagerman 1999c; chap. 8). Hyperactivity, in addition to a mood instability problem, is common in both FXS and Tourette syndrome. Although the mood problem is common in heterozygotes, as previously discussed (Freund et al. 1993; Franke et al. 1996, 1998), it is also seen in males, and it may be central to aggressive outbursts (Hagerman et al. 1994; Hagerman 1999a). There seem to be many similarities between Tourette syndrome and FXS, although the two syndromes have far more differences, including mental retardation. Since Tourette syndrome and FXS involve dysfunction in basal ganglia, limbic, and frontal areas, there may be similar neurotransmitter dysfunction in both disorders (see chap. 8; Hagerman 1999c). Tourette syndrome has also been reported in other cases of mental retardation, including autism and Down syndrome (Golden and Greenhill 1981; Barabas et al. 1986; Burd et al. 1987; Hagerman 1999c).

## Psychosis

Although psychosis is occasionally mentioned as a manifestation of FXS in males, these features have never been systematically studied. Females with the full mutation have been more thoroughly studied for schizotypal features than have males. In a psychiatric evaluation of 20 females who were cytogenetically positive, one female with schizophrenia was detected (Freund et al. 1992; Reiss et al. 1988a). Sobesky et al. (1996) showed that the presence of schizotypal features correlates with the severity of executive function deficits. Al-Semaan (1999) reported a female with the full mutation and schizoaffective psychosis who presented at age 18 years with visual hallucinations and a history of hearing voices in addition to paranoid delusions. She responded initially to risperidone, although later she required loxapine and clonazepam, with subsequent mania symptoms that required valproate and lithium (see chap. 8). This woman also had significant cognitive deficits, including an IQ of 71, and executive function deficits, including problems in organization, planning, problem solving, sequencing, flexibility of thinking, and perseveration. Neuroimaging demonstrated ventricular dilation and a mild degree of cerebral and cerebellar atrophy.

In males with FXS, psychotic ideation is seen in approximately 12% (Hagerman 1996). It is difficult to make a diagnosis of psychotic spectrum disorder in FXS because many of the typical features of FXS, such as perseveration, carrying on conversations with themselves, unusual hand mannerisms, and odd communication patterns, may look psychotic-like at first impression. However, individuals with fragile X and psychotic spectrum disorders usually develop significant delusions or hallucinations, and their functioning level and life skills often deteriorate. Silva et al. (1998) reported a 29-year-old man with FXS and an IQ of 68 who presented with delusional ideation that a former girlfriend still loved him. He believed that she communicated with him via telepathy, and he also experienced marked mood lability, anxiety, and hostility. He responded well to a tricyclic antidepressant and antipsychotic medication, and he was diagnosed with erotomania and psychotic disorder not otherwise specified.

It is important to recognize psychotic thinking in FXS because patients generally respond well to an antipsychotic, as described in chapter 8.

## Aggressive Outburst

Periodic aggressive outbursts have been a problem for approximately 50% of adolescents and men with FXS followed in Denver (table 1.4). This problem may often begin or worsen in puberty, suggesting a testosterone effect, and continue in young adulthood. Most men with FXS do not have problems with aggression in middle and late life. For a few, aggression is a problem on a daily basis, but for many it is a periodic difficulty that occurs after a reasonable period (weeks or months) of appropriate behavior. The outburst is often precipitated by excessive stimuli in the environment such that the patient is overwhelmed and cannot maintain control. Men with FXS may misperceive social approaches or confrontations by others as threatening, and their response is sometimes aggressive. Significant paranoid thinking may add to aggression, so an evaluation for psychotic thinking is necessary in the treatment of aggression. Anxiety, tactile defensiveness, and a low frustration tolerance may further exacerbate aggressive behavior. The treatment of aggressive or violent outbursts includes psychotherapy, calming techniques, and medication (discussed in chaps. 8, 9, and 10).

## Molecular Clinical Correlations

### Involvement in Individuals with the Premutation

Although individuals with the premutation have been considered unaffected cognitively (Mazzocco et al. 1993; Reiss et al. 1993), there is mounting evidence that some premutation carriers may have limited phenotypic features, which may or may not be on the continuum with the full mutation. The problem of premature ovarian failure is a feature unique to a subgroup of women with the premutation, as previously described. The problem of a progressive cerebellar tremor in a subgroup of older males with the premutation is also a unique phenotype, not typical of those with FXS. The elevated mRNA levels in those with the premutation may be the molecular marker for clinical involvement, but further mechanistic studies are necessary (chap. 12). The neuroimaging findings in those with the premutation reported by Moore et al. (2000) and Murphy et al. (1999) may represent a mild version of what is seen in those with FXS, although the brain atrophy in older men with a cerebellar tremor (fig. 1.20; Hagerman et al. 2001a) has not been seen in those with FXS. The study of older individuals with all levels of the *FMR1* mutation is needed to clarify similarities and differences between groups.

More recent studies have shown that a subgroup of individuals with the premutation have mild or severe cognitive, physical, and/or behavioral problems (Hagerman et al. 1996; Loesch et al. 1993b, 1994; Dorn et al. 1994; Hull and Hagerman 1993; Riddle et al. 1998; Steyaert et al. 1996; Tassone et al. 2000c), and these individuals are the exceptions to the typical lack of involvement in the majority of individuals with the premutation. There is limited evidence that males with the premutation may be more vulnerable to cognitive involvement than females with the premutation because mild executive function involvement has been seen in group studies of males (Hills et al. 2000) but not in females (Sobesky et al. 1996; Reiss et al. 1993) and the more severe involvement with a progressive cerebellar tremor has been seen thus far only in older men (Hagerman et al. 2001a). Emotional problems have been studied in detail only in females with the premutation, as previously described (Franke et al. 1998), although anxiety has been documented in a subgroup of males with the premutation (O'Brien et al. 1998). Dysfunction in the regulation of *FMR1* begins in the premutation range with upregulation of mRNA presumably because of a translation problem in converting mRNA into FMRP (chap. 12). Whether mild clinical involvement in some individuals with the premutation is related to mild deficits of FMRP, problems associated with elevated mRNA, or interactions of these changes with other genes will require further research.

## Molecular/Clinical Correlations in the Full Mutation Range

In males, preliminary reports suggested that the presence of mosaicism or changes in the length of the CGG repeat within the full mutation range did not make a difference in cognitive or physical involvement in FXS (Rousseau et al. 1991a; de Vries et al. 1993a). Then anecdotal reports of higher-functioning males with the full mutation, which was partially or almost completely unmethylated, appeared (Loesch et al. 1993a, 1993b; McConkie-Rosell et al. 1993; Merenstein et al. 1994; Rousseau et al. 1994b; Milà et al. 1994; fig. 1.28). Hagerman et al. (1994) carried out a study of 250 males with FXS and found that 13% of those who completed IQ testing were high functioning (defined by an IQ of ≥70). Although many individuals experienced a decrease in IQ over time, seven individuals remained high functioning into adolescence or adulthood. Three of these individuals demonstrated a full mutation that was almost completely unmethylated. All of these males demonstrated limited features of FXS including unusual mannerisms, social anxiety or shyness, and learning problems without mental retardation.

Merenstein et al. (1996) studied 218 patients with FXS and compared males with a fully methylated full mutation, males with <50% methylation of the full mutation, and males with a mosaic pattern on a variety of physical, behavioral, and IQ measures. Males with partial methylation had the highest IQ scores and the least physical involvement compared to the other groups. The CGG repeat length and the physical index score did not correlate with the degree of clinical involvement in males with the fully methylated full mutation and in mosaic males. However, after puberty mosaic males demonstrated a higher IQ (mean 60.1 ± 15) than did males with a fully methylated full mutation (41.2 ± 11.8), although males with a partial methylation had the highest IQ (88.2 ± 11.7). Further support for less involvement in mosaic males was reported by Cohen et al. (1996), who studied 51 males with FXS, of whom 27 were mosaic. The rate of adaptive skills development in nonautistic males was twice as great in mosaic cases compared to cases with the full mutation using the Vineland Adaptive Behavior Scales.

Preliminary protein studies demonstrated significant levels of FMRP using a Western blot in three high-functioning males (Hagerman et al. 1994; Merenstein et al. 1996). Over the last several years, improved technology has developed, including immunocytochemical techniques that allow better quantitation of FMRP levels by assessing lymphocytes that stain positive for the expression of FMRP (Willemsen et al. 1997; chap. 4). Tassone et al. (1999b) used this method in studying 80 individuals with FXS and found a significant correlation between IQ and FMRP levels in females with the full mutation and males with mosaicism or a partial lack of methylation. In females, the FMRP expression level in lymphocytes correlated with the overall number of typical physical features of FXS. In mosaic males, a symptom list of behavioral problems correlated inversely with FMRP (the more behavioral problems, the lower the level of FMRP), but this was not seen in other groups. Typically, males with a full mutation that was fully methylated had little (<10% of lymphocytes positive for FMRP) or no FMRP. A subsequent study by Loesch et al. (2001) demonstrated a significant correlation between FMRP and IQ, and those with >30% of FMRP had significant benefits in their IQ score. As previously mentioned,

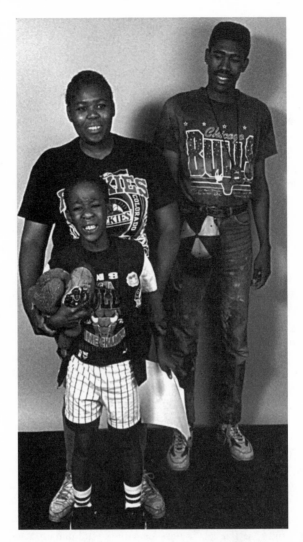

**Fig. 1.28.** A mother and her two children with fragile X syndrome. The tall young man to the right is a high-functioning male (IQ 73), whereas the younger brother has more typical features of fragile X syndrome, including long face, prominent ears and forehead, severe ADHD, and IQ < 50. The high-functioning male is producing approximately 35% of normal FMRP levels, whereas the younger brother is not producing any FMRP (Hagerman et al. 1994).

FMRP levels have now been correlated with activity on fMRI, demonstrating greater brain activity with higher FMRP levels (Menon et al. 2000; Reiss 2000; Rivera et al. 2000).

High-functioning males with FXS who do not have mental retardation have been reported by several centers (Loesch et al. 1993a; Steyaert et al. 1996; Lachiewicz et al. 1996; Smeets et al. 1995; Merenstein et al. 1994, 1996; Hagerman 1999a; Tassone et al. 1999b; Wöhrle et al. 1998; Taylor et al. 1999). Detailed neuropsychologic testing is often necessary to clarify their deficits, which usually include attentional problems, executive function deficits, mood lability, and often odd mannerisms related to FXS, including poor eye contact. Sometimes these high-functioning males are diagnosed with Asperger syndrome or schizotypal personality disorder because of odd mannerisms and social difficulties (Hagerman 1999a).

## CASE HISTORY

Jake is a 10-year 8-month-old boy who was diagnosed with fragile X syndrome one year ago when DNA testing demonstrated a mosaic pattern, with 21.2% of his cells having the premutation with 99 repeats and the rest of his cells having a full mutation with bands at 830 and 430. His FMRP level is 18% (i.e., 18% of his lymphocytes stain positive for FMRP).

He was delivered full term with a birth weight of seven pounds nine ounces, and his developmental milestones included sitting at six months, crawling at eight months, walking at fifteen months, and saying words at two years and phrases at three years of age. He had speech and language therapy from three to six years of age, and presently in his special education program he is receiving some group language therapy. He was in the regular classroom until the end of third grade, when he was expelled because of cursing, throwing things, and significant behavior problems. He was then placed in a special education program with 15 students per teacher, an aide for the classroom, and an individual aide for him. He has done remarkably well in this program, and he is now in the fifth grade. He is at grade level for reading, and he is scoring at the sixth-grade level for spelling. His social studies scores have been in the 80s and 90s; however, math is a significant problem for him, and he is receiving additional special education support for this. He has occupational therapy once a week to help with sensory integration problems. He has started attending a social skills–building group at school.

He has several friends in the classroom, although some children tend to tease or ridicule him because of his temper. At times he is uncomfortable making eye contact in social interactions. His behavioral problems include hyperactivity, which has been a difficulty for him throughout his childhood, in addition to perseveration and some obsessive-compulsive behavior. Anxiety has been a problem for him on a daily basis, and he has a panic attack during fire drills and is quite fearful of these. He hand flaps on occasion in addition to hand biting, and he may excessively chew on his clothes. He has had problems with hitting children in the past, but this rarely occurs at present. He was diagnosed in the past with pervasive developmental disorder not otherwise specified because of his unusual behaviors.

His medical history includes multiple ear infections in the first year or two, but PE tubes were never placed. He has never had a strabismus, nor apnea, nor seizures. For treatment of his hyperactivity, he took methylphenidate beginning at five years of age, and this was switched to Adderall two years ago. Tantrums increased on Adderall, so he was subsequently switched to a long-acting methylphenidate preparation, Concerta, at a dose of 36 mg/day, and this has worked well for him. He was also treated with fluvoxamine last year for his anxiety and obsessive-compulsive behavior, and this was helpful to him.

On examination, his height was in the fifteenth percentile for age, weight in the seventy-fifth percentile for age, and head circumference at the fortieth percentile for age. His blood pressure and heart rate were normal. He had a round face with mildly prominent ears that demonstrated cupping bilaterally. He had hyperextensible finger joints with MP extension to 90° bilaterally, but he was not double jointed, and his palmar creases were normal. Heart exam was normal, and his genitalia demonstrated a testicular volume of 8 ml bilaterally with Tanner stage 1 prepubertal development. Neurologic exam was normal, but he demonstrated attentional problems, distractibility, and impulsive behavior. Visual-motor coordination problems were seen, with difficulties in design copy and handwriting, although his spelling was at grade level. Cognitive testing with WISC-III demonstrated a Verbal IQ of 92, a Performance IQ of 87, and a Full-Scale IQ of 89, but his Freedom from Distractibility Score was 50, with Verbal Comprehension at 103, Perceptual Organization at 94, and Perceptual Speed at 70. On the Vineland, his overall Adaptive Behavior Composite was 74, with Communication at 91, Daily Living Skills at 76, and Socialization at 74. On the Wisconsin Card Sorting Test, he demonstrated significant executive function deficits with ADHD problems. He also perseverated on a drawing task and had unusual mannerisms, including chewing on his fingers and rubbing his hands repetitively. Because of his unusual mannerisms and obsessive thinking, along with his social deficits, he fulfills diagnostic criteria for pervasive developmental disorder not otherwise specified (PDD NOS).

His cognitive testing documents his normal intellectual abilities, but learning problems in the area of attention and concentration and visual motor coordination, in addition to academic problems in math, qualify him for special education support. He is remarkably high functioning considering that his FMRP level is only 18%, but his outstanding abilities may also be related to background gene effects and excellent environmental stimulation.

## The FXS Phenotype without the CGG Expansion

### Deletions and Point Mutations in *FMR1*

It is possible to have the phenotype of FXS without the CGG expansion. Several cases of deletions within the *FMR1* or including the *FMR1* gene have now been reported (Gedeon et al. 1992; Wöhrle et al. 1992; Tarleton et al. 1993; Albright et al. 1994; Meijer et al. 1994; Gu et al. 1994; Hirst et al. 1995; Hammond et al. 1997). These patients do not produce FMRP because of the deletion and, therefore, they have the phenotype that is typical of FXS. Hirst et al. (1995) predicted that patients with a deletion of *FMR1* would have a severe phenotype because FMRP was never available in utero in contrast to patients with the usual full mutation. There seems to be variability in the timing of methylation of the full mutation in utero such that most individuals are not methylated at the time of chorionic villus sampling (CVS) but sometime thereafter. Delayed methylation in utero would allow the benefit of FMRP production for enhancement of brain development. A more severe phenotype may also be seen when the deletion removes additional genes around *FMR1*. Quan et al. (1995) reported a large deletion in a six-year-old boy with short stature, obesity, and anal atresia in addition to features of FXS. His deletion removed Xq26.3 to Xq27.3, which presumably included other genes responsible for his anal atresia and other atypical features. The CGG repetitive sequence seems to be a hot spot for deletions, both large and small, and some just involving a back mutation to lower the CGG repeat number (de Graaff et al. 1995a; chap. 2).

De Boulle et al. (1993) described a male patient with severe mental retardation and macroorchidism who had a normal CGG repeat number and a point mutation within *FMR1* at a critical location for mRNA binding. This patient is more severely involved than the typical patient with FXS, suggesting a gain of function effect from this abnormal FMRP. Recent molecular studies have shown that the abnormal FMRP sequesters mRNAs leading to a more severe translation defect than that typically seen in FXS (Feng et al. 1997). Lugenbeel et al. (1995) subsequently reported two additional typical patients with FXS without the CGG amplification but with two different intragenic mutations. One boy has a de novo nucleotide deletion causing a frame shift and subsequently a truncated protein that is not detected in FMRP antibody studies. The second patient has an inherited two-base pair change, which also leads to premature termination and undetectable FMRP. Wang et al. (1997) reported three patients who have point mutations leading to an abnormal FMRP structure. These patients all have classical FXS, which is further evidence that the phenotype is secondary to a lack of FMRP and not related to downregulation of nearby genes caused by the CGG expansion.

## Whom to Test and Differential Diagnosis

Before the diagnosis of FXS is made, many patients have been diagnosed with general terms, such as hyperactivity (ADHD), autism, nonspecific or X-linked mental retardation, pervasive development disorder (PDD), learning disability, or emotional impairment. Any child or adult who presents with autism or autistic-like features and/or mental retardation without a specific etiology identified should undergo DNA testing for FXS (chap. 2) and, in addition, high-resolution cytogenetic testing for other structural abnormalities. Screening such patients yields a 2–5% positive rate for the *FMR1* mutation and a similar rate for other cytogenetic abnormalities (Jacky 1996; chap. 3).

Not all hyperactive patients should have DNA testing for FXS; however, individuals with additional features typical of PDD or FXS, such as poor eye contact, hand flapping, hand biting, or perseverative speech, should be tested. These behavioral features and additional physical features typical of FXS have been compiled in a fragile X checklist (table 1.6), which can be scored similarly to the Apgar score: give 2 points if the feature is present, 1 point if the feature was present in the past or is present to a borderline degree, and no points if the feature is absent (Hagerman 1987). A preliminary study screening 107 males demonstrated that 45% of those with a score of 16 or higher had FXS and 60% of those with a score of 19 or higher had FXS (Hagerman et al. 1991). A similar clinical checklist has been used by de Vries et al. (1999) and others (Maes et al. 2000) to select high-risk patients to undergo DNA testing. Lachiewicz et al. (2000b) evaluated a physical checklist of 37 items and found that 4 items were significantly different between 36 young boys with FXS and controls: adverse response to touch on the skin, difficulty touching tongue to the lips, soft skin over the dorsum of the hand, and hallucal crease.

Because FXS has been found in those with a previous diagnosis of Sotos, Asperger, Prader-Willi, FG, and Pierre Robin syndromes, individuals with these diagnoses should be reevaluated with DNA testing for FXS. Other chromosomal disorders, including Down syndrome, Klinefelter syndrome (XXY), XO, XYY, XXX, and an extra microchromosome may occur with FXS (Sutherland and Hecht 1985; Brøndum-Nielsen 1986; Fryns and Van den Berghe 1988; Fuster et al. 1988; Watson et al. 1988; Moon and Moon 1993; Lopez-Pajares et al. 1994), suggesting an increased rate of nondisjunction in heterozygotes. Therefore, individuals with these disorders but with physical and behavioral features typical of FXS should be evaluated with DNA testing.

There are a variety of X-linked disorders with physical features reminiscent of FXS, such as Coffin-Lowry syndrome, with prominent ears, coarse features, and hypotonia; Lujan syndrome, with marfanoid habitus and macroorchidism; and Atkin syndrome, with large ears, short stature, and macroorchidism (Arena and Lubs 1991). The differential diagnosis is complex, and

**Table 1.6**
**Fragile X Checklist**

| | Score | | |
|---|---|---|---|
| | *Present*<br>*0* | *Borderline*<br>*or Present in*<br>*the Past*<br>*1* | *Definitely*<br>*Present*<br>*2* |
| Mental retardation | | | |
| Hyperactivity | | | |
| Short attention span | | | |
| Tactile defensiveness | | | |
| Hand flapping | | | |
| Hand biting | | | |
| Poor eye contact | | | |
| Perseverative speech | | | |
| Hyperextensible MP joints | | | |
| Large or prominent ears | | | |
| Large testicles | | | |
| Simian crease or Sydney line | | | |
| Family history of mental retardation | | | |

an update of X-linked disorders can be found in Lubs et al. 1999, Chelly 2000, and Neri and Chiurazzi (2000).

## Why Make a Diagnosis of FXS?

It is important to diagnose children and adults with FXS for several reasons. The diagnosis benefits the family because it ends their search for reasons why their child has behavior and cognitive deficits and it focuses the family on treatment and interventions that can benefit their child (see chaps. 8, 9, 10, and 11). Parents can gain an understanding of FXS and how it modifies their child's development and behavior, and they can receive support and ideas from other parents who are struggling with the same problems. The National Fragile X Foundation has a list of parent support groups around the country and internationally, in addition to parent and professional educational materials, and they can be contacted at 1-800-688-8765 or 510-763-6030 (see appendix 1). Since FXS is a genetic disorder, counseling for the immediate family and for extended family members who are affected or who are at risk to be carriers is essential. Genetic counseling can educate family members regarding the inheritance pattern, mild forms of involvement, and the risk of having children affected by FXS. The counselor can help to inform extended family members with letters or by direct contact, with the permission of family. Prenatal diagnosis can be explained, in addition to new reproductive technology, such as egg donation and in vitro fertilization, in an effort to help the family have a normal child, if the desire for children exists (see chap. 7).

Over 90% of families diagnosed with FXS and followed at the Fragile X Treatment and Research Center in Denver have found the diagnosis beneficial (Roy et al. 1995). The majority of the families have benefited from treatment intervention, including medication, individual therapies, and educational interventions (Roy et al. 1995). Although this book focuses on the problems associated with FXS, there are also many strengths in the majority of children and adults who are affected, including a fine sense of humor, good imitation skills, a positive attitude and personality, and intense interests. Families learn from their wonderful children with FXS, and so have clinicians and researchers.

## Acknowledgments

This work was supported in part by National Institutes of Child Health and Development grant HD36071 and MCHB grant MCJ-089413. In addition, the research reported here has been partially supported by grant 5 MO1 RR00069 to our General Clinical Research Center's program; National Center for Research Resources, NIH; Children's Hospital Research Institute; Developmental Psychobiology Research Group of the University of Colorado Health Sciences Center; and M.I.N.D. Institute at University of California, Davis, Medical Center. I gratefully acknowledge the support of our team from the Fragile X Treatment and Research Center in the Child Development Unit of the Children's Hospital in Denver and our team at the M.I.N.D. Institute at the University of California at Davis Medical Center. This chapter would not have been possible without the help of Susan Harris.

## References

Abitbol, M., C. Menini, A-L. Delezoide, T. Rhyner, M. Vekemans, and J. Mallet. 1993. Nucleus basalis magnocellularis and hippocampus are the major sites of FMR-1 expression in the human fetal brain. *Nat. Genet.* 4:147–153.

Abrams, M. T., and A. L. Reiss. 1995. The neurobiology of fragile X syndrome. *Ment. Retard. Dev. Disab. Res. Rev.,*1:269–275.

Abrams, M. T., A. L. Reiss, L. S. Freund, T. Baumgardner, G. A. Chase, and M. B. Denckla. 1994. Molecular-neurobehavioral associations in females with the fragile X full mutation. *Am. J. Med. Genet.* 51:317–327.

Aicardi, J. 1986. *Epilepsy in children: The international review of child neurology.* New York: Raven Press, pp. 119–129.

Albright, S. G., A. M. Lachiewicz, J. C. Tarleton, K. W. Rao, C. E. Schwartz, R. Richie, M. B. Tennison, and A. S. Aylsworth. 1994. Fragile X phenotype in a patient with a large de novo deletion in Xq27–q28. *Am. J. Med. Genet.* 51:294–297.

Allingham-Hawkins, D. J., R. Babul-Hirji, D. Chitayat, J. J. A. Holden, K. T. Yang, C. Lee, et al. 1999. Fragile X premutation is a significant risk factor for premature ovarian failure: The international collaborative POF in fragile X study—preliminary data. *Am. J. Med. Genet.* 83:322–325.

Al-Semaan, Y., A. K. Malla, and A. Lazosky. 1999. Schizoaffective disorder in a fragile-X carrier. *Aust. N.Z. J. Psychiatry* 33:436–440.

American Psychiatric Association. 1980. *Diagnostic and statistical manual of mental disorders (DSM III),* 3d ed. Washington, D.C.: APA, pp. 87–90.

———. 1987. *Diagnostic and statistical manual of mental disorders, revised (DSM III R),* 4th ed. Washington, D.C.: APA.

Amin, V. R., and D. M. Maino. 1995. The fragile X female: A case report of the visual, visual-perceptual, and ocular health findings. *J. Am. Optom. Assoc.* 66:290–295.

Arena, J. F., and H. A. Lubs. 1991. Other disorders with X-linked mental retardation: A review of thirty-three syndromes. In R. J. Hagerman and A. C. Silverman (eds.), *Fragile X syndrome: Diagnosis, treatment, and research.* Baltimore: Johns Hopkins Univ. Press, pp. 202–227.

Arinami, Y., M. Sato, S. Nakajima, and I. Kondo. 1988. Auditory brain-stem responses in the fragile X syndrome. *Am. J. Hum. Genet.* 43:46–51.

Ashley, C. J., Jr., K. D. Wilkinson, D. Reines, and S. T. Warren. 1993. FMR-1 protein: Conserved RNP family domains and selective RNA binding. *Science* 262:563–565.

Asperger, H. 1994. Die autistischen Psychopathen im Kindesalter. *Arch. Psych. Mervenkrankh.* 117:76–136.

August, G. J., and I. H. Lockhart. 1984. Familial autism and the fragile X chromosome. *J. Autism Disord.* 14:197–204.

Bachner, D., A. Manca, P. Steinbach, D. Wöhrle, W. Just, W. Vogel, H. Hameister, and A. Poustka. 1993a. Enhanced expression of the murine FMR1 gene during germ cell proliferation suggests a special function in both the male and the female gonad. *Hum. Mol. Genet.* 2:2043–2050.

Bachner, D., P. Steinbach, D. Wöhrle, W. Just, W. Vogel, H. Hameister, A. Manca, and A. Poustka. 1993b. Enhanced Fmr-1 expression in testis [letter; comment]. *Nat. Genet.* 4:115–116.

Backes, M., B. Genç, J. Schreck, W. Doerfler, G. Lehmkuhl, and A. von Gontard. 2000. Cognitive and behavioral profile of fragile X boys: Correlations to molecular data. *Am. J. Med. Genet.* 95:150–156.

Bailey, A., P. Bolton, L. Butler, A. LeCouteur, M. Murphy, S. Scott, T. Webb, and M.

Rutter. 1993. Prevalence of the fragile X anomaly amongst autistic twins and singletons. *J. Child Psychol. Psychiatry* 34:673–688.

Bailey, D. B., G. B. Mesibov, D. D. Hatton, R. D. Clark, J. E. Roberts, and L. Mayhew. 1998. Autistic behavior in young boys with fragile X syndrome. *J. Autism Dev. Disord.* 28:499–508.

Bailey, D. B., Jr., D. D. Hatton, G. B. Mesibov, N. Ament, and M. Skinner. 2000. Early development, temperament and functional impairment in autism and fragile X syndrome. *J. Autism Dev. Disord.* 30:49–59.

Bailey, D. B., Jr., D. D. Hatton, M. Skinner, and G. B. Mesibov. 2001a. Autistic behavior, FMRP, and developmental trajectories in young males with fragile X syndrome. *J. Autism Dev. Disord.* 31:165–174.

Bailey, D. B., D. D. Hatton, F. Tassone, M. Skinner, and A. K. Taylor. 2001b. Variability in FMRP and early development in males with fragile X syndrome. *Am. J. Ment. Retard.* 106:16–27.

Bakker, C. E., C. Verheij, R. Willemsen, R. Vanderhelm, F. Oerlemans, M. Vermey, A. Bygrave, A. T. Hoogereen, B. A. Oostra, E. Reyniers, K. De Boulle, R. Dhooge, P. Cras, D. Van Velzen, G. Nagels, J. J. Martin, P. P. Dedeyn, J. K. Darby, and P. J. Willems. 1994. FMR1 knockout mice: A model to study fragile X mental retardation. *Cell* 78:23–33.

Barabas, G., B. Wardell, M. Sapiro, and W. S. Matthews. 1986. Coincident Down's and Tourette syndromes: Three case reports. *J. Child Neurol.* 1:358–360.

Baumgardner, T. L., A. L. Reiss, L. S. Freund, and M. T. Abrams. 1995. Specification of the neurobehavioral phenotype in males with fragile X syndrome. *Pediatrics* 95:744–752.

Beemer, F. A., H. Veenema, and J. M. de Pater. 1986. Cerebral gigantism (Sotos syndrome) in two patients with fra(X) chromosomes. *Am. J. Med. Genet.* 23:221–226.

Bell, M. V., J. Bloomfield, M. McKinley, N. Patterson, M. G. Darlinson, E. A. Barnard, and K. E. Davies. 1989. Physical linkage of GABA receptor subunit gene to the DXS 374 locus in human Xq28. *Am. J. Hum. Genet.* 45:883–889.

Bell, M. V., M. C. Hirst, Y. Nakahori, R. N. MacKinnon, H. Roche, T. J. Flint, P. A. Jacobs, N. Tommerup, L. Tranebjaerg, U. Froster-Iskenius, B. Kerr, G. Turner, R. H. Lindenbaum, R. Winter, M. Pembrey, S. Thibodeau, and K. E. Davies. 1991. Physical mapping across the fragile X: Hypermethylation and clinical expression of the fragile X syndrome. *Cell* 64:861–866.

Belser, R. C., and V. Sudhalter. 1995. Arousal difficulties in males with fragile X syndrome: A preliminary report. *Dev. Brain Dysfunct.* 8:270–279.

Benezech, M., and B. Noel. 1985. Fragile X syndrome and autism. *Clin. Genet.* 28:93.

Bennett, K. E., and M. P. Haggard. 1999. Behaviour and cognitive outcomes from middle ear disease. *Arch. Dis. Child.* 80:28–35.

Berkovitz, G. D., D. P. Wilson, N. J. Carpenter, T. R. Brown, and C. J. Migeon. 1986. Gonadal function in men with the Martin Bell (fragile X) syndrome. *Am. J. Med. Genet.* 23:227–239.

Berry-Kravis, E., and R. Ciurlionis. 1998. Overexpression of fragile X gene (*FMR1*) transcripts increases cAMP production in neural cells. *J. Neurosci. Res.* 51:41–48.

Berry-Kravis, E., M. Hicar, and R. Ciurlionis. 1995. Reduced cyclic AMP production in fragile X syndrome: Cytogenetic and molecular correlations. *Pediatr. Res.* 38:638–643.

Berry-Kravis, E., and P. R. Huttenlocher. 1992. Cyclic AMP metabolism in fragile X syndrome. *Am. Neurol.* 31:22–26.

Berry-Kravis, E., and P. Sklena. 1993. Demonstration of abnormal cyclic AMP production in platelets from patients with fragile X syndrome. *Am. J. Med. Genet.* 45:81–87.

Binstock, T. 1995. Fragile X and the amygdala: Cognitive, interpersonal, emotional and neuroendocrine consideration. *Dev. Brain Dys.* 8:199–217.

Black, S. H., G. Levinson, G. L. Harton, F. T. Palmer, M. E. Sisson, C. Schoener, C. Nance, E. F. Fugger, and R. A. Fields. 1995. Preimplantation genetic testing (PGT) for fragile X (fraX). *Am. J. Hum. Genet.* 57(suppl.):A31;153.

Blomquist, H. K., M. Bohman, S. O. Edvinsson, C. Gillberg, K. H. Gustavson, G. Holmgren, and J. Wahlstrom. 1985. Frequency of the fragile X syndrome in infantile autism. *Clin. Genet.* 27:113–117.

Boccia, M. L., and J. E. Roberts. 2000. Behavior and autonomic nervous system function assessed via heart period measures: The case of hyperarousal in boys with fragile X syndrome. *Behav. Res. Methods, Instruments, Computers* 32:5–10.

Bolton, P. M., M. Rutter, I. Butler, and I. Summers. 1989. Females with autism and the fragile X. *J. Autism Dev. Disord.* 19:473–476.

Borghgraef, M., J. P. Fryns, A. Dielkens, K. Dyck, and H. Van den Berghe. 1987. Fragile X syndrome: A study of the psychological profile in 23 prepubertal patients. *Clin. Genet.* 32:179–186.

Borghgraef, M., J. P. Fryns, and H. Van den Berghe. 1990. The female and the fragile X syndrome: Data on clinical and psychological findings in fragile X carriers. *Clin. Genet.* 37:341–346.

Bowen, P., B. Biederman, and K. A. Swallow. 1978. The X-linked syndrome of macroorchidism and mental retardation; further observations. *Am. J. Med. Genet.* 2:409–414.

Braat, D. D. M., A. P. T. Smits, and C. M. G. Tomas. 1999. Menstrual disorders and endocrine profiles in fragile X carriers prior to 40 years of age: A pilot study. *Am. J. Med. Genet.* 83:327–328.

Bregman, J. D., J. F. Leckman, and S. I. Ort. 1988. Fragile X syndrome: Genetic predisposition to psychopathology. *J. Autism Dev. Disord.* 18:343–354.

Bregman, J. D., J. F. Leckman, and S. I. Ort. 1990. Thyroid function in fragile-X syndrome males. *Yale J. Biol. Med.* 63:293–299.

Brøndum-Nielsen, K. 1986. Sex chromosomes anuploidy in fragile X carriers. *Am. J. Med. Genet.* 23:537–544.

———. 1988. Growth patterns in boys with fragile X syndrome. *Am. J. Med. Genet.* 30:143–147.

Brøndum-Nielsen, K., N. Tommerup, V. Dyggve, and C. Schou. 1982. Macroorchidism and fragile X in mentally retarded males: Clinical, cytogenetic and some hormonal investigations in mentally retarded males, including two with the fragile site at Xq28, fra(X) (q28). *Hum. genet.* 61:113–117.

Brøndum-Nielsen, K., N. Tommerup, B. Frills, K. Hjelt, and K. Hippe. 1983. Diagnosis of the fragile X syndrome (Martin-Bell syndrome): Clinical findings in 27 males with the fragile site at Xq28. *J. Ment. Defic. Res.* 27:211–226.

Brown, C. A., C. K. Brasington, and F. S. Grass. 1995. Paternal transmission of a full mutation in the FMR1 gene: Identification of paternal CGG repeat sizes in multiple tissues. *Am. J. Hum. Genet.* 57(suppl.):A335;1947.

Brown, W. T., E. C. Jenkins, E. Friedman, J. Brooks, K. Wisniewski, S. Raguthu, and J. French. 1982. Autism is associated with the fragile X syndrome. *J. Autism Dev. Disord.* 12:303–308.

Brown, W. T., E. C. Jenkins, I. L. Cohen, G. S. Fisch, E. G. Wolf-Schein, A. Gross, L. Waterhouse, D. Fein, A. Mason-Brothers, E. Ritvo, B. A. Rittenberg, W. Bentley, and V. Castells. 1986. Fragile X and autism: A multicenter survey. *Am. J. Med. Genet.* 23:341–352.

Brown, W. T., E. C. Jenkins, G. Neri, H. Lubs, L. R. Shapiro, K. E. Davies, S. Sherman, R. J. Hagerman, and C. Laird. 1991. Conference report: 4th International Workshop on the Fragile X and X-linked Mental Retardation. *Am. J. Med. Genet.* 38:158–172.

Burd, L., W. W. Fisher, J. Kerbeshian, and M. E. Arnold. 1987. Is development of Tourette disorder a marker for improvement in patients with autism and other pervasive developmental disorders? *J. Am. Acad. Child Psychiatry* 26:162–165.

Butler, M. G., and J. L. Najjar. 1988. Do some patients with fragile X syndrome have precocious puberty? *Am. J. Med. Genet.* 31:779–781.

Butler, M. G., A. Allen, D. Slingh, N. J. Carpenter, and B. D. Hall. 1988. Preliminary communication: Photoanthropometric analysis of individuals with the fragile X syndrome. *Am. J. Med. Genet.* 30:165–168.

Butler, M. G., M. G. Allen, J. L. Haynes, D. N. Singh, M. S. Watson, and W. R. Breg. 1991a. Anthropometric comparison of mentally retarded males with and without fragile X syndrome. *Am. J. Med. Genet.* 38:260–268.

Butler, M. G., T. Mangrum, R. Gupta, and D. N. Singh. 1991b. A 15-item checklist for screening mentally retarded males for the fragile X syndrome. *Clin. Genet.* 39:347–354.

Butler, M. G., A. Brunschwig, L. K. Miller, and R. J. Hagerman. 1992. Standards for selected anthropometric measurements in males with the fragile X syndrome. *Pediatrics* 89:1059–1062.

Cantú, J. M., H. E. Scaglia, M. Medina, M. Gonzalez-Diddi, T. Morato, M. E. Moreno, and G. Perez-Palacios. 1976. Inherited congenital normofunctional testicular hyperplasia and mental deficiency. *Hum. Genet.* 33:23–33.

Cantú, J. M., H. E. Scaglia, M. Gonzalez-Diddi, P. Hernandez-Jauregui, T. Morato, M. E. Moreno, J. Giner, A. Alcantar, D. Herrera, and G. Perez-Palacios. 1978. Inherited congenital normofunctional testicular hyperplasia and mental deficiency: A corroborative study. *Hum. Genet.* 41:331–339.

Castro-Magana, M., M. Angulo, A. Canas, A. Saharp, and B. Fuentes. 1988. Hypothalamic-pituitary gonadal axis in boys with primary hypothyroidism and macroorchidism. *J. Pediatr.* 112:397–402.

Chelly, J. 2000. MRX review. *Am. J. Med. Genet.* 94:364–366.

Christensen, A. V., and P. Krogsgaard-Larsen. 1984. GABA agonists: Molecular and behavioral pharmacology. In R. G. Fariello (ed.), *Neurotransmitters, seizures, and epilepsy II.* New York: Raven Press, pp. 109–126.

Chudley, A. E., and R. J. Hagerman. 1987. Fragile X syndrome. *J. Pediatr.* 110:821–831.

Cohen, I. L. 1995a. Behavioral profiles of autistic and nonautistic fragile X males. *Dev. Brain Dysfunct.* 8:252–269.

Cohen, I. L. 1995b. A theoretical analysis of the role of hyperarousal in the learning and behavior of fragile X males. *Ment. Retard. Dev. Disabil. Res. Rev.* 1:286–291.

Cohen, I. L., D. S. Fisch, E. G. Wolf-Schein, V. Sudhalter, D. Hanson, R. J. Hagerman, E. C. Jenkins, and W. T. Brown. 1988. Social avoidance and repetitive behavior in fragile X males: A controlled study. *Am. J. Ment. Retard.* 92:436–446.

Cohen, I. L., W. T. Brown, E. C. Jenkins, J. H. French, S. Raguthu, E. G. Wolf-Schein, V. Sudhalter, G. Fisch, and K. Wisniewski. 1989a. Fragile X syndrome in females with autism [letter to the editor]. *Am. J. Genet.* 34:302–303.

Cohen, I. L., P. M. Vietze, V. Sudhalter, E. C. Jenkins, and W. T. Brown. 1989b. Parent-child dyadic gaze patterns in fragile X males and in non-fragile X males with autistic disorder. *J. Child. Psychol. Psychiatry* 30:845–856.

Cohen, I. L., J. A. Tsiouris, and A. Pfadt. 1991a. Effects of long-acting propranolol on agonistic and stereotyped behaviors in a man with pervasive developmental disorder and fragile X syndrome: A double-blind, placebo-controlled study [letter]. *J. Clin. Psychopharmacol.* 11:398–399.

Cohen, I. L., P. M. Vietze, V. Sudhalter, E. C. Jenkins, and W. T. Brown. 1991b. Effects of age and communication level on eye contact in fragile X males and non–fragile X autistic males. *Am. J. Med. Genet.* 38:498–502.

Cohen, I. L., S. L. Nolin, V. Sudhalter, X. H. Ding, C. S. Dobkin, and W. T. Brown. 1996. Mosaicism for the FMR1 gene influences adaptive skills development in fragile X–affected males. *Am. J. Med. Genet.* 64:365–369.

Comery, T. A., J. B. Harris, P. J. Willems, B. A. Oostra, S. A. Irwin, I. J. Weiler, and W. T. Greenough. 1997. Abnormal dendritic spines in fragile X knockout mouse: Maturation and pruning deficits. *Proc. Natl. Acad. Sci. USA* 94:5401–5404.

Conners, C. K. 1973. Rating scales for use in drug studies with children. *Psychopharmacol. Bull.* (special issue):24–84, 219–222.

Conway, G. S., S. Hettiarachchi, A. Murray, and P. A. Jacobs. 1995. Fragile X premutations in familial premature ovarian failure [letter; comment]. *Lancet* 346:309–310.

Conway, G. S., N. N. Payne, J. Webb, A. Murray, and P. A. Jacobs. 1998. Fragile X premutation screening in women with premature ovarian failure [see comments]. *Hum. Reprod.* 13:1184–1187.

Cook, E. H., Jr., V. Lindgren, B. L. Leventhal, R. Courchesne, A. Lincoln, C. Shulman, and C. Lord. 1997. Autism or atypical autism in maternally but not paternally derived proximal 15q duplication. *Am. J. Hum. Genet.* 60:928–934.

Cornish, K. M., F. Munir, and G. Cross. 2001. Differential impact of the FMR-1 full mutation on memory and attentional functioning: A neuropsychological perspective. *J. Cogn. Neurosci.* 13:144–150.

Courchesne, E., J. Townsend, and O. Saitoh. 1994. The brain in infantile autism: Posterior fossa structures are abnormal. *Neurology* 44:214–223.

Crabbe, L. S., A. S. Bensky, L. Hornstein, and D. C. Schwartz. 1993. Cardiovascular abnormalities in children with fragile X syndrome. *Pediatrics* 91:714–715.

Craddock, N., J. Daniels, P. McGuffin, and M. Owen. 1994. Variation at the fragile X locus does not influence susceptibility to bipolar disease. *Am. J. Med. Genet.* 54:141–143.

Cronister, A. R., R. Schreiner, M. Wittenberger, K. Amiri, K. Harris, and R. J. Hagerman. 1991a. The heterozygous fragile X female: Historical, physical, cognitive and cytogenetic features. *Am. J. Med. Genet.* 38:269–274.

Cronister, A. R., K. Amiri, and R. J. Hagerman. 1991b. Mental impairment in fragile X positive girls. *Am. J. Med. Genet.* 38:503–504.

Crowe, R. R., L. T. Tsai, J. C. Murray, S. R. Patil, and J. Quinn. 1988. A study of autism using X chromosome DNA probes. *Biol. Psychol.* 24:473–479.

Cunningham, M., and J. D. Dickerman. 1988. Fragile X syndrome and acute lymphoblastic leukemia. *Cancer* 62:2383–2386.

Cyr, M., and C. S. Brown. 1998. Current drug therapy recommendations for the treatment of attention deficit hyperactivity disorder [erratum in *Drugs* 58(4):597, 1999]. *Drugs* 56:215–223.

Daly, E. M., C. J. Moore, G. McAlonan, K. C. Murphy, K. E. Davies, and D. G. M. Murphy. 2000. X chromosome trinucleotide repeats: Effect on brain structure. Presented at the Seventh International Fragile X Conference, Los Angeles, July 19–21.

Daniel, W. A., R. A. Feinstein, P. Howard-Peebles, and W. D. Bazley. 1982. Testicular volumes of adolescents. *J. Pediatr.* 101:1010–1012.

Davids, J. R., R. J. Hagerman, and R. E. Eilert. 1990. The orthopedist and fragile X syndrome. *J. Bone Joint Surg. Br.* 72:889–896.

De Boulle, K., A. J. M. H. Verkerk, E. Reyniers, L. Vits, J. Hendrickx, B. VanRoy, F. VanDenBos, E. de Graaff, B. A. Oostra, and P. J. Willems. 1993. A point mutation in the FMR1 gene associated with fragile X mental retardation. *Nat. Genet.* 3:31–35.

de Graaff, E., P. Rouillard, P. J. Willems, A. P. T. Smits, F. Rousseau, and B. A. Oostra. 1995a. Hotspot for deletions in the CGG repeat region of FMR1 in fragile X patients. *Hum. Mol. Genet.* 4:45–49.

de Graaff, E., R. Willemsen, N. Zhong, C. E. M. de Die-Smulders, W. T. Brown, G. Freling, and B. Oostra. 1995b. Instability of the CGG repeat and expression of the FMR1 protein in a male fragile X patient with a lung tumor. *Am. J. Hum. Genet.* 57:609–618.

DeLong, R. G., and J. Dwyer. 1988. Correlation of family history with specific autistic subgroups: Asperger's syndrome and bipolar affective disease. *J. Autism Dev. Disord.* 18:593–600.

del Pozo, B. C., and P. R. Millard. 1983. Demonstration of the fra(X) in lymphocytes, fibroblasts, and bone marrow in a patient with testicular tumor. *J. Med. Genet.* 20:225–227.

Desai, H. B., J. Donat, M. H. K. Shokeir, and D. G. Munoz. 1990. Amyotrophic lateral sclerosis in a patient with fragile X syndrome. *Neurology* 40:378–380.

de Vries, B. B. A., A. M. Wiegers, E. de Graaff, A. J. M. H. Verkerk, J. O. Van Hemel, D. T. J. Halley, J-P. Fryns, L. M. G. Curfs, M. F. Niermeijer, and P. A. Oostra. 1993a. Mental status and fragile X expression in relation to FMR-1 gene mutation. *Eur. J. Hum. Genet.* 1:72–79.

de Vries, B. B. A., J-P. Fryns, M. G. Butler, F. Canziani, E. Wesby-van Swaay, J. O. van-Hemel, B. A. Oostra, D. J. J. Halley, and M. F. Niermeyer. 1993b. Clinical and molecular studies in fragile X patients with a Prader-Willi-like phenotype. *J. Med. Genet.* 30:761–766.

de Vries, B. B. A., H. Robinson, I. Stolte-Dijkstra, C. V. T. P. Gi, D. F. Dijkstra, J. van-Doorn, D. J. J. Halley, B. A. Oostra, G. Turner, and M. F. Niermeijer. 1995. General overgrowth in the fragile X syndrome: Variability in the phenotype expression of the FMR1 gene mutation. *J. Med. Genet.* 32:764–769.

de Vries, B. B., C. C. Jansen, A. A. Duits, C. Verheij, R. Willemsen, J. O. van Hemel, A. M. van den Ouweland, M. F. Niermeijer, B. A. Oostra, and D. J. Halley. 1996a. Variable FMR1 gene methylation of large expansions leads to variable phenotype in three males from one fragile X family. *J. Med. Genet.* 33:1007–1010.

de Vries, B. B., A. M. Wiegers, A. P. Smits, S. Mohkamsing, H. J. Duivenvoorden, J. P. Fryns, L. M. Curfs, D. J. Halley, B. A. Oostra, A. M. van den Ouweland, and M. F. Niermeijer. 1996b. Mental status of females with an FMR1 gene full mutation. *Am. J. Med. Genet.* 58:1025–1032.

de Vries, B. B. A., S. Mohkamsing, A. M. W. van den Ouweland, E. Mol, K. Gelsema, M. van Rijn, A. Tibben, D. J. J. Halley, H. J. Duivenvoorden, B. A. Oostra, and M. F. Niermeijer. 1999. Screening for the fragile X syndrome among the mentally retarded: A clinical study. *J. Med. Genet.* 36:467–470.

Devys, D., V. Biancalana, F. Rousseau, J. Boue, J. L. Mandel, and I. Oberlé. 1992. Analysis of full fragile X mutations in fetal tissues and monozygotic twins indicate that abnormal methylation and somatic heterogeneity are established early in development. *Am. J. Med. Genet.* 43:208–216.

Devys, D., Y. Lutz, N. Rouyer, J. P. Bellocq, and J. L. Mandel. 1993. The FMR-1 protein is cytoplasmic, most abundant in neurons and appears normal in carriers of a fragile X premutation. *Nat. Genet.* 4:335–340.

Dorn, M., M. Mazzocco, and R. J. Hagerman. 1994. Behavioral and psychiatric disorders in adult fragile X carrier males. *J. Am. Acad. Child Adolesc. Psychiatry* 33:256–264.

Dunn, H. G., H. Renpenning, J. W. Gerrard, J. R. Miller, R. Tabata, and S. Federoff. 1963. Mental retardation as a sex-linked defect. *Am. J. Ment. Defic.* 67:827–848.

Dykens, E., and J. Leckman. 1990. Developmental issues in fragile X syndrome. In R. M. Hodapp, J. A. Buracck, and E. Zigler (eds), *Issues in the developmental approach to mental retardation.* New York: Cambridge Univ. Press, pp. 226–245.

Dykens, E., R. Hodapp, S. Ort, B. Finucane, L. Shapiro, and J. Leckman. 1989. The trajectory of cognitive development in males with fragile X syndrome. *J. Am. Acad. Child Adolesc. Psychiatry* 28:422–426.

Edwards, D. R., L. D. Keppen, J. D. Ranells, and S. M. Gollin. 1988. Autism in association with fragile X syndrome in females: Implications for diagnosis and treatment. *Neurotoxicology* 9:359–366.

Einfeld, S., H. Molony, and W. Hall. 1989. Autism is not associated with the fragile X syndrome. *Am. J. Med. Genet.* 34:187–193.

Einfeld, S. L., B. J. Tonge, and T. Florio. 1994. Behavioural and emotional disturbance in fragile X syndrome. *Am. J. Med. Genet.* 51:386–391.

Einfeld, S., B. Tonge, and G. Turner. 1999. Longitudinal course of behavioral and emotional problems in fragile X syndrome. *Am. J. Med. Genet.* 87:436–439.

Elia, M., R. Ferri, S. A. Musumeci, S. Del Gracco, M. Bottitta, C. Scuderi, G. Miano, S. Panerai, T. Bertrand, and J. Grubar. 2000. Sleep in subjects with autistic disorder: A neurophysiological and psychological study. *Brain Dev.* 22:88–92.

Escalante, J. A. 1971. Estudo genetico da deficiencia mental. Ph.D. diss., Univ. of Sao Paulo.

Escalante, J. A., H. Grunspun, and O. Frota-Pessoa. 1971. Severe sex-linked mental retardation. *J. Genet. Hum.* 19:137–140.

Farkas, L. G. 1976. Basic morphological data of external genitals in 177 healthy Central European men. *Am. J. Phys. Anthropol.* 34:325–328.

Feingold, M., and W. H. Bossert. 1974. Normal values for selected physical parameters: An aid to syndrome delineation. *Birth Defects* 10:1–15.

Feinstein, C., and A. L. Reiss. 1998. Autism: The point of view from fragile X studies. *J. Autism Dev. Disord.* 28:393–405.

Feng, Y., D. Lakkis, and S. T. Warren. 1995a. Quantitative comparison of *FMR1* gene expression in normal and premutation alleles. *Am. J. Hum. Genet.* 56:106–113.

Feng, Y., F. Zhang, L. K. Lokey, J. L. Chastain, L. Lakkis, D. Eberhart, and S. T. Warren. 1995b. Translational suppression by trinucleotide repeat expansion at FMR1. *Science* 268:731–734.

Feng, Y., D. Absher, D. E. Eberhart, V. Brown, H. E. Malter, and S. T. Warren. 1997. FMRP associates with polyribosomes as an mRNP, and the I304N mutation of severe fragile X syndrome abolishes this association. *Mol. Cell* 1:109–118.

Ferrari, A., C. Meazza, and M. Casanova. 2000. Nasopharyngeal carcinoma in a boy with fragile X syndrome. *Pediatr. Hematol. Oncol.* 17:597–600.

Ferri, R., R. M. Colognola, S. Falsone, S. A. Musumeci, M. A. Petrella, S. A. Sanfilippo, A. Viglianesi, and P. Bergonzi. 1988. Brainstem auditory and visual evoked potentials in subjects with fragile X mental retardation syndrome. In C. Barber and T. Blum (eds.), *Evoked potentials, III: The Third International Evoked Potentials Symposium.* Boston: Butterworths, pp. 167–169.

Ferri, R., S. A. Musumeci, M. Elia, S. Del Gracco, C. Scuderi, and P. Bergonzi. 1994. BIT-mapped somatosensory evoked potentials in the fragile X syndrome. *Neurophysiol. Clin.* 24:413–426.

Ferrier, L. J., A. S. Bashir, D. L. Meryash, J. Johnston, and P. Wolff. 1991. Conversational skills of individuals with fragile-X syndrome: A comparison with autism and Down syndrome. *Dev. Med. Child Neurol.* 33:776–788.

Finnelli, P. F., S. M. Pueschel, T. Padre-Mendoza, and M. M. O'Brien. 1985. Neurological findings in patients with the fragile X syndrome. *J. Neurol. Nerosurg. Psychiatry* 48:150–153.

Finucane, B. 1996. Should all pregnant women be offered carrier testing for fragile X syndrome? *Clin. Obstet. Gynecol.* 39:772–782.

Fisch, G. S., I. L. Cohen, E. C. Jenkins, and W. T. Brown. 1988. Screening developmentally disabled male populations for fragile X: The effect of sample size. *Am. J. Med. Genet.* 30:655–663.

Flood, A., and G. Sanner. 1985. Refractive errors in the fragile X syndrome. *Acta Pediatr. Scand.* 74:974.

Folsom, R. C., B. R. Weber, and G. Thompson. 1983. Auditory brainstem responses in children with early recurrent middle ear disease. *Ann. Otol. Rhinol. Laryngol.* 92:249–253.

Franke, P., W. Maier, M. Hautzinger, O. Weiffenbach, M. Gansicke, B. Iwers, F. Poustka, S. G. Schwab, and U. Froster. 1996. Fragile-X carrier females: Evidence for a distinct psychopathological phenotype? *Am. J. Med. Genet.* 64:334–339.

Franke, P., M. Leboyer, M. Gansicke, O. Weiffenbach, V. Biancalana, P. Cornillet-Lefebre, M. F. Croquette, U. Froster, S. G. Schwab, F. Poustka, M. Hautzinger, and W. Maier. 1998. Genotype-phenotype relationship in female carriers of the premutation and full mutation of FMR-1. *Psychiatry Res.* 80:113–127.

Freed, L. A., D. Levy, R. A. Levine, M. G. Larson, J. C. Evans, D. L. Fuller, B. Lehman, and E. J. Benjamin. 1999. Prevalence and clinical outcome of mitral-valve prolapse [see comments]. *N. Engl. J. Med.* 341:1–7.

Freund, L. S., A. L. Reiss, R. Hagerman, and S. Vinogradov. 1992. Chromosome fragility and psychopathology in obligate female carriers of the fragile X chromosome. *Arch. Gen. Psychiatry* 49:54–60.

Freund, L. S., A. L. Reiss, and M. Abrams. 1993. Psychiatric disorders associated with fragile X in the young female. *Pediatrics* 91:321–329.

Freund, L., C. A. Peebles, E. Aylward, and A. L. Reiss. 1995. Preliminary report on cognitive and adaptive behaviors of preschool-aged males with fragile X. *Dev. Brain Dysfunct.* 8:242–261.

Friefeld, S., and D. MacGregor. 1993. Sensory motor coordination in boys with fragile X syndrome. In J. A. Holden and B. Cameron (eds.), *Proceedings of the First Canadian Fragile X Conference, Ongwanda Resource Center, Kingston, Ontario*, pp. 59–65.

Fryns, J. P. 1984. The fragile X syndrome: A study of 83 families. *Clin. Genet.* 26:497–528.

———. 1985. X-linked mental retardation. In *Medical genetics: Past, present, and future*. New York: Alan R. Liss, pp. 309–319.

———. 1986. The female and the fragile X: A study of 144 obligate female carriers. *Am. J. Med. Genet.* 23:157–169.

———. 1989. X-linked mental retardation and the fragile X syndrome: A clinical approach. In K. Davies (ed.), *The fragile X syndrome*. Oxford: Oxford Univ. Press, pp. 1–39.

———. 1994. Massive hydrocele in postpubertal fragile X males. *Am. J. Med. Genet.* 49:259.

Fryns, J. P., and H. Van den Berghe. 1988. The concurrence of Klinefelter syndrome and fragile X syndrome. *Am. J. Med. Genet.* 30:109–113.

Fryns, J. P., J. Jacobs, A. Kleczkowska, and H. Van den Berghe. 1984. The psychological profile of the fragile X syndrome. *Clin. Genet.* 25:131–134.

Fryns, J. P., A. M. Dereymaeker, M. Hoefnagels, P. Volcke, and H. Van den Berghe. 1986. Partial fra(X) phenotype with megalotestes in fra(X) negative patients with acquired lesions of the central nervous system. *Am. J. Med. Genet.* 23:213–219.

Fryns, J. P., M. Haspeslagh, A. M. Dereymaeker, P. Volcke, and H. Van den Berghe. 1987. A peculiar subphenotype in the fra(X) syndrome: Extreme obesity, short stature, stubby hands and feet, diffuse hyperpigmentation. Further evidence of disturbed hypothalamic function in the fra(X) syndrome? *Clin. Genet.* 32:388–392.

Fryns, J. P., P. Moerman, F. Gilis, I. d'Espallier, and H. Van den Berghe. 1988. Suggestively increased incidence of infant death in children of fra(X) positive mothers. *Am. J. Med. Genet.* 30:73–75.

Fu, Y.-H., D. P. A. Kuhl, A. Pizzuti, M. Pieretti, J. S. Sutcliffe, S. Richards, A. J. M. H. Verkerk, J. J. A. Holden, R. G. Fenwick Jr., S. T. Warren, B. A. Oostra, D. L. Nelson, and C. T. Caskey. 1991. Variation of the CGG repeat at the fragile X site results in genetic instability: Resolution of the Sherman paradox. *Cell* 67:1047–1058.

Fuster, C., C. Templado, R. Miro, L. Barrios, and J. Egozcue. 1988. Concurrence of the triple-X syndrome and expression of the fragile site Xq27.3. *Hum. Genet.* 78:293.

Gedeon, A. K., E. Baker, H. Robinson, M. W. Partington, B. Gross, A. Manca, B. Korn, A. Poustka, S. Yu, G. R. Sutherland, and J. C. Mulley. 1992. Fragile X syndrome without CGG amplification has an FMR1 deletion. *Nat. Genet.* 1:341–344.

Gillberg, C. 1983. Identical triplets with infantile autism and the fragile X syndrome. *Br. J. Psychiatry* 143:256–260.

———. 1985. Asperger's syndrome and recurrent psychosis—a case study. *J. Autism Dev. Disord.* 15:389–396.

Gillberg, C., and J. Wahlstrom. 1985. Chromosome abnormalities in infantile autism and other childhood psychoses: A population study of 66 cases. *Dev. Med. Child Neurol.* 127:293–304.

Gillberg, C., E. Persson, and J. Wahlstrom. 1986. The autism-fragile X syndrome (AFRAX): A population based study of ten boys. *J. Ment. Defic. Res.* 30:27–39.

Gillberg, C., S. Steffenburg, and G. Jakobson. 1987. Neurobiological findings in 20 relatively gifted children with Kanner-type autism or Asperger syndrome. *Dev. Med. Child Neurol.* 29:641–649.

Gillberg, C., V. A. Ohlson, J. Wahlstrom, S. Steffenburg, and K. Blix. 1988. Monozygotic female twins with autism and the fragile-X syndrome (AFRAX). *J. Child Psychol. Psychiatry* 29:447–451.

Giovannucci Uzielli, M. L., S. Guarducci, E. Lapi, A. Cecconi, U. Ricci, G. Ricotti, C. Biondi, B. Scarselli, F. Vieri, P. Scarnato, F. Gori, and A. Sereni. 1999. Premature ovarian failure (POF) and fragile X premutation females: From POF to fragile X carrier identification, from fragile X carrier diagnosis to POF association data. *Am. J. Med. Genet.* 84:300–303.

Glesby, M. J., and R. E. Pyeritz. 1989. Association of mitral valve prolapse and systemic abnormalities of connective tissue. *JAMA* 262:523–528.

Godfraind, J. M., E. Reyniers, K. De Boulle, D. H. R. P. P. De Deyn, C. E. Bakker, B. A. Oostra, R. F. Kooy, and P. J. Willems. 1996. Long-term potentiation in the hippocampus of fragile X knockout mice. *Am. J. Med. Genet.* 64:246–251.

Golden, G. S., and L. Greenhill. 1981. Tourette syndrome in mentally retarded children. *J. Ment. Retard.* 19:17–19.

Goldfine, P. E., P. M. McPherson, G. A. Heath, V. A. Hardesty, L. J. Beauregard, and B. Gordon. 1985. Association of fragile X syndrome with autism. *Am. J. Psychiatry* 142:108–110.

Goldfine, P. E., P. M. McPherson, V. A. Hardesty, G. A. Heath, L. J. Beauregard, and A. A. Baker. 1987. Fragile-X chromosome associated with primary learning disability. *J. Am. Acad. Child Adolesc. Psychiatry* 26:589–592.

Goldson, E., and R. J. Hagerman. 1993. Fragile X syndrome and failure to thrive. *Am. J. Dis. Child.* 147:605–607.

Gould, E. L., D. Z. Loesch, M. J. Martin, R. J. Hagerman, S. M. Armstrong, and R. M. Huggins. 2000. Melatonin profiles and sleep characteristics in boys with fragile X syndrome: A preliminary study. *Am. J. Med. Genet.* 95:307–315.

Greco, C., R. J. Hagerman, F. Tassone, A. Chudley, M. Del Bigio, S. Jacquemont, M. Leehey, and P. J. Hagerman. 2001. Neuronal intranuclear inclusions in a new cerebellar/ataxia syndrome among fragile X carriers. *Brain.* Submitted.

Grigsby, J., K. Kaye, J. Kowalsky, and A. M. Kramer. 2001. Association of behavioral self-regulation with concurrent functional capacity among stroke rehabilitation patients. *J. Clin. Geropsychol.* In press.

Gu, Y., K. A. Lugenbeel, J. G. Vockley, W. W. Grody, and D. L. Nelson. 1994. A de novo deletion in FMR1 in a patient with a developmental delay. *Hum. Mol. Genet.* 3:1705–1706.

Guerreiro, M. M., E. E. Camargo, M. Kato, A. P. Marques-De-Faria, S. M. Ciasca, C. A. M. Guerreiro, J. R. Menezes Netto, and M. V. L. Moura-Ribeiro. 1998. Fragile X syndrome: Clinical, electroencephalographic, and neuroimaging characteristics. *Arq. Neuropsiquiatr.* 56:18–23.

Hagerman, R. J. 1987. Fragile X syndrome. *Curr. Probl. Pediatr.* 17:627–674.

———. 1990. Chromosomes, genes, and autism. In C. Gilbert (ed.), *Autism—diagnosis and treatment: The state of the art.* New York: Plenum Press, pp. 105–131.

———. 1991. Physical and behavioral phenotype. In R. J. Hagerman and A. C. Silverman (eds.), *Fragile X syndrome: Diagnosis, treatment, and research.* Baltimore: Johns Hopkins Univ. Press, pp. 3–68.

———. 1992. Annotation: Fragile X syndrome. Advances and controversy. *J. Child Psychol. Psychiatry* 33:1127–1139.

———. 1996. Physical and behavioral phenotype. In R. J. Hagerman and A. Cronister (eds.), *Fragile X syndrome: Diagnosis, treatment, and research,* 2d ed. Baltimore: Johns Hopkins Univ. Press, pp. 3–87.

———. 1999a. Fragile X syndrome. In: *Neurodevelopmental disorders: Diagnosis and treatment.* New York: Oxford Univ. Press, pp. 61–132.

———. 1999b. Psychopharmacological interventions in fragile X syndrome, fetal alcohol syndrome, Prader-Willi syndrome, Angelman syndrome, Smith-Magenis syndrome, and velocardiofacial syndrome. *Ment. Retard. Dev. Disabil. Res. Rev.* 5:305–313.

———. 1999c. Tourette syndrome. In: *Neurodevelopmental disorders: Diagnosis and treatment.* New York: Oxford Univ. Press, pp. 133–172.

Hagerman, R. J., and A. R. Falkenstein. 1987. An association between recurrent otitis media in infancy and later hyperactivity. *Clin. Pediatr.* 26:253–257.

Hagerman, R. J., and P. J. Hagerman. 2001. Fragile X syndrome: A model of gene-brain-behavior relationships. *Mol. Genet. Metab.* In press.

Hagerman, R. J., and A. C. M. Smith. 1983. The heterozygous female. In R. J. Hagerman and P. McBogg (eds.), *The fragile X syndrome: Diagnosis, biochemistry, and intervention.* Dillon, Colo.: Spectra Publishing, pp. 83–94.

Hagerman, R. J., and W. E. Sobesky. 1989. Psychopathology in fragile X syndrome. *Am. J. Orthopsychiatry* 59:142–152.

Hagerman, R. J., A. C. M. Smith, and R. Mariner. 1983. Clinical features of the fragile X syndrome. In R. J. Hagerman and P. McBogg (eds.), *The fragile X syndrome: Diagnosis, biochemistry, and intervention.* Dillon, Colo.: Spectra Publishing, pp. 17–53.

Hagerman, R. J., K. Van Housen, A. C. M. Smith, and L. McGavran. 1984. Consideration of connective tissue dysfunction in the fragile X syndrome. *Am. J. Med. Genet.* 17:111–121.

Hagerman, R. J., M. Kemper, and M. Hudson. 1985. Learning disabilities and attentional problems in boys with the fragile X syndrome. *Am. J. Dis. Child* 139:674–678.

Hagerman, R. J., A. E. Chudley, J. H. Knoll, A. W. Jackson, M. Kemper, and R. Ahmad. 1986a. Autism in fragile X females. *Am. J. Med. Genet.* 23:375–380.

Hagerman, R. J., A. W. Jackson, A. Levitas, B. Rimland, and M. Braden. 1986b. An analysis of autism in 50 males with the fragile X syndrome. *Am. J. Med. Genet.* 23:359–370.

Hagerman, R. J., D. Altshul-Stark, and P. McBogg. 1987. Recurrent otitis media in boys with the fragile X syndrome. *Am. J. Dis. Child.* 141:184–187.

Hagerman, R. J., R. Berry, A. W. Jackson III, J. Campbell, A. Smith, and L. McGavran. 1988. Institutional screening for the fragile X syndrome. *Am. J. Dis. Child.* 142: 1216–1221.

Hagerman, R. J., R. A. Schreiner, M. B. Kemper, M. D. Wittenberger, B. Zahn, and K. Habicht. 1989. Longitudinal IQ follow-up in fragile X males. *Am. J. Med. Genet.* 33:513–518.

Hagerman, R. J., K. Amiri, and A. Cronister. 1991. The fragile X checklist. *Am. J. Med. Genet.* 38:283–287.

Hagerman, R. J., C. Jackson, K. Amiri, A. C. Silverman, R. O'Connor, and W. E. Sobesky. 1992. Fragile X girls: Physical and neurocognitive status and outcome. *Pediatrics* 89:395–400.

Hagerman, R. J., C. E. Hull, J. F. Safanda, I. Carpenter, L. W. Staley, R. O'Connor, C. Seydel, M. M. Mazocco, K. Snow, S. Thibodeau, D. Kuhl, D. L. Nelson, C. T. Caskey, and A. Taylor. 1994. High-funcitoning fragile X males: Demonstration of an unmethylated, fully expanded FMR-1 mutation associated with protein expression. *Am. J. Med. Genet.* 51:298–308.

Hagerman, R. J., J. E. Riddle, L. S. Roberts, K. Brease, and M. Fulton. 1995. A survery of the efficacy of clonidine in fragile X syndrome. *Dev. Brain Dys.* 8:336–344.

Hagerman, R. J., L. W. Staley, R. O'Conner, K. Kugenbeel, D. Nelson, S. McLean, and A. Taylor. 1996. Learning disabled males with a fragile X CGG expansion in the upper premutation size range. *Pediatrics* 97:122–126.

Hagerman, R. J., L. T. Kimbro, and A. K. Taylor. 1998. Fragile X syndrome: A common cause of mental retardation and premature menopause. *Contemp. OB/GYN* 43:47–70.

Hagerman, R. J., J. Hills, S. Scharfenaker, and H. Lewis. 1999. Fragile X syndrome and selective mutism. *Am. J. Med. Genet.* 83:313–317.

Hagerman, R. J., M. Leehey, W. Heinrichs, F. Tassone, R. Wilson, J. Hills, J. Grigsby, B. Gage, and P. J. Hagerman. 2001a. Intention tremor, Parkinsonism and generalized brain atrophy in older male carriers of fragile X. *Neurology* 57:127–130.

Hagerman, R. J., L. J. Miller, J. McGrath-Clarke, K. Riley, E. Goldson, S. W. Harris, J.

Simon, K. Church, J. Bonnell, and D. McIntosh. 2001b. The influence of stimulants on electrodermal studies in fragile X syndrome. *Microsc. Res. Tech.* In press.

Hammond, L. S., M. M. Macias, J. C. Tarleton, and G. S. Pai. 1997. Fragile X syndrome and deletions in FMR1: New case and review of the literature. *Am. J. Med. Genet.* 72:430–434.

Hanzlik, A. J., H. M. Osemlak, M. A. Hanser, and D. M. Kurnit. 1993. A recombination-based assay demonstrates that the fragile X sequence is transcribed widely during development. *Nat. Genet.* 3:44–48.

Harner, D. H., S. Hu, V. L. Magnuson, N. Hu, and A. M. L. Pattatucci. 1993. A linkage between DNA markers on the X chromosome and the male sexual orientation. *Science* 261:321–327.

Harris, S. W., K. E. Brown, J. L. Hills, F. Tassone, P. J. Hagerman, A. K. Taylor, and R. J. Hagerman. 2000. Adaptive functioning and molecular relationships in individuals with fragile X syndrome. Presented at the Seventh International Fragile X Conference, Los Angeles, July 19–23.

Hartman, N., R. Kramer, W. T. Brown, and R. B. Devereaux. 1982. Panic disorder in patients with mitral valve prolapse. *Am. J. Psychiatry* 139:669–670.

Harvey, J., C. Judge, and S. Weiner. 1977. Familial X-linked mental retardation with an X chromosome abnormality. *J. Med. Genet.* 14:46–50.

Hatton, D. D., E. G. Buckley, A. Lachiewicz, and J. Roberts. 1998. Ocular status of young boys with fragile X syndrome: A prospective study. *J. Am. Assoc. Pediatr. Ophthalmol. Strabismus* 2:298–301.

Hatton, D. D., D. B. Bailey Jr., M. Q. Hargett-Beck, M. Skinner, and R. D. Clark. 1999. Behavioral style of young boys with fragile X syndrome. *Dev. Med. Child Neurol.* 41:625–632.

Hill Karrer, J., D. Fitzpatrick, R. S. Karrer, R. J. Hagerman, J. Vavold, and J. Gora. 2000a. Movement-readiness brain potentials (MRPs) illuminate subtle prefrontal cognitive dysfunction among premutation female carriers of fragile X syndrome. Presented at the Seventh International Fragile X Conference, Los Angeles, July 19–23.

Hill Karrer, J., R. J. Hagerman, R. S. Karrer, D. Fitzpatrick, J. Vavold, L. Chaney, and J. Gora. 2000b. Electrophysiological characterization of early neurocognitive development in fragile X syndrome: Event related brain potential studies among infants and toddlers during visual recognition memory. Presented at the Seventh International Fragile X Conference, Los Angeles, July 19–23.

Hills, J. L., R. Wilson, W. Sobesky, S. W. Harris, J. Grigsby, E. Butler, D. Loesch, and R. J. Hagerman. 2000. Executive functioning deficits in adult males with the fragile X premutation: An emerging phenotype. Presented at the Seventh International Fragile X Foundation Conference, Los Angeles, July 19–22.

Hinds, H. L., C. T. Ashley, J. S. Sutcliffe, D. L. Nelson, S. T. Warren, D. E. Housman, and M. Schalling. 1993. Tissue specific expression of FMR1 provides evidence for a functional role in fragile X syndrome. *Nat. Genet.* 3:36–43.

Hinton, V. J., W. T. Brown, K. Wisniewski, and R. D. Rudelli. 1991. Analysis of neocortex in three males with fragile X syndrome. *Am. J. Med. Genet.* 41:289–294.

Hirst, M. D., A. Barnicoat, G. Flynn, Q. Wang, M. Daker, V. J. Buckle, K. E. Davies, and M. Bobrow. 1993. The identification of a third fragile site, FRAXF, in Xq27-q28 distal to both FRAXA and FRAXE. *Hum. Mol. Genet.* 2:197–200.

Hirst, M. D., P. Grewal, A. Flannery, R. Slatter, E. Maher, D. Barton, J. P. Fryns, and K. Davies. 1995. Two new cases of FMR1 deletion associated with mental impairment. *Am. J. Hum. Genet.* 56:67–74.

Hjalgrim, H., T. B. Jacobsen, K. Norgaard, H. C. Lou, K. Brøndum-Nielsen, and O. Jonassen. 1999. Frontal-subcortical hypofunction in the fragile X syndrome [letter]. *Am. J. Med. Genet.* 83:140–141.

Hjalgrim, H., B. F. Hansen, K. Brøndum-Nielsen, D. Nolting, and I. Kjær. 2000. Aspects of skeletal development in fragile X syndrome fetuses. *Am. J. Med. Genet.* 95:123–129.

Ho, H. H., and D. K. Kalousek. 1989. Brief report: Fragile X syndrome in autistic boys. *J. Autism Dev. Disord.* 19:343–347.

Hockey, A., and J. Crowhurst. 1988. Early manifestations of the Martin-Bell syndrome based on a series of both sexes from infancy. *Am. J. Med. Genet.* 30:61–71.

Hodapp, R. M., J. Leckman, E. Kykens, S. Sparrow, D. Zelinsky, and S. Ort. 1992. K-ABC profiles in children with fragile X syndrome, Down syndrome and nonspecific mental retardation. *Am. J. Ment. Retard.* 97:39–46.

Hull, C., and R. J. Hagerman. 1993. A study of the physical, behavioral, and medical phenotype, including anthropometric measures of females with fragile X syndrome. *Am. J. Dis. Child.* 147:1236–1241.

Hundscheid, R. D., E. A. Sistermans, C. M. Thomas, D. D. Braat, H. Straatman, L. A. Kiemeney, B. A. Oostra, and A. P. Smits. 2000. Imprinting effect in premature ovarian failure confined to paternally inherited fragile X premutations. *Am. J. Hum. Genet.* 66:413–418.

Irwin, S. A., R. Galvez, and W. T. Greenough. 2000. Dendritic spine structural anomalies in fragile-X mental retardation syndrome. *Cereb. Cortex* 10:1038–1044.

Jacky, P. 1996. Cytogenetics. In R. J. Hagerman and A. Cronister (eds.), *Fragile X syndrome: Diagnosis, treatment, and research,* 2d ed. Baltimore: Johns Hopkins Univ. Press, pp. 114–164.

Jacobs, P. A., M. Mayer, J. Matsuura, F. Rhoades, and S. C. Yu. 1983. Cytogenetic study of a population of mentally retarded males with special reference to the marker X chromosome. *Hum. Genet.* 63:139–148.

Jakala, P., T. Hanninen, M. Ryynanen, M. Laakso, K. Partanen, A. Mannermaa, and H. Soininen. 1997. Fragile-X: Neuropsychological test performance, CGG triplet repeat lengths, and hippocampal volumes. *J. Clin. Invest.* 100:331–338.

Jayakar, P., A. E. Chudley, M. Ray, J. Evans, J. Perlov, and R. Wand. 1986. Fra(2)(q13) and inv(9)(p11q12) in autism: Casual relationship? *Am. J. Med. Genet.* 23:381–392.

Jeffries, F. M., A. L. Reiss, W. T. Brown, D. A. Meyers, A. C. Glicksman, and S. Bandyopadhyay. 1993. Bipolar spectrum disorder and fragile X syndrome: A family study. *Biol. Psychiatry* 33:213–216.

Jenkins, E. C., W. T. Brown, J. Brooks, C. J. Duncan, R. D. Rudelli, and H. M. Wisniewski. 1984. Experience with prenatal fragile X detection. *Am. J. Med. Genet.* 17:215–239.

Johannisson, R., H. Rehder, V. Wendt, and E. Schwinger. 1987. Spermatogenesis in two patients with fragile X syndrome. *Hum. Genet.* 76:141–147.

Jorgensen, O. S., K. Brøndum-Nielsen, T. Isagar, and S. E. Mouridsen. 1984. Fragile X-chromosome among child psychiatric patients with disturbances of language and social relationships. *Acta Psychiatr. Scand.* 70:514.

Kandel, E. R., and J. H. Schwartz. 1982. Molecular biology of learning: Modulation of transmitter release. *Science* 218:433–443.

Kano, Y., M. Ohta, Y. Nagai, K. Yokota, and Y. Shimizu. 1988. Tourette's disorder coupled with infantile autism: A prospective study of two boys. *Jpn. J. Psychiatry Neurol.* 42:49–57.

Kates, W. R., M. T. Abrams, W. E. Kaufmann, S. N. Breiter, and A. L. Reiss. 1997. Reliability and validity of MRI measurement of the amygdala and hippocampus in children with fragile X syndrome. *Psychiatry Res. Neuroimaging Section* 75:31–48.

Kau, A. S. M., E. E. Reider, L. Payne, W. A. Meyer, and L. S. Freund. 2000. Early behavior signs of psychiatric phenotypes in fragile X syndrome. *Am. J. Ment. Retard.* 105:266–299.

Kaufmann, W. E., M. T. Abrams, W. Chen, and A. L. Reiss. 1999. Genotype, molecular phenotype, and cognitive phenotype: Correlations in fragile X syndrome. *Am. J. Med. Genet.* 83:286–295.

Kerbeshian, J., and L. Burd. 1986. Asperger's syndrome and Tourette syndrome: The case of the pinball wizard. *Br. J. Psychiatry* 148:731–736.

Kerbeshian, J., L. Burd, and J. T. Martsoff. 1984. Fragile X syndrome associated with Tourette symptomatology in a male with moderate mental retardation and autism. *J. Dev. Behav. Pediatr.* 5:201–203.

Kerby, D. S., and B. L. Dawson. 1994. Autistic features, personality, and adaptive behavior in males with the fragile X syndrome and no autism. *Am. J. Ment. Retard.* 98:455–462.

Kermadi, I., and D. Boussaoud. 1995. Role of the primate striatum in attention and sensorimotor processes: Comparison with premotor cortex. *NeuroReport* 6:1177–1181.

Khandijan, E. W., A. Fortin, A. Thibodeau, S. Tremblay, F. Cote, D. Devys, J. Mandel, and F. Rousseau. 1995. A heterogeneous set of FMRI proteins is widely distributed in mouse tissues and is modulated in cell culture. *Hum. Mol. Genet.* 4:783–789.

King, R. A., R. J. Hagerman, and M. Houghton. 1995. Ocular findings in fragile X syndrome. *Dev. Brain Dys.* 8:223–229.

Kluger, G., I. Bohm, M. C. Laub, and C. Waldenmaier. 1996. Epilepsy and fragile X gene mutations. *Pediatr. Neurol.* 15:358–360.

Knight, S. J. L., M. A. Voelchel, M. C. Hirst, A. V. Flannery, A. Moncla, and K. E. Davis. 1994. Triplet repeat expansion at the FRAXE locus and X-linked mild mental handicap. *Am. J. Hum. Genet.* 55:81–86.

Kooy, R. F., E. Reyniers, M. Verhoye, J. Sijbers, C. E. Bakker, B. A. Oostra, P. J. Willems, and A. Van Der Linden. 1999. Neuroanatomy of the fragile X knockout mouse brain studied using in vivo high resolution magnetic resonance imaging. *Eur. J. Hum. Genet.* 7:526–532.

Kopp, S., and C. Gillberg. 1997. Selective mutism: A population-based study. A research note. *J. Child Psychol. Psychiatry* 38:257–262.

Kotilainen, J., and S. Pirinen. 1999. Dental maturity is advanced in fragile X syndrome. *Am. J. Med. Genet.* 83:298–301.

Kowalczyk, C. L., E. Schroeder, V. Pratt, J. Conard, K. Wright, and G. L. Feldman. 1996. An association between precocious puberty and fragile X syndrome? *J. Pediatr. Adolesc. Gynecol.* 9:199–202.

Kranjc, B. S., A. Brezigar, and B. Peterlin. 1998. Bilateral macular dysplasia in fragile X syndrome. *Optom. Vis. Sci.* 75:856–859.

Kruyer, H., M. Mila, G. Glover, P. Carbonell, F. Ballesta, and X. Estivill. 1993. Fragile X syndrome and the $(CGG)_n$ mutation: Two families with discordant MZ twins. *Am. J. Hum. Genet.* 54:437–442.

Lachiewicz, A. M., and D. V. Dawson. 1994a. Behavioral problems of young girls with fragile X syndrome: Factor scores on the Conner's parent questionnaire. *Am. J. Med. Genet.* 15:364–369.

———. 1994b. Do young boys with fragile X syndrome have macroorchidism? *Pediatrics* 93:992–995.

Lachiewicz, A. M., C. Gullion, G. Spiridigliozzi, and A. Aylsworth. 1987. Declining IQs of young males with the fragile X syndrome. *Am. J. Ment. Retard.* 92:272–278.

Lachiewicz, A. M., S. F. Hoegerman, G. Holmgren, E. Holmberg, and K. Arinbjarnarson. 1991. Association of the Robin sequence with the fragile X syndrome. *Am. J. Med. Genet.* 41:275–278.

Lachiewicz, A. M., G. A. Spiridigliozzi, C. M. Gullion, S. N. Ransford, and K. Rao. 1994. Aberrant behaviors of young boys with fragile X syndrome. *Am. J. Ment. Retard.* 98:567–579.

Lachiewicz, A. M., G. A. Spiridigliozzi, A. McConkie-Rosell, and J. Tarleton. 1995. A fragile X male with a broad smear on Southern blot of 100 to 500 CGG repeats and no methylation. Poster presented at the 7th International Workshop on the Fragile X and X-Linked Mental Retardation, Aug. 2–5, Tromsø, Norway.

Lachiewicz, A. M., G. A. Spiridigliozzi, A. McConkie-Rosell, D. Burgess, Y. Feng, S. T. Warren, and J. Tarleton. 1996. A fragile X male with a broad smear on Southern blot analysis representing 100–500 CGG repeats and no methylation at the EagI site of the FMR-1 gene. *Am. J. Med. Genet.* 64:278–282.

Lachiewicz, A., D. V. Dawson, A. McConkie-Rosell, and G. A. Spiridigliozzi. 2000a. Mathematics weakness in premutation females wtih the fragile X syndrome. Presented at the Seventh International Fragile X Conference, July 19–23, Los Angeles.

Lachiewicz, A. M., D. V. Dawson, and G. A. Spiridigliozzi. 2000b. Physical characteristics of young boys with fragile X syndrome: Reasons for difficulties in making a diagnosis in young males. *Am. J. Med. Genet.* 92:229–236.

Lalande, M. 1994. In and around SNRPN. *Nat. Genet.* 8:5–7.

Largo, R. H., and A. Schinzel. 1985. Developmental and behavioral disturbances in 13 boys with fragile X syndrome. *Eur. J. Pediatr.* 143:269–275.

Le Couteur, A., M. Rutter, D. Summers, and L. Butler. 1988. Fragile X in female autistic twins. *J. Autism. Dev. Disord.* 18:458–460.

Levitas, A., R. J. Hagerman, M. Braden, B. Rimland, P. McBogg, and I. Matus. 1983. Autism and the fragile X syndrome. *J. Dev. Behav. Pediatr.* 4:151–158.

Li, S-Y., Y-C. J. Chen, T-J. Lai, C-Y. Hsu, and Y-C. Wang. 1993. Molecular and cytogenetic analysis of autism in Taiwan. *Hum. Genet.* 92:441–445.

Libb, J. W., A. Dahle, K. Smith, F. P. McCollister, and C. McLain. 1985. Hearing disorder and cognitive function of individuals with Down syndrome. *Am. J. Ment. Deficien.* 90:353–356.

Lisik, M., K. Szymanska-Parkieta, and U. Galecka. 2000. The comparison of anthropometric variables in mentally retarded boys with and without fragile X syndrome [letter]. *Clin. Genet.* 57:456–458.

Loehr, J. P., D. P. Synhorst, R. R. Wolfe, and R. J. Hagerman. 1986. Aortic root dilatation and mitral valve prolapse in the fragile X syndrome. *Am. J. Med. Genet.* 23:189–194.

Loesch, D. Z., and D. A. Hay. 1988. Clinical features and reproductive patterns in fragile X female heterozygotes. *J. Med. Genet.* 25:407–414.

Loesch, D. Z., and R. M. Huggins. 1992. Fixed and random effects in the variation of the finger ridge count: A study of fragile X families. *Am. J. Hum. Genet.* 50:1067–1076.

Loesch, D. Z., and M. Sampson. 1993. Effect of the fragile X anomaly on body proportions estimated by pedigree analysis. *Clin. Genet.* 44:82–88.

Loesch, D. Z., D. A. Hay, G. R. Sutherland, J. Halliday, C. Judge, and G. C. Webb. 1987. Phenotypic variation in male-transmitted fragile X: Genetic inferences. *Am. J. Med. Genet.* 27:401–417.

Loesch, D. Z., M. Lafranchi, and D. Scott. 1988. Anthropometry in Martin-Bell syndrome. *Am. J. Med. Genet.* 30:149–164.

Loesch, D. Z., D. A. Hay, and M. Leversha. 1991. Problems in ascertainment of transmitting males in Martin-Bell syndrome. *Am. J. Med. Genet.* 41:410–416.

Loesch, D. Z., D. A. Hay, and L. Sheffield. 1992. Fragile X family with unusual digital and facial abnormalities. *Am. J. Med. Genet.* 44:543–550.

Loesch, D. Z., R. Huggins, D. A. Hay, A. K. Gedeon, J. C. Mulley, and G. R. Sutherland. 1993a. Genotype-phenotype relationships in fragile X syndrome: A family study. *Am. J. Med. Genet.* 53:1064–1073.

Loesch, D. Z., R. M. Huggins, and W. F. Chin. 1993b. Effect of fragile X on physical and intellectual traits estimated by pedigree analysis. *Am. J. Med. Genet.* 46:415–422.

Loesch, D. Z., D. A. Hay, and J. Mulley. 1994. Transmitting males and carrier females in fragile X—revisited. *Am. J. Med. Genet.* 51:392–399.

Loesch, D. Z., R. M. Huggins, and N. H. Hoang. 1995. Growth in stature in fragile X families: A mixed longitudinal study. *Am. J. Med. Genet.* 58:249–256.

Loesch, D. Z., R. M. Huggins, E. Butler, A. K. Taylor, and R. J. Hagerman. 2001. Effect of the fragile X status and the FMRP levels on cognitive profiles of fragile X males and females with special consideration of the full mutation high functioning subjects. *Am. J. Med. Genet.* Submitted.

Lopez-Pajares, I., A. Delicade, I. Pascual-Castroviejo, V. Lopez-Martin, F. Moreno, and J. A. Garcia-Marcos. 1994. Fragile X syndrome with extra microchromosome. *Clin. Genet.* 45:186–189.

Lubs, H., P. Chiurazzi, J. Arena, C. Schwartz, L. Tranebjaerg, and G. Neri. 1999. XLMR genes: Update 1998. *Am. J. Med. Genet.* 83:237–247.

Lugenbeel, K. A., A. M. Peier, N. L. Carson, A. E. Chudley, and D. L. Nelson. 1995. Intragenic loss of function mutations demonstrate the primary role of FMR1 in fragile X syndrome. *Nat. Genet.* 10:483–485.

Maes, B., J. P. Fryns, M. van Walleghem, and H. van den Berghe. 1993. Fragile X syndrome and autism: A prevalent association or a misinterpreted connection. *Genet. Couns.* 4:245–263.

Maes, B., J. P. Fryns, P. Ghesquière, and M. Borghgraef. 2000. Phenotypic checklist to screen for fragile X syndrome in people with mental retardation. *Ment. Retard.* 38:207–215.

Maino, D. M., D. Schlange, J. H. Maino, and B. Caden. 1990. Ocular anomalies in fragile X syndrome. *J. Am. Optom. Assoc.* 61:316–323.

Maino, D. M., M. Wesson, D. Schlange, G. Cibis, and J. H. Maino. 1991. Optometric findings in the fragile X syndrome. *Optom. Vis. Sci.* 68:634–640.

Malter, H. E., J. C. Iber, R. Willemsen, E. de Graaff, J. C. Tarleton, J. Leisti, S. T. Warren, and B. A. Oostra. 1997. Characterization of the full fragile X syndrome mutation in fetal gametes. *Nat. Genet.* 15:165–169.

Mandokora, H., S. Ohdo, T. Sonoda, and K. Ohba. 1986. Frequency of the fragile X syndrome in infantile autism. *Acta Pediatr. Jpn.* 90:316–323.

Mariner, R., A. W. Jackson, A. Levita, R. J. Hagerman, M. Braden, P. M. McBogg, R. Berry, and A. C. M. Smith. 1986. Autism, mental retardation and chromosomal abnormalities. *J. Autism Develop. Disord.* 16:425–440.

Marozzi, A., W. Vegetti, E. Manfredini, M. G. Tibiletti, G. Testa, P. G. Crosignani, E. Ginelli, R. Meneveri, and L. Dalpra. 2000. Association between idiopathic premature ovarian failure and fragile X premutation. *Hum. Reprod.* 15:197–202.

Martin, J. P., and J. Bell. 1943. A pedigree of mental defect showing sex-linkage. *J. Neurol. Psychiatry* 6:154–157.

Matsuishi, T., Y. Shiotsuki, N., Niikawa, Y. Katafuchi, E. Otaki, H. Ando, Y. Yamashita, M. Horikawa, F. Urabe, N. Kuriya, and F. Yamashita. 1987. Fragile X syndrome in Japanese patients with infantile autism [review]. *Pediatr. Neurol.* 3:284–287.

Mattei, J. F., M. G. Mattei, C. Aumeras, M. Auger, and F. Giraud. 1981. X-linked mental retardation with the fragile X: A study of 15 families. *Hum. Genet.* 59:281–289.

Mazzocco, M. M. M. 2000. Advances in research on fragile X syndrome. *Ment. Retard. Dev. Disabil. Res. Rev.* 6:96–106.

Mazzocco, M. M. M., B. Pennington, and R. J. Hagerman. 1993. The neurocognitive phenotype of female carriers of fragile X: Further evidence for specificity. *J. Dev. Behav. Pediatr.* 14:328–335.

Mazzocco, M. M. M., L. S. Freund, T. L. Baumgardner, L. Forman, and A. L. Reiss. 1995. The neurobehavioral and neuroanatomical effects of the FMR1 full mutation: Monozygotic twins dyscordant for fragile X syndrome. *Neuropsychology* 9:470–480.

Mazzocco, M. M. M., W. R. Kates, T. L. Baumgardner, L. S. Freund, and A. L. Reiss. 1997a. Autistic behaviors among girls with fragile X syndrome. *J. Autism Dev. Disord.* 27:415–435.

Mazzocco, M. M. M., N. L. Sonna, J. T. Teisl, A. Pinit, B. K. Shapiro, N. Shah, and A. L. Reiss. 1997b. The FMR1 and FMR2 mutations are not common etiologies of academic difficulty among school-age children. *Dev. Behav. Pediatr.* 18:392–398.

McConkie-Rosell, A., A. Lachiewicz, G. A. Spiridigliozzi, J. Tarleton, S. Schoenwald, M. C. Phelan, P. Goonewardena, X. Ding, and W. T. Brown. 1993. Evidence that methylation of the FMR-1 locus is repsonsible for variable phenotypic expression of the fragile X syndrome. *Am. J. Hum. Genet.* 53:800–809.

McDermott, A., R. Walters, R. T. Howell, and A. Gardner. 1983. Fragile X chromosome: Clinical and cytogenetic studies on cases from seven families. *J. Med. Genet.* 20:169–178.

McGillivray, B. C., D. S. Herbst, F. J. Dill, H. J. Sandercock, and B. Tischler. 1986. Infantile autism: An occasional manifestation of fragile (X) mental retardation. *Am. J. Med. Genet.* 23:353–358.

Meijer, H., E. de Graaff, D. M. Merckx, R. J. Jongbloed, C. E. de Die-Smulders, J. J. Engelen, J. P. Fryns, P. M. Curfs, and B. A. Oostra. 1994. A deletion of q1.6Kb proximal to the CGG repeat of the FMR1 gene causes the clinical phenotype of the fragile X syndrome. *Hum. Med. Genet.* 3:615–620.

Mendlewicz, J., and D. Hirsch. 1991. Bipolar manic depressive illness and the fragile X syndrome. *Biol. Psychiatry* 29:298–299.

Menon, V., H. Kwon, S. Eliez, A. K. Taylor, and A. L. Reiss. 2000. Functional brain activation during cognition is related to FMR1 gene expression. *Brain Res.* 877:367–370.

Merenstein, S. A., V. Shyu, W. E. Sobesky, L. W. Staley, A. K. Taylor, and R. J. Hagerman. 1994. Fragile X syndrome in a normal IQ male with learning and emotional problems. *J. Am. Acad. Child. Adolesc. Psychiatry* 33:1316–1321.

Merenstein, S. A., W. E. Sobesky, A. K. Taylor, J. E. Riddle, H. X. Tran, and R. J. Hagerman. 1996. Molecular-clinical correlations in males with an expanded FMR1 mutation. *Am. J. Med. Genet.* 64:388–394.

Meryash, D. L., L. S. Szymanski, and P. S. Gerald. 1982. Infantile autism associated with the fragile-X syndrome. *J. Autism Dev. Disord.* 12:295–301.

Meryash, D. L., C. E. Cronk, B. Sachs, and P. S. Gerald. 1984. An anthropometric study of males with the fragile-X syndrome. *Am. J. Med. Genet.* 17:159–174.

Miezejeski, C. M., and V. J. Hinton. 1992. Fragile X learning disability: Neurobehavioral research, diagnostic models and treatment options. In R. J. Hagerman and P. McKenzie (eds.), *The 1992 International Fragile X Conference Proceedings.* Denver: National Fragile X Foundation and Spectra Publishing, pp. 85–98.

Miezejeski, C. M., G. Heaney, R. Belser, W. T. Brown, E. C. Jenkins, and E. A. Sersen. 1997. Longer brainstem auditory evoked response latencies of individuals with fragile X syndrome related to sedation. *Am. J. Med. Genet.* 74:167–171.

Milà, M., H. Kruyer, G. Glover, A. Sánchez, P. Carbonell, S. Castellví-Bel, V. Volpini, J. Rosell, J. Gabarrón, I. López, M. Villa, F. Ballestra, and X. Estivill. 1994. Molecular analysis of the $(CGG)_n$ expansion in the FMR-1 gene in 59 Spanish families. *Hum. Genet.* 94:395–400.

Miller, L. J., D. N. McIntosh, J. McGrath, V. Shyu, M. Lampe, A. K. Taylor, F. Tassone, K. Neitzel, T. Stackhouse, and R. J. Hagerman. 1999. Electrodermal responses to sensory stimuli in individuals with fragile X syndrome: A preliminary report. *Am. J. Med. Genet.* 83:268–279.

Miller, K., J. Miller, and R. J. Hagerman. 2000. Selective mutism in a male with fragile X syndrome. Presented at the Seventh International Fragile X Conference, Los Angeles, July 19–23.

Moon, H. R., and S. Y. Moon. 1993. Fragile site chromosomes in mentally retarded boys. *J. Korean Med. Sci.* 8:192–196.

Moore, P. S. J., A. E. Chudley, and S. D. Winter. 1990. True precocious puberty in a girl with the fragile X syndrome. *Am. J. Med. Genet.* 37:265–267.

Moore, C. J., E. M. Daly, G. McAlonan, K. Davis, K. C. Murphy, and D. G. M. Murphy. 2000. X-chromosome trinucleotide repeats: Effects on brain structure. *J. Med. Genet.* 37:S58.

Mostofsky, S. H., M. M. M. Mazzocco, G. Aakalu, I. S. Warsofsky, M. B. Denckla, and A. L. Reiss. 1998. Decreased cerebellar posterior vermis size in fragile X syndrome. *Am. Acad. Neurol.* 50:121–130.

Munir, F., K. M. Cornish, and J. Wilding. 2000. A neuropsychological profile of attention deficits in young males with fragile X syndrome. *Neuropsychologia* 38:1261–1270.

Murphy, D. G. M., M. J. Mentis, P. Pietrini, C. L. Grady, C. J. Moore, B. Horwitz, V. Hinton, C. S. Dobkin, M. B. Schapiro, and S. I. Rapoport. 1999. Premutation female carriers of fragile X syndrome: A pilot study on brain anatomy and metabolism. *J. Am. Acad. Child Adolesc. Psychiatry* 38:1294–1301.

Murray, A., J. Webb, S. Grimley, G. Conway, and P. Jacobs. 1998. Studies of FRAXA and FRAXE in women with premature ovarian failure. *J. Med. Genet.* 35:637–640.

Murray, A., J. Webb, F. MacSwiney, E. L. Shipley, N. E. Morton, and G. S. Conway. 1999. Serum concentrations of follicle stimulating hormone may predict premature ovarian failure in FRAXA premutation women. *Hum. Reprod.* 14:1217–1218.

Murray, A., S. Ennis, F. MacSwiney, J. Webb, and N. E. Morton. 2000a. Reproductive and menstrual history of females with fragile X expansions. *Eur. J. Hum. Genet.* 8:247–252.

Murray, A., S. Ennis, and N. Morton. 2000b. No evidence for parent of origin influencing premature ovarian failure in fragile X premutation carriers [letter; see comments]. *Am. J. Hum. Genet.* 67:253–254; discussion 256–258.

Murray, K. F., S. P. Ryan, and M. C. Hough. 1995. Radiological case of the month. *Arch. Pediatr. Adolesc. Med.* 149:460–461.

Musumeci, S. A., P. Bergonzi, and G. L. Gigli. 1985. Patologia malformative come fattore eziopatogenetico dell 'epilessia nel bambino. *Boll. Lega Ital. Epelessia* 51/52:55–57.

Musumeci, S. A., R. Ferri, R. M. Colognola, G. Neri, S. Sanfilippo, and P. Bergonzi. 1988a. Prevalence of a novel epileptogenic EEG pattern in the Martin-Bell syndrome. *Am. J. Med. Genet.* 30:207–212.

Musumeci, S. A., R. M. Colognola, R. Ferri, G. L. Gigli, M. A. Petrella, S. Sanfilippo, P. Bergonzi, and C. A. Tassinari. 1988b. Fragile-X syndrome: A particular epileptogenic EEG pattern. *Epilepsia* 29:41–47.

Musumeci, S. A., R. Ferri, M. Viglianesi, M. Elia, R. M. Ragusa, and P. Bergonzi. 1991a. Cutis verticis gyrata and chromosomal fragile sites. *Am. J. Med. Genet.* 38:249–250.

Musumeci, S. A., R. Ferri, M. Elia, R. M. Colognola, P. Bergonzi, and C. A. Tassinari. 1991b. Epilepsy and fragile X syndrome: A follow-up study. *Am. J. Med. Genet.* 38:511–513.

Musumeci, S. A., M. Elia, R. Ferri, C. Scuderi, and S. Del Gracco. 1994. Evoked spikes and giant somatosensory evoked potentials in a patient with fragile-X syndrome. *Ital. J. Neurol. Sci.* 15:365–368.

Musumeci, S. A., R. Ferri, M. Elia, S. Del Gracco, C. Scuderi, M. C. Stefanini, A. Castano, and G. Azan. 1995. Sleep neurophysiology in fragile X syndrome patients. *Dev. Brain Dysf.* 8:218–222.

Musumeci, S. A., R. Ferri, M. Elia, S. Del Gracco, C. Scuderi, and M. C. Stefanini. 1996. Normal respiratory pattern during sleep in young fragile X-syndrome patients [letter]. *J. Sleep Res.* 5:272.

Musumeci, S. A., R. J. Hagerman, R. Ferri, P. Bosco, K. Dalla Bernardina, C. A. Tassinari, G. B. DeSarro, and M. Elia. 1999. Epilepsy and EEG findings in males with fragile X syndrome. *Epilepsia* 40:1092–1099.

Musumeci, S. A., P. Bosco, G. Calabrese, C. Bakker, G. B. De Sarro, M. Elia, R. Ferri, and B. A. Oostra. 2000. Audiogenic seizures susceptibility in transgenic mice with fragile X syndrome. *Epilepsia* 41:19–23.

Neri, G., and P. Chiurazzi. 2000. X-linked mental retardation. *Semin. Med. Genet.* 97:173.

Newell, K., B. Sanborn, and R. J. Hagerman. 1983. Speech and language dysfunction in the fragile X syndrome. In R. J. Hagerman and P. M. McBogg (eds.), *The fragile X syndrome.* Dillon, Colo.: Spectra Publishing, pp. 175–200.

Nistal, M., F. Martinez-Garcia, J. Regadera, P. Cobo, and R. Paniagua. 1992. Macroorchidism: Light and electron microscopic study of four cases. *Hum. Pathol.* 23:1011–1018.

Nolin, S. L., D. A. Snider, E. C. Jenkins, W. T. Brown, M. Krawczun, D. Stetka, G. Houck, C. S. Dobkin, G. Strong, G. Smith-Dobransky, A. Victor, K. Hughes, D. Kimpton, A. Little, U. Nagaraja, B. Kenefick, and C. Sullivan. 1991. Fragile X screening program in New York State. *Am. J. Med. Genet.* 38:251–255.

O'Brien, G., K. Bretherton, A. Alcorn, M. Gale, and J. Goodship. 1998. A controlled psychiatric study of fragile X low-expressing males. Presented at the Fifth International Symposium of the Society for the Study of Behavioural Phenotypes, November 19–21, Baltimore.

O'Hare, J. P., I. A. D. O'Brien, J. Arendt, P. Astley, W. Ratcliffe, H. Andrews, R. Walters, and R. J. M. Corrall. 1986. Does melatonin deficiency cause the enlarged genitalia of the fragile X syndrome? *Clin. Endocrinol.* 24:327–333.

Opitz, J. M., and G. R. Sutherland. 1984. Conference report: International Workshop on the Fragile X and X-Linked Mental Retardation. *Am. J. Med. Genet.* 17:5–94.

Opitz, J. M., J. M. Westphal, and A. Daniel. 1984. Discovery of a connective tissue dysplasia in the Martin-Bell syndrome. *Am. J. Med. Genet.* 17:101–109.

Ornitz, E. M. 1989. Autism at the interface between sensory and information processing. In G. Dawson (ed.), *Autism: Nature, diagnosis and treatment.* New York: Guilford Press, pp. 174–207.

Ornitz, E. M., and E. R. Ritvo. 1968. Perceptual inconstancy in early infantile autism. *Arch. Gen. Psychiatry* 18:76–98.

Paradee, W., H. E. Melikian, D. L. Rasmussen, A. Kenneson, P. J. Conn, and S. T. Warren. 1999. Fragile X mouse strain effects of knock out phenotype and evidence suggesting deficient amygdala function. *Neuroscience* 94:185–192.

Paradise, J. L., C. A. Dollaghan, T. F. Campbell, H. M. Feldman, B. S. Bernard, D. K. Colborn, H. E. Rockette, J. E. Janosky, D. L. Pitcairn, D. L. Sabo, M. Kurs-Lasky, and C. G. Smith. 2000. Language, speech sound production, and cognition in three-year-old children in relation to otitis media in their first three years of life. *Pediatrics* 105:1119–1130.

Partington, M. W. 1984. The fragile X syndrome II: Preliminary data on growth and development in males. *Am. J. Med. Genet.* 17:175–194.

Partington, M. W., D. Y. Moore, and G. M. Turner. 1996. Confirmation of early menopause in fragile X carriers. *Am. J. Med. Genet.* 64:370–372.

Paul, R., E. Dykens, J. Leckman, M. Watson, W. Breg, and D. Cohen. 1987. A comparison of language characteristics of mentally retarded adults with fragile X syndrome and those with non-specific mental retardation and autism. *J. Autism Dev. Disord.* 17:454–468.

Pauls, D. L., K. E. Towbin, J. F. Leckman, G. E. Zahner, and D. J. Cohen. 1986. Gilles de la Tourette's syndrome and obsessive-compulsive disorder: Evidence supporting a genetic relationship. *Arch. Gen. Psychiatry* 43:1180–1182.

Payton, J. B., M. W. Steele, S. L. Wenger, and N. J. Minshew. 1989. The fragile X marker and autism in perspective. *J. Am. Acad. Child. Adolesc. Psychiatry* 28:417–421.

Pesso, R., M. Berkenstadt, H. Cuckle, E. Gak, L. Peleg, M. Frydman, and G. Barkai. 2000. Screening for fragile X syndrome in women of reproductive age. *Prenat. Diagn.* 20:611–614.

Phelan, M. C., R. E. Stevenson, J. L. Collins, and H. E. Trent. 1988. Fragile X syndrome and neoplasia. *Am. J. Med. Genet.* 30:77–82.

Pieretti, M., F. Zhang, Y-H. Fu, S. T. Warren, B. A. Oostra, C. T. Caskey, and D. L. Nelson. 1991. Absence of expression of the FMR-1 gene in fragile X syndrome. *Cell* 66:817–822.

Piussan, C., M. Mathieu, P. Berquin, and J. P. Fryns. 1996. Fragile X mutation and FG syndrome-like phenotype. *Am. J. Med. Genet.* 64:395–398.

Prader, A. 1966. Testicular size: Asessment and clinical importance. *Triangle* 7:240–243.

Prasad, C., A. N. Prasad, B. N. Chodirker, C. Lee, A. K. Dawson, L. J. Jocelyn, and A. E. Chudley. 2000. Genetic evaluation of pervasive developmental disorders: The terminal 22q13 deletion syndrome may represent a recognizable phenotype. *Clin. Genet.* 57:103–109.

Primrose, D. A., R. el-Matmati, E. Boyd, C. Gosden, and M. Newton. 1986. Prevalence of the fragile X syndrome in an institution for the mentally handicapped. *Br. J. Psychiatry* 148:655–657.

Prior, T. W., A. C. Papp, P. J. Snyder, M. S. Sedra, M. Guida, and B. G. Enrile. 1995. Germline mosaicism at the fragile X locus. *Am. J. Med. Genet.* 55:384–386.

Proops, R., and T. Webb. 1981. The "fragile" X chromosome in the Martin-Bell-Renpenning syndrome and in males with other forms of familial mental retardation. *J. Med. Genet.* 18:366–373.

Prouty, L. A., R. C. Rogers, R. E. Stevenson, J. H. Dean, K. K. Palmer, R. J. Simensen, G. N. Coston, and C. E. Schwartz. 1988. Fragile X syndrome: Growth, development, and intellectual function. *Am. J. Med. Genet.* 30:123–142.

Pueschel, S. M., and R. Herman. 1985. Brief report: screening children with autism for fragile-X syndrome and phenylketonuria. *J. Autism Dev. Disord.* 15:335–338.

Puzzo, A., G. Fiamma, V. E. Rubino, P. A. Gagliano, G. Giordano, L. Russo, B. Aloisi, and U. Manzoli. 1990. Cardiovascular aspects of Martin-Bell syndrome. *Cardiologia* 35:857–862.

Quan, F., J. Zonana, K. Gunter, K. L. Peterson, R. E. Magenis, and B. W. Popovich. 1995. An atypical case of fragile X syndrome caused by a deletion that includes the FMR1 gene. *Am. J. Hum. Genet.* 56:1042–1051.

Rasmusson, D. D. 1993. Cholinergic modulation of sensory information. *Prog. Brain Res.* 98:357–363.

Rees, M., U. Diebold, K. Parker, H. Doose, R. M. Gardiner, and W. P. Whitehouse. 1993. Benign childhood epilepsy with centrotemporal spikes and the focal sharp wave trait is not linked to the fragile X region. *Neuropediatrics* 24:211–213.

Reiss, A. L. 2000. Neuroimaging workshop. Presented at the Seventh International Fragile X Conference, Los Angeles, July 19–23.

Reiss, A. L., and L. Freund. 1990. Fragile X syndrome, DSM-III-R, and autism. *J. Am. Acad. Child Adolesc. Psychiatry* 29:885–891.

———. 1992. Behavioral phenotype of fragile X syndrome: DSM-III-R autistic behavior in male children. *Am. J. Med. Genet.* 43:35–46.

Reiss, A. L., R. J. Hagerman, S. Vinogradov, M. Abrams, and R. J. King. 1988a. Psychiatric disability in female carriers of the fragile X chromosome. *Arch. Gen. Psychiatry* 45:25–30.

Reiss, A. L., S. Patel, A. J. Kumar, and L. Freund. 1988b. Preliminary communication: Neuroanatomical variations of the posterior fossa in men with the fragile X (Martin-Bell) syndrome. *Am. J. Med. Genet.* 31:407–414.

Reiss, A. L., L. Freund, S. Vinogradov, R. Hagerman, and A. Cronister. 1989. Parental inheritance and psychological disability in fragile X females. *Am. J. Hum. Genet.* 45:697–705.

Reiss, A. L., E. Aylward, L. S. Freund, P. K. Joshi, and R. N. Bryan. 1991a. Neuroanatomy of the fragile X syndrome: The posterior fossa. *Ann. Neurol.* 29:26–32.

Reiss, A. L., L. Freund, J. E. Tseng, and P. K. Joshi. 1991b. Neuroanatomy in fragile X females: The posterior fossa. *Am. J. Hum. Genet.* 49:279–288.

Reiss, A. L., L. Freund, M. T. Abrams, C. Boehm, and H. Kazazian. 1993. Neurobehavioral effects of the fragile X premutation in adult women: A controlled study. *Am. J. Hum. Genet.* 52:884–894.

Reiss, A. L., J. Lee, and L. Freund. 1994. Neuroanatomy of fragile X syndrome: The temporal lobe. *Neurology* 44:1317–1324.

Reiss, A., M. Abrams, R. Greenlaw, L. Freund, and M. Denckla. 1995a. Neurodevelopmental effects of the FMR-1 full mutation in humans. *Nat. Med.* 1:159–167.

Reiss, A. L., L. S. Freund, T. L. Baumgardner, M. T. Abrams, and M. B. Denckla. 1995b. Contribution of the FMR1 gene mutation to human intellectual dysfunction. *Nat. Genet.* 11:331–334.

Reyniers, E., L. Vits, K. De Boulle, B. Van Roy, D. Van Velzen, E. de Graaff, A. J. M. H. Verkerk, H. Z. J. Jorens, J. K. Darby, B. Oostra, and P. Willems. 1993. The full mutation in the FMR-1 gene of male fragile X patients is absent in their sperm. *Nat. Genet.* 4:143–146.

Reyniers, E., J. J. Martin, P. Cras, E. Van Marck, I. Handig, H. Z. Jorens, B. A. Oostra, R. F. Kooy, and P. J. Willems. 1999. Postmortem examination of two fragile X brothers with an FMR1 full mutation. *Am. J. Med. Genet.* 84:245–249.

Rhoads, F. A. 1984. Fragile-X syndrome in Hawaii: A summary of clinical experience. *Am. J. Med. Genet.* 17:209–214.

Riddle, J. E., A. Cheema, W. E. Sobesky, S. C. Gardner, A. K. Taylor, B. F. Pennington, and R. J. Hagerman. 1998. Phenotypic involvement in females with the FMR1 gene mutation. *Am. J. Ment. Retard.* 102:590–601.

Rivera, S. M., V. Menon, C. D. White, G. Glover, and A. L. Reiss. 2000. Functional brain activation during arithmetic processing in females with fragile X syndrome. Presented at the Seventh International Fragile X Conference, Los Angeles, July 19–21.

Rivera, S. M., V. Menon, C. D. White, B. Glaser, and A. L. Reiss. 2001. Functional brain activation during arithmetic processing in females with fragile X syndrome. *Hum. Brain Mapping.* Submitted.

Rodewald, L., D. C. Miller, L. Sciorra, G. Barabas, and M. L. Lee. 1987. Central nervous system neoplasm in a young man with Martin-Bell syndrome—fra(X)-XLMR. *Am. J. Med. Genet.* 26:7–12.

Rogers, S. J., E. A. Wehner, and R. Hagerman. 2001. The behavioral phenotype in fragile X syndrome: Symptoms of autism in very young children with fragile X syndrome, idiopathic autism, and other developmental disorders. *J. Dev. Behav. Pediatr.* In press.

Rojas, D. C., T. Benkers, S. J. Rogers, P. D. Teale, M. L. Reite, and R. J. Hagerman. 2001. Auditory evoked magnetic fields in adults with fragile X syndrome. *Neuroreport.* 12:2573–2576.

Rousseau, F., D. Heitz, V. Biancalana, S. Blumenfeld, C. Kretz, J. Boue, N. Tommerup, C. van der Hagen, C. DeLozier-Blanchet, M.-F. Croquette, S. Gilgenkrantz, P. Jalbert, M. A. Voelckel, I. Oberle, and J-L. Mandel. 1991a. Directdiagnosis by DNA analysis of the fragile X syndrome of mental retardation. *N. Engl. J. Med.* 325:1673–1681.

Rousseau, F., D. Heitz, I. Oberle, and J-L. Mandel. 1991b. Selection in blood cells from female carriers responsible for variable phenotypic expression of the fragile X syndrome: Inverse correlation between age and proportion of active X carrying the full mutation. *J. Am. Genet.* 28:830–836.

Rousseau, F., D. Heitz, J. Tarleton, J. MacPherson, H. Malmgren, N. Dahl, A. Barnicost, C. Mathew, E. Mornet, I. Teuada, A. Maddalena, R. Spiegel, A. Schinzel, J. A. G. Marcos, D. F. Schorderet, T. Schaap, L. Maccioni, S. Russo, P. A. Jacobs, C. Schwartz, and J. L. Mandel. 1994a. A multicenter study on genotype-phenotype correlations in fragile X syndrome, using direct diagnosis with probe StB12.3: The first 2253 cases. *Am. J. Hum. Genet.* 55:225–237.

Rousseau, F., L. J. Robb, P. Rouillard, and V. M. der Kaloustian. 1994b. No mental retardation in a man with 40% abnormal methylation at the FMR1 locus and transmission of sperm cell mutations as premutations. *Hum. Mol. Genet.* 6:927–930.

Roy, J. C., J. Johnson, K. Breese, and R. Hagerman. 1995. Fragile X syndrome: What is the impact of diagnosis on families? *Dev. Brain Dysfunct.* 8:327–335.

Rudelli, R. D., W. T. Brown, K. Wisniewski, E. C. Jenkins, M. Laure-Kamionowska, F. Connell, and H. M. Wisniewski. 1985. Adult fragile X syndrome: Clinico-neuropathologic findings. *Acta Neuropathol.* 67:289–295.

Ruvalcaba, R. H., S. A. Myhre, E. C. Roosen-Runge, and J. B. Beckwith. 1977. X-linked mental deficiency megalotestes syndrome. *JAMA* 238:1646–1650.

Sabaratnam, M. 2000. Pathological and neuropathological findings in two males with fragile X syndrome. *J. Intellect. Disabil. Res.* 44:81–85.

Sanfilippo, S., R. M. Ragusa, S. Musumeci, and G. Neri. 1986. Fragile X mental retardation: Prevalence in a group of institutionalized patients in Italy and description of a novel EEG pattern. *Am. J. Med. Genet.* 23:589–595.

Saxon, S. A., and E. Witriol. 1976. Down's syndrome and intellectual development. *J. Pediatr. Psychol.* 1:45–47.

Schapiro, M., G. Murphy, R. Hagerman, N. Azari, G. Alexander, C. Miezejeski, V. Hinton, B. Horowitz, J. Haxby, A. Kumar, B. White, and C. Grady. 1995. Adult fragile X syndrome: Neuropsychology, brain anatomy and metabolism. *Am. J. Med. Genet.* 60:480–493.

Schepis, C., R. Palazzo, R. M. Ragusa, E. Spina, and E. Barletta. 1989. Association of cutis verticis gyrata with fragile X syndrome and fragility of chromosome 12. *Lancet* 2:279.

Schinzel, A., and R. H. Largo. 1985. The fragile X syndrome (Martin-Bell syndrome): Clinical and cytogenetic findings in 16 prepubertal boys and in 4 of their 5 families. *Helvetica Paediatr. Acta* 40:133–152.

Schopmeyer, B. B., and F. Lowe (eds.). 1992. *The fragile X child.* San Diego: Singular Publishing Co.

Schrander-Stumpel, C., W-T. Gerver, H. Meyer, J. Engelen, H. Mulder, and J-P. Fryns. 1994. Prader-Willi-like phenotype in fragile X syndrome. *Clin. Genet.* 45:175–180.

Schwartz, C. E., J. Dean, P. N. Howard-Peebles, M. Bugge, M. Mikkelsin, N. Tommerup, C. E. Hull, R. J. Hagerman, J. J. A. Holden, and R. E. Stevenson. 1994. Obstetrical and gynecolocial complication in fragile X carriers: A multicenter study. *Am. J. Med. Genet.* 51:400–402.

Shapiro, L. R., P. L. Wilmot, R. A. Omar, M. M. Davidian, and P. N. Chander. 1986. Prenatal onset of macroorchidism in the fragile X syndrome: Significance in prenatal diagnosis. *Am. J. Hum. Genet.* 39:A265.

Sherman, S. L. 2000. Premature ovarian failure among fragile X premutation carriers: Parent-of-origin effect? [comment; editorial]. *Am. J. Hum. Genet.* 67:11–13.

Sherman, S. L., P. A. Jacobs, N. E. Morton, U. Froster-Iskenius, P. N. Howard-Peebles, K. B. Nielsen, M. W. Partington, G. R. Sutherland, G. Turner, and M. Watson. 1985. Further segregation analysis of the fragile X syndrome with special reference to transmitting males. *Hum. Genet.* 69:289–299.

Silva, J. A., M. M. Ferrari, and G. B. Leong. 1998. Erotomania in a case of fragile X syndrome. *Gen. Hosp. Psychiatry* 20:126–127.

Simko, A., L. Hornstein, S. Soukup, and N. Bagamery. 1989. Fragile X syndrome: Recognition in young children. *Pediatrics* 83:547–552.

Simon, E. W., and B. M. Finucane. 1996. Facial emotion identification in males with fragile X syndrome. *Am. J. Med. Genet.* 67:77–80.

Simpson, N. E., B. J. Newman, and M. W. Partington. 1984. Fragile-X syndrome III: Dermatoglyphic studies in males. *Am. J. Med. Genet.* 17:195–207.

Singh, R., G. R. Sutherland, and J. Manson. 1999. Partial seizures with focal epileptogenic electroencephalographic patterns in three related female patients with fragile-X syndrome. *J. Child Neurol.* 14:108–112.

Slegtenhorst-Eegdeman, K. E., D. G. de Rooij, M. Verhoef-Post, H. J. van de Kant, C. E. Bakker, B. A. Oostra, J. A. Grootegoed, and A. P. Themmen. 1998. Macroorchidism in FMR1 knockout mice is caused by increased Sertoli cell proliferation during testicular development. *Endocrinology* 139:156–162.

Smeets, H., A. Smits, C. E. Verheij, J. Theelen, R. Willemsen, I. van de Burgt, A. T. Hoogeveen, J. C. Oosterwijk, and B. A. Oostra. 1995. Normal phenotype in two brothers with a full FMR1 mutation. *Hum. Mol. Genet.* 4:2103–2108.

Sobesky, W. E., C. E. Hull, and R. J. Hagerman. 1992. The emotional phenotype in mildly affected carriers. In R. J. Hagerman and P. McKenzie (eds.), *1992 International Fragile X Conference Proceedings.* Denver: Spectra Publishing and the National Fragile X Foundation, pp. 99–106.

———. 1994a. Symptoms of schizotypal personality disorder in fragile X females. *J. Am. Acad. Child. Adolesc. Psychiatry* 33:247–255.

Sobesky, W. E., B. F. Pennington, D. Porter, C. E. Hull, and R. J. Hagerman. 1994b. Emotional and neurocognitive deficits in fragile X. *Am. J. Med. Genet.* 51:378–384.

Sobesky, W. E., D. Porter, B. F. Pennington, and R. J. Hagerman. 1995. Dimensions of shyness in fragile X females. *Dev. Brain Dysfunct.* 8:280–292.

Sobesky, W. E., A. K. Taylor, B. F. Pennington, L. Bennetto, D. Porter, J. Riddle, and R. J. Hagerman. 1996. Molecular/clinical correlations in females with fragile X. *Am. J. Med. Genet.* 64:340–345.

Solanto, M. V. 1998. Neuropsychopharmacological mechanisms of stimulant drug action in attention-deficit hyperactivity disorder: A review and integration. *Behav. Brain Res.* 94:127–152.

Sreeram, N., C. Wren, M. Bhate, P. Robertson, and S. Hunter. 1989. Cardiac abnormalities in the fragile X syndrome. *Br. Heart J.* 61:289–291.

Staley, L., C. Hull, M. M. Mazzocco, S. Thibodeau, K. Snow, V. Wilson, A. Taylor, L. McGavran, J. E. Riddle, R. O'Connor, and R. J. Hagerman. 1993. Molecular-clinical correlations in fragile X children and adults. *Am. J. Dis. Child.* 147:723–726.

Steinbach, P., D. Wöhrle, G. Tarierdian, I. Kennerknecht, G. Barbi, J. Edlinger, H. Enders, M. Gotz-Sothmann, H. Heilbonner, D. H. Hosenfeld, R. Kircheisen, F. Majewski, P. Meinecke, E. Passarge, A. Schmidt, H. Seidel, G. Wolff, and M. Zankl. 1993. Molecular analysis of mutations in the gene FMR1 segregating in fragile X families. *Hum. Genet.* 92:491–498.

Steyaert, J., M. Borghgraef, E. Legius, and J. P. Fryns. 1996. Molecular-intelligence correlations in young fragile X males with a mild CGG repeat expansion in the FMR1 gene. *Am. J. Med. Genet.* 64:274–277.

Storm, R. L., R. PeBenito, and C. Ferretti. 1987. Ophthalmologic findings in the fragile X syndrome. *Arch. Ophthalmol.* 105:1099–1102.

Sudhalter, V., I. L. Cohen, W. Silverman, and E. G. Wolf-Schein. 1990. Conversational analyses of males with fragile X, Down syndrome and autism: A comparison of the emergence of deviant language. *Am. J. Ment. Retard.* 94:431–441.

Sutherland, G. R., and F. Hecht. 1985. *Fragile sites on human chromosomes.* New York: Oxford Univ. Press.

Syrrou, M., I. Georgiou, P. C. Patsalis, I. Bouba, G. Adonakis, and G. N. Pagoulatos. 1999. Fragile X premutations and (TA)n estrogen receptor polymorphism in women with ovarian dysfunction. *Am. J. Med. Genet.* 84:306–308.

Tantam, D. 1988. Lifelong eccentricity and social isolation: I. Psychiatric, social, and forensic aspects. *Br. J. Psychiatry* 153:777–782.

Tarleton, J. C., R. Richie, C. Schwartz, K. Rao, A. S. Aylsworth, and A. Lachiewicz. 1993. An extensive de novo deletion removing FMR1 in a patient with mental retardation and the fragile X syndrome phenotype. *Hum. Mol. Genet.* 2:1973–1974.

Tassone, F., R. J. Hagerman, L. W. Gane, and A. K. Taylor. 1999a. Strong similarities of the FMR1 mutation in multiple tissues: Postmortem studies of a male with the full mutation and a male carrier of a premutation. *J. Med. Genet.* 84:240–244.

Tassone, F., R. J. Hagerman, D. Ikle, P. N. Dyer, M. Lampe, R. Willemsen, B. A. Oostra, and A. K. Taylor. 1999b. FMRP expression as a potential prognostic indicator in fragile X syndrome. *Am. J. Med. Genet.* 84:250–261.

Tassone, F., R. J. Hagerman, W. D. Chamberlain, and P. J. Hagerman. 2000a. Transcription of the FMR1 gene in individuals with fragile X syndrome. *Semin. Med. Genet.* 97:195–203.

Tassone, F., R. J. Hagerman, A. K. Taylor, L. W. Gane, T. E. Godfrey, and P. J. Hagerman. 2000b. Elevated levels of *FMR1* mRNA in carrier males: A new mechanism of involvement in fragile X syndrome. *Am. J. Hum. Genet.* 66:6–15.

Tassone, F., R. J. Hagerman, A. K. Taylor, J. B. Mills, S. W. Harris, L. W. Gane, and P. J. Hagerman. 2000c. Clinical involvement and protein expression in individuals with the *FMR1* premutation. *Am. J. Med. Genet.* 91:144–152.

Taylor, A. K., J. F. Safanda, K. A. Lugenbeel, D. L. Nelson, and R. J. Hagerman. 1994a. Molecular and phenotypic studies of fragile X males with variant methylation of the FMR1 gene reveal that the degree of methylation influences clinical severity. *Am. J. Hum. Genet.* 55:A18;85.

Taylor, A. K., J. F. Safanda, M. Z. Fall, C. Quince, K. A. Lang, C. E. Hull, I. Carpenter, L. W. Staley, and R. J. Hagerman. 1994b. Molecular predictors of involvement in fragile X females. *JAMA* 271:507–514.

Taylor, A. K., F. Tassone, P. M. Dyer, S. M. Hersch, J. B. Harris, W. T. Greenough, and R. J. Hagerman. 1999. Tissue heterogeneity of the FMR1 mutation in a high functioning male with fragile X syndrome. *Am. J. Med. Genet.* 84:233–239.

Teele, D. W., J. O. Klein, B. Rosner, L. Bratton, G. R. Risch, O. R. Mathieu, P. J. Porter, S. G. Starobin, L. D. Tarlin, and R. P. Younes. 1983. Middle ear disease and the practice of pediatrics: Burden during the first five years of life. *JAMA* 249:1026–1029.

Tejada, M. I., E. Mornet, E. Tizzano, M. Molina, M. Biaget, and A. Boue. 1993. Identification by molecular diagnosis of mosaic Turner's syndrome in an obligate carrier female for fragile X syndrome. *J. Med. Genet.* 31:76–78.

Tharapel, A. T., K. P. Anderson, J. L. Simpson, P. R. Martens, R. S. Wilroy Jr., J. S. Uerena Jr., and C. E. Schwartz. 1993. Deletion (X) (q26.1-q28) in a proband and her mother: Molecular consideration and phenotypic-karyotypic deductions. *Am. J. Hum. Genet.* 52:463–471.

Theobald, T. M., D. A. Hay, and C. Judge. 1987. Individual variation and specific cognitive deficits in the fra(X) syndrome. *Am. J. Med. Genet.* 28:1–11.

Thompson, N. M., G. A. Rogeness, E. McClure, R. Clayton, and C. Johnson. 1996. Influence of depression on cognitive functioning in fragile X females. *Psychiatry Res.* 64:97–104.

Tirosh, E., and Z. Borochowitz. 1992. Sleep apnea in fragile X syndrome. *Am. J. Med. Genet.* 43:124–127.

Towbin, J. A. 1999. Toward an understanding of the cause of mitral valve prolapse [editorial; comment]. *Am. J. Hum. Genet.* 65:1238–1241.

Turk, J. 1998. Fragile X syndrome and attentional deficits. *J. Appl. Res. Int. Disabil.* 11:175–191.

Turk, J., and P. Graham. 1997. Fragile X syndrome, autism, and autistic features. *Autism* 1:175–197.

Turk, J., and K. Cornish. 1998. Face recognition and emotion perception in boys with fragile-X syndrome. *J. Intellect. Disabil. Res.* 42:490–499.

Turner, G. 1983. Historical overview of X-linked mental retardation. In R. J. Hagerman and P. M. McBogg (eds.), *The fragile X syndrome: Diagnosis, biochemistry, and intervention.* Dillon, Colo.: Spectra Publishing, pp. 1–16.

Turner, G., C. Eastman, J. Casey, A. McLeay, P. Procopis, and B. Turner. 1975. X-linked mental retardation associated with macro-orchidism. *J. Med. Genet.* 12:367–371.

Turner, G., R. Till, and A. Daniel. 1978. Marker X chromosomes, mental retardation and macroorchidism [letter]. *N. Engl. J. Med.* 299:1472.

Turner, G., A. Daniel, and M. Frost. 1980. X-linked mental retardation, macroorchidism, and the Xq27 fragile site. *J. Pediatr.* 96:837–841.

Turner, G., J. M. Opitz, W. T. Brown, K. E. Davies, P. A. Jacobs, E. C. Jenkins, M. Mikkelsen, M. W. Partington, and G. R. Sutherland. 1986. Conference report: Second International Workshop on the Fragile X and on X-linked Mental Retardation. *Am. J. Med. Genet.* 23:11–67.

Turner, G., H. Robinson, S. Laing, M. Van den Berk, A. Colley, A. Goddard, S. Sherman, and M. Partington. 1992. Population screening for fragile X syndrome. *Lancet* 339:1210–1213.

Turner, G., H. Robinson, S. Wake, and N. Martin. 1994. Dizygous twinning and premature menopause in fragile X syndrome. *Lancet* 344:1500.

Turner, W. J. 1995. Homosexuality, type I: An Xq28 phenomenon. *Arch. Sex. Behav.* 24:109–134.

Varley, C. K., V. A. Holm, and M. O. Eren. 1985. Cognitive and psychiatric variability in three brothers with fragile X syndrome. *J. Dev. Behav. Pediatr.* 6:87–90.

Venter, P. A., J. Op't Hof, D. J. Coetzee, C. Van der Walt, and A. E. Retief. 1984. No marker (X) syndrome in autistic children. *Hum. Genet.* 67:107.

Verheij, C., C. E. Bakker, E. de Graaff, J. Keulemans, R. Willemsen, A. J. Verkerk, H. Galjaard, A. J. Reuser, A. T. Hoogeveen, and B. A. Oostra. 1993. Characterization and localization of the FMR1 gene product associated with fragile X syndrome. *Nature* 363:722–724.

Verkerk, A. J., M. Pieretti, J. S. Sutcliffe, Y-H. Fu, D. P. Kuhl, A. Pizzuti, O. Reiner, S. Richards, M. F. Victoria, F. Zhang, B. E. Eussen, G. J. van Ommen, L. A. J. Blonden, G. J. Riggins, J. L. Chastain, C. B. Kunst, H. Galjaard, C. T. Caskey, D. L. Nelson, B. A. Oostra, and S. T. Warren. 1991. Identification of a gene (FMR-1) containing a CGG repeat coincident with a breakpoint cluster region exhibiting length variation in fragile X syndrome. *Cell* 65:905–914.

Verma, I. C., and R. Elango. 1994. Variable expression of clinical features of Martin Bell syndrome in younger patients. *Indian Pediatr.* 31:433–438.

Vianna-Morgante, A. M. 1999. Twinning and premature ovarian failure in premutation fragile X carriers [letter]. *Am. J. Med. Genet.* 83:326.

Vianna-Morgante, A. M., and S. S. Costa. 2000. Premature ovarian failure is associated with maternally and paternally inherited premutation in Brazilian families with fragile X [letter; see comments]. *Am. J. Hum. Genet.* 67:254–255; discussion 256–258.

Vianna-Morgante, A. M., I. Armando, and O. Frota-Pessoa. 1982. Escalante syndrome and the marker X chromosome [letter]. *Am. J. Med. Genet.* 12:237–240.

Vianna-Morgante, A. M., S. S. Costa, A. S. Pares, and I. T. Verreschi. 1996. FRAXA premutation associated with premature ovarian failure. *Am. J. Med. Genet.* 64:373–375.

Vieregge, P., and U. Froster-Iskenius. 1989. Clinico-neurological investigations in the fra X form of mental retardation. *J. Neurol.* 236:85–92.

Vincent, S., D. Heitz, C. Petit, C. Kretz, I. Oberle, J. L. Mandel. 1991. Abnormal pattern detected in fragile-X patients by pulsed-field gel electrophoresis. *Nature* 349:674–676.

Voelckel, M. A., M. G. Mattei, C. N. Guyen, N. Philip, F. Birg, and J. F. Mattei. 1988. Dissociation between mental retardation and fragile site expression in a family with fragile X-linked mental retardation. *Hum. Genet.* 80:375–378.

Voelckel, M. A., N. Philip, C. Piquet, M. C. Pellissier, I. Oberle, F. Birg, M. G. Mattei, and J. F. Mattei. 1989. Study of a family with a fragile site of the X chromosome at Xq27-27 without mental retardation. *Hum. Genet.* 81:353–357.

von Gontard, A., M. Backes, C. Laufersweiler-Plass, C. Wendland, G. Lehmkuhl, K. Zerres, and S. Rudnik-Schöneborn. 2001. Psychopathology and familial stress: Comparison of boys with fragile X syndrome and spinal muscular atrophy. In press.

Vorst, E. J., N. A. Levene, R. Nisani, and A. Berrebi. 1993. Fragile X syndrome and myelodysplasia discovered during pregnancy. *Br. J. Haematol.* 85:415–416.

Waldstein, G., and R. Hagerman. 1988. Aortic hypoplasia and cardiac valvular abnormalities in a boy with fragile X syndrome. *Am. J. Med. Genet.* 30:83–98.

Waldstein, G., G. Mierau, R. Ahmad, S. N. Thibodeau, R. J. Hagerman, and S. Caldwell. 1987. Fragile X syndrome: Skin elastin abnormalities. *Birth Defects: Original Article Ser.* 23:103–114.

Waller, B. F. 1985. Exercise related sudden death in young (age ≤ 30 years) and old (age > 30 years) conditioned subjects. *Cardiovasc. Clin.* 15:9–73.

Wang, Y. C., M. L. Lin, S. J. Lin, Y. C. Li, and S. Y. Li. 1997. Novel point mutation within intron 10 of FMR-1 gene causing fragile X syndrome [see comments]. *Hum. Mutat.* 10:393–399.

Watson, M. S., J. F. Leckman, B. Annex, W. R. Breg, D. Boles, F. R. Volkmar, D. J. Cohen, and C. Carter. 1984. Fragile X in a survey of 75 autistic males [letter]. *N. Engl. J. Med.* 310:1462.

Watson, M. S., W. R. Breg, D. Pauls, W. T. Brown, A. J. Carroll, P. N. Howard-Peebles, D. Meryash, and L. R. Shapiro. 1988. Aneuploidy and the fragile X syndrome. *Am. J. Med. Genet.* 30:115–121.

Webb, T. P., A. Thake, and J. Todd. 1986. Twelve families with fragile Xq27. *Med. Genet.* 23:400–406.

Weiler, I. J., and W. T. Greenough. 1999. Synaptic synthesis of the fragile X protein: Possible involvement in synapse maturation and elimination. *Am. J. Med. Genet.* 83:248–252.

Weiler, I. J., S. A. Irwin, A. Y. Klintsova, C. M. Spencer, A. D. Brazelton, K. Miyashiro, T. A. Comery, B. Patel, J. Eberwine, and W. T. Greenough. 1997. Fragile X mental retardation protein is translated near synapses in response to neurotransmitter activation. *Proc. Natl. Acad. Sci. USA* 94:5395–5400.

Wenstrup, R. J., S. Murad, and S. R. Pinnelli. 1989. Ehlers-Danlos syndrome type VI: Clinical manifestations of collagen lysyl hydroxylate deficiency. *J. Pediatr.* 115:405–409.

Werry, J. S., R. L. Sprague, and M. N. Cohen. 1975. Conners' Teacher Rating Scale for use in drug studies with children: An empirical study. *J. Abnorm. Child Psychol.* 3:217–229.

Wiegers, A. M., L. M. G. Curfs, E. L. M. H. Vermeer, and J. P. Fryns. 1993. Adaptive behavior in the fragile X syndrome. *Am. J. Med. Genet.* 47:216–220.

Wilhelm, D., U. Froster-Iskenius, J. Paul, and E. Schwinger. 1988. Fra(X) frequency on the active X-chromosome and phenotype in heterozygous carriers of the fra(X) form of mental retardation. *Am. J. Med. Genet.* 30:407–415.

Willems, P. J., B. VanRoy, K. De Boulle, L. Vits, E. Reyniers, O. Beck, J. E. Dumon, A. Verkerk, and B. Oostra. 1992. Segregation of the fragile X mutation from an affected male to his normal daughter. *Hum. Mol. Genet.* 1:511–515.

Willemsen, R., S. Mohkemsing, B. de Vries, D. Devys, A. Van den Ouweland, J. L. Mandel, H. Galjaard, and B. A. Oostra. 1995. Rapid antibody test for fragile X syndrome. *Lancet* 345:1147–1148.

Willemsen, R., A. Smits, S. Mohkamsing, H. van Beerendonk, A. de Haan, B. de Vries, A. van den Ouweland, E. Sistermans, H. Galjaard, and B. A. Oostra. 1997. Rapid antibody test for diagnosing fragile X syndrome: A validation of the technique. *Hum. Genet.* 99:308–311.

Wilson, D. P., N. J. Carpenter, and G. Berkovitz. 1988. Thyroid function in men with fragile X-linked MR [letter]. *Am. J. Med. Genet.* 31:733–734.

Wing, L. 1981. Asperger's syndrome: A clinical account. *Psychol. Med.* 11:115–129.

Wisbeck, J. M., L. C. Huffman, L. Freund, M. Gunnar, E. P. Davis, and A. L. Reiss. 2000. Cortisol and social stressors in children with fragile X: A pilot study. *J. Dev. Behav. Pediatr.* 21:278–282.

Wisniewski, K. E., J. H. French, W. T. Brown, E. C. Jenkins, and C. M. Miezejeski. 1989.

The fragile X syndrome and developmental disabilities. In J. French and C. P. Harels (eds.), *Child neurology and developmental disabilities: Selected proceedings of the Fourth International Child Neurology Congress.* Baltimore: Paul H. Brookes Publishing, pp. 11–20.

Wisniewski, K. E., S. M. Segan, C. M. Miezejeski, E. A. Sersen, and R. D. Rudelli. 1991. The fra(X) syndrome: Neurological, electrophysiological, and neuropathological abnormalities. *Am. J. Med. Genet.* 38:476–480.

Witt, R. M., B. K. Kaspar, A. D. Brazelton, T. A. Comery, A. M. Craig, I. J. Weiler, and W. T. Greenough. 1995. Developmental localization of fragile X mRNA in rat brain. *Soc. Neurosci. Abstr.* 21:1;293.6.

Wöhrle, D., D. Kotzot, M. C. Hirst, A. Manca, B. Korn, A. Schmidt, G. Barbi, H-D. Rott, A. Poustka, K. E. Davies, and P. Steinbach. 1992. A microdeletion of less than 250 kb, including the proximal part of the FMR-1 gene and the fragile X site, in a male with the clinical phenotype of fragile X syndrome. *Am. J. Hum. Genet.* 51:299–306.

Wöhrle, D., I. Hennig, W. Vogel, and P. Steinbach. 1993. Mitotic stability of fragile X mutations in differentiated cells indicates early post-conceptional trinucleotide repeat expansion. *Nat. Genet.* 4:140–142.

Wöhrle, D., U. Salat, D. Glaser, J. Mucke, M. Meisel-Stosiek, D. Schindler, W. Vogel, and P. Steinbach. 1998. Unusual mutations in high functioning fragile X males: Apparent instability of expanded unmethylated CGG repeats. *J. Med. Genet.* 35:103–111.

Wolff, P. H., J. Gardner, J. J. Paccia, and J. Lappen. 1989. The greeting behavior of fragile X males. *Am. J. Ment. Retard.* 93:406–411.

Wright, H. H., S. R. Young, J. G. Edwards, R. K. Abramson, and J. Duncan. 1986. Fragile X syndrome in a population of autistic children. *J. Am. Acad. Child Psychiatry* 25:641–644.

Wright-Talamante, C., A. Cheema, J. E. Riddle, D. W. Luckey, A. K. Taylor, and R. J. Hagerman. 1996. A controlled study of longitudinal IQ changes in females and males with fragile X syndrome. *Am. J. Med. Genet.* 64:350–355.

Yu, S., M. Pritchard, E. Kermer, M. Lynch, J. Nancarrow, E. Baker, K. Holman, J. C. Mulley, S. T. Warren, D. Schlessinger, G. R. Sutherland, and R. I. Richards. 1991. Fragile X genotype characterized by an unstable region of DNA. *Science* 252:1179–1181.

Zachmann, M., A. Prader, H. P. Kind, H. Hafliger, and H. Budliger. 1974. Testicular volume during adolescence: Cross-sectional and longitudinal studies. *Helv. Paediatr. Acta* 29:61–72.

# CHAPTER 2

# The Molecular Biology of the Fragile X Mutation

W. Ted Brown, M.D., Ph.D.

## DNA and the Fragile X Syndrome

The molecular biology of the fragile X mutation is an area of very active investigation and research. New information is appearing frequently. This chapter covers DNA studies of the fragile X gene, molecular diagnostic methods, and likely future directions in the investigation of the fragile X locus. Recent developments in the use of recombinant DNA technology have led to new methods for diagnosis of genetic diseases in general and fragile X syndrome in particular. The new techniques allow diagnosis by direct analysis of DNA and have largely replaced cytogenetics as a means of accurate diagnosis of fragile X. This approach has also been applied to carrier identification and prenatal testing. Recommendations regarding who should be tested and how results should be reported are discussed. Questions concerning the ancestral history of the fragile X mutation have been the subject of numerous studies. Finally, the fragile X mutation is now recognized as similar to several mutations that involve trinucleotide repeats, and lessons learned from these other mutations may offer insights into the fragile X mutation as well. We begin with a review of basic information about DNA techniques.

## The Basics of Recombinant DNA Technology

The development of recombinant DNA technology has depended on two basic discoveries: endonucleases and gene cloning. In 1970, it was observed that some bacterial enzymes called *restriction endonucleases* degrade foreign DNA.

*Fragile X Syndrome: Diagnosis, Treatment, and Research,* third edition, ed. Randi Jenssen Hagerman and Paul J. Hagerman (Baltimore: Johns Hopkins University Press, 2002), © The Johns Hopkins University Press.

The first such enzyme to be discovered was found in the bacteria *Haemophilus influenzae* by Smith and Wilcox (1970). This enzyme recognizes a specific sequence of six base pairs in the DNA molecule. Since their initial discovery in 1970, more than four hundred different restriction enzymes have been isolated from different strains of bacteria. These enzymes generally recognize a specific sequence of four or six DNA base pairs (bps). The enzymes are named for the bacterial species from which they are isolated. The convention has been adopted that the host bacterial organism is identified by the letter of the genus name and the first two letters of the second name to form a letter abbreviation. For example, the enzyme from *Haemophilus influenzae* is known as *Hin* and that from *Escherichia coli* is known as *Eco*. A strain identification follows the genus abbreviation, for example, *Eco*R. When more than one restriction enzyme system has been identified within a given bacterial strain, these are identified separately by roman numerals, such as *Eco*RI and *Hin*dIII. By use of such restriction enzymes, DNA can be cut at specific and reproducible sites. Restriction enzymes cut DNA into pieces generally averaging 1,000 to 10,000 bps long. As the human genome contains about $3 \times 10^9$ bps, 300,000 to 3,000,000 pieces are produced when human DNA is digested with such an enzyme.

The discovery of restriction enzymes allowed the development of gene cloning. In this process a fragment of cut DNA can be inserted into bacterial host carriers known as *vectors*. Vectors include plasmids, bacteriophages, and cosmids. These vectors generally live and reproduce in the cytoplasm of bacteria. On specific sites, a restriction enzyme can cut a vector and a foreign piece of DNA can be inserted. Thus, DNA from two species can be recombined. The various fragments produced by a restriction enzyme digestion of a sample of human DNA can each be individually cloned into vectors. A collection of clones (e.g., all fragments from a given chromosome) is called a *library*. From this library, individual clones can be selected and grown up to a very large quantity. The cloned DNA fragment can be isolated from the vector using the restriction enzyme that cuts the exact site where the DNA from the two species is joined. In this manner, a pure quantity of given gene or DNA fragment of interest can be isolated for further study. Because these vectors and their host bacteria can be grown quickly in the laboratory, large quantities of a DNA sequence can be isolated to be further studied with speed and efficiency.

To study the gene or DNA sequence of interest from a given individual, one needs a method to visualize DNA. The most widely used method for visualizing the gene of interest is the method of Southern blotting (Southern 1975). DNA from an individual is isolated from an available tissue source such as white blood cells. The DNA is cut by one of the restriction enzymes. The millions of fragments of various sizes that are produced can be separated by electrophoresis in an agarose gel. The movement of the various fragments in the gel is a function of their length. The DNA is then transferred by blotting from the agarose gel onto a supporting membrane such as nitrocellulose paper, to which the DNA can be covalently bound. The position of the DNA fragments on the paper is the same as was their position in the agarose gel. For visualization of the position of a particular DNA sequence among the millions of fragments on the paper, a vector containing a cloned DNA sequence is radioactively labeled. This labeled DNA sequence is complementary to a sequence that is on the filter paper. The radioactive DNA is used to detect its complementary sequence. It hybridizes under conditions that allow the complementary sequence to be recognized. The position of the radioactive probe is visualized after exposure to X-ray film. This method allows one to detect a given sequence of DNA among the millions of sequences of DNA that are produced when a sample of human DNA is cut with a restriction enzyme.

Polymerase chain reaction (PCR) analysis is a significant technology invented in the late 1980s, which is being used for analysis of a variety of human genetic mutations (Erlich and Arnheim 1992). It is fast, efficient, and inexpensive and can be performed with very small amounts of DNA. The principle of the technique is that a gene region can be rapidly synthesized in the laboratory such that millions of copies of the sequence of interest can be made in a few hours. Then mutations can be easily visualized. The procedure involves the use of two primers, which are stretches of 20 base pairs that correspond to the DNA sequences that flank the sequence of interest. Native DNA is heated to the point that the two strands separate. On cooling, the primers that are in large excess concentration will hybridize to their matching sequences. Then, using DNA polymerase and free nucleotide bases, new DNA for the region between the primers is synthesized. This newly synthesized double-stranded DNA is heated again to separate the single strands, and the process is repeated. Each such cycle results in a doubling of the amount of DNA present for the specific region between the primers. Since each cycle approximately doubles the amount of DNA of the sequence of interest, after 30 cycles approximately $2^{30}$ copies $(1,000,000,000\times)$ are present for each original molecule.

## Identification of the Fragile X Gene

After many attempts to identify the exact location of the fragile X gene, in the spring of 1991 the studies of several laboratories resulted in the much-hoped-for discovery. The laboratories of Mandel and Davies independently cloned a region located at the apparent fragile site (Bell et al. 1991; Vincent et al. 1991). The region included a CpG island, often indicating the presence of a promoter and usually found near expressed gene sequences. DNA in this region was overmethylated in samples from affected fragile X males but not so in samples from normal or nonpenetrant (carrier) males. Mandel's laboratory reported the isolation of a large (425 kb) cloned DNA fragment in a yeast artificial chromosome (YAC) that contained sequences previously shown to be located on either side of the fragile site (Heitz et al. 1991). Near the middle of the YAC clone was the CpG island that was hypermethylated in fragile X–positive males. Thus, the cloning of the fragile X site had been achieved. The investigators used a small (7 kb) subclone located adjacent to the CpG island to show that fragile X males had a significantly increased number of base sequences within this region. Sutherland's laboratory nearly simultaneously also reported similar findings using a separately isolated subclone (Yu et al. 1991).

These studies showed that nonpenetrant males have an insertion of 100 to 500 bps. They transmit this insertion to their normal daughters, who then can transmit it to affected sons. These sons typically have a further enlargement to a size of 600 to 4,000 bps. Thus, the fragile X mutation was found to involve first a small insertion or a "premutation," which did not affect methylation, but when transmitted to affected sons underwent enlargement to a much bigger size that did affect methylation. In summary, individuals with the full mutation generally exhibit the chromosomal fragile site at Xq27.3 and cytogenetic frequencies correlate with the average size of the amplification (Yu et al. 1992).

Oostra, Nelson, and Warren's laboratories collaborated to clone the fragile X gene (Verkerk et al. 1991). They used a cosmid clone from within the unstable region to isolate an expressed gene from a cDNA library. The gene was named *FMR1* (fragile X mental retardation 1), assuming that this was the first of an unknown number of future genes that might be isolated from the X chromosome involving fragility and mental retardation. *FMR1* had many remarkable properties. Near its 5' beginning was a long stretch of a variable number of trinucleotide repeats consisting mostly of CGG. This long repeat region offered a possible site for the apparent size enlargement seen in affected males. At first, since the CGG repeat region was part of the cDNA obtained from a messenger RNA, it was assumed to be coding for protein. Later, it was recognized that, although the CGG region was transcribed into RNA, the site where protein translation is initiated was located 69 bps downstream of the CGG repeat region (Ashley et al. 1993a). The *FMR1* gene was found to be highly conserved in structure across a number of species. The human cDNA cross-hybridized with genomic DNA from chimpanzees, gorillas, monkeys, pigs, cows, hamsters, rabbits, and chickens. The gene was noted to have a nuclear import signal indicating that it could be involved in movement between the cell cytoplasm and the nucleus. The structure of the gene initially could not be related to any known gene, and its function was unknown. Two years later, it was noticed that the gene has sequences characteristic of proteins that bind to RNA, several KH domains, and RGG boxes. Ashley et al. (1993b) showed that the isolated protein does bind to about 4% of brain messenger RNA, including its own message. It seems to be evolutionarily related to several other genes that have a high degree of sequence homology and are termed *FXR1* and *FXR2* (see chap. 5). A nuclear export signal was also identified in the *FMR1* sequence, suggesting the FMR1 protein (FMRP) may shuttle in and out of the cell nucleus and modify the translation of a set of other gene transcripts to which it binds (Eberhart et al. 1996). Further understanding of the function of *FMR1* and the related *FXR* genes will undoubtedly lead to insights into the genetics of mental function and, it is hoped, the development of specific therapies for affected individuals.

## The Fragile X Mutation

The length of the repeat region was found to be highly polymorphic in normal individuals, with lengths ranging from approximately 6 to 55 CGGs (Fu et al. 1991; Brown et al. 1993; Snow et al. 1993). As illustrated in figure 2.1, the most frequent control repeat number is 30, followed by 29, 31, 20, and 23. Approximately 5% of normal alleles are 40 or greater, 2% are more than 45, and 0.5% are more than 50. Carrier females and transmitting males have an enlargement of the region to a range of approximately 55 to 200 repeats, which is referred to as a *premutation*. Offspring of carrier females can show small increases or decreases of the repeat or can expand to have enlargements to values ranging from 200 to over 2,000 repeats, which is referred to as the *full mutation*. The daughters of transmitting males are all carriers of the premutation. In general, none of the daughters of transmitting males is affected and none has an expanded full mutation. In this regard, affected full-mutation males have fathered normal daughters who carry only a premutation-sized allele. Analysis of sperm samples from full-mutation males reveals only premutation-sized alleles, suggesting that the amplification process occurs postzygotically (Reyniers et al. 1993). Analysis of single sperm repeats of premutation males has shown a large range of sizes, further indicating that instability occurs after conception (Nolin et al. 1999).

A minority of affected individuals have a mosaic pattern with some proportion of cells showing sizes of less than 200 repeats and partially active gene expression (Rousseau et al. 1991). Methylation mosaicism (i.e., a full mutation showing only partial methylation) has also been observed. Using a sensitive Southern blotting method and heavily loaded DNA samples, we found about 40% of fragile X males to be mosaics. About 20% of affected males show a strong mosaic pattern, and another 20% show a faint mosaic pattern (Nolin et al. 1994). Evidence indicates that mosaicism is correlated with higher functioning and a better prognosis (McConkie-Rosell et al. 1993; Cohen et al. 1996).

Based on studies of 30 female carriers, Fu et al. (1991) demonstrated that the risk of a premutation allele being passed on as a full mutation was related

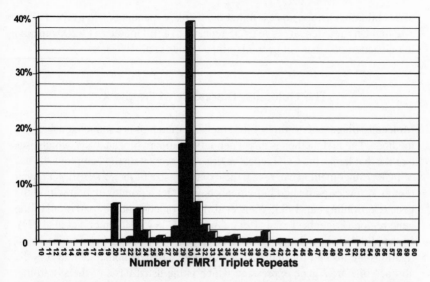

**Fig. 2.1.** Percentages of *FMR1* triplet repeat length alleles in a series of 2,500 controls. The alleles were selected to have repeat numbers <60 and were from a random population from the New York area. None of the individual X chromosomes was directly related to any individual with fragile X syndrome. Repeat lengths were sized according to the PCR method of Brown et al. (1993, 1994).

to the premutation size. Female carriers of the premutation who have had affected children have between 59 and 200 repeats, based on a survey of 20 laboratories (Nolin et al., unpublished). Thus, repeat alleles in the range 50–58, occasionally present in individuals within fragile X families, were not observed to progress in one generation to the full mutation. However, a 37% progression was observed for alleles in the 59–69 range, 65% for the 70–79 range, 70% for the 80–89 range, 93% in the 90–99 range, and repeat alleles of over 100 in nearly all cases studied (Nolin et al. 1996). As the premutation is transmitted through subsequent generations within families, it demonstrates *anticipation,* which means that greater numbers of affected individuals are observed in later generations than in earlier ones. This phenomenon, specifically, that the brothers of transmitting males are less likely to be affected than the sons of their daughters, was termed the *Sherman paradox* by Opitz (1986). The size-related risk of expansion helped to explain this paradox. In addition to the size-related risk of expansion, we have noted that there is a strong familial clustering of repeat size expansion. The offspring of some mothers tend to be full mutations, whereas those of others tend to be only premutations (Nolin et al. 1994, 1996). No carriers of less than 59 repeats have yet been found to have had affected male children. Further, no new mutation, that is, expanding from a repeat allele size in the normal repeat range (<55 repeats) to a full mutation (>200 repeats) in one generation, has yet been identified (Smits et al. 1993).

## The Molecular Diagnosis of Fragile X

Molecular diagnostic testing of the fragile X mutation is conducted using two methods. The first method is direct genomic Southern blot analysis, which uses a probe that flanks the CGG repeat region. The second method employs the use of PCR. Either method can reveal the expanded size of the *FMR1* triplet repeat region. A few rare affected individuals have either a point mutation within the gene (De Boulle et al. 1993; Wang et al. 1997) or a deletion of part or all of the gene region (Lugenbeel et al. 1995; Quan et al. 1995; Hammond et al. 1997). If one of these rare deletion types is suspected, more detailed molecular investigations are needed for diagnosis. These rare cases demonstrate that it is the absence of *FMR1* gene expression which is the usual basis of the syndrome. The repeat amplification mutation is far and away (>99%) the most common molecular basis of the syndrome. In addition, protein testing for FMRP levels (see chap. 4) is currently conducted in certain research settings but is not routinely available. The test, rather than a quantitation of protein, involves scoring cells as either expressing (positive) or nonexpressing (negative) and determining a percentage of positive cells. Testing of protein has been proposed as a prognostic indicator of the severity of the fragile X syndrome (Tassone et al. 1999), and further progress in this area of testing may be expected (see chap. 12).

For Southern blot analysis of fragile X mutations, several useful probes have been developed (Oostra et al. 1993). A commonly used probe, StB12.3, employs a double digestion with two restriction enzymes. With StB12.3 (Oberlé et al. 1991), a *Pst* I–derived 1.1 kb fragment located a few hundred bps downstream from the CGG repeat region, both the methylation and amplification could be seen in a single sample after an *Eco*RI + *Eag* I (methylation-sensitive) double digest. As illustrated in figures 2.2 and 2.3, digestion with the first enzyme (*Eco*RI) produces a 5.2 kb band on a Southern blot. The second methylation-sensitive enzyme (*Eag* I) cuts unmethylated DNA at the CpG island, producing a 2.8 kb band, but leaves methylated DNA uncut. Thus, a normal female produces both a 2.8 kb band, reflecting her active unmethylated X chromosome, and a 5.2 kb band, reflecting her inactive, methylated X chromosome. Premutation alleles generally produce bands in the range of 2.9 to 3.2 kb for the active X, as are present in transmitting males, and 5.3 to 5.7 kb for the inactive X. Normal carrier females generally have two doublets on analysis. Affected males generally have bands or smears in the 5.8 to 9 kb range, reflecting a large

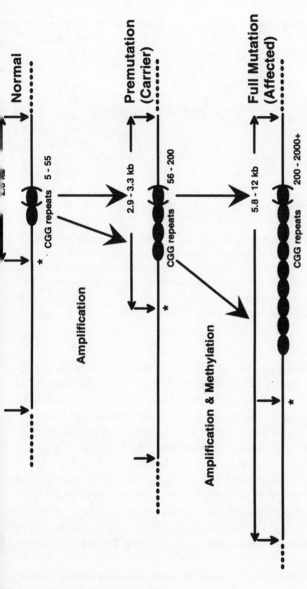

**Fig. 2.2.** The fragile X gene *FMR1* contains a mutable CGG repeat region. This repeat is amplified to a premutation in carriers and undergoes further amplification and methylation to result in the full mutation in affected individuals. Using a flanking probe and following a double digest with the restriction enzymes *Eco*RI and *Eag*I, fragments are generated by cleavage at the *small vertical arrows*. Only the fragments containing the CGG repeat region are detected. DNA methylation prevents cleavage by *Eag*I at the position marked * (a CpG island). In normal individuals, a 5.2 kb fragment is detected in methylated chromosomes and a 2.8 kb fragment is detected in unmethylated chromosomes. The amplification of the CGG repeat region leads to an increase in the size of these fragments. In affected individuals, not only is the CGG repeat region amplified, but the DNA is also methylated, including the CpG island. This methylation prevents cleavage at the methylation-sensitive (*) restriction site.

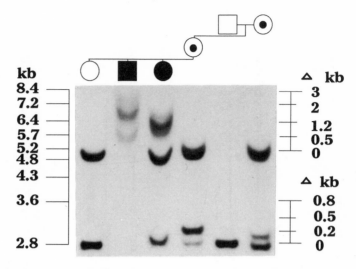

**Fig. 2.3.** Direct Southern blot analysis of a fragile X family using probe StB12.3. The lanes correspond to the individuals in the pedigree at the *top,* with males as *squares* and females as *circles.* The carrier grandmother has bands of approximately 2.8 and 2.9 kb (the active chromosomes) and 5.2 and 5.3 (the inactive chromosomes). Her carrier daughter has a premutation that is slightly larger. The affected son and daughter have full mutations with smears ranging from about 5.7 kb to 8.4 kb.

amplification with an increased size of 500 to 6,000 bps above controls and corresponding to CGG repeats of approximately 200 to 2,000 (Rousseau et al. 1991). The frequency of mental retardation in persons with premutations (60 to 200 repeats) seems to be no different from that in the general population. Approximately 95% of males and about 50% of females with the full mutation have mental retardation (i.e., a measured IQ below 70). There definitely are carrier females with the full mutation who are intellectually normal. A notable example is that of identical twin females, both diagnosed as cytogenetically positive (implying full mutations) and yet one was retarded whereas the other had above average intelligence (Tuckerman et al. 1985). This example points out that the random inactivation pattern of the X chromosome in the developing brain is likely to contribute substantially to the resulting full-mutation female phenotype.

The number of CGG repeats usually undergoes an amplification during transmission from carrier mother to offspring. Expansion of repeat numbers to more than about 200 is usually associated with methylation of the upstream CpG island. All affected individuals thus far studied, with the exception of rare point mutation and deletion patients, have had a mother who carried a premutation. Every carrier mother of an affected child thus far tested has inherited the premutation from one of her parents, and no one has yet identified a new mutation (Smits et al. 1993).

PCR analysis for fragile X mutations is rapid and uses small amounts of starting DNA for analysis. However, because the region is high in CG content, special methods are needed for successful amplification of full mutations. Initial attempts to PCR amplify the CGG repeat region in the fragile X locus by PCR were unsuccessful (Kremer et al. 1991). Fu et al. (1991) developed a PCR method that successfully amplified normal-sized alleles and many premutation alleles but failed to amplify full mutations with over 200 CGGs. We developed a method that allows successful amplification of most full mutations as well as a high resolution of normal allele sizes (Pergolizzi et al. 1992; Erster et al. 1992; Brown et al. 1993; Brown 1994). The method replaces dGTP with 100% deaza-dGTP. The use of 100% deaza-dGTP inhibits visualization with ethidium bromide. Lowering the ratio of deaza-dGTP:dGTP from 100% to 50%:50% or to 25%:75% has been reported to allow for direct visualization with ethidium bromide (Chong et al. 1994; Wang et al. 1995). However, with less than 100% deaza-dGTP, not all premutation alleles amplify successfully. Our protocol uses short denaturing polyacrylamide gels and commonly available electrophoresis apparatus. The small gel size allows rapid electroblotting. The protocol uses a sensitive, stable, nonradioactive, chemiluminescent probe detection system, which is convenient and faster than alternatives, such as radioactive probes or internal labeling. We have been able to visualize the PCR products with our protocol using single cell samples of DNA. After DNA isolation and PCR amplification, the analysis can be completed in fewer than eight hours. Because nanogram amounts of DNA are sufficient for PCR analysis, prenatal samples can be studied directly. The protocol allows accurate resolution of alleles within the normal repeat range of 10–50, as illustrated in figure 2.4, and approximate sizing of the larger premutation and full-mutation allele sizes, as illustrated in figure 2.5. In our experience, approximately 10% of full-mutation alleles fail to amplify successfully. Hence, there is a need to have both methods available for routine diagnostic and prenatal testing purposes.

As summarized in table 2.1, PCR and Southern blot analysis each has several different advantages. The main advantages to the use of Southern blot analysis are that it is more reliable in detecting the large expansions seen in full mutations and can be used to detect the methylation status of the CpG island. On the other hand, PCR is faster and generally less expensive, only minimal DNA is needed, and the size resolution of normal alleles is greater. The PCR product length of a normal allele is approximately 150 bps, whereas Southern blots of restriction enzyme-digested DNA generally are best used to analyze fragments several kilobases (kb) long (Oostra et al. 1993). The small PCR size allows improved size resolution, an advantage for detecting carriers of small

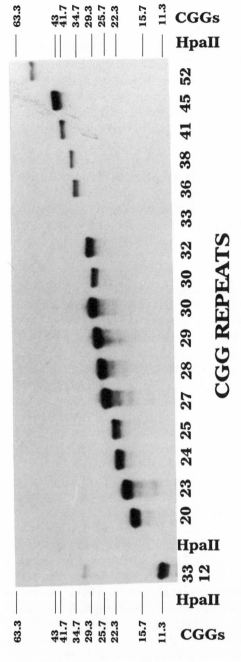

**CGG REPEATS**

**Fig. 2.4.** PCR analysis of alleles within the normal size range of CGG repeats. The sizes range from 12 to 52. Sizes were calibrated using *Hpa*II digests of pBR322 as markers, with the use of the method of Brown et al. (1993, 1994).

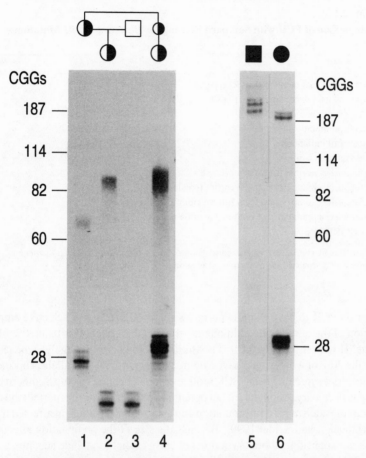

**Fig. 2.5. PCR** analysis of premutations and full mutations. Three related premutation carriers are on the *left*. Two full-mutation individuals, a male and a female, are on the *right*. Markers are as in figure 2.4. Above the top marker of 187, there is considerable compression of the size bands, where the largest bands may not amplify well in the presence of smaller bands. *Source:* Data from Nolin and Brown.

premutations. The number of CGG repeats in the normal population is highly variable (fig. 2.1). As a consequence, approximately 80% of normal women will be heterozygous, with two different CGG repeat alleles. Among the 20% who are homozygous, a common size is usually seen, since 75% will have a 30-repeat size and 15% a 29-repeat. The female carriers of a premutation will usually have a pattern with the premutation allele (56–200) and the normal-sized allele (7–55) clearly separated. Women with the full-mutation pattern may ap-

**Table 2.1**

**Comparison of PCR with Southern Blotting for Detecting *FMR1* Mutation**

| Test Feature | PCR | Southern |
|---|---|---|
| Determines exact number of CGG repeats | +++ | − |
| Rapid and uses small amounts of DNA | +++ | + |
| Detects methylation | − | +++ |
| Detects premutations | ++ | + |
| Detects full mutations | + | ++ |
| Detects mosaicism | + | ++ |
| Distinguishes normal from carrier females | ++ | +[a] |
| Distinguishes homozygous from carrier females | ++ | + |
| Distinguishes homozygous from full-mutation females | ± | ++ |
| Distinguishes premutation from full-mutation males | ++ | + |
| Detects deletions | − | ± |

[a]Alleles that are close in size may be indistinguishable (i.e., 50 and 60 repeats); likewise, normal alleles may be widely separated and misinterpreted as carriers (i.e., 20 and 50).

pear on PCR to have a single normal-sized band because of selective amplification of the normal allele. In our experience, this occurs less than 10% of the time. However, because of this possibility, a Southern blot analysis is needed for the 20% of women who have a homozygous normal-sized allele. This means that carrier screening using PCR is quite efficient but that backup Southern blotting is necessary. Another rare but potential problem has been reported: the finding of mosaicism for a full-mutation and a normal-sized allele in affected males (Schmucker and Seidel 1999). Because the size of the premutation affects the risk of expansion, laboratory reports of carriers should include accurate sizing of alleles. In cases of affected individuals, the presence or absence of mosaicism should also be reported, since it may have prognostic significance.

## Indications for Fragile X Testing

It is clear that a clinical suspicion of FXS is an indication to pursue *FMR1* testing. A family history of unexplained developmental problems or mental retardation along with some of the characteristic physical and behavioral features is the most common reason for detecting the family with *FMR1* mutations. However, in our experience, only one individual is affected with FXS in up to one-third of recognized families. Further, as the phenotype can be very subtle and nonspecific, some individuals with FXS have physical features that do not suggest FXS even to the trained observer. Because molecular *FMR1* analysis is relatively fast and inexpensive, we recommend that all developmentally delayed children should be screened. If a positive diagnosis is made, such individuals will benefit from early intervention and their relatives would benefit from genetic counseling. Furthermore, in principle, all pregnant women could be screened for fragile X carrier status in programs similar to current maternal alpha-fetoprotein analysis. Since all affected full-mutation individuals have a mother who carries a premutation with more than 58 repeats, screening of all pregnant women could be done efficiently and not result in an excess of false positives. Preconceptual screening would be preferable to allow adequate time for genetic counseling of identified carriers.

A large-scale prospective screening program among 9,459 women of reproductive age with no known family history of fragile X, including 80% that were pregnant, has been reported from Israel (Pesso et al. 2000). Among this total, 134 (1/70) carriers were detected and 108 pregnancies were monitored by prenatal diagnosis. The success of this program indicated that screening for fragile X should be widely available. Routine monitoring of amniotic samples could also be carried out. Fragile X population screening programs in Australia have been successful in identifying cases and at-risk carriers, thereby leading to a significant reduction in the burden of familial mental retardation (Turner et al. 1997).

## Prenatal Diagnosis

Before the identification of the *FMR1* gene in 1991, prenatal diagnosis of the fragile X chromosome by cytogenetic means was difficult and not entirely reliable because of occasional false-negative results (Jenkins et al. 1995). Improved reliability was achieved by combined use of cytogenetics and DNA linkage analysis. However, family studies were also necessary, and because linkage analysis was an indirect test of the inheritance of the fragile X chromosome, there were still occasional discrepancies. The availability of direct gene assays for *FMR1* mutations greatly improved the ability to offer prenatal diagnosis.

Beginning in 1991, direct *FMR1* testing and prenatal diagnosis on amniotic fluid and chorionic villus samples was accomplished (Dobkin et al. 1991; Hirst et al. 1991; Sutherland et al. 1991). Preliminary PCR sizing of parent samples assists with interpretation of fetal specimen results. For a male fetus, if the mother's normal allele is identified by PCR of the fetal sample, then a normal outcome is predicted. For a female fetus, if both the maternal and paternal alleles are normal and distinct, as occurs approximately 80% of the time, then a normal outcome is predicted. On the other hand, if only the father's normal allele is seen, then the female fetus has presumably inherited the fragile X chromosome. Premutation alleles are generally seen as a distinct band, and full-mutation alleles are seen as an enlarged band or smear. Follow-up with confirmatory Southern blotting is needed to securely distinguish between homozygous allele sizes and females with full mutations that may have selective-normal size allele amplifications. The reliability of this approach is high (Brown et al. 1993, 1996). Maternal cell contamination is a potential complicating factor known to occur in 1% to perhaps 15% of samplings (Batanian et al. 1998) and must be guarded against. Mosaicism is also a potential problem. Chorionic villus sampling (CVS) does not show the methylation of full mutations in approximately half of the cases at the usual time of sampling at 10 weeks. However, since very few carrier alleles have sizes of greater than 140 repeats, the distinction between a typical premutation allele size of 70 to 100 repeats and an allele with a high risk of expansion to the full mutation is usually straightforward. As of 2000, our group had analyzed prenatal samplings from 230 known fragile X carriers by prenatal diagnosis with both PCR and direct testing. Among these, 98 full mutations and 16 premutations have been correctly identified.

## AGGs and the Basis of Repeat Instability

The specific molecular mechanisms that result in triplet repeat mutational expansions are still unclear, but occurrence of a form of DNA slippage error or alternative DNA helix formation during replication seems most likely (Bowater and Wells 2000; Jin and Warren 2000). Within the normal CGG repeat region, there usually are one or more interrupting AGGs. These seem to stabilize the sequence and prevent slippage during replication. The AGGs interspersed within the CGG repeat region and the length of pure repeat seem to be the major factors determining allele stability. The normal *FMR1* allele that was first sequenced showed 30 CGG repeats interrupted with two AGGs (Verkerk et al. 1991). Although the high CG content of the *FMR1* $(CGG)_n$ repeat has made it difficult to sequence through the region using conventional approaches, several alternative strategies have been attempted (Hirst et al. 1994; Kunst and Warren 1994; Snow et al. 1994). Methods have also been developed to analyze the repeat sequence variations by using a restriction enzyme (*Mnl* I) that cuts at the AGG site within a CGG background (Eichler et al. 1994; Zhong et al. 1995). These studies have shown that the highest variability of pure repeat lengths occurs at the 3' end. Analysis of sets of two related males with premutations showed that repeat instability has been observed to occur only within the 3' region (Eichler et al. 1994; Zhong et al. 1995). Thus, instability is polar and occurs within the 3' region. This supports the hypothesis that it is the loss of the AGG within the 3' end that acts to destabilize the CGG repeat region and leads to its expansion to the full mutation. A new mutation could be the result of the mutational change of an AGG to a CGG resulting in a long 3′ pure CGG repeat of more than 35.

Predicting whether alleles within the range of 35–60 (the so-called gray zone) are likely to be stable will depend on their AGG interspersion pattern. Most control size alleles have multiple AGGs, as illustrated in figure 2.6. Unstable or premutation alleles have a pure CGG region, which is usually more than 40 repeats. In our experience, the majority of premutation alleles (two-thirds) lack any AGG, while the rest have but one. The threshold for instability seems to be approximately 35 pure CGG repeats (Eichler et al. 1994). Since no fragile X–affected child has yet been identified who was born to a mother with fewer than 59 repeats, the threshold for expansion to the full mutation is probably around 59 pure repeats. A few alleles with repeats in the range of 35 to 52 may be unstable but are unlikely to present a significant risk of expansion to the full mutation within a single generation. An analysis of 16 intermediate-sized alleles with repeats of 45 to 55 showed that 50% had zero or one interspersed AGG, which suggests that half of alleles of this size are likely to be unstable (Zhong et al. 1996b). Thus far, no convenient method has been developed to separate the two female alleles for separate AGG analysis.

## New Mutations and Founder Effects in Fragile X

It is of both theoretical and practical interest to determine whether new fragile X mutations occur and how frequently. No one has yet identified what might be considered a new mutation, which might be reflected as a change in size from a definite normal allele size to a definite fragile X size. Because full-mutation fragile X males generally do not reproduce and pass on their fragile X gene to subsequent generations, their genes are lost from the human gene pool. Assuming that the frequency of the condition is neither increasing nor decreasing in the population leads to the conclusion that there must be a new mutation rate equal to the rate of loss of their genes. The Haldane equation states that for an X-linked condition in which affected males essentially do not reproduce, the new mutation rate should be equal to one-third the frequency of the gene in the population. Since no new fragile X mutations have been identified, this has been a puzzling situation. Rather than having a sharp mutational jump from normal size to full mutation, models of the mutational process suggest that there may be a gradual increase in CGG repeat size and that the rate of increase may be a function of the length of the repeat (Kolehmainen 1994). Once the threshold of around 50 repeats is exceeded (perhaps 35–40 pure repeats), there may be a much more rapid rate of increase. This may explain why identification of a new mutation is unlikely.

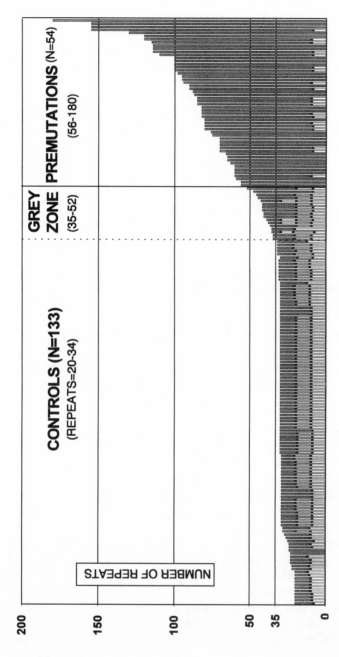

**Fig. 2.6.** AGG organization of *FMR1* alleles. The number of repeats is indicated on the *left*. The first *unshaded bar* from the bottom of each column is the position of the 5′ first CGG repeat segment, *black bars* are AGGs, and *shaded bars* are additional CGG repeat segments. Shown are the analyses of 117 controls with <35 repeats, 16 gray zone controls with 35–52 repeats, and 54 premutations. *Source:* Data from Zhong and Brown.

An alternative way of analyzing the new mutation frequency is to look for founder effects. Founder effects are present if there exists one or very few original mutations for a disease within a population. Founder effects are demonstrated by analysis of the set of background polymorphisms found in the genomic region where the mutation is located. A class of polymorphisms known as microsatellites or short tandem repeats is conveniently used for founder effect analyses, and microsatellites typically consist of repeats of $(CA)_n$ with $n$ values often in the range of 10 to 30 (Weber 1990). Two microsatellite markers—*FRAXAC1* (Richards et al. 1992) and *DXS548* (Riggins et al. 1992) located proximal at about 7 kb and 150 kb, respectively, to the *FMR1* $(CGG)_n$ repeat region—and one microsatellite—*FRAXAC2* (Zhong et al. 1993) located approximately 12 kb distal—have been widely used for studies of founder effects in fragile X. A single dinucleotide A/G polymorphism located 5.6 kb distal has also been identified (Gunter et al. 1998). These studies have shown that fragile X mutations tend to be associated (i.e., in linkage disequilibrium) with a different set of markers than are controls. This probably reflects the mutational history of the expansion, rather than a mutational mechanism or pathway, although cis- or trans-acting factors have not been entirely excluded (Crawford et al. 2000).

Because the present-day population of Finland is believed to have originated from a small tribe of settlers some 2000 years ago, founder effects for several Finnish genetic diseases have been identified. Studies flanking microsatellite alleles in Finland showed a striking founder effect: 90–95% fragile X chromosomes had a DXS548 allele found in less than 20% of controls (Oudet et al. 1993b; Haataja et al. 1994; Zhong et al. 1996a). Including *FRAXAC1* and the more distantly located triplet repeat *FRAXE*, we have found that the predominant haplotype in Finland accounts for more than 80% of mutations, while two less common types account for the remaining. This suggests that one ancient and two more recent fragile X founder mutations may have occurred in this population (Zhong et al. 1996a). These studies tend to suggest that, over relatively short times of fewer than 100 generations, definite founder effects are likely to be present but that some low frequency of new mutations may be occurring.

## Nearby Genes and FRAXE

The nearest known neighboring genes to fragile X are surprisingly far away. The proximal region to *FMR1* is very sparsely populated with genes. This is based on available results of the completion of the Human Genome Sequencing Project. Approximately 3 million bps upstream is the nearest presumptive gene (an open reading frame), labeled *CXORF1*. Approximately 6.5 million bps upstream is the closest of a set of melanoma antigen family C genes, or

*MAGEC2* (Lucas et al. 1998). It is estimated that on average there are some 20 or 30 genes per million bps in the human genome. Thus, with only two genes within 6.5 million bps, the region proximal to *FMR1* is extremely gene-poor relative to the rest of the genome. Distally, the closest gene that has been identified and characterized, other than *FRAXE* as discussed below, is approximately 1 million base pairs away. It is the iduronate 2-sulfatase (IDS) gene, which is mutated in an X-linked lysosomal storage disease causing Hunter syndrome (Wilson et al. 1990). Thus, the immediate distal region is also very gene-poor. Further on down from *IDS* are many genes with a high density.

At about 600 kb distal to *FMR1* and proximal to *IDS* is another fragile site, *FRAXE*. This folate-sensitive fragile site has been found in several families whose members selectively showed some degree of developmental delay but who turned out negative on molecular testing for *FMR1*. The fragile site was cloned (Knight et al. 1993) and found to have a trinucleotide repeat sequence of $(GCC)_n$. Controls had from 6 to about 25 copies, while individuals with the mutation had more than 200 copies. They also had a methylated CpG island similar to *FMR1*. The gene was cloned and identified as *FMR2* (Gecz et al. 1997). It is a large gene composed of 22 exons spanning over 500 kb. The gene product translates into a 1,311-amino acid nuclear protein with properties of a transcriptional factor.

Because only a handful of families with *FRAXE/FMR2* mutations have yet been identified and their phenotype is as yet not well defined, it is unclear whether this represents a rare but true syndrome of mental delay. The phenotype of the individuals with this fragile site is without distinguishing physical features, and the cognitive deficit is highly variable, with some showing no apparent affects and others more severely disabled. Most IQ tests of identified males have been reported to be low normal to mildly retarded, with an average of approximately 70 (Mulley et al. 1995). Surveys of some 2,184 males with mental delays found 3 with *FRAXE* mutations (Brown 1996). A recent survey of 3,738 boys with developmental disabilities revealed 20 with fragile X syndrome and one with a *FRAXE* mutation (Youings et al. 2000). We estimate that the ratio of *FMR2* mutations to *FMR1* mutations is likely to be on the order of 1:25 (Brown 1996).

## Lessons from Other Triplet Repeat Diseases

Fragile X was the first to be identified of a new class of human genetic mutations that involve amplification of triplet repeats and show *anticipation*. This is defined as increasing severity or frequency of the disorder over succeeding generations. Instability is observed in all, in both germline and somatic tissues. Further, the sex of the parent from whom the mutation is inherited usually has a major influence on the degree of expansion. At least 14 diseases involving trinucleotide repeat sequences, including fragile X and *FRAXE* syndrome, have now been identified (Cummings and Zoghbi 2000). A primary distinction is whether the repeat is in a noncoding region, as in fragile X and *FRAXE,* myotonic dystrophy, Friedreich ataxia, and spinocerebellar ataxia types 8 and 12 (*SCA8* and *SCA12*), or in a part of the gene that is coding. Coded sequences usually involve polyglutamine tracts and produce dominant negative gain-of-function effects, as in Huntington disease, X-linked spinal and bulbar muscular atrophy (Kennedy disease), dentatorubral-pallidoluysian atrophy, and the spinocerebellar ataxias types 1, 2, 3, 6, and 7. Two other fragile sites, *FRAXF* and *FRA16A,* also include trinucleotide repeats but have not yet been associated with genetic diseases (Parrish et al. 1994; Nancarrow et al. 1994). Any disease in which anticipation may be present is now a candidate for having an underlying triplet repeat mutation. In this regard both anticipation and a larger triplet repeat size distribution have been reported for bipolar affective disorder and schizophrenia (O'Donovan et al. 1995).

The threshold for instability of around 40 pure repeats in fragile X is similar to other triplet repeat disorders as well. In spinocerebellar ataxia 1 (SCA1), 100% of normal alleles with 22 to 40 repeats have imperfect interruptions, whereas mutant alleles, which are always larger than 40 repeats, have no interruptions (Chung et al. 1993). The underlying basis for the threshold of approximately 40 repeats may be the upper size limit of Okazaki fragments (Brown et al. 1993; Eichler et al. 1994; Kunst and Warren 1994). These have an average size of 105 bps, corresponding to 35 repeats (Burhans et al. 1990). When a pure repeat exceeds the normal Okazaki fragment length by some threshold amount, then the probability of slippage may greatly increase.

## References

Ashley, C. T., J. S. Sutcliffe, C. B. Kunst, H. A. Leiner, E. E. Eichler, D. L. Nelson, and S. T. Warren. 1993a. Human and murine *FMR-1:* Alternative splicing and translational initiation downstream of the CGG-repeat. *Nat. Genet.* 4:244–251.

Ashley, C. T., K. D. Wilkinson, D. Reines, and S. T. Warren. 1993b. *FMR1* protein: Conserved RPN family domains and selective RNA binding. *Science* 262:563–566.

Batanian, J. R., D. H. Ledbetter, and R. G. Fenwick. 1998. A simple VNTR-PCR method for detecting maternal cell contamination in prenatal diagnosis. *Genet. Test* 2:347–350.

Bell, M. V., M. C. Hirst, Y. Nakahori, R. N. MacKinnon, A. Roche, T. J. Flint, P. A. Jacobs, N. Tommerup, L. Tranebjaerg, U. Froster-Iskenius, B. Kerr, G. Turner, R. H. Lindenbaum, R. Winter, M. Pembrey, S. Thibodeau, and K. E. Davies. 1991. Physical mapping across the fragile X: Hypermethylation and clinical expression of the fragile X syndrome. *Cell* 64:861–866.

Bowater, R. P., and R. D. Wells. 2000. The intrinsically unstable life of DNA triplet repeats associated with human hereditary disorders. *Prog. Nucleic Acid Res. Mol. Biol.* 66:159–202.

Brown, W. T. 1994. Molecular analysis of fragile X syndrome. In: *Current Protocols in Human Genetics.* New York: John Wiley & Sons, pp. 9.5.1–9.5.14.

———. 1996. The *FRAXE* syndrome: Is it time for routine screening? *Am. J. Hum. Genet.* 58:903–905.

Brown, W. T., G. Houck Jr., A. Jeziorowska, F. Levinson, X-H. Ding, C. Dobkin, N. Zhong, J. Henderson, S. Sklower-Brooks, and E. C. Jenkins. 1993. Rapid fragile X carrier screening and prenatal diagnosis by a non-radioactive PCR test. *JAMA* 270:1569–1575.

Brown, W. T., S. Nolin, G. Houck Jr., X-H. Ding, A. Glicksman, S-Y. Li, S. Stark-Houck, P. Brophy, C. Duncan, C. Dobkin, and E. Jenkins. 1996. Prenatal diagnosis and carrier screening by PCR. *Am. J. Med. Genet.* 64:191–195.

Burhans, W. C., L. T. Vassilev, M. S. Caddle, N. H. Heintz, and M. L. DePamplilis. 1990. Identification of an origin of bidirectional DNA replication in mammalian chromosomes. *Cell* 62:955–965.

Buyle, S., E. Reyniers, L. Vits, K. De Boulle, I. Handig, F. L. E. Wuyts, W. Deelen, D. J. J. Halley, B. A. Oostra, and P. J. Willems. 1993. Founder effect in a Belgian-Dutch fragile X population. *Hum. Genet.* 92:269–272.

Chong, S. S., E. E. Eichler, D. L. Nelson, and M. R. Hughes. 1994. Robust amplification and ethidium-visible detection of the fragile X syndrome CGG repeat using *Pfu* polymerase. *Am. J. Med. Genet.* 51:522–526.

Chung, M. Y., L. P. W. Ranum, L. A. Duvick, A. Servadio, H. Y. Zoghbi, and H. T. Orr. 1993. Evidence for a mechanism predisposing to intergenerational CAG repeat instability in spinocerebellar ataxia type I. *Nat. Genet.* 5:254–258.

Cohen, I. L., S. L. Nolin, V. Sudhalter, X. Ding, C. S. Dobkin, and W. T. Brown. 1996. Mosaicism for the *FMR1* gene influences adaptive skills development in fragile X affected males. *Am. J. Med. Genet.* 64:365–369.

Crawford, D. C., C. E. Schwartz, K. L. Meadows, J. L. Newman, L. F. Taft, C. Gunter, W. T. Brown, N. J. Carpenter, P. N. Howard-Peebles, K. G. Monaghan, S. L. Nolin, A. L. Reiss, G. L. Feldman, E. M. Rohlfs, S. T. Warren, and S. L. Sherman. 2000. Survey of the fragile X syndrome CGG repeat and the short-tandem-repeat and single-nucleotide-polymorphism haplotypes in an African American population. *Am. J. Hum. Genet.* 66:480–493.

Cummings, C. J., and H. Y. Zoghbi. 2000. Fourteen and counting: Unraveling trinucleotide repeat diseases. *Hum. Mol. Genet.* 9:909–916.

De Boulle, K. A., J. M. H. Verkerk, E. Reyniers, L. Vits, J. Hendrickx, B. Van Roy, F. Van Den, F. Bos, E. de Graaffe, B. A. Oostra, and P. J. Willems. 1993. A point mutation in the *FMR-1* gene associated with the fragile X mental retardation. *Nat. Genet.* 3:31–35.

Dobkin, C. S., X-H. Ding, E. C. Jenkins, M. S. Krawczun, W. T. Brown, P. Goonewardena, J. Willner, C. Benson, D. Heitz, and F. Rousseau. 1991. Prenatal diagnosis of fragile X syndrome. *Lancet* 338:957–958.

Eberhart, D. E., H. E. Malter, Y. Feng, and S. T. Warren. 1996. The fragile X mental retardation protein is a ribonucleoprotein containing both nuclear localization and nuclear export signals. *Hum. Mol. Genet.* 5:1083–1091.

Eichler, E. E., J. J. A. Holden, B. W. Popovich, A. L. Reiss, K. Snow, S. N. Thibodeau, S. Richards, P. A. Ward, and D. L. Nelson. 1994. Length of uninterrupted CGG repeats determines instability in the *FMR1* gene. *Nat. Genet.* 8:88–94.

Erlich, H. A., and N. Arnheim. 1992. Genetic analysis using the epolymerase chain reaction. *Annu. Rev. Genet.* 26:479–506.

Erster, S. H., W. T. Brown, P. Goonewardena, C. S. Dobkin, E. C. Jenkins, and R. G. Pergolizzi. 1992. Polymerase chain reaction analysis of fragile X-mutations. *Hum. Genet.* 90:55–61.

Fu, Y. H., D. P. A. Kuhl, A. Pizzuti, M. Pieretti, J. S. Sutcliffe, S. Richards, A. Verkerk, J. J. A. Holden, R. G. Fenwick Jr., S. T. Warren, B. A. Oostra, D. L. Nelson, and C. T. Caskey. 1991. Variation of the CGG repeat at the fragile X site results in genetic instability: Resolution of the Sherman paradox. *Cell* 67:1047–1058.

Gecz, J., S. Bielby, G. R. Sutherland, and J. C. Mulley. 1997. Gene structure and subcellular localization of *FMR2,* a member of a new family of putative transcription activators. *Genomics* 44:201–213.

Gedeon, Á. K., M. Meinänen, L. C. Adès, H. Kääriäinen, J. Gécz, E. Baker, S. G. R. Sutherland, and J. C. Mulley. 1995. Overlapping submicroscopic deletions in Xq28 in two unrelated boys with developmental disorders: Identification of a gene near FRAXE. *Am. J. Hum. Genet.* 56:907–914.

Gunter, C., W. Paradee, D. C. Crawford, K. A. Meadows, J. Newman, C. B. Kunst, D. L. Nelson, C. Schwartz, A. Murray, J. N. Macpherson, S. L. Sherman, and S. T. Warren. 1998. Re-examination of factors associated with expansion of CGG repeats using a single nucleotide polymorphism in *FMR1. Hum. Mol. Genet.* 7:1935–1946.

Haataja, R., M-J. Väisänen, M. Li, and L. J. Ryynänen. 1994. The fragile X syndrome in Finland: Demonstration of a founder effect by analysis of microsatellite haplotypes. *Hum. Genet.* 94:479–483.

Hammond, L. S., M. M. Macias, J. C. Tarleton, A. Shashidhar, and G. Pai. 1997. Fragile X syndrome and deletions in *FMR1:* New case and review of the literature. *Am. J. Med. Genet.* 72:430–434.

Heitz, D., F. Rousseau, D. Devys, S. Saccone, H. Abderrahim, D. LePaslier, D. Cohen, A. Vincent, D. Oniolo, G. Della Valle, S. Johnson, D. Schlessinger, I. Oberle, and J. L. Mandel. 1991. Isolation of sequences that span the fragile X and identification of a fragile X–related CpG island. *Science* 251:1236–1239.

Hirst, M., S. Knight, K. Davies, G. Cross, K. Ocraft, S. Raeburn, S. Heeger, D. Eunpu, E. C. Jenkins, and R. Lindenbaum. 1991. Prenatal diagnosis of the fragile X syndrome. *Lancet* 338:956–957.

Hirst, M. C., P. K. Grewal, and K. E. Davies. 1994. Precursor arrays for triplet repeat expansion at the fragile X locus. *Hum. Mol. Genet.* 3:1553–1560.

Jenkins, E. C., G. E. Houck Jr., X-H. Ding, S-Y. Li, S. L. Stark-Houck, J. Salerno, M. Genovese, A. Glicksman, S. L. Nolin, N. Zhong, S. L. Sklower Brooks, C. S. Dobkin, and W. T. Brown. 1995. An update on fragile X prenatal diagnosis: End of the cytogenetics testing era. *Dev. Brain Dysfunct.* 8:293–301.

Jin, P., and S. T. Warren. 2000. Understanding the molecular basis of fragile X syndrome. *Hum. Mol. Genet.* 9:901–908.

Knight, S. J. L., A. V. Flannery, M. C. Hirst, L. Campbell, Z. Christodoulou, S. R. Phelps, J. Pointon, H. R. Middleton-Price, A. Barnicoat, M. E. Pembrey, J. Holland, B. A. Oostra, M. Bobrow, and K. E. Davis. 1993. Trinucleotide repeat amplification and hypermethylation of a CpG island in *FRAXE* mental retardation. *Cell* 74:127–134.

Kolehmainen, K. 1994. Population genetics of fragile X: A multiple allele model with variable risk of CGG repeat expansion. *Am. J. Med. Genet.* 51:428–435.

Kremer, E. J., M. Pritchard, M. Lynch, S. Yu, K. Holman, E. Baker, S. T. Warren, D. Schlessinger, G. R. Sutherland, and R. I. Richard. 1991. Mapping of DNA instability at the fragile X to a trinucleotide repeat sequence p(CCG)*n*. *Science* 252:1711–1714.

Kunst, C. B., and S. T. Warren. 1994. Cryptic and polar variation of the fragile X repeat could result in predisposing normal alleles. *Cell* 77:853–861.

Lucas, S., C. De Smet, K. C. Arden, C. S. Viars, B. Lethe, C. Lurquin, and T. Boon. 1998. Identification of a new MAGE gene with tumor-specific expression by representational difference analysis. *Cancer Res.* 58:743–752.

Lugenbeel, K. A., A. M. Peier, N. L. Carson, A. E. Chudley, and D. L. Nelson. 1995. Intragenic loss of function mutations demonstrate the primary role of *FMR1* in fragile X syndrome. *Nat. Genet.* 10:483–485.

McConkie-Rosell, A., A. M. Lachiewicz, G. A. Spiridigliozzi, J. Tarleton, S. Schoenwald, M. C. Phelan, P. Goonewardena, X-H. Ding, and W. T. Brown. 1993. Evidence that methylation of the *FMR-1* locus is responsible for variable phenotypic expression of the fragile X syndrome. *Am. J. Hum. Genet.* 53:800–809.

Mulley, J. C., S. Yu, D. Z. Loesch, D. A. Hay, A. Donnelly, A. K. Gedeon, P. Carbonell, et al. 1995. *FRAXE* and mental retardation. *J. Med. Genet.* 32:162–169.

Nancarrow, J. K., E. Kreme, K. Holman, et al. 1994. Implications of *FRA16A* structure for the mechanism of chromosomal fragile site genesis. *Science* 264:1938–1940.

Nolin, S. L., A. Glicksman, G. E. Houck Jr., W. T. Brown, and C. S. Dobkin. 1994. Mosaicism in fragile X affected males. *Am. J. Med. Genet.* 51:509–512.

Nolin, S. L., A. Lewis French III, L. L. Ye, G. E. Houck Jr., A. E. Glicksman, P. Limprasert, S-Y. Li, N. Zhong, A. E. Ashley, E. Feingold, S. L. Sherman, and W. T. Brown. 1996. Familial transmission of the *FMR1* CGG repeat. *Am. J. Hum. Genet.* 59:1252–1261.

Nolin, S. L., G. E. Houck Jr., A. D. Gargano, H. Blumstein, C. S. Dobkin, and W. T. Brown. 1999. *FMR1* CGG-repeat instability in single sperm and lymphocytes of fragile-X premutation males. *Am. J. Hum. Genet.* 65:680–688.

Oberlé, I., F. Rousseau, D. Heitz, C. Kretz, D. Devys, A. Hanauer, J. Boué, M. F. Bertheas, and J. L. Mandel. 1991. Instability of a 550-base pair DNA segment and abnormal methylation in fragile X syndrome. *Science* 52:1097–1102.

O'Donovan, M. C., C. Guy, N. Craddock, K. C. Murphy, A. G. Cardno, L. A. Jones, M. J. Owen, and P. McGuffin. 1995. Expanded CAG repeats in schizophrenia and bipolar disorder. *Nat. Genet.* 10:380–381.

Oostra, B. A., P. B. Jacky, W. T. Brown, and F. Rousseau. 1993. Guidelines for the diagnosis of fragile X syndrome. *J. Med. Genet.* 30:410–413.

Opitz, J. 1986. On the gates of hell and a most unusual gene. *Am. J. Med. Genet.* 23:1–10.

Oudet, C., E. Mornet, J. L. Serrel, F. Thomas, S. Lentes-Zengerling, C. Kretz, C. Deluchat, I. Tejada, J. Boué, et al. 1993a. Linkage disequilibrium between the fragile X mutation and two closely linked CA repeats suggests that fragile X chromosomes are derived from a small number of founder chromosomes. *Am. J. Hum. Genet.* 52:297–304.

Oudet, C., H. von Koskull, A. M. Nordstrom, M. Peippo, and J-L. Mandel. 1993b. Striking founder effect for the fragile X syndrome in Finland. *Eur. J. Hum. Genet.* 1:181–189.

Parrish, J. E., B. A. Oostra, A. J. M. H. Verkerk, C. S. Richards, J. Reynolds, A. S. Skipes, L. G. Shaffer, and D. L. Nelson. 1994. Isolation of a GCC repeat showing expansion in *FRAXF,* a fragile site distal to FRAXA and *FRAXE. Nat. Genet.* 8:229–235.

Pergolizzi, R. G., S. H. Erster, P. Goonewardena, and W. T. Brown. 1992. Detection of full fragile X mutation. *Lancet* 339:271–272.

Pesso, R., M. Berkenstadt, H. Cuckle, E. Gak, L. Peleg, M. Frydman, and G. Barkai. 2000. Screening for fragile X syndrome in women of reproductive age. *Prenat. Diagn.* 20:611–614.

Pieretti, M., F. Zhang, Y. H. Fu, S. T. Warren, B. A. Oostra, C. T. Caskey, and D. L. Nelson. 1991. Absence of expression of the *FMR-1* gene in fragile X syndrome. *Cell* 66:1–20.

Quan, F., J. Zonana, K. Gunter, K. L. Peterson, R. E. Magenis, and B. W. Popovich. 1995. An atypical case of fragile X syndrome caused by a deletion that includes the *FMR1* gene. *Am. J. Hum. Genet.* 56:1042–1051.

Reyniers, E., L. Lits, K. De Boulle, B. Van Roy, D. Van Velzen, E. de Graaff, A. J. M. H. Verker, H. Z. J. Jorens, J. K. Darby, B. A. Oostra, and P. J. Willems. 1993. The full mutation in the *FMR-1* gene of male fragile X patients is absent in their sperm. *Nat. Genet.* 4:143–146.

Richards, R. I., K. Holman, K. Friend, E. Kremer, D. Hillen, A. Staples, W. T. Brown, P. Goonewardena, J. Tarleton, C. Schwartz, and G. R. Sutherland. 1992. Evidence of founder chromosomes in fragile X syndrome. *Nat. Genet.* 1:257–260.

Riggins, G. J., S. L. Sherman, B. A. Oostra, J. S. Sutcliffe, D. Feitell, D. L. Nelson, B. A. van Oost, et al. 1992. Characterization of a highly polymorphic dinucleotide repeat 150 kb proximal to the fragile X site. *Am. J. Med. Genet.* 43:237–243.

Rousseau, F., D. Heitz, V. Biancalana, S. Blumenfeld, C. Kretz, J. Boué, T. N. Tommerup, C. Van Der Hagen, C. DeLozier-Blanchet, M-F. Croquette, S. Gilgenkrantz, P. Jalbert, M-A. Voelckel, I. Oberlé, and J-L. Mandel. 1991. Direct diagnosis by DNA analysis of the fragile X syndrome of mental retardation. *N. Engl. J. Med.* 325:1673–1681.

Schmucker, B., and J. Seidel. 1999. Mosaicism for a full mutation and a normal size allele in two fragile X males. *Am. J. Med. Genet.* 84:221–225.

Smith, H., and K. W. Wilcox. 1970. A restriction enzyme from *Haemophilus influenzae:* I. Purification and general properties. *J. Mol. Biol.* 51:379–391.

Smits, A. P. T., J. C. F. M. Dreesen, J. G. Post, D. F. C. M. Smeets, C. de Die-Smulders, T. Spaans-van der Bijl, L. C. P. Govaerts, S. T. Warren, B. A. Oostra, and B. A. Bam van Oost. 1993. The fragile X syndrome: No evidence for any recent mutations. *J. Med. Genet.* 30:94–96.

Snow, K., L. K. Doud, R. Hagerman, R. G. Pergolizzi, S. H. Erster, and S. N. Thibodeau. 1993. Analysis of a CGG sequence at the *FMR-1* locus in fragile X families and in the general population. *Am. J. Hum. Genet.* 53:1217–1228.

Snow, K., D. J. Tester, K. E. Kruckeberg, D. J. Schaid, and S. N. Thibodeau. 1994. Sequence analysis of the fragile X trinucleotide repeat: Implications for the origin of the fragile X mutation. *Hum. Mol. Genet.* 3:1543–1551.

Southern, E. M. 1975. Detection of specific sequences among DNA fragments separated by gel electrophoresis. *J. Mol. Biol.* 98:503–517.

Sutherland, G. R., A. Gedeon, L. Kornman, A. Donnelly, R. W. Byard, J. C. Mulley, M. Lynch, M. Pritchard, Y. Sui, and R. I. Richards. 1991. Prenatal diagnosis of fragile X syndrome by direct detection of the unstable DNA sequence. *N. Engl. J. Med.* 325:1720–1722.

Tassone, F., R. J. Hagerman, D. N. Ikle, P. N. Dyer, M. Lampe, R. Willemsen, B. A. Oostra, and A. K. Taylor. 1999. FMRP expression as a potential prognostic indicator in fragile X syndrome. *Am. J. Med. Genet.* 84:250–261.

Tuckerman, E., T. Webb, S. E. Bundy. 1985. Frequency and replication status of the fragile X, fra(X)(q27–28), in a pair of monozygotic twins of markedly differing intelligence. *J. Med. Genet.* 22:85–91.

Turner, G., H. Robinson, S. Wake, S. Laing, and M. C. Partington. 1997. Case finding for the fragile X syndrome and its consequences. *Br. Med. J.* 315:1223–1226.

van den Ouweland, A. M. W., W. H. Deelen, C. B. Kunst, M. L. G. Uziell, D. L. Nelson, S. T. Warren, B. A. Oostra, and D. J. J. Halley. 1994. Loss of mutation at the *FMR1* locus through multiple exchanges between maternal X chromosomes. *Hum. Mol. Genet.* 3:1823–1827.

Verkerk, A. J. M. H., M. Pleretti, J. S. Sutcliffe, Y-H. Fu, D. P. A. Kuhl, A. Pizzuti, O. Reiner, S. Richards, M. F. Victoria, F. Zhang, B. E. Eussen, G-J. B. van Ommen, L. A. J. Blonden, G. J. Riggins, J. L. Chastain, C. B. Kunst, H. Galjaard, C. T. Caskey, D. L. Nelson, B. A. Oostra, and S. T. Warren. 1991. Identification of a gene (*FMR-1*) containing a CGG repeat coincident with a breakpoint cluster region exhibiting length variation in fragile X syndrome. *Cell* 65:905–914.

Vincent, A., D. Heitz, C. Petit, C. Kretz, I. Oberle, and J. L. Mandel. 1991. Abnormal pattern detected in fragile X patients by pulsed-field gel electrophoresis. *Nature* 349:624–626.

Wang, Q., E. Green, M. Bobrow, and C. G. Mathew. 1995. A rapid, non-radioactive screening test for fragile X mutations at the FRAXA and *FRAXE* loci. *J. Med. Genet.* 32:170–173.

Wang, Y. C., M. L. Lin, S. J. Lin, Y. C. Li, and S. Y. Li. 1997. Novel point mutation within intron 10 of *FMR-1* gene causing fragile X syndrome. *Hum. Mutat.* 10:393–399.

Warren, S. T., and D. L. Nelson. 1994. Advances in molecular analysis of fragile X syndrome. *JAMA* 271:536–542.

Weber, J. L. 1990. Informativeness of human $(dC-dA)_n \cdot (dG-dT)_n$ polymorphisms. *Genomics* 7:524–530.

Wilson, P. J., C. P. Morris, D. S. Hanson, T. Occhiodoro, J. Bielicki, P. R. Clements, and J. J. Hopwood. 1990. Hunter syndrome: Isolation of an iduronate-2-sulfate cDNA clone and analysis of patient DNA. *Proc. Natl. Acad. Sci. USA* 87:8531–8535.

Youings, S. A., A. Murray, N. Dennis, S. Ennis, C. Lewis, N. McKechnie, M. Pound, A. Sharrock, and P. Jacobs. 2000. FRAXA and *FRAXE*: The results of a five year survey. *J. Med. Genet.* 37:415–421.

Yu, S., M. Pritchard, E. Kremer, M. Lynch, J. Nancarrow, E. Baker, K. Holman, J. C. Mulley, S. T. Warren, D. Schlessinger, G. R. Sutherland, and R. I. Richards. 1991. Fragile X genotype characterized by an unstable region of DNA. *Science* 252:1179–1181.

Yu, S., J. Mulley, D. Loesch, G. Turner, A. Donnelly, A. Gedeon, D. Hillen, E. Kremer, M. Lynch, M. Pritchard, G. R. Sutherland, and R. I. Richards. 1992. Fragile-X syndrome: Unique genetics of the heritable unstable element. *Am. J. Hum. Genet.* 50: 968–980.

Zhong, N., C. Dobkin, and W. T. Brown. 1993. A complex mutable polymorphism located within the fragile X gene. *Nat. Genet.* 5:248–253.

Zhong, N., W. Yang, C. Dobkin, and W. T. Brown. 1995. Fragile X gene instability: Anchoring AGGs and linked microsatellites. *Am. J. Hum. Genet.* 57:351–361.

Zhong, N., E. Kajanoja, B. Smits, J. Pietrofesa, D. Curley, D. Wang, W. Ju, S. L. Nolin, C. Dobkin, M. Ryynanen, and W. T. Brown. 1996a. Fragile X founder effects and new mutations in Finland. *Am. J. Med. Genet.* 64:226–233.

Zhong, N., W. Ju, J. Pietrofesa, D. Wang, C. Dobkin, W. T. Brown. 1996b. Fragile X "gray zone" alleles: AGG patterns, expansion risks and associated haplotypes. *Am. J. Med. Genet.* 64:261–265.

# CHAPTER 3

# Epidemiology

## Stephanie Sherman, Ph.D.

### Recognition of the Fragile X or Martin-Bell Syndrome

An excess of males among the mentally retarded has been recognized since the late 1800s. In 1897, Johnson (1897) mentioned a 24% excess of retarded males relative to females according to U.S. census figures but gave no explanation for this excess. In 1938, Penrose also noted the high male:female ratio in the Colchester survey of institutionalized individuals and suggested that the male majority resulted from biases in ascertainment. Males were more often identified as mentally retarded because of the higher expectation for males than for females, and males exhibited aggressive behavior more often than females and therefore were more likely to be institutionalized. No genetic explanation for the excess of males was considered for many years. Lehrke, in his Ph.D. thesis written in 1969, was the first to argue persuasively that the preponderance of mentally retarded males was due to X-linked genes and that X-linked mental retardation (XLMR) may be responsible for a substantially large proportion of mental retardation (MR). He suggested that the contribution of XLMR had gone largely unnoticed because obvious clinical symptoms were absent (Lehrke 1974).

In 1971, Turner et al. suggested that XLMR in individuals with no other clinical signs should be considered as a distinct diagnostic category. They suggested that one of the earliest XLMR pedigrees published by Martin and Bell (1943) as well as others (Losowsky 1961; Renpenning et al. 1962; Dunn et al. 1963; Snyder and Robinson 1969) fit into this category. Thus, by the mid-1970s the importance of nonspecific XLMR had been recognized, but it was appreciated that this group was etiologically heterogeneous.

In 1969, Lubs reported a unique cytogenetic marker on the X chromosome,

*Fragile X Syndrome: Diagnosis, Treatment, and Research,* third edition, ed. Randi Jenssen Hagerman and Paul J. Hagerman (Baltimore: Johns Hopkins University Press, 2002), © The Johns Hopkins University Press.

which was seen in four retarded males in a family with XLMR. However, this was thought to be an isolated finding and was not considered relevant to the diagnosis of XLMR. It was not until 1973 that a second XLMR family with a cytogenetic marker was reported, but the report was written in Portuguese and published in Brazil (Escalante and Frota-Pessoa 1973) and, unfortunately, largely went unnoticed. However, by the late 1970s it was realized that nonspecific XLMR associated with a cytogenetic marker located on the end of the long arm of the X chromosome was not uncommon (Giraud et al. 1976; Harvey et al. 1977) and, moreover, that the cytogenetic marker may be a useful diagnostic tool. Confirmation of the original observation was delayed primarily because expression of the marker depends on culturing cells under particular conditions. In 1977, Sutherland showed that the cell culture medium must be deficient in folic acid or thymidine to stimulate expression. This marker is known as the fragile X site because of its appearance as a gap or break in the chromosome arm.

Macroorchidism was shown to be associated with some forms of XLMR in 1971 by Escalante et al. and subsequently by others (Turner et al. 1975; Cantú et al. 1976). Endocrine and germinal functions of the large testes were shown to be normal (Ruvalcaba et al. 1977). In 1978, Turner et al. showed that macroorchidism was also associated with some XLMR families segregating for the cytogenetic marker.

Finally, the pedigree originally published by Martin and Bell (1943) was reevaluated by Richards and Webb (1982) and found to show both macroorchidism and the cytogenetic marker on the X chromosome. In recognition of the first published pedigree, XLMR associated with the X chromosome cytogenetic marker originally was named the Martin-Bell syndrome. Now it is usually called the fragile X syndrome (FXS), referring to the association of the unique cytogenetic marker, the fragile X site. It has become routine to use the term *Martin-Bell phenotype* to refer to the classical facial characteristics associated with FXS.

## The Fragile X Mental Retardation Gene

In 1991, the mutation leading to FXS was identified and the gene isolated. In over 95% of cases, FXS is caused by a single type of mutation, an unstable CGG trinucleotide repeat sequence mutation found in the 5′ untranslated region of the X-linked, fragile X mental retardation gene (*FMR1*) (Fu et al. 1991; Verkerk et al. 1991). There are essentially four allelic forms of the *FMR1* gene with respect to the repeat length found in the population, and they are referred to as *normal, intermediate* or *gray zone, premutation,* and *full mutation.* The normal form contains, on average, 29–31 CGG repeats and is usually interspersed with

1 to 3 single AGG sequences found approximately every 9 to 10 CGG repeats (Yu et al. 1991; Fu et al. 1991; Eichler et al. 1994; Kunst and Warren 1994; Snow et al. 1993, 1994; Hirst et al. 1994; Zhong et al. 1995; chap. 2). The region is highly polymorphic with respect to the number of repeats (ranging from 6 to 50 repeats) and the number and position of the interspersed AGG sequences.

Normally, the repeat region is stable when transmitted from parent to child. Loss of the AGG interspersed sequences and/or an increase in the number of perfect 3' CGG repeats is suggested to cause the repeat region to become unstable and to expand in size when transmitted from parent to child (Kunst and Warren 1994; Eichler et al. 1994; Hirst et al. 1994; Snow et al. 1994; Zhong et al. 1995). This unstable form of the gene is called a *premutation* and usually consists of 55 to 200 repeats. Female premutation carriers are at high risk for having offspring with the fragile X syndrome, as premutation alleles of greater than 60 repeats frequently expand in size during transmission (see chaps. 2 and 7).

Premutation carriers, male and female, do not usually exhibit overt cognitive deficits or behavioral problems. However, mounting evidence suggests that premutation carriers may be at risk for specific disorders not present among full-mutation carriers (see chap. 1 and below).

There is obvious overlap between the so-called normal and premutation allele size ranges. Alleles in this overlap, between 40 and 60 repeats, are called *intermediate* or *gray zone alleles.* Some proportion of these alleles is unstable and will expand a few repeats during transmission. The instability seems to be related to the length of the pure 3' repeat sequence; unstable alleles have at least 34–50 pure 3' CGG repeats (Eichler et al. 1994; Murray et al. 1997; Nolin et al. 1996). In most populations, the frequency of intermediate alleles is about 2–4% (Crawford et al. 1999; Murray et al. 1996; Patsalis et al. 1999). The frequency of unstable intermediate alleles is thought to be about 1% of the general population, although extensive studies have not been done to confirm this figure.

The full mutation form of the *FMR1* gene consists of over 200 repeats and is abnormally hypermethylated. Consequently, little or no messenger RNA (mRNA) is produced (Pieretti et al. 1991; Sutcliffe et al. 1992; McConkie-Rosell et al. 1993; chap. 12), and the lack of the gene product FMRP, an RNA-binding protein, is responsible for the mental retardation (Ashley et al. 1993). Because of X-linkage, males have more severe expression of the phenotype associated with the syndrome than do females. Thus, almost all males carrying the full mutation exhibit some type of significant cognitive deficit, whereas only 50–60% of the full-mutation females show cognitive impairment, usually ranging from learning disabilities to mild mental retardation (Wolff et al. 1988;

Rousseau et al. 1994; chap. 6). In addition, almost all males exhibit a characteristic phenotype including a long, narrow face, large ears, and macroorchidism (see chap. 1).

Full mutations show instability in both the germ line and somatic cell lines. The evidence for somatic instability is based on Southern blotting analyses of DNA extracted from peripheral blood. The full mutation can appear as a single band, discrete multiple bands, or, most often, a smear (Rousseau et al. 1991). In addition, some full-mutation carriers have unmethylated, premutation-sized bands that presumably produce FMRP. These are referred to as *mosaics*. The frequency of such carriers depends on the technique used to detect the small proportion of premutation alleles and ranges from 6% to 41% in full-mutation males (Rousseau et al. 1991; Nolin et al. 1994). Last, another class of full-mutation alleles is those with more than 200 repeats but that are only partially methylated or completely unmethylated. This class is rare and is usually found in a mosaic state in DNA from peripheral blood. Among individuals with reduced methylation, FMRP levels seemed to be reduced in nonneuronal biopsy tissues in a few cases (Feng et al. 1995; Lachiewicz et al. 1996; chap. 12). Also, Feng et al. (1995) showed that large expansions might inhibit translation in lymphoblastoid and fibroblast clones, and Tassone et al. (2000) presented evidence that a protein deficit may extend into the high-premutation range.

Until 1992, chromosome analysis was the only available diagnostic tool to detect the fragile X syndrome–associated fragile site located at Xq27.3. Once a diagnosis was confirmed, cytogenetics was used in conjunction with linkage analysis to examine the carrier status of the extended family of an affected individual. The cytogenetic test was limited for several reasons. First, it lacked the sensitivity to detect the mutation in nonexpressing heterozygous females and premutation carrier males. Second, the presence of nearby fragile sites unrelated to FXS sometimes led to false-positive results. Finally, chromosome analysis is extremely labor-intensive and expensive, and it prohibits large-scale population testing. In terms of the sensitivity of the test with respect to FXS (i.e., the probability of fragile X expression given that an individual has FXS), the presence of the fragile X site is a good diagnostic marker for fragile X–related MR in males and a relatively good one for fragile X–related MR in females (Jacobs and Sherman 1985).

DNA-based testing is now routinely used, allows identification of both expressing and nonexpressing carriers, and is inexpensive relative to cytogenetic testing. The diagnostic test determines the size of the repeat region relative to that of a noncarrier. Thus, it can be used to identify individuals with the premutation and full mutation. This test is close to 100% specific and is about 98% sensitive, missing only those cases with point mutations or small deletions. It is now the test of choice in a clinical setting.

## Epidemiology

The goal of epidemiologic studies of FXS is to obtain accurate estimates of the various forms of *FMR1* with specific attention to those forms that lead to increased risk of specific morbid phenotypes or increased risk for having offspring with FXS. The prevalence estimates obtained to date have been based on surveys of targeted populations (e.g., mentally impaired or learning disabled). Subsequent estimates for the general population have been extrapolated from vital statistics of the population from which the target population was drawn. To provide some historical perspective, I will review the early studies that estimated the prevalence of nonspecific X-linked mental retardation and four population-based studies of FXS based on the cytogenetic diagnosis. Next, estimates of the prevalence of the FXS and premutation forms of the *FMR1* gene will be summarized from studies that used the DNA diagnostic test and obtained point estimates of the prevalence. Last, studies that obtained estimates of the prevalence of premature ovarian failure among premutation carriers will be reviewed, as this phenotype can potentially lead to significant morbidity. Because of space limitations, only those studies conducted since 1996 or that surveyed a large sample size will be reviewed.

## Prevalence Studies

### The Prevalence of Nonspecific X-Linked Mental Retardation

Nonspecific X-linked mental retardation (XLMR) accounts for a significant proportion of retarded males in the population. The measurement of this proportion or a direct measurement of the population frequency of XLMR is impossible, since the feature that distinguishes XLMR from nonspecific mental retardation (MR), the pattern of inheritance, is not always revealed in small families. Therefore, XLMR cannot be completely separated from the heterogeneous group of nonspecific MR. One indirect way to measure the frequency of XLMR is to identify families with two or more affected siblings, as multiple affected siblings are an indication of a genetic cause. Then, the number of affected brother pairs is compared to the number of affected sister pairs, and the excess of brother pairs is assumed to be caused by X-linked genes. Most studies have shown a 2:1 ratio of families with male:female affected sibling pairs (Wright et al. 1959; Priest et al. 1961; Wortis et al. 1966; Davison 1973). Using this same strategy in a population-based study in New South Wales, Australia, Turner and Turner (1974) found that the prevalence of carrier females of X-linked moderate MR (IQ 30–55) was 0.74/1000. If it is assumed that XLMR is caused by an X-linked recessive lethal gene, these data suggest that the frequency of males with moderate MR caused by X-linked genes is 0.55/1,000 (for specific calculations, see Turner and Turner 1974). The authors concluded that approximately 20% of the moderate retardation in males was caused by X-linked genes.

Herbst and Miller (1980) undertook a similar study in British Columbia, Canada, during a 20-year period and included all types of nonspecific MR. They found that the prevalence of carrier females was 2.44/1,000, which suggests that the prevalence of affected males caused by X-linked genes is about 1.83/1,000. Two reasons for the higher prevalence in the British Columbia study may be considered: Individuals ascertained included those with all levels of MR who were either dead or alive at the time of study, whereas those ascertained in the New South Wales study included only moderately retarded individuals who were living at the time of the study. More recent studies suggest that these prevalence estimates reflect over 200 forms of XLMR (Neri and Chiurazzi 1999, 2000).

## The Prevalence of FXS Using the Cytogenetic Test

Once FXS could be distinguished from the heterogeneous group of nonspecific XLMR, it was possible to estimate the disease frequency of this particular type of XLMR. The earliest estimate of prevalence was extrapolated from data obtained from the affected brothers study of Herbst and Miller (1980). Based on the literature at that time (Jacobs et al. 1979; Howard-Peebles and Stoddard 1980; Jacobs et al. 1980; Turner et al. 1980), Herbst and Miller assumed that approximately 50% of XLMR was caused by the fragile X mutation; thus, they estimated the prevalence of FXS in males to be one-half of 1.83/1,000, or 0.92/1,000 male births.

A more direct approach was taken by Fishburn et al. (1983). They reexamined the moderately retarded brother pairs ascertained in the study of Turner and Turner (1974) for the fragile X site and macroorchidism. They estimated the prevalence of FXS to be 0.19/1,000 male births, the prevalence of XLMR and macroorchidism and no fragile X to be 0.09/1,000, and the prevalence of other forms of XLMR to be 0.28/1,000. Thus, approximately one-third of moderate XLMR was due to the FXS.

Table 3.1 shows the estimates of prevalence of fragile X–related MR obtained from four studies that attempted to ascertain all individuals with FXS in a defined population. In each, mentally retarded individuals were identified and screened for the fragile X site, and prevalence figures were then estimated on the basis of vital statistics. The two Scandinavian studies were based on registries, whereas the other two studies were based on screening of school-aged children.

In 1977, Gustavson et al. studied an unselected series of children with an IQ of less than 50 in a northern Swedish county born between 1959 and 1970 and found the prevalence of moderate to severe MR to be 3.5/1,000. In this same

**Table 3.1**

**Prevalence of the Fragile X Syndrome Obtained from Population-based Studies**

| Country Studied | Population Size | Number Studied | Prevalence | Percentage of Individuals with FXS | | Reference |
|---|---|---|---|---|---|---|
| | | | | Severe MR | Mild MR | |
| *Males* | | | | | | |
| Sweden | 40,871[a] | 89 | 0.6/1,000 | 7.3 | 4.5 | Gustavson et al. 1986 |
| Finland | 6,594 | 61 | 0.8/1,000 | 8.7 | 0 | Kähkönen et al. 1987 |
| Australia | 58,094 | 472 | 0.4/1,000 | 2.6 | 1.0 | Turner et al. 1986b |
| U.K. | 28,611 | 219 | 0.7/1,000 | 4.4 | 3.2 | Webb et al. 1986 |
| *Females* | | | | | | |
| Finland | 6,288 | 50 | 0.4/1,000 | 0 | 5.4 | Kähkönen et al. 1987 |
| Australia | 54,641 | 203 | 0.2/1,000 | 1.0 | 2.9 | Turner et al. 1986b |
| U.K. | 26,945 | 128 | 0.6/1,000 | 3.2 | 5.2 | Webb et al. 1986 |

[a]Includes both males and females.

population, Blomquist et al. (1981) found the prevalence of mild retardation (IQ between 50 and 69) to be 3.8/1,000. Later, this population was screened for FXS, and 7.3% of moderate to severely retarded males and 4.5% of mildly retarded males were fragile X positive (Blomquist et al. 1982; Blomquist et al. 1983). Extrapolating to the total population, Gustavson et al. (1986) estimated that the prevalence of fragile X–related MR in males was 0.6/1,000 in this Swedish county.

Kähkönen et al. (1987) studied FXS in the province of Kuopio in Finland by screening MR individuals identified through a registry and through achievement tests in normal schools. They found that 8.7% of severely retarded males and no severely retarded females had FXS and that none of the mildly retarded males and 5.4% of mildly retarded females had FXS. Overall, they estimated the prevalence to be 0.8/1,000 and 0.4/1,000 in males and females, respectively.

Turner et al. (1986b) surveyed one area of Sydney, Australia, to evaluate the potential public health application of cytogenetic screening for FXS among mentally impaired individuals. They found a prevalence of 0.4/1,000 males and 0.2/1,000 females. In a subsequent study, they surveyed all of New South Wales, a population of about 5.6 million (Turner et al. 1986a). Their intent was not to determine a prevalence but to identify previously unidentified individuals with the syndrome so that their extended families could be properly informed of the risks before making decisions about childbearing. Of the 253 individuals found to have FXS in the program, 70% had not been previously diagnosed.

Webb et al. (1986) surveyed schools for the educationally subnormal including children between the ages of 11 and 16 in the county of Coventry in the United Kingdom. The prevalence of FXS was 0.7/1,000 males and almost the same in females, 0.6/1,000.

Based on the mentioned studies using the cytogenetic diagnostic tool, prevalence estimates of FXS in a predominantly Caucasian population ranged from 0.4/1,000 to 0.8/1,000 in males and from 0.2/1,000 to 0.6/1,000 in females.

## The Prevalence of FXS Using the DNA Diagnostic Test

The limitation of the cytogenetic test to determine the prevalence of FXS was recognized when studies of Turner et al. (1986b) and Webb et al. (1986) were reanalyzed by testing the fragile X–positive males using the DNA diagnostic test for FXS (Turner et al. 1996). They found a high false-positive rate in both studies and attributed most to the expression of other fragile X sites. On final analysis, the prevalence of FXS was estimated to be approximately 1/4,000 males.

Subsequent studies using the DNA diagnostic test have surveyed target populations (i.e., those with some defined intellectual disability) and extrapolated to the general population using the assumption that individuals with FXS would be identified only in that target population. The validity of this assumption clearly depends on the phenotype among the individuals of the target population.

To date, the fragile X syndrome has been identified in every racial/ethnic group that has been studied. Studies to compare the prevalence among ethnic groups are limited. One study conducted in Israel found that the majority of families diagnosed with FXS were Tunisian Jews (Falik-Zaccai et al. 1997); although a prevalence was not estimated, this finding suggests that the prevalence may vary in more isolated populations. However, in larger admixed populations, the confidence limits of the estimates of the prevalence of FXS overlap (e.g., Crawford et al. 2000). A representative set of studies of males published since 1996 and providing a prevalence estimate in the general population is summarized in table 3.2. The prevalence in the general population ranges from 1/2,359 to 1/6,045, with most being around 1/4,000. If we assume that about 50% of female carriers show clinical symptoms of FXS and that the frequency of carriers of the full mutation is equal in males and females (for review, see Sherman 1995), we would expect the prevalence of FXS in females to be approximately 1/8,000. Studies to date have not been based on a large enough sample size to determine whether this inference is correct.

**Table 3.2**
**Studies since 1996 using DNA Testing Providing Prevalence Estimates of FXS among Males in the General Population**

| Study | Country | Target Population | No. Positive/ No. Tested | Estimate Prevalence Target Population | Estimate Prevalence General (95% CI[a]) |
|---|---|---|---|---|---|
| de Vries et al. 1997 | Southwest Netherlands | Schools and institutes for mentally retarded, no known etiology | Mild MR: 4/333 Mod/sev.: 5/533 | Mild MR: 2.0% Mod/sev.: 2.4% | 1/6,045 (1/9,981–1/3,851) |
| Patsalis et al. 1999 | Hellenic population of Greece and Cyprus | Referred clinical population of idiopathic mental retardation | 8/611 | MR: 1.3% | 1/4,246 (1/16,440–1/1,333) |
| Elbaz et al. 1998 | Guadeloupe, French West Indies | SEN school population of unknown etiology | 11/163 | SEN: 6.7% | 1/2,359 (1/4,484–1/1,276) |
| Youings et al. 2000 | U.K. (Wessex) | SEN school population of unknown etiology, ages 5–18 | 20/3,738 | SEN: 0.5% | 1/5,530 (1/8,922–1/4,007) |
| Crawford et al. 2000 | U.S. (Atlanta, GA) | SEN school population, ages 7–10 | Caucasian: 4/1,572 African Am.: 3/752 | SEN Caucasian: 0.3% SEN African Am.: 0.4% | Caucasian: 1/3,717 (1/7,143–1/1,869) African Am.: 1/2,545 (1/5,208–1/289) |

*Note:* MR, mental retardation; Mod/sev., moderate to severe; SEN, special education needs; Am., American.
[a]Confidence limits were based on the total number of individuals in the general population, not on the tested population. Thus, these confidences are underestimates (more narrow) and provide only a guide.

Comparisons of studies of the prevalence among specific types of target populations cannot be made because of differences in the definitions of MR and because of the method of ascertainment (e.g., clinical referral vs. surveys). For example, most estimates among males labeled as having MR are 2–3% (e.g., de Vries et al. 1997; Turner et al. 1996; Haddad et al. 1999; Tan et al. 2000; Millan et al. 1999), although sometimes such estimates are as high as 5–8% (e.g., Goldman et al. 1997; Arrieta et al. 1999; Ruangdaraganon et al. 2000). Probably the proportion of MR males with FXS does not exceed 8% and is more likely about 2–5%.

## The Prevalence of Premutation Carriers of FXS

Representative studies that provide estimates of the prevalence of premutation male and female carriers—defined as those with >60 repeat alleles—are summarized in table 3.3. The largest surveys to date have been conducted by Rousseau et al. (1995, 1996). They surveyed a large, anonymous sample of males and females from a population of more than 600,000 individuals in the Québec City metropolitan area. They used blood samples left over from a consecutive series of routine hemoglobin/hematocrit or complete blood counts (CBCs) from 10,572 males and 10,624 female outpatients who attended a general hospital in Québec. Forty-one females with 55 repeats or more were identified, leading to a heterozygote carrier frequency of 1/259 (95% confidence interval [CI]: 1/373 to 1/198) (Rousseau et al. 1995). Fourteen males with 54 repeats or more were identified, leading to a hemizygote carrier frequency of 1/755 (95% CI: 1/1,327–1/138).

Using a lower bound of 60 repeats, the frequencies of premutations found in the Quebec study are similar to those found in other large admixed populations (table 3.3). If we estimate that approximately 1/1,000 males and 1/350 females carry a premutation, the female:male ratio (2.85:1) is higher than the ratio of 2:1 expected for a simple X-linked disorder but fits models of inheritance of a dynamic repeat sequence (for review, see Sherman 1995).

## Epidemiologic Studies of the Phenotype Consequence of High-Repeat Alleles

In chapter 1, the phenotype consequence of high-repeat alleles that are not abnormally methylated (those in the intermediate range and those in the premutation range) is reviewed. Here we will discuss the prevalence of the one phenotype among premutation carrier females that has been convincingly established, namely, premature ovarian failure. In addition, we will review two large studies that have examined the frequency of high-repeat alleles among children in special education schools and among controls to determine whether there is a cognitive and/or behavioral consequence of carrying such alleles.

**Table 3.3**
**Studies That Estimate the Prevalence of Males and Females with 60 or More CGG Repeats**

| Study | Country | Target Population | No. Positive/No. Tested Males | No. Positive/No. Tested Females | Estimated Prevalence in Males (95% CI) | Estimated Prevalence in Females (95% CI) |
|---|---|---|---|---|---|---|
| | | *Population selected for cognitive impairment* | | | | |
| Hagerman et al. 1994 | U.S. (CO) | Children considered "high risk" for FXS, ages 2–18 | 1/299 | 0/140 | 1/299 (1/5,727–1/63) | |
| Mazzocco et al. 1997 | U.S. (Baltimore, MD) | Children with learning or school difficulties, ages 5–18 | 1/673 | 0/341 | 1/673 (1/12,892–1/141) | |
| Syrrou et al. 1998 | Hellenic population of Greece and Cyprus | Referred clinical population of idiopathic MR | 1/257 | 0/176 | 1/257 (1/4,923–1/54) | |
| Youings et al. 2000 | Wessex, U.K. | SEN school boys, ages 5–18 | 2/3,732 | | 1/1,866 (1/5,376–1/288) | |
| Crawford et al. 2000 | U.S. (Atlanta, GA) | SEN schoolchildren, ages 7–10 | Caucasians: 2/2,045 African Am.: 0/805 | Caucasians: 2/670 African Am.: 0/321 | Caucasian: 1/1,022 African Am.: (1/5,917–1/254) | Caucasian: 1/335 (1/1,934–1/84) |

| | | Population not selected for cognitive impairment | | | |
|---|---|---|---|---|---|
| Reiss et al. 1994 | U.S. (Baltimore, MD) | Families referred for genetic disorders | 0/416 | 1/561 | 1/561 (1/10,741–1/118) |
| Rousseau et al. 1995 | Canada (Quebec) | Consecutive series of outpatients from a public hospital | | 28/10,624 | 1/354 (1/515–1/248) |
| Dawson et al. 1995 | Canada (Manitoba) | Consecutive births | 1/778 | 0/735 | 1/778 (1/14,904–1/120) |
| Holden et al. 1995 | Canada (Ontario) | Consecutive births | 1/1,000 | | 1/1,000 (1/19,157–1/155) |
| Rynanen et al. 1999 | Finland | Pregnant women seeking prenatal care | | 6/1,447 | 1/246 (1/605–1/107) |
| Drasinover et al. 2000 | Israel | Screening women with no history of FXS or MR | | 39/10,587 | 1/271 (1/377–1/201) |

*Note:* FXS, fragile X syndrome; MR, mental retardation; SEN, special education needs.

## Premature Ovarian Failure

The premutation allele was originally not considered detrimental; that is, there did not seem to be a phenotype consequence of the long repeat tract. However, in the late 1980s and early 1990s, preliminary findings suggested that nonimpaired heterozygotes were at risk for early menopause (Cronister et al. 1991; Schwartz et al. 1994) and increased rates of twinning (Fryns 1986; Turner et al. 1994), both indications of ovarian failure.

Once premutation carriers could be distinguished from full-mutation carriers, this phenotype was found to be restricted to premutation carriers only. Results from a large collaborative study confirmed the increased rate of premature ovarian failure (POF) among premutation carriers only: the estimate for POF among premutation carriers ($n = 395$) ranged from 16% (inclusion of all women >18 years) to 24% (inclusion of women >40 years), whereas those for full ($n = 128$) and noncarrier ($n = 237$) relatives were similar to the general population risk, 1% (Allingham-Hawkins et al. 1999).

Four recent studies with large sample sizes and conducted at single sites using personal interviews are summarized in table 3.4. Using the combined information from women interviewed at age 40 or greater, the best estimate of the rate of POF among premutation carriers is 21% (95% CI: 15–27%), or a relative risk of 21 assuming the general population rate of 1%.

The question remains whether all women with premutations have some level of reduced ovarian function or whether only a subset of women with premutations have ovarian dysfunction. Hundsheid et al. (2000b) found evidence for a parent-of-origin effect of the premutation: carriers who received the premutation from their fathers were at higher risk for POF (28%) compared with those who received the premutation from their mothers (4%). Although two subsequent reports could not confirm this finding (Murray et al. 2000a; Vianna-Morgante and Costa 2000), there were enough differences between study populations to warrant further investigation into this possible effect (Hundscheid et al. 2000a; Sherman 2000a).

The overall mean age at menopause for premutation carriers has been reported from two studies that extracted full information using survival analysis: 47.87 years among premutation carriers compared with 52.96 in controls (Murray et al. 2000b) and 45 years among premutation carriers (Hundscheid et al. 2000a). Interestingly, in a random subset of premutation women from the study of Murray et al. (1999), a significant increase in serum follicle-stimulating hormone (FSH) was found among women who were still cycling. This suggests that, as a group, premutation carriers may enter menopause before full-mutation carriers and unaffected controls.

Another approach to assessment of the effect of the *FMR1* premutation allele on POF is to determine the frequency of premutation carriers among

**Table 3.4**
**Summary of Studies That Examined the Rate of POF among Women Ascertained through Families with Fragile X Syndrome at a Single Site Using Personal Interviews**

| Study | Method/Subjects | Rate of POF among Women Who Were Interviewed at ≥40 yr | | Comments |
|---|---|---|---|---|
| Giovannucci-Uzielli et al. 1999 | Women ≥ 18 yr | FM | 0% (0/25) | |
| | 63 FM | PM | 14% (6/42) | |
| | 170 PM | Control | 0% (0/44) | |
| | 118 noncarrier relatives | | | |
| Hundscheid et al. 2000 | Women ≥ 18 yr | PM | 22% (24/109) | Significant difference between PIP and |
| | 148 PM (106 PIP, | PIP | 28% (23/82) | MIP using only women ≥40 and using |
| | 42 MIP) | MIP | 4% (1/27) | survival analysis on all women |
| Vianna-Morgante and Costa 2000 | Women ≥25 yr | PM | 28% (7/25) | No parent-of-origin effect |
| | 113 PM (32 PIP, | PIP | 33% (5/15) | |
| | 42 MIP) | MIP | 20% (2/10) | |
| Murray et al. 2000a, 2000b | Women ≥ 18 yr | FM | 18% (2/11) | Sample size among full mutations |
| | 31 FM | PM | 15% (10/66) | too small to draw conclusions |
| | 116 PM (51 PIP, | PIP | 17% (2/12) | Significant differences in mean age |
| | 40 MIP) | MIP | 28% (5/18) | at menopause between premutation and |
| | 205 noncarrier relatives | Control | 2% (2/92) | controls using survival analysis |
| | | | | No parent-of-origin effect using women |
| | | | | ≥40 or using survival analysis on all |
| | | | | women |

*Note:* POF, premature ovarian failure; FM, full mutation carriers; PM, premutation carriers; PIP, paternally inherited premutation carriers; MIP, maternally inherited premutation carriers.

women with idiopathic POF. This frequency can be compared with the expected frequency of carriers in the general population, approximately 1/350. Conway et al. (1995) were the first to take this approach and found no fragile X mutations among 37 women with sporadic POF but found 2 premutation carriers among 9 women with familial POF. This series was expanded in two subsequent reports, and the frequency of premutations among sporadic and familial cases of POF was found to be 1.6% and 8%, respectively. Both estimates were significantly increased over the general population (Murray et al. 1998; Conway et al. 1998). No full mutations were identified. The size of premutations ranged from 80 to 175 repeats, and the age of menopause varied from 11 to 30 years.

Since the original survey of Conway et al. (1995), others have examined various series of women with POF ascertained through infertility clinics, obstetrics and gynecology clinics, genetic laboratories, and general surveys (e.g., Kenneson et al. 1997; Patsalis 1999; Giovannucci-Uzielli et al. 1999; Marozzi et al. 2000). Overall, the frequency of premutation carriers among women with POF depends on the age of onset of POF ascertained through each series and the proportion of sporadic and familial cases. Using the two studies that ascertained women primarily through a reproductive endocrinology clinic and clearly separated familial and sporadic POF (Conway et al. 1998; Marozzi et al. 2000), the estimate of premutation carriers is 13.8% and 2.1%, respectively. No full-mutation carriers were identified in any of the series reported to date. Because the relative risk of POF is as high as 21, these estimates of 13.8% and 2.1% approximate the fraction of idiopathic familial or sporadic POF, respectively, that can be uniquely attributed to the premutation allele (i.e., the attributable risk).

Data supporting increased twinning rates are conflicting and need to be resolved (for review, see Sherman 2000b). Neither the underlying cellular pathophysiology of POF caused by the premutation allele nor the molecular mechanism underlying the presence of the long repeat tract of the premutation allele is understood. Women who carry the premutation allele should have not only genetic counseling but also fertility counseling to ensure that they reach their goals for reproduction.

### The Prevalence of High-Repeat Alleles among Children with Special Needs

Evidence for a phenotype consequence of high-repeat alleles is inconsistent, with some studies having shown an increased frequency of high-repeat alleles among populations with cognitive problems (Youings et al. 2000; Haddad et al. 1998) while others have not (Crawford et al. 1999; Mazzocco et al. 1997, 1998; Mornet et al. 1998). Two studies with the largest sample sizes—one conducted in metropolitan Atlanta, Georgia (Crawford et al. 1999, 2000), and that of

Youings et al. (2000) conducted in Wessex, Britain—used the same study design and found different results. The Atlanta study did not find an increased frequency of high-repeat alleles among a special education needs (SEN) population compared with maternal control X chromosomes, while the study in Wessex did find a statistically significant increase in frequency (4.45% vs. 2.97%, $p = 0.001$). Again, differences in study populations were significant. In addition to the recognized differences in criteria for entry into SEN classes between the two sites, the Atlanta population was younger (7–10 years old compared with 5–18 years old) and was more heterogeneous (included girls and boys of two major ethnic groups compared with only Caucasian boys in the Wessex study). Thus, if there is an effect of long repeat tracts, it may be evident only in males and may be more overt in older individuals. Since the frequency of high-repeat carrier males and females is approximately 4% and 8%, respectively, follow-up studies are important to confirm or refute the possibility of a phenotype consequence of high-repeat alleles.

## Genetic Epidemiology

Genetic epidemiology is the study of the familial distribution of a disorder with the goal of understanding the possible genetic basis. This task seemed simple for FXS: Fragile X–related mental retardation was known to be transmitted as an X-linked trait and to cosegregate with the marker on the X chromosome, the fragile X site. However, several observations were exceptions to the simple rules of X-linked inheritance, and these were noted even before the FXS was fully delineated. Martin and Bell (1943) reported two apparently normal brothers who both had affected grandsons. Losowsky (1961) reported a family with a normal male who had an affected brother and affected grandsons and great-grandsons. In 1963, Dunn et al. posed several genetic epidemiologic questions based on the inheritance pattern observed in a large XLMR pedigree: (1) Through whom did the defect enter the pedigree? (2) Why is there a deficiency of affected males? (3) Do the males and females of low-normal intelligence have the disease in a mild form? (4) Can we be sure that this defect is inherited by sex-linked recessive rather than dominant sex-limited transmission? In 1978, Wolff et al. were some of the first to speculate on how males could carry a mutation on the X chromosome and not express it. They suggested that the unaffected male carrier noted in their pedigree may be a mosaic with normal cells and mutant cells that carry the X-linked defect. They proposed three mechanisms for the mosaicism: (1) a half-chromatid mutation in the maternal gamete, (2) an early embryonic mutation, or (3) a mutation in the primordial germ cell.

Using segregation analysis of families with FXS, Sherman et al. (1984, 1985) identified specific characteristics of the inheritance pattern of fragile X–related MR that made it different from other X-linked traits. First, no new mutations were predicted; thus, all mothers of affected sons were carriers. Second, 20% of males who carried the mutation and transmitted it to their daughters did not express any clinical or cognitive symptoms. Third, a relatively high proportion of female carriers expressed the mutation, although they were usually more mildly affected than were males. Four, the risk of FXS in offspring depended on the sex and phenotype of the carrier parent: (1) daughters of nonexpressing carrier males were rarely, if ever, mentally impaired, whereas daughters of non-expressing carrier females had about a 30% risk of having daughters with FXS, and (2) cognitively impaired female carriers had a higher risk of having offspring with FXS than had those who were cognitively normal. Last, the risk of having an offspring with FXS increased in each succeeding generation, a phenomenon called *anticipation.*

Once the FXS mutation was identified and found to be a "dynamic" trinucleotide repeat mutation, the biological basis for the unusual inheritance pattern of the fragile X–related mental retardation was provided. Although the exact mechanism that causes expansion of the CGG repeats is unknown, it has been observed that the number of repeats most often increases as it is passed from parent to offspring, although contractions are observed (Fu et al. 1991; Yu et al. 1992); irrespective, all full mutations are derived from premutations. This explains why no new mutation has been observed (i.e., the normal form of the *FMR1* gene becoming a premutation gene), as ancestors of several previous generations are not available for study. The dynamic mutation process also explains why the risk for FXS increases in each generation: the number of repeats expands through every transmission until it exceeds 200 repeats and causes the gene to be silenced. The magnitude of the increase in repeat number is greater when transmitted by a female carrier than when transmitted by a male carrier. A female carrier has a 50% chance of passing the unstable *FMR1* gene to her offspring, as is true for any X-linked gene. The risk of expansion from the female carrier's premutation to the full mutation is high and depends on her repeat number (Heitz et al. 1992; Fu et al. 1991; Snow et al. 1993; Yu et al. 1992; Sherman et al. 1996; Nolin et al. 1996). For example, less than 5% of premutation alleles with less than 60 repeats expand to the full mutation, whereas about 50% of those with 60–80 and almost all of those with 90 repeats expand to the full mutation. A male premutation carrier has a 100% chance of passing his premutation to all of his daughters and to none of his sons. His *FMR1* repeat region does not change dramatically when transmitted to his daughters; in fact, the repeat size decreases or remains the same in about 30–40% of transmissions (Fisch et al. 1995; Nolin et al. 1996). Interestingly, the rate of contraction is correlated with increasing repeat size in the carrier father (Nolin et al. 1996; Ashley-Koch et al. 1998). The risk of expansion to the full mutation is extremely small, if any.

The pattern of instability of premutation alleles explains the unusual inheritance pattern observed in early segregation studies of fragile X–related mental retardation (Sherman et al. 1984, 1985). The decreased risk of having offspring with FXS among mothers of transmitting males compared with mothers of affected males can be explained by the fact that mothers of transmitting males will carry, on average, smaller premutation alleles than those of affected males. Although not understood, the observation that transmitting males do not have FXS daughters is accounted for by the fact that the premutation is rather stable in paternal transmissions compared with maternal transmissions. This may be due to severe selection against sperm with full mutations compared with a lack of or minimal selection against eggs with full mutations. Other factors that influence the expansion of the premutation, in addition to repeat size and sex of the carrier parent, have been examined, including parental age, origin of the grandparental allele, sex of the offspring (Ashley-Koch et al. 1998), and a familial factor (Nolin et al. 1996). Only some yet unidentified familial factor was found to significantly influence rates of expansion. That is, offspring within sibships of premutation carriers had more similar repeat expansions than among sibships (Nolin et al. 1996). Also, there was a trend for increased rates of expansion to the full mutation among premutation carrier females who received their mutation from fathers compared with mothers (Ashley-Koch et al. 1998), although more data need to be collected to confirm this finding. Observed associations with parental age and sex of the offspring could be explained by an apparent bias resulting from somatic selection against full mutations and timing of the diagnostic test and by an apparent bias of incomplete testing of sibships, respectively (Ashley-Koch et al. 1998).

## Screening for the Fragile X Mutation

Population screening for FXS has been a topic of consideration since the *FMR1* gene was identified and an accurate test was developed to identify increased repeat length, the mutation occurring in over 98% of individuals with FXS. Advances in understanding the molecular basis of the syndrome have elicited new prospects for identifying a greater number of individuals at risk for the disorder or at risk for transmitting the disorder. In the mid-1990s, four potential target populations for screening were reviewed and the advantages and limitations in each were discussed (Meadows and Sherman 1996). The target populations included women considering pregnancy, pregnant women (prenatal screening), newborns, and children with developmental delay. More recently, Murray et al.

(1997) provided a review of the literature concerning screening for FXS and considered the information necessary for health planners.

Here, we will briefly describe some of the important issues pertaining to screening for FXS to provide a framework for future work. Two types of economic evaluations at a basic level can be considered for screening any target population: cost-effectiveness and cost-benefit. Cost-effectiveness analysis examines the most efficient way of achieving the goals of a screening program, whereas cost-benefit analysis examines whether the goals of the program are worthwhile. Only two of the many target populations will be discussed, newborns and women of reproductive age, representing the two extremes with respect to available options once a diagnosis is made. Only issues of population screening that are specific to the fragile X mutation will be considered. Other issues, such as access to results and resources needed to implement a program, are general to screening of any genetic disorder.

## The Significance of the Fragile X Mutation

The first issue to consider in the cost benefit analysis is the significance of the disorder. Components to assess significance include the seriousness, frequency, and clinical utility of the diagnosis of the disorder. Using the information outlined in table 3.5, two possible scenarios for screening for fragile X mutations are highlighted: (1) screening newborn males for the full mutation and (2) screening females for the premutation or full-mutation alleles.

Several important issues must be considered related to screening newborns for FXS. All males with the full mutation have significant cognitive and behavioral disorders, whereas only 50–70% of full mutation females have such deficits and, most times, the deficits are milder than those found among males (chaps. 1 and 6). Currently, there is no prognostic test for severity of expression among full-mutation females. Many have suggested that screening for the absence of FMRP among males, and perhaps females if a quantitative test can be developed, may be the best strategy for newborn screening. The major disadvantage of screening newborns is that there is no cure to date. Thus, the significant costs related to the upbringing of the child with FXS, both monetary and emotional costs, are not prevented.

Screening females of reproductive age has significant advantages. Each identified female would be informed about the risks of having a child with significant MR, and all options for family planning would be available. Also, a woman would be informed about the risk for POF, a significant disorder for women who want a family. In most cases, the effect of POF can be minimized if a woman begins her family earlier in life, in her young to mid 20s. Several reports have assessed screening woman at the time of pregnancy (e.g., Ryynanen et al. 1999; Spence et al. 1996). Although a screening program may be easier to implement at this time, since most women seek prenatal care, few options are open with respect to family planning—only the choice of whether or not to terminate an affected fetus. Of course, subsequent family planning includes all options.

The disadvantage of screening at any stage is the potential for stigmatization or loss of self-esteem related to being a carrier of a mutation. Attitudes related to carrier testing for FSX have been examined by McConkie-Rosell and her colleagues from several different perspectives: attitudes and opinions of obligate carrier females (McConkie-Rosell et al. 1997), parental attitudes regarding carrier testing in children at risk for FXS (McConkie-Rosell et al. 1999), and the effect of carrier testing on a woman's self-concept (McConkie-Rosell et al. 2000). Their work reinforces the importance of assessing the feasibility of population screening of women of reproductive age. In their most recent work, which examined self-concept, they assessed women who were at 50% risk of carrying the fragile X mutation at two time points, before and after learning about their carrier testing results (McConkie-Rosell et al. 2000). There were no differences initially between carriers and noncarriers and no changes between the two time points on measures related to self-concept. Analysis of a scale specifically related to FXS indicated that the total sample (i.e., all women at risk) had a reduction in positive feelings about self at the initial time point. After finding out results (after a six-month period), noncarriers reported improved feelings about self, while carriers had no change in feelings about self. Further study suggested that feelings about self with respect to genetic testing are not related to global self-concept. Instead, they are related to the implications of a positive carrier test for themselves and their relatives. In the study among obligate carriers, the women did not feel guilty about being a carrier; instead, they had feelings of anger, depression, or lowered self-esteem related to having an affected child (McConkie-Rosell et al. 1997). Last, the overwhelming majority of obligate carrier parents wanted their children to know their carrier status before becoming sexually active and wanted their children to be able to marry informed of their genetic risk (McConkie-Rosell et al. 1999).

These results emphasize the importance of screening women of or even before reproductive age to ensure that all possible options for family planning are available. The studies to date have been performed only on individuals who are in families with FXS. No assessment of attitudes has been performed on individuals at low risk for carrying the fragile X mutation (i.e., the general population). Furthermore, no studies have been conducted concerning the effect of learning ambiguous results related to the risk of having affected offspring (i.e., women who carry alleles with 50–60 repeats). Thus, more studies in this area are needed before implementing a population-based screening program.

**Table 3.5**
**Significance of the Fragile X Mutation**

| | Premutation | Full mutation |
|---|---|---|
| | | **Males** |
| **Frequency of carriers** | 1/1,000 | 1/4,000 |
| **Seriousness** | | |
| symptoms | none/mild | moderate MR, behavioral problems (range of severity) |
| risk of FXS in offspring | ~0 | ~0 |
| **Clinical utility** | | |
| advantages of an early diagnosis | early intervention for subgroup with clinical involvement | **For the child** early intervention targeted education based on FXS knowledge **For the family** eliminates cost of finding a diagnosis permits progress to next phase of rearing the child provides parents with information about their child; regain confidence about parenting informed about genetic risks before next pregnancy diagnosis before symptoms (parent-child bonding?) no treatment specific to FXS third-party discrimination |
| disadvantages of an early diagnosis | stigmatization based on carrier status third-party discrimination | |

|  | | Females |
|---|---|---|
| **Frequency of carriers** | 1/350[a] | 1/4,000 |
| **Seriousness** | | |
| symptoms | 21% at risk for premature ovarian failure (POF) | 50% at risk for mild MR (range of severity) |
| risk of FXS in offspring | up to 50%—depends on repeat size | 50% |
| **Clinical utility** | | |
| advantages of an early diagnosis | informed about genetic risks before next pregnancy<br>all options available for family planning<br>informed about POF and risks associated with delaying family planning | for expressing females, same as for symptomatic males<br>for nonexpressing females, same as for premutation females, although they have no risk for POF |
| disadvantages of an early diagnosis | stigmatization based on carrier status<br>third-party discrimination | no prognostic test to determine whether a female will express FXS symptoms—only 50% at risk for FXS diagnosis before symptoms, if any at all<br>no treatment specific to FXS<br>stigmatization based on carrier status<br>third-party discrimination |

[a]This is the frequency of carriers with 61–199 repeats. If 55 repeats is used for the definition of a premutation, the frequency is estimated to be approximately 1/250.

## The Screening Test

The analysis of the screening test is one component of cost-effectiveness. When determining the best test for screening, the validity, the cost, and the ability to ensure quality control for the test must be assessed with respect to the target population and the phenotype being screened (e.g., FXS, risk for affected offspring, risk for affected relatives, risk for POF). Two types of molecular tests are available for screening: (1) those that determine repeat size and (2) those that determine FMRP levels. The latter tests are still under development but offer great potential for quickly screening newborn blood spots at low cost. In contrast, the former tests are well established and accurate but more expensive.

For newborn screening, the strategy that seems most valid would be testing for presence/absence of the full mutation (or FMRP) among males. Such tests could be done using blood spots. This test would have >98% sensitivity (would miss mutations in the coding region), about 100% specificity, and 100% positive predicted value (PPV). Testing newborn females would reduce the PPV to 50%.

For screening women of reproductive age, determination of repeat size would be necessary. The validity of the test would depend on the number of repeats that would be considered as a positive result. One scenario may be to define a positive test result as >60 repeats and the condition as the increased risk of FXS among offspring. Under these conditions, the test is 98% sensitive, 100% specific, and 100% PPV. Of course, the magnitude of the increased risk will depend on the repeat number (Sherman et al. 1996). However, if this cutoff point is decreased to 50 repeats, the specificity and PPV are reduced. Thus, careful consideration must made with respect to the definition of a positive result. As research is continuing to determine factors leading to instability on repeats in the intermediate range, follow-up tests will become available to categorize alleles as stable or unstable (e.g., determining the repeat structure to assay the number of 3' pure repeats). With respect to POF, all parameters would be reduced, as only 21% of premutation carriers have POF. Based on current data, there does not seem to be a correlation of risk with repeat size within the premutation range.

## Feasibility

Cost-effectiveness analysis must also evaluate acceptability, yield, and the ability to implement the program and follow up positive results. Studies related to acceptability for the two target populations being considered here, newborns and women of reproductive age, have not been done. The yield of the screening test depends on the strategy being taken. For the two conservative approaches outlined above, the yield would be high relative to other genetic disorders. For screening newborn males, full-mutation carriers would be identified at about 1/4,000. For screening women, premutation carriers would be identified at about 1/350.

The implementation of a newborn screening program for FXS would be straightforward as the infrastructure already exists. Implementation of a program to screen women in the general population is more difficult because of the absence of a preconceptional consultation system. Thus, high coverage is difficult. Suggested time points for consideration have included the high school setting and routine gynecologic or primary physician visits.

## Summary

Cost-benefit and cost-effectiveness are important components of any screening program, and only some of the issues are described here. Genetic screening programs need to be subjected to cost analysis and can be implemented only when the cost of service is equal to the financial savings. At least two groups have initiated screening programs for the fragile X mutation in women of reproductive age, one in Israel (Pesso et al. 2000) and one in Finland (Ryynanen et al. 1999) and have concluded that such programs are economically feasible. Wildhagen et al. (1998) provide a comprehensive evaluation of the costs, effects, and savings of screening for female carriers of the fragile X mutation prenatally and preconceptionally. They found no economic obstacle to screening under either scenario and suggest that the decision to screen should concentrate on the discussion of medical, social, psychologic, and ethical considerations.

## Conclusion

Many years of intensive research have begun to unravel the genetics of FXS. The trinucleotide repeat sequence mutation process that was originally thought to be unique to FXS is now known to be the underlying etiology for many disorders. Efforts to understand this mutational process as well as efforts to determine the function of the gene product are well under way. With the collaboration of many scientific and medical disciplines and with the enthusiasm and cooperation of concerned families, progress continues to be made to understand this perplexing disorder.

## References

Allingham-Hawkins, D. J., R. Babul, D. Chitayat, J. J. A. Holden, K. T. Yang, C. Lee, R. Hudson, H. Gorwill, S. L. Nolin, A. Glicksman, E. C. Jenkins, W. T. Brown, P. N.

Howard-Peebles, C. Becchi, E. Cummings, L. Fallon, S. Seitz, S. H. Black, A. M. Vianna-Morgante, S. S. Costa, P. A. Otto, R. Mingroni-Netto, A. Murray, J. Webb, F. MacSwinney, N. Dennis, P. A. Jacobs, M. Syrrou, I. Georgiou, P. C. Patsalis, M. L. Giovannucci-Uzielli, S. Guarducci, E. Lapi, A. Cecconi, U. Ricci, G. Ricotti, C. Biondi, B. Scarselli, and F. Vieri. 1999. Fragile X premutation is a significant risk factor for premature ovarian failure. *Am. J. Med. Genet.* 83:322–325.

Arrieta, I., B. Criado, B. Martinez, M. Telez, T. Nunez, O. Penagarikano, B. Ortega, and C. M. Lostao. 1999. A survey of fragile X syndrome in a sample from Spanish Basque country. *Ann. Genet.* 42:197–201.

Ashley, C. T., K. D. Wilkinson, D. Reines, and S. T. Warren. 1993. FMR1 protein: Conserved RNP family domains and selective RNA binding. *Science* 262:563–566.

Ashley-Koch, A. E., H. Robinson, A. E. Glicksman, S. L. Nolin, C. E. Schwartz, W. T. Brown, G. Turner, and S. L. Sherman. 1998. Examination of factors associated with instability of the *FMR1* CGG repeat. *Am. J. Hum. Genet.* 63:776–785.

Blomquist, H. K., K. H. Gustavson, and G. Holmgren. 1981. Mild mental retardation in children in a northern Swedish county. *J. Ment. Defic. Res.* 25:169–186.

Blomquist, H. K., K. H. Gustavson, G. Holmgren, I. Nordenson, and A. Sweins. 1982. Fragile site X chromosomes and X-linked mental retardation in severely retarded boys in a northern Swedish county: A prevalence study. *Clin. Genet.* 21:209–214.

Blomquist, H. K., K. H. Gustavson, G. Holmgren, I. Nordenson, and U. Palsson-Strae. 1983. Fragile X syndrome in mildly mentally retarded children in a northern Swedish county: A prevalence study. *Clin. Genet.* 24:393–398.

Cantú, J. M., H. E. Scaglia, M. Medina, M. Gonzalez-Diddi, T. Morato, M. E. Moreno, G. Perez-Palacios, and G. Needa. 1976. Inherited congenital normofunctional testicular hyperplasia and mental deficiency. *Hum. Genet.* 33:23–33.

Conway, G. S., S. Hettiarachchi, A. Murray, and P. A. Jacobs. 1995. Fragile X premutations in familial premature ovarian failure [letter; comment]. *Lancet* 346:309–310.

Conway, G. S., N. N. Payne, J. Webb, A. Murray, and P. A. Jacobs. 1998. Fragile X premutation screening in women with premature ovarian failure. *Hum. Reprod.* 13:1184–1187.

Crawford, D. C., K. L. Meadows, J. L. Newman, L. F. Taft, D. L. Pettay, L. B. Gold, J. S. Hersey, P. Homgreen, M. Yeargin-Allsopp, C. Boyle, and S. L. Sherman. 1999. Examining the prevalence and phenotype consequence of FRAXA and FRAXE alleles in a large, ethnically diverse special education needs population. *Am. J. Hum. Genet.* 64:495–507.

Crawford, D. C., K. L. Meadows, J. L. Newman, L. F. Taft, M. Leslie, L. Shubek, P. Homgreen, M. Yeargin-Allsopp, C. Boyle, and S. L. Sherman. 2000. Survey of the fragile X syndrome CGG repeat and the short-tandem-repeat and single-nucleotide-polymorphism haplotypes in an African American population. *Am. J. Hum. Genet.* 66:480–493.

Cronister, A., R. Schreiner, M. Wittenberger, K. Amiri, K. Harris, and R. J. Hagerman. 1991. The heterozygous fragile X female: Historical, physical, cognitive and cytogenetic features. *Am. J. Med. Genet.* 38:269–274.

Davison, B. C. C. 1973. Genetic studies in mental subnormality: I. Familial idiopathic severe subnormality: The question of a contribution by X-linked genes. *Br. J. Psychiatry,* special publ., 8:1–60.

Dawson, A. J., B. N. Chodirker, and A. E. Chudley. 1995. Frequency of *FMR1* premutations in a consecutive newborn population by PCR screening of Guthrie blood spots. *Biochem. Mol. Med.* 56:63–69.

de Vries, B. B., A. M. van den Ouweland, S. Mohkamsing, H. J. Duivenvoorden, E. Mol, K. Gelsema, M. van Rijn, D. J. Halley, L. A. Sandkuijl, B. A. Oostra, A. Tibben, and M. F. Niermeijer. 1997. Screening and diagnosis for the fragile X syndrome among the mentally retarded: An epidemiological and psychological survey. Collaborative Fragile X Study Group. *Am. J. Hum. Genet.* 61:660–667.

Drasinover, V., S. Ehrlich, N. Magal, E. Taub, V. Libman, T. Shohat, G. J. Halpern, and M. Shohat. 2000. Increased transmission of intermediate alleles of the *FMR1* gene compared with normal alleles among female heterozygotes. *Am. J. Med. Genet.* 93: 155–157.

Dunn, H. G., H. Renpenning, J. W. Gerrard, J. R. Miller, T. Tabata, and S. Federoff. 1963. Mental retardation as a sex-linked defect. *Am. J. Ment. Defic.* 67:827–848.

Eichler, E. E., J. A. Holden, B. W. Popovich, A. L. Reiss, K. Snow, S. N. Thibodeau, C. S. Richards, P. A. Ward, and D. L. Nelson. 1994. Length of uninterrupted CGG repeats determines instability in the *FMR1* gene. *Nat. Genet.* 8:88–94.

Elbaz, A., J. Suedois, M. Duquesnoy, C. Beldjord, C. Berchel, and G. Merault. 1998. Prevalence of fragile-X syndrome and FRAXE among children with intellectual disability in a Caribbean island, Guadeloupe, French West Indies. *J. Intellect. Disabil. Res.* 42 (pt. 1): 81–89.

Escalante, J. A., and O. Frota-Pessoa. 1973. Retardamento mental. In W. Becak and O. Frota-Pessoa (eds.), *Genetica Medica.* Sao Paulo: Sarvier, pp. 300–308.

Escalante, J. A., H. Grunspun, and O. Frota-Pessoa. 1971. Severe sex-linked mental retardation. *J. Genet. Hum.* 19:137–140.

Falik-Zaccai, T. C., E. Shachak, M. Yalon, Z. Lis, Z. Borochowitz, J. N. Macpherson, D. L. Nelson, and E. E. Eichler. 1997. Predisposition to the fragile X syndrome in Jews of Tunisian descent is due to the absence of AGG interruptions on a rare Mediterranean haplotype. *Am. J. Hum. Genet.* 60:103–112.

Feng, Y., L. Lakkis, D. Devys, and S. T. Warren. 1995. Quantitative comparison of *FMR1* gene expression in normal and premutation alleles. *Am. J. Hum. Genet.* 56: 106–113.

Fisch, G. S., K. Snow, S. N. Thibodeau, M. Chalifaux, J. J. A. Holden, D. L. Nelson, P. N. Howard-Peebles, and A. Maddalena. 1995. The fragile X premutation in carriers and its effect on mutation size in offspring. *Am. J. Hum. Genet.* 56:1147–1155.

Fishburn, J., G. Turner, A. Daniel, and R. Brookwell. 1983. The diagnosis and frequency of X-linked conditions in a cohort of moderately retarded males with affected brothers. *Am. J. Med. Genet.* 14:713–724.

Fryns, J. P. 1986. The female and the fragile X: A study of 144 obligate female carriers. *Am. J. Med. Genet.* 23:157–169.

Fryns, J. P., A. Kleczkowska, A. Dereymaeker, M. Hoefnagels, G. Heremans, J. Marien, and H. van den Berghe. 1986. A genetic-diagnostic survey in an institutionalized population of 173 severely mentally retarded patients. *Clin. Genet.* 30:315–323.

Fu, Y. H., D. P. A. Kuhl, A. Pizzuti, M. Pieretti, J. S. Sutcliffe, S. Richards, A. J. M. H. Verkerk, J. J. A. Holden, R. G. Fenwick, S. T. Warren, B. A. Oostra, D. L. Nelson, and C. T. Caskey. 1991. Variation of the CGG repeat at the fragile X site results in genetic instability: Resolution of the Sherman paradox. *Cell* 67:1047–1058.

Giovannucci-Uzielli, M-L., S. Guarducci, E. Lapi, A. Cecconi, U. Ricci, G. Ricotti, C. Biondi, B. Scarselli, F. Vieri, P. Scarnato, F. Gori, and A. Sereni. 1999. Premature ovarian failure (POF) and fragile X premutation females: From POF to fragile X carrier identification, from fragile X carrier diagnosis to POF association data. *Am. J. Med. Genet.* 84:300–303.

Giraud, F., S. Ayme, and M. G. Mattei. 1976. Constitutional chromosomal breakage. *Hum. Genet.* 34:125–136.

Goldman, A., A. Krause, and T. Jenkins. 1997. Fragile X syndrome occurs in the South African black population [editorial]. *S. Afr. Med. J.* 87:418–420.

Gustavson, K. H., G. Holmgren, R. Jonsell, and H. K. Blomquist. 1977. Severe mental retardation in children in a northern Swedish county. *J. Ment. Defic. Res.* 21:161–180.

Gustavson, K. H., H. K. Blomquist, and G. Holmgren. 1986. Prevalence of the fragile-X syndrome in mentally retarded boys in a Swedish county. *Am. J. Med. Genet.* 23:581–587.

Haddad, L. A., M. J. Aguiar, S. S. Costa, R. C. Mingroni-Netto, A. M. Vianna-Morgante, and S. D. Pena. 1999. Fully mutated and gray-zone FRAXA alleles in Brazilian mentally retarded boys. *Am. J. Med. Genet.* 84:198–201.

Hagerman, R. J., P. Wilson, L. W. Staley, K. A. Lang, T. Fan, C. Uhlhorn, S. Jewell-Smart, C. Hull, J. Drisko, K. Flom, and A. K. Taylor. 1994. Evaluation of school children at high risk for fragile X syndrome utilizing buccal cell FMR-1 testing. *Am. J. Med. Genet.* 51:474–481.

Harvey, J., C. Judge, and S. Weiner. 1977. Familial X-linked mental retardation with an X chromosome abnormality. *J. Med. Genet.* 14:46–50.

Heitz, D., D. Devys, G. Imbert, C. Kretz, and J. L. Mandel. 1992. Inheritance of the fragile X syndrome: Size of the fragile X premutation is a major determinant of the transition to full mutation. *J. Med. Genet.* 29:794–801.

Herbst, D. S., and J. R. Miller. 1980. Nonspecific X-linked mental retardation: II. The frequency in British Columbia. *Am. J. Med. Genet.* 7:461–469.

Hirst, M. C., P. K. Grewal, and K. E. Davies. 1994. Precursor arrays for triplet repeat expansion at the fragile X locus. *Hum. Mol. Genet.* 3:1553–1560.

Holden, J. A., M. Chalifaux, M. Wing, C. Julien-Inalsingh, J. S. Lawson, J. V. Higgins, S. Sherman, and B. N. White. 1995. Distribution and frequency of *FMR1* CGG repeat numbers in the general population. *Dev. Brain Dysfunct.* 8:405–407.

Howard-Peebles, P. N., and G. R. Stoddard. 1980. Race distribution in X-linked mental retardation with macro-orchidism and fragile site in Xq. *Am. J. Hum. Genet.* 32:629–630.

Hundscheid, R. D. L., E. A. Sistermans, C. M. G. Thomas, D. D. M. Braat, H. Straatman, L. A. L. M. Kiemeney, B. A. Oostra, and A. P. T. Smits. 2000a. Imprinting effect in premature ovarian failure confined to paternally inherited fragile X premutations. *Am. J. Hum. Genet.* 66:413–418.

Hundscheid, R. D. L., C. M. G. Thomas, D. D. M. Braat, B. A. Oostra, and A. P. T. Smits.

2000b. Call for verification of imprinting effect in premature ovarian failure in fragile X premutations. *Am. J. Hum. Genet.* 67:256–258.

Jacobs, P. A., and S. L. Sherman. 1985. The fragile(X): A marker for the Martin-Bell syndrome. *Dis. Markers* 3:9–25.

Jacobs, P. A., M. Mayer, and E. Rudak. 1979. More on marker X chromosomes, mental retardation and macro-orchidism. *N. Engl. J. Med.* 300:737–738.

Jacobs, P. A., T. W. Glover, M. Mayer, P. Fox, J. W. Gerrard, H. Dunn, and D. S. Herbst. 1980. X-linked mental retardation: A study of 7 families. *Am. J. Med. Genet.* 7:471–489.

Johnson, G. E. 1897. Contribution to the psychology and pedagogy of feeble-minded children. *J. Psycho-asthenics* 2:26–32.

Kähkönen, M., T. Alitalo, E. Airaksinen, R. Matilainen, K. Launiala, S. Autio, and J. Leisti. 1987. Prevalence of the fragile X syndrome in four birth cohorts of children of school age. *Hum. Genet.* 77:85–87.

Kenneson, A., D. W. Cramer, and S. T. Warren. 1997. Fragile X premutations are not a major cause of early menopause. *Am. J. Hum. Genet.* 61:1362–1369.

Kunst, C. B., and S. T. Warren. 1994. Cryptic and polar variation of the fragile X repeat could result in predisposing normal alleles. *Cell* 77:853–861.

Lachiewicz, A. M., G. A. Spiridigliozzi, A. McConkie-Rosell, D. Burgess, Y. Feng, S. T. Warren, and J. Tarleton. 1996. A fragile X male with a broad smear on Southern blot analysis representing 100–500 CGG repeats and no methylation at the *Eag* I site of the *FMR-1* gene. *Am. J. Med. Genet.* 64:278–282.

Lehrke, R. G. 1974. X-linked mental retardation and verbal disability. In D. Bergsma (ed.), *Birth defects: Original article series.* New York: National Foundation, pp. 1–100.

Losowsky, M. S. 1961. Hereditary mental defect showing the pattern of sex influence. *J. Ment. Defic. Res.* 5:60–62.

Lubs, H. A. 1969. A marker X chromosome. *Am. J. Hum Genet.* 21:231–244.

Marozzi, A., W. Vegetti, E. Manfredini, M. G. Tibiletti, G. Testa, P. G. Crosignani, E. Ginelli, R. Meneveri, and L. Dalpra. 2000. Association between idiopathic premature ovarian failure and fragile X premutation. *Hum. Reprod.* 15:197–202.

Martin, J. P., and J. Bell. 1943. A pedigree of mental defect showing sex linkage. *J. Neurol. Psychiatry* 6:154–157.

Mazzocco, M. M., N. L. Sonna, J. T. Teisl, A. Pinit, B. K. Shapiro, N. Shah, and A. L. Reiss. 1997. The *FMR1* and *FMR2* mutations are not common etiologies of academic difficulty among school-age children. *J. Dev. Behav. Pediatr.* 18:392–398.

Mazzocco, M. M., G. F. Myers, J. L. Hamner, R. Panoscha, B. K. Shapiro, and A. L. Reiss. 1998. The prevalence of the *FMR1* and *FMR2* mutations among preschool children with language delay. *J. Pediatr.* 132:795–801.

McConkie-Rosell, A., A. M. Lachiewicz, G. A. Spiridigliozzi, J. Tarleton, S. Schoenwald, M. C. Phelan, P. Goonewardena, X. Ding, and W. T. Brown. 1993. Evidence that methylation of the FMR-1 locus is responsible for variable phenotypic expression of the fragile X syndrome. *Am. J. Hum. Genet.* 53:800–809.

McConkie-Rosell, A., G. A. Spiridigliozzi, T. Iafolla, J. Tarleton, and A. M. Lachiewicz. 1997. Carrier testing in the fragile X syndrome: Attitudes and opinions of obligate carriers. *Am. J. Med. Genet.* 68:62–69.

McConkie-Rosell, A., G. A. Spiridigliozzi, K. Rounds, D. V. Dawson, J. A. Sullivan, D. Burgess, and A. M. Lachiewicz. 1999. Parental attitudes regarding carrier testing in children at risk for fragile X syndrome. *Am. J. Med. Genet.* 82:206–211.

McConkie-Rosell, A., G. A. Spiridigliozzi, J. A. Sullivan, D. V. Dawson, and A. M. Lachiewicz. 2000. Carrier testing in the fragile X syndrome: Effect on self-concept. *Am. J. Med. Genet.* 92:336–342.

Meadows, K. L., and S. L. Sherman. 1996. Fragile X syndrome: Examination of issues pertaining to population-based screening. *Screening* 4:175–192.

Millan, J. M., F. Martinez, A. Cadroy, J. Gandia, M. Casquero, M. Beneyto, L. Badia, and F. Prieto. 1999. Screening for *FMR1* mutations among the mentally retarded: Prevalence of the fragile X syndrome in Spain [letter]. *Clin. Genet.* 56:98–99.

Mornet, E., B. Simon-Bouy, and J. L. Serre. 1998. The intermediate alleles of the fragile X CGG repeat in patients with mental retardation [abstract]. *Clin. Genet.* 53:200–201.

Morton, N. E., D. C. Rao, H. Lang-Brown, C. J. Maclean, R. D. Bart, and R. Lew. 1977. Colchester revisited: A genetic study of mental defect. *J. Med. Genet.* 14:1–9.

Mulley, J. C., and G. R. Sutherland. 1987. Letter to the editor: Fragile X transmission and the determination of carrier probabilities for genetic counseling. *Am. J. Med. Genet.* 26:987–990.

Murray, A., S. Youings, N. Dennis, L. Latsky, P. Linehan, N. McKechnie, J. Macpherson, M. Pound, and P. Jacobs. 1996. Population screening at the FRAXA and FRAXE loci: Molecular analyses of boys with learning difficulties and their mothers. *Hum. Mol. Genet.* 5:727–735.

Murray, A., J. N. Macpherson, M. C. Pound, A. Sharrock, S. A. Youings, N. R. Dennis, N. McKechnie, P. Linehan, N. E. Morton, and P. A. Jacobs. 1997. The role of size, sequence and haplotype in the stability of FRAXA and FRAXE alleles during transmission. *Hum. Mol. Genet.* 6:173–184.

Murray, A., J. Webb, S. Grimley, G. Conway, and P. Jacobs. 1998. Studies of FRAXA and FRAXE in women with premature ovarian failure. *J. Med. Genet.* 35:637–640.

Murray, A., J. Webb, F. MacSwiney, E. L. Shipley, N. E. Morton, and G. S. Conway. 1999. Serum concentrations of follicle stimulating hormone may predict premature ovarian failure in FRAXA premutation women. *Hum. Reprod.* 14:1217–1218.

Murray, A., S. Ennis, and N. Morton. 2000a. No evidence for parent of origin influencing premature ovarian failure in fragile X premutation carriers. *Am. J. Hum. Genet.* 67:253–254.

Murray, A., S. Ennis, F. MacSwiney, J. Webb, and N. E. Morton. 2000b. Reproductive and menstrual history of females with fragile X expansions. *Eur. J. Hum. Genet.* 8:247–252.

Murray, J., H. Cuckle, G. Taylor, and J. Hewison. 1997. Screening for fragile X syndrome: Information needs for health planners. *J. Med. Screen.* 4:60–94.

Neri, G., and P. Chiurazzi. 1999. X-linked mental retardation. *Adv. Genet.* 41:55–94.

———. 2000. X-linked mental retardation. *Am. J. Med. Genet. (Semin. Med. Genet.)* 97:173.

Nolin, S. L., A. Glicksman, G. E. J. Houck, W. T. Brown, and C. S. Dobkin. 1994. Mosaicism in fragile X affected males. *Am. J. Med. Genet.* 51:509–512.

Nolin, S. L., F. A. Lewis, L. L. Ye, G. E. Houck, A. E. Glicksman, P. Limprasert, S. Y. Li, N. Zhong, A. E. Ashley, E. Feingold, S. L. Sherman, and W. T. Brown. 1996. Familial transmission of the *FMR1* CGG repeat. *Am. J. Hum. Genet.* 59:1252–1261.

Patsalis, P. C. 1999. *FMR1* repeat analysis in patients with ovarian dysfunction or failure. *Am. J. Med. Genet.* 83:329–330.

Patsalis, P. C., C. Sismani, J. A. Hettinger, I. Boumba, I. Georgiou, G. Stylianidou, V. Anastasiadou, R. Koukoulli, G. Pagoulatos, and M. Syrrou. 1999. Molecular screening of fragile X (FRAXA) and FRAXE mental retardation syndromes in the Hellenic population of Greece and Cyprus: Incidence, genetic variation and stability. *Am. J. Med. Genet.* 84:184–190.

Penrose, L. S. 1938. A clinical and genetic study of 1,280 cases of mental defect. *Ment. Res. Council Special Report Ser.* 229.

Pesso, R., M. Berkenstadt, H. Cuckle, E. Gak, L. Peleg, M. Frydman, and G. Barkai. 2000. Screening for fragile X syndrome in women of reproductive age. *Prenat. Diagn.* 20:611–614.

Pieretti, M., F. Zhang, Y. H. Fu, S. T. Warren, B. A. Oostra, C. T. Caskey, and D. L. Nelson. 1991. Absence of expression of the FMR-1 gene in fragile X syndrome. *Cell* 66:817–822.

Priest, J. H., H. C. Thuline, G. D. LaVeck, and D. B. Jarvis. 1961. An approach to genetic factors in mental retardation. *Am. J. Ment. Defic.* 66:42–50.

Reiss, A. L., H. H. Kazazian, C. M. Krebs, A. McAughan, C. D. Boehm, M. T. Abrams, and D. L. Nelson. 1994. Frequency and stability of the fragile X premutation. *Hum. Mol. Genet.* 3:393–398.

Renpenning, H., J. W. Gerrard, W. A. Zaleski, and T. Tabata. 1962. Familial sex-linked mental retardation. *Can. Med. Assoc. J.* 87:954–956.

Richards, B. W., and T. Webb. 1982. The Martin-Bell-Renpenning syndrome. *J. Med. Genet.* 19:79.

Rousseau, F., D. Heitz, V. Biancalana, S. Blumenfeld, C. Kretz, J. Boue, N. Tommerup, C. Van Der Hagen, C. DeLozier-Blanchet, and M. F. Croquette. 1991. Direct diagnosis by DNA analysis of the fragile X syndrome of mental retardation [see comments]. *N. Engl. J. Med.* 325:1673–1681.

Rousseau, F., D. Heitz, J. Tarleton, J. Macpherson, H. Malmgren, N. Dahl, A. Barnicoat, et al. 1994. A multicenter study on genotype-phenotype correlations in fragile X syndrome, using direct diagnosis with probe StB128: The first 2,253 cases. *Am. J. Hum. Genet.* 55:225–237.

Rousseau, F., P. Rouillard, M-L. Morel, E. W. Khandjian, and K. Morgan. 1995. Prevalence of carriers of premutation-sized alleles of the FMR1 gene—and implications for the population genetics of the fragile X syndrome. *Am. J. Hum. Genet.* 57:1006–1018.

Rousseau, F., M. L. Morel, P. Rouillard, E. W. Khandjian, and K. Morgan. 1996. Surprisingly low prevalence of *FMR1* premutations among males from the general population [abstract]. *Am. J. Hum. Genet.* 59 (suppl.): A188;1069.

Ruangdaraganon, N., P. Limprasert, T. Sura, T. Sombuntham, N. Sriwongpanich, and N. Kotchabhakdi. 2000. Prevalence and clinical characteristics of fragile X syndrome at child development clinic, Ramathibodi Hospital. *J. Med. Assoc. Thai.* 83:69–76.

Ruvalcaba, R. H. A., S. A. Myhre, E. C. Roosen-Runge, and J. B. Beckwith. 1977. X-linked mental deficiency megalotestes syndrome. *JAMA* 238:1646–1650.

Ryynanen, M., S. Heinonen, M. Makkonen, E. Kajanoja, A. Mannermaa, and K. Pertti. 1999. Feasibility and acceptance of screening for fragile X mutations in low-risk pregnancies. *Eur. J. Hum. Genet.* 7:212–216.

Schwartz, C. E., J. Dean, P. N. Howard-Peebles, M. Bugge, M. Mikkelsen, N. Tommerup, C. Hull, R. Hagerman, J. J. Holden, and R. E. Stevenson. 1994. Obstetrical and gynecological complications in fragile X carriers: A multicenter study. *Am. J. Med. Genet.* 51:400–402.

Sherman, S. 1995. Modeling the natural history of the fragile X gene. *Ment. Retard. Dev. Disabil. Res. Rev.* 1:263–269.

Sherman, S. L. 2000a. Premature ovarian failure among fragile X premutation carriers: Parent-of-origin effect? *Am. J. Hum. Genet.* 67:11–13.

Sherman, S. L. 2000b. Seminars in Genetics: Premature ovarian failure in the fragile X syndrome. *Am. J. Med. Genet.* 97:189–194.

Sherman, S. L., N. E. Morton, P. A. Jacobs, and G. Turner. 1984. The marker (X) syndrome: A cotygenetic and genetic analysis. *Ann. Hum. Genet.* 48:21–37.

Sherman, S. L., P. A. Jacobs, N. E. Morton, U. Froster-Iskenius, P. N. Howard-Peebles, K. B. Nielsen, M. W. Partington, G. R. Sutherland, G. Turner, and M. Watson. 1985. Further segregation analysis of the fragile X syndrome with special reference to transmitting males. *Hum. Genet.* 69:289–299.

Sherman, S. L., K. L. Meadows, and A. E. Ashley. 1996. Examination of factors that influence the expansion of the fragile X mutation in a sample of conceptuses from known carrier females. *Am. J. Med. Genet.* 64:256–260.

Snow, K., L. K. Doud, R. Hagerman, R. G. Pergolizzi, S. H. Erster, and S. N. Thibodeau. 1993. Analysis of a CGG sequence at the FMR-1 locus in fragile X families and in the general population. *Am. J. Hum. Genet.* 53:1217–1228.

Snow, K., D. J. Tester, K. E. Kruckeberg, D. J. Schaid, and S. N. Thibodeau. 1994. Sequence analysis of the fragile X trinucleotide repeat: Implications for the origin of the fragile X mutation. *Hum. Mol. Genet.* 3:1543–1551.

Snyder, R. D., and A. Robinson. 1969. Recessive sex-linked mental retardation in the absence of other recognizable abnormalities. *Clin. Pediatr.* 8:669–674.

Spence, W. C., S. H. Black, L. Fallon, A. Maddalena, E. Cummings, G. Menapace-Drew, D. P. Bick, G. Levinson, J. D. Schulman, and P. N. Howard-Peebles. 1996. Molecular fragile X screening in normal populations. *Am. J. Med. Genet.* 64:181–183.

Sutcliffe, J. S., D. L. Nelson, F. Zhang, M. Pieretti, C. T. Caskey, D. Saxe, and S. T. Warren. 1992. DNA methylation represses FMR-1 transcription in fragile X syndrome. *Hum. Mol. Genet.* 1:397–400.

Sutherland, G. R. 1977. Fragile sites on human chromosomes: Demonstration of their dependence on the type of tissue culture medium. *Science* 197:265–266.

Syrrou, M., I. Georgiou, M. Grigoriadou, M. B. Petersen, S. Kitsiou, G. Pagoulatos, and P. C. Patsalis. 1998. FRAXA and FRAXE prevalence in patients with nonspecific mental retardation in the Hellenic population. *Genet. Epidemiol.* 15:103–109.

Tan, B. S., H. Y. Law, Y. Zhao, C. S. Yoon, and I. S. Ng. 2000. DNA testing for fragile

X syndrome in 255 males from special schools in Singapore. *Ann. Acad. Med. Singapore* 29:207–212.

Tassone, F., R. J. Hagerman, A. K. Taylor, L. W. Gane, T. E. Godfrey, and P. J. Hagerman. 2000. Elevated levels of *FMR1* mRNA in carrier males: A new mechanism of involvement in the fragile X syndrome. *Am. J. Hum. Genet.* 66:6–15.

Turner, G., and B. Turner. 1974. X-linked mental retardation. *J. Med. Genet.* 11:109–113.

Turner, G., B. Turner, and E. Collins. 1971. X-linked mental retardation without physical abnormality: Renpenning's syndrome. *Dev. Med. Child Neurol.* 13:71–78.

Turner, G., C. Eastman, J. Casey, A. McLeary, P. Procopis, and B. Turner. 1975. X-linked mental retardation associated with macro-orchidism. *J. Med. Genet.* 12:367–371.

Turner, G., R. Till, and A. Daniel. 1978. Marker X chromosomes, mental retardation and macro-orchidism. *N. Engl. J. Med.* 299:1472.

Turner, G., A. Daniel, and M. Frost. 1980. X-linked mental retardation, macro-orchidism, and the Xq27 fragile site. *J. Pediatr.* 96:837–841.

Turner, G., J. Opitz, W. Brown, K. Davies, P. Jacobs, E. Jenkins, M. Mikkelsen, M. Partington, and G. Sutherland. 1986a. Conference report: Second International Workshop in the Fragile X and X-linked Mental Retardation. *Am. J. Med. Genet.* 23:11–67.

Turner, G., H. Robinson, S. Laing, and S. Purvis-Smith. 1986b. Preventive screening for the fragile X syndrome. *N. Engl. J. Med.* 315:607–609.

Turner, G., H. Robinson, S. Wake, and N. Martin. 1994. Dizygous twinning and premature menopause in fragile X syndrome [letter; see comments]. *Lancet* 344:1500.

Turner, G., T. Webb, S. Wake, and H. Robinson. 1996. Prevalence of fragile X syndrome. *Am. J. Med. Genet.* 64:196–197.

Verkerk, A. J. M. H., M. Pieretti, J. S. Sutcliffe, Y. Fu, D. P. A. Kuhl, A. Pizzuti, O. Reiner. S. Richards, M. F. Victoria, F. Zhang, B. E. Eussen, G. B. van Ommen, L. A. J. Blonden, G. J. Riggins, J. L. Chastain, C. B. Kunst, H. Galjaard, C. T. Caskey, D. L. Nelson, B. A. Oostra, and S. A. Warren. 1991. Identification of a gene (FMR-1) containing a CGG repeat coincident with a breakpoint cluster region exhibiting length variation in fragile X syndrome. *Cell* 65:905–914.

Vianna-Morgante, A. M., and S. S. Costa. 2000. Premature ovarian failure is associated with maternally and paternally inherited premutation in Brazilian fragile X families. *Am. J. Hum. Genet.* 67:254–255.

Webb, T. P., S. Bundey, A. Thake, and J. Todd. 1986. The frequency of the fragile X chromosome among school children in Coventry. *J. Med. Genet.* 23:396–399.

Wildhagen, M. F., T. A. M. van Os, J. J. Polder, L. P. ten Kate, and J. D. F. Habbema. 1998. Explorative study of costs, effects and savings of screening for female fragile X premutation and full mutation carriers in the general population. *Community Genet.* 1:36–47.

Wolff, G., H. Hameister, and H. H. Ropers. 1978. X-linked mental retardation: Transmission of the trait of an apparently unaffected male. *Am. J. Med. Genet.* 2:217–224.

Wolff, P. H., J. Gardner, J. Lappen, J. Paccia, and D. Meryash. 1988. Variable expression of the fragile X syndrome in heterozygous females of normal intelligence. *Am. J. Med. Genet.* 30:213–225.

Wortis, H., M. Pollack, and J. Wortis. 1966. Families with two or more mentally retarded or mentally disturbed siblings: The preponderance of males. *Am. J. Ment. Defic.* 70: 745–752.

Wright, S. W., G. Tarjan, and L. Eyer. 1959. Investigation of families with two or more mentally retarded siblings. *Am. J. Dis. Child.* 97:445–463.

Youings, S. A., A. Murray, N. Dennis, S. Ennis, C. Lewis, N. McKechnie, M. Pound, A. Sharrock, and P. Jacobs. 2000. FRAXA and FRAXE: The results of a five year survey. *J. Med. Genet.* 37:415–421.

Yu, S., M. Pritchard, E. Kermer, M. Lynch, J. Nancarrow, E. Baker, K. Holman, J. C. Mulley, S. T. Warren, D. Schlessinger, G. R. Sutherland, and R. I. Richards. 1991. Fragile X genotype characterized by an unstable region of DNA. *Science* 252:1179–1181.

Yu, S., J. Mulley, D. Loesch, G. Turner, A. Donnelly, A. Gedeon, D. Hillen, E. Kremer, M. Lynch, M. Pritchard, G. R. Sutherland, and R. I. Richards. 1992. Fragile-X syndrome: Unique genetics of the heritable unstable element. *Am. J. Hum. Genet.* 50: 968–980.

Zhong, N., W. Yang, C. Dobkin, and W. T. Brown. 1995. Fragile X gene instability: Anchoring AGGs and linked microsatellites [see comments]. *Am. J. Hum. Genet.* 57: 351–361.

# CHAPTER 4

# *FMR1* Protein Studies and Animal Model for Fragile X Syndrome

Ben A. Oostra, Ph.D., and Andre T. Hoogeveen, Ph.D.

Since the identification of the *FMR1* gene in 1991, much has become known about its gene expression. The polymorphic CGG repeat resides within the first exon of the gene and is located 250 bp downstream of the CpG island that may serve as the promoter of the *FMR1* gene (Eichler et al. 1993; Hwu et al. 1993). The fragile X syndrome is caused by a mutation in the *FMR1* gene resulting in a loss of function of the *FMR1* gene product. The *FMR1* gene is silenced in most fragile X patients because of methylation of the CpG island (Pieretti et al. 1991; Sutcliffe et al. 1992; see chap. 12). Although the two main clinical features of fragile X syndrome, mental retardation and macroorchidism, indicate that brain and testis are tissues where the *FMR1* RNA is present, in situ RNA hybridization has revealed a widespread distribution of *FMR1* transcripts in human and mouse tissues (Abitbol et al. 1993; Hinds et al. 1993). The *FMR1* gene is expressed as a 4.4 kb transcript in most tissues, albeit at different levels. On Northern analysis of human tissues, high expression is observed in brain, placenta, testis, lung, and kidney (Hinds et al. 1993). Low expression was found in liver, skeletal muscle, and pancreas.

## The Characterization of *FMR1* Gene Product

For the characterization of the FMR1 protein (FMRP), different monoclonal and polyclonal antibodies have been used (Devys et al. 1993; Siomi et al. 1993; Verheij et al. 1993). As a result of alternative splicing, multiple FMRP bands were detected with these antibodies, which were FMRP specific as demonstrated by their absence in male fragile X patients, as illustrated in figure 4.1

*Fragile X Syndrome: Diagnosis, Treatment, and Research,* third edition, ed. Randi Jenssen Hagerman and Paul J. Hagerman (Baltimore: Johns Hopkins University Press, 2002), © The Johns Hopkins University Press.

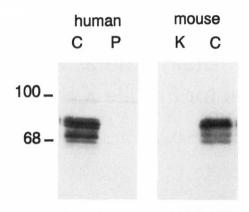

**Fig. 4.1.** The expression of *FMR1* protein. Imunoprecipitation and Western blotting of human lymphoblastoid cell lines or mouse brain tissues with polyclonal antibodies (Verheij et al. 1993) against FMRP. *C*, control; *P,* fragile X patient; *K,* knockout mouse.

(Devys et al. 1993; Verheij et al. 1993). The antibodies recognize proteins with apparent molecular weights ranging from 67 to 80 kDa.

The CGG repeat, which is confined to the 5′ untranslated region of the *FMR1* gene and is located 69 bases in front of the start ATG, has also been conserved during evolution in many species (Ashley et al. 1993b; Deelen et al. 1994). This might point to an important regulatory role at the DNA and/or RNA level. The CGG repeat in the *FMR1* gene is possibly a protein binding motif and has been shown to bind a protein denoted CCG-BP1 (Richards et al. 1993). This protein has not yet been characterized further. The CGG repeat-binding protein (CGGBP1 or p20) binds specifically to nonmethylated, but not to methylated, 5′-(CGG)(n)-3′ repeats in the promoter of the *FMR1* gene (Deissler et al. 1996). The CGG binding protein is targeted to the nucleus and affects the activity of the *FMR1* promoter (Muller-Hartmann et al. 2000).

The multiple FMRP bands represent different isoforms generated by alternative splicing (Ashley et al. 1993b; Verheij et al. 1993; Verkerk et al. 1993). Because of alternative splicing of the precursor messenger RNA (mRNA) at three different locations in the gene, the *FMR1* gene can give rise to as many as 12 partially different molecules and thus 12 possible proteins, which differ in various internal segments. The alternative splicing in *FMR1* does not seem to be tissue specific, for no differences were detected between various tissues analyzed (Verkerk et al. 1993). In these splicing events, involving exons 12, 15, and 17, the open reading frame is maintained (fig. 4.2*A*). This results in different proteins that share the same N- and C-terminus. The longest possible tran-

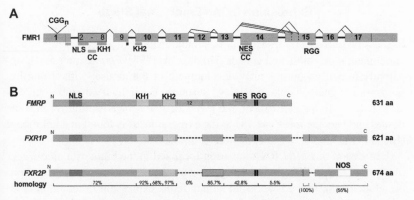

**Fig. 4.2.** Schematic drawing of the *FMR1* gene and the *FMR1, FXR1,* and *FXR2* proteins. *A:* Part of the genomic structure of the *FMR1* gene showing the introns as *lines* and exons as *boxes.* Places of alternative splicing are indicated. The positions of the KH domains, RGG box, NES, NLS, and cc (coiled-coiled domain) are given. *B:* Alignment of the *FMR1, FXR1,* and *FXR2* proteins. The percentage of homology is given at the *bottom.* The positions of the domains are given.

script codes for a protein of 631 amino acids, the smallest for 568 amino acids. In addition, alternative splicing involving exon 14 was identified in both human and mouse. The exclusion of exon 14 causes a frameshift in the open reading frame. Exon 13 can be joined to several splice acceptor sites in exon 15. As a result of skipping exon 14, multiple protein isoforms are predicted with new amino acid sequences at the C-terminus. Skipping of exon 14 is a minor event, as all protein bands seen in figure 4.1 are recognized by antibodies that are raised against the C-terminus of the longest open reading frame, containing exon 17 (Verheij et al. 1993).

The *FMR1* gene is highly conserved among different species (Verkerk et al. 1991). The murine homolog Fmrp shows about 97% identity in the predicted amino acid sequence with the human FMRP (Ashley et al. 1993b). Also, in mouse and monkey a heterogeneous subset of proteins with apparent molecular weight between 67 and 80 kDa was observed, as is illustrated in figure 4.1 (Khandjian et al. 1995; Verheij et al. 1995). In some human, monkey, and murine tissues, low molecular mass *FMR1* proteins (33–52 kDA) were found, which have the same N-terminus as the 67–80 kDa isoforms but differ in their C-terminus. These proteins are most likely the results of carboxy-terminal proteolytic cleavage. Using high-resolution two-dimensional gel electrophoresis, it was shown that at least 10 independent isoforms could be detected in the mouse (Khandjian et al. 1995).

## Expression in the Embryonal Stage

Expression of the *Fmr1* transcripts was found in early mouse embryos with an enrichment in the brain and gonads (Hinds et al. 1993). *Fmr1* expression is apparently turned on during early development of the mouse, with strong hybridization signals visible at 10 days gestation throughout all embryonic tissues. Later during development, the levels of *Fmr1* mRNA diminish in some tissues and become more specific to the expression, as is found in adult mouse (Bakker et al. 2000a; De Diego Otero et al. 2000).

Expression of *FMR1* RNA has been localized in the brain of a nine-week-old fetus in the proliferating and migrating tissues of the nervous system (Abitbol et al. 1993). In a 25-week-old human fetus, expression in the brain is restricted mainly to cholinergic neurons, with highest expression being present in nucleus basalis magnocellularis and the pyramidal neurons of the hippocampus.

It is not yet clear at what point in development the methylation and subsequent loss of *FMR1* expression in fragile X patients occurs. The majority of chorion villus samples of a male fetus have been found to be undermethylated when carrying a full mutation (Rousseau et al. 1991). In one chorion villus sample obtained early during pregnancy (11 weeks), the *FMR1* gene was not methylated and the gene was transcribed, whereas in fetal tissues obtained at 13 weeks of gestation, nearly complete *FMR1* methylation was demonstrated and hardly any mRNA and protein could be detected (Losekoot et al. 1997; Sutcliffe et al. 1992; Willemsen et al. 1996b). It may be that methylation of the *FMR1* gene takes place relatively late in the embryo and that the *FMR1* gene is expressed from conception onward during early development, even of an affected fetus. However, no obvious differences were found between affected males with a full mutation and males who have a deletion in the *FMR1* gene (Gedeon et al. 1992; Wöhrle et al. 1992). As a result, no FMRP was produced during embryonal development, suggesting no crucial role for FMRP in early embryonic development.

## Expression in the Adult Stage

In situ RNA expression studies in adult mice tissues showed high levels of *Fmr1* mRNA in brain, testis, ovaries, thymus, esophagus, and spleen. Moderate levels of expression were detected in kidney, liver, and lung, while no expression was observed in heart, aorta, and muscle tissues (Hinds et al. 1993). Similar levels of expression were described by Khandjian et al. by testing the presence of Fmrp in different murine tissues using immunoblot analysis (Khandjian et al. 1995). However, they found very low expression of Fmrp in heart and muscle.

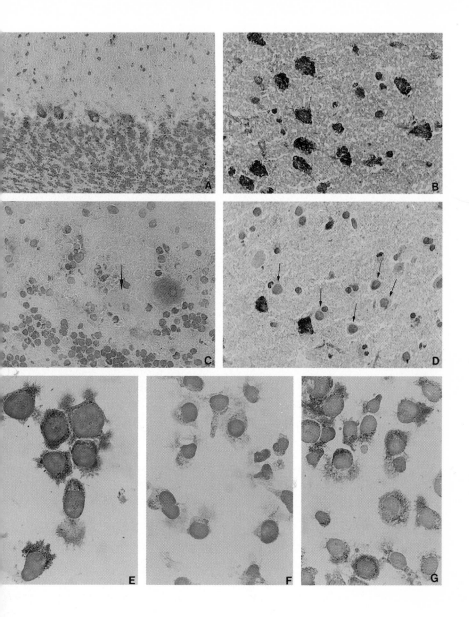

**Fig. 4.3.** The expression of FMRP in different tissues using monoclonal 1A1 (Devys et al. 1993). Immunostaining for *FMR1* protein in cerebellum (*A* and *C*), cortex (*B* and *D*), and EBV-transformed lymphocytes (*E–G*) from healthy individuals (*A, B,* and *E*) and patients with the fragile X syndrome (*C, D, F,* and *G*). *G:* A patient with a point mutation. *Arrows* indicate the absence of FMRP in Purkinje cells (*C*) and neurons of the cortex (*D*) in a fragile X patient.

No differences in the expression pattern of Fmrp isoforms were observed in different murine tissues (Khandjian et al. 1995; Verheij et al. 1995).

In mouse brain, expression was predominantly found in neurons, while no expression was found in the white matter or glial cells (Hinds et al. 1993). Expression was most intense in the granular layers of the hippocampus and cerebellum (Bakker et al. 2000a). Intermediate expression was found in the cerebral cortex. In the rat frontal cortical neurons in vivo, immunostaining of FMRP has been shown to be distributed in perikaryon and through dendrites (Feng et al. 1997b). In addition, some axonal staining has also been detected. In the mouse testis, expression was observed in the tubuli (Bächner et al. 1993b).

The expression of FMRP in neurons (fig. 4.3*B*) and not in the supporting cells in a human brain was confirmed by immunohistochemical analysis (Devys et al. 1993; Tamanini et al. 1997). In the cerebellum Purkinje cells also show high expression of FMRP (fig. 4.3*A*). Expression can sometimes be found in neurons of fragile X patients because of the mosaic nature of the fragile X mutation. The percentage of cells that express FMRP depends on the percentage of cells that have a premutation allele, which is, in the example shown, only 1% of the neurons of the cerebellum and the cortex. Only a small section of the cerebellum and the cortex is shown in figure 4.3, *C* and *D*. In human testis, FMRP is observed in the tubuli, in the spermatogonia (Devys et al. 1993; Tamanini et al. 1997). In male fragile X patients with a full mutation in somatic tissues, a premutation is found in sperm cells (Reyniers et al. 1993). In the testis of a fragile X patient, FMRP expression was observed in the early spermatogonia, at the same location where it is present in normal males (De Graaff et al. 1995). Therefore, it was suggested (Bächner et al. 1993a) that FMRP has a special function in the male gonad. However, this could be rejected, as normal spermatogenesis was observed in a male with a deletion in the *FMR1* gene (Meijer et al. 1994), and mice that lack Fmrp show normal fertility (Bakker et al. 1994).

## FMRP Is an RNA Binding Protein

Analysis of the predicted amino acids of FMRP revealed sequences characteristic of RNA binding proteins. FMRP contains two KH domains in the middle of the protein at amino acid positions 222–251 and 285–314, respectively (fig. 4.2*A*) (Ashley et al. 1993a; Siomi et al. 1993). KH domains were found originally in the heterogeneous nuclear ribonucleoprotein (hnRNP) K protein that is involved in the biogenesis of mRNA. The KH domain has been identified in several other proteins that are known to be RNA binding proteins. These include the archaebacterial ribosomal protein S3 and the yeast meiosis-specific splicing regulator *MER*1. The two FMRP KH domains show 100% identity among the human, mouse, and chicken homologs (Ashley et al. 1993a). In an RNA homopolymer binding assay, FMRP showed strong binding to polyguanylic acid [poly(G)] and polyuridylic acid [poly(U)]. Ashley et al. showed that FMRP is binding in vitro to approximately 4% of human fetal brain messages, including its own message (Ashley et al. 1993a). None of these RNAs has been characterized yet. A 2:1 stoichiometry of binding of RNA:protein is reported, which implies that each *FMR1* protein molecule has the potential to interact with two RNA molecules. Important evidence that the KH domain is critical for the FMRP function is the finding of a patient with the fragile X phenotype, lacking a CGG repeat amplification, who has an I304N (sometimes referred to as I364N) point mutation in one of the most highly conserved residues of the second KH domain (Ashley et al. 1993a; De Boulle et al. 1993; Siomi et al. 1993). This amino acid substitution in an in vitro produced FMRP interferes with RNA homopolymer binding under high salt concentrations (Siomi et al. 1994; Verheij et al. 1995). This I304N substitution in the FMRP did not alter the translation, processing, and localization of FMRP in lymphoblastoid cells from the patient (Verheij et al. 1995). All of the high molecular mass *FMR1* proteins in lymphoblastoid cells from this patient were able to bind RNA but had a reduced affinity for RNA binding at high salt concentrations in comparison with control (Verheij et al. 1995). The structure of the first KH module of FMRP was solved by nuclear magnetic resonance (NMR) (Musco et al. 1996). This information has important consequences for the interpretation of published mutants and in demonstrating conclusively that a KH motif is autonomously able to bind to RNA. The effect of an I304N mutation (that occurs in the second KH of FMRP), mapped at the N-terminus of the second helix of the KH fold, leads to disrupture of the domain with consequent impairment of RNA binding.

In addition, FMRP shows two RGG boxes toward the carboxyl end (Ashley et al. 1993a; Siomi et al. 1993) (Fig. 4.2*A*). The RGG boxes have been demonstrated to have RNA binding activity and are found in several nuclear RNA binding proteins. The involvement of the RGG box in the RNA binding ability of FMRP has been shown by the inability of FMRP, lacking the RGG box, to bind RNA (Siomi et al. 1993). These studies suggest that FMRP has an RNA binding function in the cell and that FMRP by its interaction with a selective number of RNAs in the cell could play a role in the pleiotropic phenotype of the fragile X syndrome. The severe fragile X phenotype seen in a patient with the point mutation in the *FMR1* gene can be explained by a possible gain-of-function of FMRP. However, it must be stressed that, under physiologic conditions, normal RNA binding was demonstrated. Therefore, it is important to know which mRNAs are binding to the FMRP, the physiologic significance of this RNA binding, and how the lack of FMRP and the subsequent absence of binding to these RNAs can lead to mental retardation.

## Nuclear-Cytoplasmic Shuttling

FMRP contains a functional nuclear localization signal (NLS) and a nuclear export signal (NES) (Bardoni et al. 1997; Eberhart et al. 1996; Fridell et al. 1996; Sittler et al. 1996) (Fig. 4.2*A*). The leucine-rich FMRP NES motif is similar to the Rev/PKI-type NES (Fischer et al. 1995; Wen et al. 1995). This type of NES has been identified in an increasing number of nucleocytoplasmic shuttling proteins. The presence of these localization signals suggests that FMRP may shuttle between cytoplasm and nucleus and is involved in the transport of a subset of RNAs from the nucleus to the ribosomes. This is supported by immuno-electron microscopic studies, on both neurons and COS cells overexpressing FMRP, showing that a minor part of the protein is also detected in the nucleus (Feng et al. 1997a; Fridell et al. 1996; Tamanini et al. 1999a; Willemsen et al. 1996a). When a mutation is introduced into the NES, FXR2P is found in the nucleolus (Fig. 4.4).

# NUCLEAR-CYTOPLASMIC SHUTTLING AND DISTINCT TARGETTING OF FMRP AND FXR2P

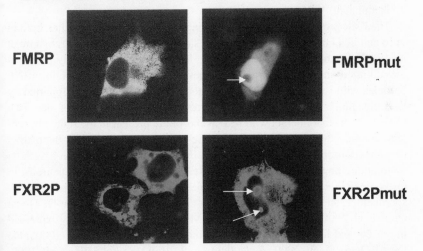

**Fig. 4.4.** Immunohistochemical staining of FMRP and FXR2P using specific antibodies in COS cells transfected with *FMR1* and *FXR2* expression vectors shows nuclear-cytoplasmic shuttling and distinct targeting of FMRP and FXR2P. Two different types of clones were used: normal clones (FMRP and FXR2P) and clones with a mutation in the NES (FMRPmut and FXR2Pmut). The *arrows* indicate the position of the nucleolus, which is empty for FMRPmut but contains FXR2P in the mutated clone.

Recent studies showed that the mutated FMRP (FMRPI304N) is incorporated into smaller (600–150 kDa) ethylenediaminetetraacetic acid (EDTA)-resistant messenger ribonucleoprotein (mRNP) particles and is shuttling faster between cytoplasm and nucleus, most likely because the mutated FMRP is less associated to ribosomes than is the normal FMRP (Feng et al. 1997a; Tamanini et al. 1999a).

## Homology

FXR1P and FXR2P, two proteins homologous with FMRP, have been identified and characterized (Siomi et al. 1995; Zhang et al. 1995) (Fig. 4.2*B*). The amino acid sequence of FMRP is highly similar to FXR1P and FXR2P in the amino-terminal (86% and 70% identity, respectively). This region includes the NLS, dimerization domain (Siomi et al. 1996), KH domains, and leucine-rich NES (fig. 4.4). The RGG box in the carboxy-terminal is also conserved between the three proteins. Like FMRP, FXR1P and FXR2P are detected predominantly in the cytoplasm associated with the ribosomal 60S subunit (Devys et al. 1993; Eberhart and Warren 1996; Feng et al. 1997b; Khandjian et al. 1995; Tamanini et al. 1996).

The FXR proteins can interact with themselves and with each other, both in vitro and in an overexpressed cellular system (Ceman et al. 1999; Tamanini et al. 1999b; Zhang et al. 1995). However, in vivo they preferentially form homomultimers in mammalian cells, suggesting that they participate in mRNP particles with separate function (Tamanini et al. 1999b). This is supported by the intracellular distribution of the different proteins in different tissues. Two other proteins that interact with FMRP and/or are present in the same big protein complex, which includes FMRP, are NUFIP (nuclear-FMRP-interacting protein) (Bardoni et al. 1999) and nucleolin (Ceman et al. 1999).

In brain, the three proteins are coexpressed in the cytoplasm of neurons. In testis, FMRP is expressed mainly in spermatogonia, FXR1P in postmeiotic spermatides, and FXR2P in all testicular cells (Bakker et al. 2000a; De Diego Otero et al. 2000; Tamanini et al. 1997). Moreover, FXR1P is highly expressed in muscle and heart, where FMRP is almost absent (Bakker et al. 2000a; De Diego Otero et al. 2000; Khandjian et al. 1998; Kirkpatrick et al. 1999; Tamanini et al. 1997). The distribution of the FXR proteins was investigated in humans and mice during early development. The expression pattern of the FXR proteins exhibits high similarities; however, during late development and in the neonate, a more differential expression is observed, especially in some non-neural tissues (Agulhon et al. 1999; De Diego Otero et al. 2000; Tamanini et al. 1997).

## Subcellular Localization

Recent studies showed that, like the *FMR1* gene, the *FXR1* gene is alternatively spliced. At least seven spliced forms (iso-a to iso-g) have been identified (Kirkpatrick et al. 1999). In contrast to *FMR1,* the mechanism of alternative splicing appears to be tissue specific for *FXR1,* with different isoforms expressed preferentially in different tissues (Khandjian et al. 1998; Kirkpatrick et al. 1999; Tamanini et al. 2000).

FXR1P and FXR2P can shuttle between cytoplasm and nucleus. The nuclear export of the FXR proteins is mediated by the export receptor exportin1, since its functional inhibition with leptomycin B results in the nuclear accumulation of the FXR proteins (Tamanini et al. 1999a). In addition, FMRP shuttles between cytoplasm and nucleoplasm, while FXR2P and some of the FXR1P spliceforms (e-g) shuttle between cytoplasm and nucleolus (Tamanini et al. 1999a, 2000). When the NES is mutated, FMRP is found in the nucleus and FXR2P is found in the nucleolus (fig. 4.4). The presence of a specific nucleolar-targeting signal (NoS) in both FXR2P and the FXR1P spliceforms e-g suggests that the presence or absence of this new functional motif determines the shuttling of the FXR proteins to different subnuclear compartments. Therefore, in contrast with FMRP, the individual FXR1P proteins display a specific tissue distribution. In particular, *FXR1* iso e and f are almost exclusively found in heart and skeletal muscle (Kirkpatrick et al. 1999; Tamanini 2000). This tissue specificity and the fact that FXR1P spliceforms (iso e-g) contain functional nucleolar targeting signals suggest a tissue-specific function for the individual *FXR1* splice-products.

## The Influence of CGG Repeat Length on Translation

As mentioned above, the CGG repeat of the *FMR1* gene is not translated into protein. Transcription of *FMR1* alleles with repeat lengths within the premutation range was demonstrated to be qualitatively normal (Feng et al. 1995), although more recent, quantitative measurements (Tassone et al. 2000a) demonstrated mRNA levels that are elevated by as much as fivefold (see chap. 12). Premutation transcripts have been shown to have a normal turnover, with an mRNA half-life estimated to be 9–12 h (Feng et al. 1995; Tassone et al. 2000a). For premutation alleles with fewer than 110 repeats, no significant reduction in FMRP levels has been noted, indicating that there is no major effect of repeat length on translation of the *FMR1* mRNA in that range. For alleles with more than 110 repeats, FMRP levels were moderately reduced (Tassone et al. 2000a). Feng et al. (1995) showed that translation was suppressed from transcripts with more than 200 repeats. They demonstrated that transcripts with more than 200 repeats were associated with stalled 40S ribosomes, which can be explained by the inability of ribosomes to pass such a long repeat. This resulted in loss of protein expression. On the other hand, Smeets et al. (1995) described two apparently normal brothers with large expanded CGG repeats and cytogenetically visible fragile sites. The *FMR1* promoter in these alleles was unmethylated, and both RNA and protein were detectable in all cells analyzed, although the level of FMRP seemed to be reduced. Further data about the possible translation of *FMR1* mRNAs containing large CGG repeats comes from chorionic villi. Chorionic villi of a male fetus with a full mutation are not methylated, if they are taken in the 10th week of pregnancy, and they also express FMRP (Losekoot et al. 1997; Willemsen et al. 1996a). Further evidence for expression came from experiments in which in a cell line of a patient with a full mutation of the *FMR1* gene was partially demethylated, resulting in modest expression of FMRP (Chiurazzi et al. 1998, 1999; Coffee et al. 1999). If transcription and translation are possible for a gene with a large expansion, therapeutic strategies might be set up that are based on demethylation of the *FMR1* gene of patients in order to restore *FMR1* protein production.

## The Diagnostic Antibody Test

Since the discovery of the *FMR1* gene, the molecular diagnosis of fragile X syndrome has been made via Southern blot hybridization (Oostra et al. 1993; Rousseau 1994) or polymerase chain reaction (PCR) analysis (Brown et al. 1993; Fu et al. 1991; chap. 2). The availability of antibodies directed against FMRP stimulated the development of a new diagnostic test to identify fragile X patients (Willemsen et al. 1995). The test is based on the presence of FMRP in cells from unaffected individuals and the absence of FMRP in cells from fragile X patients. Initially, an antibody test that detects the presence of FMRP in blood smears was developed (fig. 4.3) (Willemsen et al. 1995).

Fragile X patients can be identified by the absence of FMRP or, in the case of female fragile X patients, by the diminished percentage of cells that express FMRP. This test can also identify patients who do not produce *FMR1* protein due to a small deletion in the *FMR1* gene, but patients with a missense mutation might be missed (fig. 4.3). Frequently, FMRP expression has been observed in some lymphocytes from affected males, suggesting the presence of a premutation or an unmethylated full mutation in these positively stained cells. For males, the diagnostic power of the test is high because there is no overlap between the values of unaffected individuals and of affected males with the full mutation. The cutoff point of the diagnostic test for males has been determined to be 42% (Willemsen et al. 1997b). Recently, a cutoff point of 50% has been suggested because this percentage has more potential as a prognostic indicator of nonretarded IQ in males (Tassone et al. 2000b). This noninvasive test can be used for screening large groups of mentally retarded people for fragile X syndrome; however, the test is less specific in identifying females with the full mutation.

Until now, several antibody tests for prenatal and postnatal detection of fragile X syndrome have been described, using different biopsy material, including chorionic villi, amniotic fluid cells, blood (fetal), and, most recently, hair roots (Lambiris et al. 1999; Willemsen et al. 1995, 1996b, 1997a, 1999). Plucked hairs contain the inner root sheath, a large part of the outer root sheath, and the upper part of the bulb. The cells in the hair bulb express especially high levels of FMRP. A low percentage of FMRP-stained hair roots is diagnostic of fragile X syndrome. For males, the diagnostic power of this new noninvasive test is high, and it can be readily used to identify male patients. In a recent validation study, Willemsen found a high diagnostic power for females with the full mutation (Willemsen, submitted). A first example of the use of FMRP expression in hair roots as an indicator for mental status in females with the full mutation has been reported in monozygotic twin sisters. One twin is affected (showing low expression in hair roots), and the other is intellectually normal (showing high expression in hair roots) (Willemsen et al. 2000). Furthermore, the power of this new technique was further illustrated by the identification of four fragile X patients who could not be diagnosed by DNA analysis (Willemsen et al. 1999; unpublished results). The new test on hair roots is extremely suitable for use in large screening programs among males, illustrated by a recent study in Turkey (Tuncbilek et al. 2000).

## An Animal Model

### Transgenic Mice

The *FMR1* gene is highly conserved among species (Verkerk et al. 1991), and the murine homolog *Fmr1* shows 95% sequence identity at the nucleic level and 97% identity in amino acid sequence (Ashley et al. 1993b). The murine *Fmr1* gene also contains a CGG repeat that is polymorphic between different mouse strains, with an average repeat length of 10 CGG repeats. The expression pattern of *FMR1* at the mRNA and protein level is almost identical in various tissues of humans and mice (Abitbol et al. 1993; Bächner et al. 1993a, 1993b; Devys et al. 1993; Hinds et al. 1993), which makes the mouse a good animal model in which to study the fragile X syndrome. No naturally occurring animal model for the trinucleotide diseases has been described. The development of an animal model has major advantages. First, the unlimited supply of tissues gives the opportunity to study the effects on the morphologic and mol-

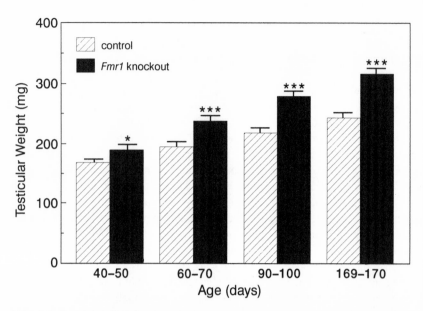

**Fig. 4.5.** Testis size. Combined testicular weight of both testes of knockout versus control mice. The data are derived at age 40–50 days, 60–70 days, 90–100 days, and 160–170 days. The *error bars* display SEM. *Asterisks* indicate statistical differences between the mutant and age-matched normal littermates (*, $0.01 < p < 0.05$; ***, $p < 0.001$), calculated by Student's *t*-test.

ecular level. Second, the phenotype and behavior of mice can be studied to understand the development of the disease phenotype in human patients.

A mouse has been developed in which the *Fmr1* gene has been inactivated (Bakker et al. 1994). The knockout mouse has been generated by homologous recombination in embryonic stem cells, using a vector in which exon 5 of the *Fmr1* gene was interrupted. As in fragile X patients, these knockout mice lack normal *Fmr1* RNA and protein (fig. 4.1). The knockout mice are perfectly viable and healthy and have a normal fertility, as was apparent from normal litter size.

## The Phenotype and Pathology of Knockout Mice

By visual inspection no differences between control and knockout animals have been found, and no significant difference in body weight has been observed. One of the most obvious phenotypic characteristics of fragile X patients is macroorchidism; sometimes this is manifested in childhood, but it is present in almost all fragile X patients after puberty. A nearly 30% increase in testicular weight confirms macroorchidism in the knockout mouse (Bakker et al. 1994; Kooy et al. 1996) (fig. 4.5). As in patients, there is a gradual enlargement of the testes over time. The increase in testicular weight of the knockout mice was found to be the result of an increased rate of Sertoli cell division within the normal period of cell proliferation, between embryonic day 12 and day 15 postnatally (Slegtenhorst-Eegdeman et al. 1998). During this developmental period, FMRP is expressed in the primordial germ cells of normal testes (Tamanini et al. 1997), but it is not clear whether the increased testicular weight of the knockout mouse is the result of absence of FMRP expression locally in the testes or in the brain.

Examination of kidney, spleen, liver, lung, and heart of mutant mice revealed no abnormalities, consistent with the absence of abnormalities in human patients. Immunohistologic studies of brain and testis did not show any pathologic abnormalities in the mutant mice (Bakker et al. 1994). For further discussion of the ultrastructure of the brain, see chapter 5.

## Behavior and Cognitive Function

The mutant mice show mild cognitive impairment in the form of deficits in learning, as was shown in Morris water maze experiments (Bakker et al. 1994; D'Hooge et al. 1997; Peier et al. 2000). In this test the mice are placed in a large circular pool filled with opaque water, where they are trained to find a hidden platform. Knockouts experienced difficulties in learning to locate the hidden platform when, after a period of intensive acquisition training, the platform's position was changed during the reversal trials. In a recent publication, Paradee et al. (1999) were able to replicate only part of these results, which could be attributed to the influence of strain differences between C57BL/6 and 129Re/J on the *Fmr1* knockout phenotype.

A state of social anxiety has been reported in fragile X patients (Franke et al. 1998; chap. 1). Interestingly, Paradee et al. (1999) did observe deficits in conditioned fear responses in *Fmr1* knockouts. It was recently shown that the *Fmr1* mouse displayed reduced anxiety-related responses with increased exploratory behavior (Peier et al. 2000).

Spontaneous epileptic seizures, occurring in roughly 20% of fragile X patients (Musumeci et al. 1999), have not been observed in control or knockout mice. However, on audiogenic induction, the knockout mouse shows increased susceptibility to seizures when compared with control littermates (Musumeci et al. 2000). This might indicate increased cortical excitability because of the lack of FMRP.

To answer the question of whether reintroduction of the Fmrp protein can restore the disease phenotype, investigators constructed a transgenic mouse that expressed the human FMRP (Bakker et al. 2000b). The *FMR1* transgene was under the control of a cytomegalovirus (CMV) promoter in order to obtain ubiquitous expression of FMRP. The rescue mouse did express the FMR1 protein, but did not show a reversal of the phenotype, most likely because the level of FMRP expressed from the transgene in the rescue mouse is inadequate or not time or cell specific. A different approach was taken by Peier et al. (2000), who generated transgenic mice containing yeast artificial chromosome (YAC) to determine whether the *Fmr1* knockout mouse phenotype could be rescued. *FMR1* YAC transgenic mice overexpressing the human protein did produce opposing behavioral responses, and additional abnormal behaviors were also observed (Peier et al. 2000). These findings have significant implications for gene therapy for fragile X syndrome, since overexpression of the gene may harbor its own phenotype.

## The Pathogenesis of Fragile X Syndrome in the Knockout Mouse Model

It was suggested that FMRP is important for normal synaptic function, as the lack of full-length FMRP in fragile X patients and in knockout mice results in immature dendritic spine morphology and density (Comery et al. 1997; Hinton et al. 1991; Rudelli et al. 1985; see chap. 5). Recently, mutations of *oligophrenin-1* (Billuart et al. 1998), *GDI1* (D'Adamo et al. 1998), and *PAK3* (Allen et al. 1998) genes have been shown to be associated with nonsyndromic forms of X-linked mental retardation. Together, this suggests that defects in synaptic maturation may underlie some forms of mental retardation. These genes are regulators of pre- and postsynaptic function (Antonarakis and Van Aelst 1998).

A subset of mRNAs that neurons express is transported from the neuronal cell body into dendrites (Steward 1997). The local synthesis of these mRNAs into specific proteins in the subsynaptic cytoplasm is thought to be important for the synaptic function. Weiler et al. (Weiler and Greenough 1999; Weiler et al. 1997) detected *FMR1* mRNA in synaptoneurosome preparations and showed that synthesis of FMRP at synaptic sites is increased by synaptic activity (see chap. 5). Not only FMRP but also its homologs, FXR1P and FXR2P, are present at the same locations. FMRP is co-localized with synaptophysin in presynaptic terminals of hippocampal neurons, which is consistent with the role of FMRP in the synaptic pathology (Castren et al. 2001; Tamanini et al. 1997). If FMRP does play a role in targeting, one would expect that normal patterns of mRNA localization in dendrites and/or dendritic transport of mRNA would be disrupted in *Fmr1* knockout mice. However, the localization of the mRNAs for MAP2 and CAMII kinase and the migration of recently synthesized ARC mRNA were indistinguishable from normal in *Fmr1* knockout mice. This indicates that FMRP does not play an obligatory role in the localization of at least these representatives of the family of dendritically localized mRNAs or in the dendritic transport of ARC mRNA after induction. It might be that FMRP is involved in targeting other dendritic mRNAs yet to be identified.

The abnormalities found in the *Fmr1* knockout mouse (Bakker et al. 1994) may indicate the significance of an intracellular routing for FMRP. Abnormalities in Morris water-maze testing are commonly attributed to abnormalities in the hippocampus, a highly specialized brain structure consisting almost exclusively of interconnecting neurons. However, in subsequent electrophysiologic experiments, no evidence for altered efficiency of synaptic transmission in the hippocampus has been demonstrated (Godfraind et al. 1996). It remains to be seen whether the synaptic abnormalities resulting from the *Fmr1* null mutation can be explained by the disruption of the local synthesis of a key functional molecule of the synaptic junction, as suggested by Weiler et al. (1997), or by the loss of mRNA binding functions of the molecule, as proposed by Feng et al. (1997a).

Recently, a knockout mouse for *Fxr2* has been developed (unpublished data). Experiments showed that these mice have behavior and cognitive deficits similar to those seen in the *Fmr1* knockout mice. The observation of a similar set of defects in both mutant mice suggests that these mice can be used as a model to study (fragile X) mental retardation.

## Conclusion

Although the *FMR1* protein has been shown to contain RNA binding domains and domains involved in shuttling, many questions remain to be answered:

—What is the specific function of this RNA binding domain?

—What is the profile of mRNAs that are involved in mental retardation?

—Does FMRP have functions other than RNA binding?

—How does a loss of FMRP lead to mental retardation?

—What is the role of the *FXR1* and *FXR2* proteins?

## Acknowledgments

The authors thank their coworkers in the fragile X research groups of Rotterdam and Antwerp. This research was supported by the FRAXA Research Foundation, BIOMED BMH4-CT91663, and NIH grant HD388038.01.

## References

Abitbol, M., C. Menini, A. L. Delezoide, T. Rhyner, M. Vekemans, and J. Mallet. 1993. Nucleus basalis magnocellularis and hippocampus are the major sites of *FMR-1* expression in the human fetal brain. *Nat. Genet.* 4:147–153.

Agulhon, C., P. Blanchet, A. Kobetz, D. Marchant, N. Faucon, P. Sarda, C. Moraine, A. Sittler, V. Biancalana, A. Malafosse, and M. Abitbol. 1999. Expression of *FMR1, FXR1,* and *FXR2* genes in human prenatal tissues. *J. Neuropathol. Exp. Neurol.* 58: 867–880.

Allen, K. M., J. G. Gleeson, S. Bagrodia, M. W. Partington, J. C. MacMillan, R. A. Cerione, J. C. Mulley, and C. A. Walsh. 1998. PAK3 mutation in nonsyndromic X-linked mental retardation. *Nat. Genet.* 20:25–30.

Antonarakis, S. E., and L. Van Aelst. 1998. Mind the GAP, Rho, Rab and GDI [news; comment]. *Nat. Genet.* 19:106–108.

Ashley, C., Jr., K. D. Wilkinson, D. Reines, and S. T. Warren. 1993a. *FMR1* protein: Conserved RNP family domains and selective RNA binding. *Science* 262:563–568.

Ashley, C. T., J. S. Sutcliffe, C. B. Kunst, H. A. Leiner, E. E. Eichler, D. L. Nelson, and S. T. Warren. 1993b. Human and murine *FMR-1:* Alternative splicing and translational initiation downstream of the CGG-repeat. *Nat. Genet.* 4:244–251.

Bächner, D., A. Manca, P. Steinbach, D. Wöhrle, W. Just, W. Vogel, H. Hameister, and A. Poustka. 1993a. Enhanced expression of the murine *FMR1* gene during germ cell proliferation suggests a special function in both the male and the female gonad. *Hum. Mol. Genet.* 2:2043–2050.

Bächner, D., P. Steinbach, D. Wöhrle, W. Just, W. Vogel, H. Hameister, A. Manca, and A. Poustka. 1993b. Enhanced *Fmr-1* expression in testis. *Nat. Genet.* 4:115–116.

Bakker, C. E., C. Verheij, R. Willemsen, R. Vanderhelm, F. Oerlemans, M. Vermey, A. Bygrave, A. T. Hoogeveen, B. A. Oostra, E. Reyniers, K. Deboulle, R. Dhooge, P. Cras, D. Van Velzen, G. Nagels, J. J. Martin, P. P. Dedeyn, J. K. Darby, and P. J. Willems. 1994. *Fmr1* knockout mice: A model to study fragile X mental retardation. *Cell* 78:23–33.

Bakker, C. E., Y. de Diego Otero, C. Bontekoe, P. Raghoe, T. Luteijn, A. T. Hoogeveen, B. A. Oostra, and R. Willemsen. 2000a. Immunocytochemical and biochemical characterization of FMRP, FXR1P, and FXR2P in the mouse. *Exp. Cell Res.* 258:162–170.

Bakker, C. E., R. F. Kooy, R. D'Hooge, F. Tamanini, R. Willemsen, I. Nieuwenhuizen, B. B. A. De Vries, E. Reyniers, A. T. Hoogeveen, P. J. Willems, P. P. De Deyn, and B. A. Oostra. 2000b. Introduction of a *FMR1* transgene in the fragile X knockout mouse. *Neurosci. Res. Commun.* 26:265–277.

Bardoni, B., A. Sittler, Y. Shen, and J. L. Mandel. 1997. Analysis of domains affecting intracellular localization of the FMRP protein. *Neurobiol. Dis.* 4:329–336.

Bardoni, B., A. Schenck, and J. L. Mandel. 1999. A novel RNA-binding nuclear protein that interacts with the fragile X mental retardation (*FMR1*) protein. *Hum. Mol. Genet.* 8:2557–2566.

Billuart, P., T. Bienvenu, N. Ronce, V. des Portes, M. C. Vinet, R. Zemni, H. R. Crollius, A. Carrie, F. Fauchereau, M. Cherry, S. Briault, B. Hamel, J. P. Fryns, C. Beldjord, A. Kahn, C. Moraine, and J. Chelly. 1998. Oligophrenin-1 encodes a rhoGAP protein involved in X-linked mental retardation. *Nature* 392:923–926.

Brown, W. T., G. E. Houck, A. Jeziorowska, F. N. Levinson, X. Ding, C. Dobkin, N. Zhong, J. Henderson, S. S. Brooks, and E. C. Jenkins. 1993. Rapid fragile-X carrier screening and prenatal diagnosis using a nonradioactive PCR test. *JAMA* 270:1569–1575.

Castren, M., A. Haapasalo, B. A. Oostra, and E. Castren. 2001. Subcellular localization of fragile X mental retardation protein and its I304N mutated form in cultured hippocampal neurons. *Cell. Mol. Neurobiol.* 21:29–38.

Ceman, S., V. Brown, and S. T. Warren. 1999. Isolation of an FMRP-associated messenger ribonucleoprotein particle and identification of nucleolin and the fragile X-related proteins as components of the complex. *Mol. Cell. Biol.* 19:7925–7932.

Chiurazzi, P., M. G. Pomponi, R. Willemsen, B. A. Oostra, and G. Neri. 1998. In vitro reactivation of the *FMR1* gene involved in fragile X syndrome. *Hum. Mol. Genet.* 7:109–113.

Chiurazzi, P., M. G. Pomponi, A. Sharrock, J. Macpherson, S. Lormeau, M. L. Morel, and F. Rousseau. 1999. DNA panel for interlaboratory standardization of haplotype studies on the fragile X syndrome and proposal for a new allele nomenclature. *Am. J. Med. Genet.* 83:347–349.

Coffee, B., F. Zhang, S. T. Warren, and D. Reines. 1999. Acetylated histones are associated with *FMR1* in normal but not fragile X-syndrome cells. *Nat. Genet.* 22:98–101.

Comery, T. A., J. B. Harris, P. J. Willems, B. A. Oostra, S. A. Irwin, I. J. Weiler, and W. T. Greenough. 1997. Abnormal dendritic spines in fragile X knockout mice: Maturation and pruning deficits. *Proc. Natl. Acad. Sci. USA* 94:5401–5404.

D'Adamo, P., A. Menegon, C. Lo Nigro, M. Grasso, M. Gulisano, F. Tamanini, T. Bienvenu, A. K. Gedeon, B. Oostra, S. K. Wu, A. Tandon, F. Valtorta, W. E. Balch, J. Chelly, and D. Toniolo. 1998. Mutations in *GDI1* are responsible for X-linked nonspecific mental retardation. *Nat. Genet.* 12:134–139.

De Boulle, K., A. J. Verkerk, E. Reyniers, L. Vits, J. Hendrickx, B. Van Roy, F. Van den Bos, E. de Graaff, B. A. Oostra, and P. J. Willems. 1993. A point mutation in the *FMR-1* gene associated with fragile X mental retardation. *Nat. Genet.* 3:31–35.

De Diego Otero, Y., C. E. Bakker, P. Raghoe, L. W. F. M. Severijnen, A. Hoogeveen, B. A. Oostra, and R. Willemsen. 2000. Immunocytochemical characterization of FMRP, FXR1P and FXR2P during embryonic development in the mouse. *Gene Funct. Dis.* 1:28–37.

Deelen, W., C. Bakker, D. Halley, and B. A. Oostra. 1994. Conservation of CGG region in *FMR1* gene in mammals. *Am. J. Med. Genet.* 51:513–516.

De Graaff, E., R. Willemsen, N. Zhong, C. E. M. De Die-Smulders, W. T. Brown, G. Freling, and B. A. Oostra. 1995. Instability of the CGG repeat and expression of the *FMR1* protein in a male fragile X patient with a lung tumour. *Am. J. Hum. Genet.* 57:609–618.

Deissler, H., A. Behn-Krappa, and W. Doerfler. 1996. Purification of nuclear proteins from human HeLa cells that bind specifically to the unstable tandem repeat (CGG)n in the human *FMR1* gene. *J. Biol. Chem.* 271:4327–4334.

Devys, D., Y. Lutz, N. Rouyer, J. P. Bellocq, and J. L. Mandel. 1993. The *FMR-1* protein is cytoplasmic, most abundant in neurons and appears normal in carriers of a fragile X premutation. *Nat. Genet.* 4:335–340.

D'Hooge, R., G. Nagels, F. Franck, C. E. Bakker, E. Reyniers, K. Storm, R. F. Kooy, B. A. Oostra, P. J. Willems, and P. P. Dedeyn. 1997. Mildly impaired water maze performance in male Fmr1 knockout mice. *Neuroscience* 76:367–376.

Eberhart, D. E., and S. T. Warren. 1996. The molecular basis of fragile X syndrome. *Cold Spring Harb. Symp. Quant. Biol.* 61:679–687.

Eberhart, D. E., H. E. Malter, Y. Feng, and S. T. Warren. 1996. The fragile X mental retardation protein is a ribosonucleoprotein containing both nuclear localization and nuclear export signals. *Hum. Mol. Genet.* 5:1083–1091.

Eichler, E. E., S. Richards, R. A. Gibbs, and D. L. Nelson. 1993. Fine structure of the human *FMR1* gene. *Hum. Mol. Genet.* 2:1147–1153.

Feng, Y., D. Lakkis, and S. T. Warren. 1995. Quantitative comparison of *FMR1* gene expression in normal and premutation alleles. *Am. J. Hum. Genet.* 56:106–113.

Feng, Y., D. Absher, D. E. Eberhart, V. Brown, H. E. Malter, and S. T. Warren. 1997a. FMRP associates with polyribosomes as an mRNP, and the I304N mutation of severe fragile X syndrome abolishes this association. *Mol. Cell* 1:109–118.

Feng, Y., C. A. Gutekunst, D. E. Eberhart, H. Yi, S. T. Warren, and S. M. Hersch. 1997b. Fragile X mental retardation protein: Nucleocytoplasmic shuttling and association with somatodendritic ribosomes. *J. Neurosci.* 17:1539–1547.

Fischer, U., J. Huber, W. C. Boelens, I. W. Mattaj, and R. Luhrmann. 1995. The HIV-1 Rev activation domain is a nuclear export signal that accesses an export pathway used by specific cellular RNAs. *Cell* 82:475–483.

Franke, P., M. Leboyer, M. Gansicke, O. Weiffenbach, V. Biancalana, P. Cornillet-Lefebre, M. F. Croquette, U. Froster, S. G. Schwab, F. Poustka, M. Hautzinger, and W. Maier. 1998. Genotype-phenotype relationship in female carriers of the premutation and full mutation of *FMR-1*. *Psychiatry Res.* 80:113–127.

Fridell, R. A., R. E. Benson, J. Hua, H. P. Bogerd, and B. R. Cullen. 1996. A nuclear role for the fragile X mental retardation protein. *EMBO J.* 15:5408–5414.

Fu, Y. H., D. P. Kuhl, A. Pizzuti, M. Pieretti, J. S. Sutcliffe, S. Richards, A. J. Verkerk, J. J. Holden, R. Fenwick Jr., S. T. Warren, B. A. Oostra, D. L. Nelson, and C. T. Caskey. 1991. Variation of the CGG repeat at the fragile X site results in genetic instability: Resolution of the Sherman paradox. *Cell* 67:1047–1058.

Gedeon, A. K., E. Baker, H. Robinson, M. W. Partington, B. Gross, A. Manca, B. Korn, A. Poustka, S. Yu, G. R. Sutherland, and J. C. Mulley. 1992. Fragile X syndrome without CCG amplification has an *FMR1* deletion. *Nat. Genet.* 1:341–344.

Godfraind, J. M., E. Reyniers, K. Deboulle, R. Dhooge, P. P. Dedeyn, C. E. Bakker, B. A. Oostra, R. F. Kooy, and P. J. Willems. 1996. Long-term potentiation in the hippocampus of fragile X knockout mice. *Am. J. Med. Genet.* 64:246–251.

Hinds, H. L., C. T. Ashley, J. S. Sutcliffe, D. L. Nelson, S. T. Warren, D. E. Housman, and M. Schalling. 1993. Tissue specific expression of *FMR-1* provides evidence for a functional role in fragile X syndrome. *Nat. Genet.* 3:36–43.

Hinton, V. J., W. T. Brown, K. Wisniewski, and R. D. Rudelli. 1991. Analysis of neocortex in three males with the fragile X syndrome. *Am. J. Med. Genet.* 41:289–294.

Hwu, W-L., Y-M. Lee, S-C. Lee, and T-R. Wang. 1993. In vitro DNA methylation inhibits *FMR1* promoter. *Biochem. Biophys. Res. Commun.* 193:324–329.

Khandjian, E. W., A. Fortin, A. Thibodeau, S. Tremblay, F. Cote, D. Devys, J. L. Mandel, and F. Rousseau. 1995. A heterogeneous set of *FMR1* proteins is widely distributed in mouse tissues and is modulated in cell culture. *Hum. Mol. Genet.* 4:783–790.

Khandjian, E. W., B. Bardoni, F. Corbin, A. Sittler, S. Giroux, D. Heitz, S. Tremblay, C. Pinset, D. Montarras, F. Rousseau, and J. Mandel. 1998. Novel isoforms of the fragile X related protein FXR1P are expressed during myogenesis. *Hum. Mol. Genet.* 7:2121–2128.

Kirkpatrick, L. L., K. A. McIlwain, and D. L. Nelson. 1999. Alternative splicing in the murine and human *FXR1* genes. *Genomics* 59:193–202.

Kooy, R. F., R. Dhooge, E. Reyniers, C. E. Bakker, G. Nagels, K. Deboulle, K. Storm, G. Clincke, P. P. Dedeyn, B. A. Oostra, and P. J. Willems. 1996. Transgenic mouse model for the fragile X syndrome. *Am. J. Med. Genet.* 64:241–245.

Lambiris, N., H. Peters, R. Bollmann, G. Leschik, J. Leisti, R. Salonen, G. Cobet, B. A. Oostra, and R. Willemsen. 1999. Rapid *FMR1*-protein analysis of fetal blood: An enhancement of prenatal diagnostics. *Hum. Genet.* 105:258–260.

Losekoot, M., E. Hoogendoorn, R. Olmer, C. Jansen, J. C. Oosterwijk, A. M. W. Vandenouweland, D. J. J. Halley, S. T. Warren, R. Willemsen, B. A. Oostra, and E. Bakker. 1997. Prenatal diagnosis of the fragile X syndrome: Loss of mutation owing to a double recombinant or gene conversion event at the *FMR1* locus. *J. Med. Genet.* 34:924–926.

Meijer, H., E. De Graaff, D. M. L. Merckx, R. J. E. Jongbloed, C. E. M. De Die-Smulders, J. J. M. Engelen, J. P. Fryns, P. M. G. Curfs, and B. A. Oostra. 1994. A deletion of 1.6 kb proximal to the CGG repeat of the *FMR1* gene causes the clinical phenotype of the fragile X syndrome. *Hum. Mol. Genet.* 3:615–620.

Muller-Hartmann, H., H. Deissler, F. Naumann, B. Schmitz, J. Schroer, and W. Doerfler. 2000. The human 20-kDa 5′-(CGG)(n)-3′-binding protein is targeted to the nucleus and affects the activity of the *FMR1* promoter. *J. Biol. Chem.* 275:6447–6452.

Musco, G., G. Stier, C. Joseph, M. A. Castilioni Morelli, M. Nilges, T. J. Gibson, and A. Pastore. 1996. Three-dimensional structure and stability of the KH domain: Molecular insights into the fragile X syndrome. *Cell* 85:237–245.

Musumeci, S. A., R. J. Hagerman, R. Ferri, P. Bosco, B. Dalla Bernardina, C. A. Tassinari, G. B. De Sarro, and M. Elia. 1999. Epilepsy and EEG findings in males with fragile X syndrome. *Epilepsia* 40:1092–1099.

Musumeci, S. A., P. Bosco, G. Calabrese, C. Bakker, G. B. De Sarro, M. Elia, R. Ferri, and B. A. Oostra. 2000. Audiogenic seizures susceptibility in transgenic mice with fragile X syndrome. *Epilepsia* 41:19–23.

Oostra, B. A., P. B. Jacky, W. T. Brown, and F. Rousseau. 1993. Guidelines for the diagnosis of fragile X syndrome. *J. Med. Genet.* 30:410–413.

Paradee, W., H. E. Melikian, D. L. Rasmussen, A. Kenneson, P. J. Conn, and S. T. Warren. 1999. Fragile X mouse: Strain effects of knockout phenotype and evidence suggesting deficient amygdala function. *Neuroscience* 94:185–192.

Peier, A. M., K. L. McIlwain, A. Kenneson, S. T. Warren, R. Paylor, and D. L. Nelson.

2000. (Over)correction of *FMR1* deficiency with YAC transgenics: Behavioral and physical features. *Hum. Mol. Genet.* 9:1145–1159.

Pieretti, M., F. P. Zhang, Y. H. Fu, S. T. Warren, B. A. Oostra, C. T. Caskey, and D. L. Nelson. 1991. Absence of expression of the *FMR-1* gene in fragile X syndrome. *Cell* 66:817–822.

Reyniers, E., L. Vits, K. De Boulle, B. Van Roy, D. Van Velzen, E. de Graaff, A. J. M. H. Verkerk, H. Z. Jorens, J. K. Darby, B. A. Oostra, and P. J. Willems. 1993. The full mutation in the *FMR-1* gene of male fragile X patients is absent in their sperm. *Nat. Genet.* 4:143–146.

Richards, R. I., K. Holman, S. Yu, and G. R. Sutherland. 1993. Fragile X syndrome unstable element, p(CCG)n, and other simple tandem repeat sequences are binding sites for specific nuclear proteins. *Hum. Mol. Genet.* 2:1429–1435.

Rousseau, F. 1994. The fragile X syndrome: Implications of molecular genetics for the clinical syndrome. *Eur. J. Clin. Invest.* 24:1–10.

Rousseau, F., D. Heitz, V. Biancalana, S. Blumenfeld, C. Kretz, J. Boue, N. Tommerup, C. Van Der Hagen, C. DeLozier-Blanchet, M. F. Croquette, S. Gilgenkranz, P. Jalbert, M. A. Voelckel, I. Oberlé, and J. L. Mandel. 1991. Direct diagnosis by DNA analysis of the fragile X syndrome of mental retardation. *N. Engl. J. Med.* 325:1673–1681.

Rudelli, R. D., W. T. Brown, K. Wisniewski, E. C. Jenkins, M. Laure-Kamionowska, F. Connell, and H. M. Wisniewski. 1985. Adult fragile X syndrome: Clinico-neuropathologic findings. *Acta Neuropathol. (Berl.)* 67:289–295.

Siomi, H., M. C. Siomi, R. L. Nussbaum, and G. Dreyfuss. 1993. The protein product of the fragile X gene, *FMR1*, has characteristics of an RNA-binding protein. *Cell* 74:291–298.

Siomi, H., M. Choi, M. C. Siomi, R. L. Nussbaum, and G. Dreyfuss. 1994. Essential role for KH domains in RNA binding: Impaired RNA binding by a mutation in the KH domain of *FMR1* that causes fragile X syndrome. *Cell* 77:33–39.

Siomi, M. C., H. Siomi, W. H. Sauer, S. Srinivasan, R. L. Nussbaum, and G. Dreyfuss. 1995. *FXR1,* an autosomal homolog of the fragile X mental retardation gene. *EMBO J.* 14:2401–2408.

Siomi, M. C., Y. Zhang, H. Siomi, and G. Dreyfuss. 1996. Specific sequences in the fragile X syndrome protein *FMR1* and the FXR proteins mediate their binding to 60S ribosomal subunits and the interactions among them. *Mol. Cell. Biol.* 16:3825–3832.

Sittler, A., D. Devys, C. Weber, and J-L. Mandel. 1996. Alternative splicing of exon 14 determines nuclear or cytoplasmic localisation of *FMR1* protein isoforms. *Hum. Mol. Genet.* 5:95–102.

Slegtenhorst-Eegdeman, K. E., H. J. G. van de Kant, M. Post, A. Ruiz, J. T. J. Uilenbroek, C. E. Bakker, B. A. Oostra, J. A. Grootegoed, D. G. de Rooij, and A. P. N. Themmen. 1998. Macro-orchidism in *FMR1* knockout mice is caused by increased Sertoli cell proliferation during testis development. *Endocrinology* 139:156–162.

Smeets, H., A. Smits, C. E. Verheij, J. Theelen, R. Willemsen, M. Losekoot, I. Van de Burgt, A. T. Hoogeveen, J. Oosterwijk, and B. A. Oostra. 1995. Normal phenotype in two brothers with a full *FMR1* mutation. *Hum. Mol. Genet.* 4:2103–2108.

Steward, O. 1997. mRNA localization in neurons: A multipurpose mechanism? *Neuron* 18:9–12.

Sutcliffe, J. S., D. L. Nelson, F. Zhang, M. Pieretti, C. T. Caskey, D. Saxe, and S. T. Warren. 1992. DNA methylation represses *FMR-1* transcription in fragile X syndrome. *Hum. Mol. Genet.* 1:397–400.

Tamanini, F., N. Meijer, C. Verheij, P. J. Willems, H. Galjaard, B. A. Oostra, and A. T. Hoogeveen. 1996. FMRP is associated to the ribosomes via RNA. *Hum. Mol. Genet.* 5:809–813.

Tamanini, F., R. Willemsen, L. van Unen, C. Bontekoe, H. Galjaard, B. A. Oostra, and A. T. Hoogeveen. 1997. Differential expression of *FMR1, FXR1* and *FXR2* proteins in human brain and testis. *Hum. Mol. Genet.* 6:1315–1322.

Tamanini, F., C. Bontekoe, C. E. Bakker, L. van Unen, B. Anar, R. Willemsen, M. Yoshida, H. Galjaard, B. A. Oostra, and A. T. Hoogeveen. 1999a. Different targets for the fragile X–related proteins revealed by their distinct nuclear localizations. *Hum. Mol. Genet.* 8:863–869.

Tamanini, F., L. Van Unen, C. Bakker, N. Sacchi, H. Galjaard, B. A. Oostra, and A. T. Hoogeveen. 1999b. Oligomerization properties of fragile-X mental-retardation protein (FMRP) and the fragile-X–related proteins FXR1P and FXR2P. *Biochem. J.* 343:517–523.

Tamanini, F., L. L. Kirkpatrick, J. Schonkeren, L. Unen, C. Bontekoe, C. Bakker, D. L. Nelson, H. Galjaard, B. A. Oostra, and A. T. Hoogeveen. 2000. The fragile X–related proteins FXR1P and FXR2P contain a functional nucleolar-targeting signal equivalent to the HIV-1 regulatory proteins. *Hum. Mol. Genet.* 9:1487–1493.

Tassone, F., R. J. Hagerman, A. K. Taylor, L. W. Gane, T. E. Godfrey, and P. J. Hagerman. 2000a. Elevated levels of *FMR1* mRNA in carrier males: A new mechanism of involvement in the fragile X syndrome. *Am. J. Hum. Genet.* 66:6–15.

Tassone, F., R. J. Hagerman, A. K. Taylor, J. B. Mills, S. W. Harris, L. W. Gane, and P. J. Hagerman. 2000b. Clinical involvement and protein expression in individuals with the *FMR1* premutation. *Am. J. Med. Genet.* 91:144–152.

Tuncbilek, E., M. Alikasifoglu, D. Aktas, F. Duman, H. Yanik, B. Anar, R. Willemsen, and B. A. Oostra. 2000. Screening for the fragile X syndrome among mentally retarded males by hair root analysis. *Am. J. Med. Genet.* 95:105–107.

Verheij, C., C. E. Bakker, E. de Graaff, J. Keulemans, R. Willemsen, A. J. Verkerk, H. Galjaard, A. J. Reuser, A. T. Hoogeveen, and B. A. Oostra. 1993. Characterization and localization of the *FMR-1* gene product associated with fragile X syndrome. *Nature* 363:722–724.

Verheij, C., E. De Graaff, C. E. Bakker, R. Willemsen, P. J. Willems, N. Meijer, H. Galjaard, A. J. J. Reuser, B. A. Oostra, and A. T. Hoogeveen. 1995. Characterization of *FMR1* proteins isolated from different tissues. *Hum. Mol. Genet.* 4:895–901.

Verkerk, A. J., M. Pieretti, J. S. Sutcliffe, Y. H. Fu, D. P. Kuhl, A. Pizzuti, O. Reiner, S. Richards, M. F. Victoria, F. P. Zhang, B. E. Eussen, G. J. B. Van Ommen, L. A. J. Blonden, G. J. Riggins, J. L. Chastain, C. B. Kunst, H. Galjaard, C. T. Caskey, D. L. Nelson, B. A. Oostra, and S. T. Warren. 1991. Identification of a gene (*FMR-1*) containing a CGG repeat coincident with a breakpoint cluster region exhibiting length variation in fragile X syndrome. *Cell* 65:905–914.

Verkerk, A. J., E. De Graaff, K. De Boulle, E. E. Eichler, D. S. Konecki, E. Reyniers, A. Manca, A. Poustka, P. J. Willems, D. L. Nelson, and B. A. Oostra. 1993. Alternative splicing in the fragile X gene *FMR1*. *Hum. Mol. Genet.* 2:399–404.

Weiler, I. J., and W. T. Greenough. 1999. Synaptic synthesis of the fragile X protein: Possible involvement in synapse maturation and elimination. *Am. J. Med. Genet.* 83:248–252.

Weiler, I. J., S. A. Irwin, A. Y. Klintsova, C. M. Spencer, A. D. Brazelton, K. Miyashiro, T. A. Comery, B. Patel, J. Eberwine, and W. T. Greenough. 1997. Fragile X mental retardation protein is translated near synapses in response to neurotransmitter activation. *Proc. Natl. Acad. Sci. USA* 94:5395–5400.

Wen, W., J. L. Meinkoth, R. Y. Tsien, and S. S. Taylor. 1995. Identification of a signal for rapid export of proteins from the nucleus. *Cell* 82:463–473.

Willemsen, R., S. Mohkamsing, B. De Vries, D. Devys, A. Van den Ouweland, J. L. Mandel, H. Galjaard, and B. Oostra. 1995. Rapid antibody test for fragile X syndrome. *Lancet* 345:1147–1148.

Willemsen, R., C. Bontekoe, F. Tamanini, H. Galjaard, A. T. Hoogeveen, and B. A. Oostra. 1996a. Association of FMRP with ribosomal precursor particles in the nucleolus. *Biochem. Biophys. Res. Commun.* 225:27–33.

Willemsen, R., J. C. Oosterwijk, F. J. Los, H. Galjaard, and B. A. Oostra. 1996b. Prenatal diagnosis of fragile X syndrome. *Lancet* 348:967–968.

Willemsen, R., F. Los, S. Mohkamsing, A. Vandenouweland, W. Deelen, H. Galjaard, and B. Oostra. 1997a. Rapid antibody test for prenatal diagnosis of fragile X syndrome on amniotic fluid cells: A new appraisal. *J. Med. Genet.* 34:250–251.

Willemsen, R., A. Smits, S. Mohkamsing, H. Vanbeerendonk, A. Dehaan, B. Devries, A. Vandenouweland, E. Sistermans, H. Galjaard, and B. A. Oostra. 1997b. Rapid antibody test for diagnosing fragile X syndrome: A validation of the technique. *Hum. Genet.* 99:308–311.

Willemsen, R., B. Anar, Y. de Diego Otero, B. B. de Vries, Y. Hilhorst-Hofstee, A. Smits, E. van Looveren, P. J. Willems, H. Galjaard, and B. A. Oostra. 1999. Noninvasive test for fragile X syndrome, using hair root analysis. *Am. J. Hum. Genet.* 65:98–103.

Willemsen, R., R. Olmer, Y. De Diego Otero, and B. A. Oostra. 2000. Twin sisters: Monozygotic with the fragile X mutation, but with a different phenotype. *J. Med. Genet.* 37:603–604.

Wöhrle, D., D. Kotzot, M. C. Hirst, A. Manca, B. Korn, A. Schmidt, G. Barbi, H. D. Rott, A. Poustka, K. E. Davies, and P. Steinbach. 1992. A microdeletion of less than 250 kb, including the proximal part of the *FMR-1* gene and the fragile-X site, in a male with the clinical phenotype of fragile-X syndrome. *Am. J. Hum. Genet.* 51:299–306.

Zhang, Y., J. P. O'Connor, M. C. Siomi, S. Srinivasan, A. Dutra, R. L. Nussbaum, and G. Dreyfuss. 1995. The fragile X mental retardation syndrome protein interacts with novel homologs FXR1 and FXR2. *EMBO J.* 14:5358–5366.

# CHAPTER 5

# Brain Structure and the Functions of *FMR1* Protein

Scott Irwin, M.D., Roberto Galvez,
Ivan Jeanne Weiler, Ph.D.,
Andrea Beckel-Mitchener, Ph.D., and
William Greenough, Ph.D.

This chapter focuses on the brain structural phenotype in fragile X syndrome (FXS) and the ways in which the normal function of *FMR1* protein (FMRP) might lead to these abnormalities in its absence. Both gross brain morphologic abnormalities and dendritic structure abnormalities that suggest impaired development of neurons have been described in association with FXS, and dendritic abnormalities have similarly been described in the leading animal model, the fragile X knockout mouse.

## Gross Brain Morphology in Fragile X Syndrome

Gross brain abnormalities have been described in structural magnetic resonance imaging (MRI) studies of patients with FXS. Reiss et al. (1991) and Mostofsky et al. (1998) reported that fragile X males exhibit a reduction in the size of the posterior cerebellar vermis and an enlargement of the fourth ventricle as compared to controls. Reduced cerebellar vermis volume has also been reported in autism, along with pathology and cell loss in both vermis and hemispheres of the cerebellum (e.g., Bailey et al. 1998; Carper and Courchesne 2000; Ritvo et al. 1986). In addition, an increased volume in fragile X patients was also reported in the hippocampus (Reiss et al. 1994; Kates et al. 1997), the caudate nucleus (Reiss et al. 1995), and the lateral ventricles (Reiss et al. 1995) as com-

*Fragile X Syndrome: Diagnosis, Treatment, and Research,* third edition, ed. Randi Jenssen Hagerman and Paul J. Hagerman (Baltimore: Johns Hopkins University Press, 2002), © The Johns Hopkins University Press.

pared to controls. An age-related increase in the volume of the hippocampus and decrease in the volume of the superior temporal gyrus were also found in fragile X patients (Reiss et al. 1994). The gross volumetric changes found by MRI in fragile X patients were not observed in a separate study of two fragile X patients, which used physical measurement of autopsy material (Reyniers et al. 1999), nor were volumetric changes found with MRI in the mouse model of FXS (Kooy et al. 1999). However, increases in human brain volumes seem to be consistent with the findings of increased spine density and increased spine length in FXS, which are described below.

## Neuronal Structure in Fragile X Syndrome

Several studies indicate impaired neuronal development in clinical cases of FXS. Rudelli et al. (1985) and Wisniewski et al. (1991) both described long, thin, tortuous dendritic spines with prominent heads and irregular dilations on apical dendrites of pyramidal cells in Golgi-impregnated cerebral cortex of the same fragile X patient. Reduced mean synaptic contact area was also reported; however, no other major neuropathologic findings were noted. Hinton et al. (1991) reported similar dendritic spine characteristics and no differences in neuronal density in two additional fragile X patients, as well as the one studied by Rudelli et al. and Wisniewski et al., compared to controls. Figure 5.1 illustrates tissue examined by Irwin et al. (2001). There were no differences in neuronal density (number of neurons per unit tissue volume), suggesting normal neurogenesis and cell migration in fragile X patients; however, the stereologic method used would have overcounted relatively larger cells, and cell size was not measured. The bias toward an overcount occurs because larger cells will, on average, appear in more tissue sections of any given thickness, so knowledge of cell size is required for interpreting these data.

**A.**               **B.**

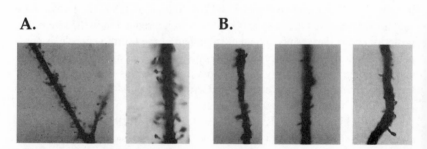

**Fig. 5.1.** Golgi-impregnated dendrites from a human afflicted by fragile X syndrome (*A*) and an unaffected control (*B*). These photos illustrate spine morphology but are not accurate indicators of spine density.

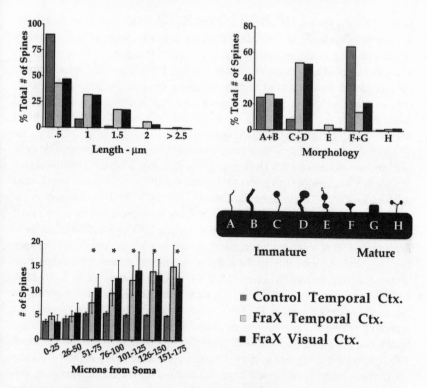

**Fig. 5.2.** Fragile X (*FraX*) patients exhibit elongated dendritic spines (*top left*), a higher density of spines along dendrites (*bottom left*), and a more immature morphology (*right*) compared with a matched sample of unaffected individuals. Control tissue from temporal cortex (*Ctx.*) did not impregnate properly. *Source:* Irwin et al. 2001. Reprinted by permission of Wiley-Liss, Inc., a subsidiary of John Wiley & Sons, Inc.

The previous studies of spine morphology used largely qualitative observations. As illustrated in figure 5.2, a quantitative neuroanatomic study of Golgi-Kopsch prepared human autopsy temporal and occipital cortex reported significantly more, long dendritic spines and fewer, short spines. Those investigators also observed more spines with immature shapes and correspondingly fewer with mature shapes in fragile X patients as compared to matched controls (Irwin et al. 2001). These effects were consistent across multiple dendritic branch types in both visual and temporal cortex. The results for spine shape, in particular, suggested an arrest of normal spine maturation in FXS. Perhaps most important to this interpretation was the finding that fragile X patients exhibited a significantly greater spine density on distal segments of apical dendritic shafts and the same tendency on apical oblique and basilar dendrites in both brain regions. This suggests a persistent failure of normal synapse pruning processes, another possible indicator of delayed or arrested maturation. However, overly active synaptogenesis, or simply a higher rate of synapse stabilization in development, could also account for this finding. If the increased spine number reflects greater numbers of excitatory synapses, this could contribute to the increased tendency toward seizure phenomena seen in children with FXS and might account for some aspects of attentional dysfunction, perceptual disorders, and motor impairments often seen in FXS.

Many of these findings have been supported by animal studies. A "knockout" mouse model of FXS (KO mice) was developed by the Dutch-Belgian Fragile X Consortium (Bakker et al. 1994) (see chap. 4). In initial brain morphology studies of these animals, Comery et al. (1997) demonstrated an increase in spine density and spine length on layer V pyramidal cells in the visual cortex in adult KO mice compared with wild-type (WT) mice, further suggesting impairment of spine maturation and pruning in FXS. Although this has been the only brain abnormality in these mice thus far published, with other measures appearing normal (Bakker et al. 1994; Godfraind et al. 1996; Kooy et al. 1996), it may involve a mitigating circumstance. An unknown number of the mice used in the Comery et al. (1997) study may have been homozygous for a recessive retinal degeneration gene found in the FVB strain into which the knock-out gene had been crossed from the 129 source strain (Bowes et al. 1990). Retinal dysfunction is likely to affect cell morphology in the visual cortex of these animals and could have differentially affected the knockout animals. This finding of a possible interaction between sensory deprivation and the absence of FMRP suggests that some phenotypic consequences of the knockout might be exacerbated by inadequate experience. This finding also raises the possibility that an experience-rich environment might have ameliorative effects in FXS patients.

To assess differences between KO and wild-type mice in the absence of sensory defects, a quantitative neuroanatomic study of mice genetically screened for intact retinae demonstrated that adult KO mice have longer, more immature-appearing dendritic spines than do wild-type control mice (Irwin et al. 1999, 2000a). KO mice have a greater percentage of spines than do controls on segments of apical dendritic shafts, apical oblique dendrites, and basilar dendrites. Similarly, KO mice exhibit more immature-appearing spine shapes and fewer mature-shaped spines on segments of apical dendritic shafts and apical oblique dendrites. Two independent groups have confirmed these results in vitro, demonstrating a larger relative number of longer spines resembling an immature morphology in cultured hippocampal neurons from KO mice compared to wild-type mice (Warren and Torre 2000; Nimchinsky et al. 2000). In both cases, the differences in spine length decreased with increasing time that the neurons were maintained in culture. Unlike humans affected with FXS, KO mice lacking retinal degeneration did not exhibit any statistically significant spine density increases, relative to wild-type mice, along any of the branch types (Warren and Torre 2000). Results do suggest a trend toward a higher spine density in KO relative to wild-type mice. These characteristics might be associated with the behavioral deficits described in chapter 1. Not all studies have shown a persistent increase in spine density into adulthood. A transient increase in spine density that diminishes after 2 weeks has been reported in both hippocampal cultured neurons and pyramidal cells in the barrel cortex (Nimchinsky et al. 2001; Warren and Torre 2000). These observations were based on methods different from those that generated the data presented above.

Since dendrites of some cell populations also undergo an overproduction and developmental pruning process (Falls and Gobel 1979; Brunjes et al. 1982; Murphy and Magness 1984; Greenough and Chang 1988b), dendritic tree branching complexity and total amount of dendritic material were assessed in KO mice. No significant differences in the number of branches at each branch order, the probability of bifurcation at each branch order, or the amount of dendritic material at fixed intervals away from the soma were found between KO and wild-type mice for layer V pyramidal visual cortical cells (Irwin et al. 1999, 2000a). These results do not agree with some in vitro studies conducted on young cultured hippocampal neurons. In vitro cell culture studies done on 7- and 21-day-old hippocampal neurons found that KO mice exhibited shorter dendrites, fewer spines, and no significant difference in spine length when compared to wild-type mice (Braun and Segal 2000). Furthermore, in vitro cell culture studies on gestational day 16 hippocampal neurons found that KO mice exhibited fewer primary dendrites and shorter dendrites when compared to wild-type mice (Warren and Torre 2000). The above study also found, as reported and referenced above, that KO mice exhibited a larger number of longer spines then did wild-type mice, a result consistent with the in vivo studies. Though some of these data seem to contradict the above findings, it is important to note that the age of the neurons differed between the in vivo and in vitro studies (adult vs. 7 and 21 days or gestational day 16) and that the two studies were conducted not only in different regions of the brain (cortex vs. hippocampus), but also using different preparations (in vivo vs. in vitro). The fact that KO mice do not show any dendritic arborization abnormalities in the cortex suggests that the effects of the absence of FMRP in cortical neurons in vivo may be limited to spine/synaptic structure and that it does not play an essential role affecting overall neuronal morphology of pyramidal neurons in the cerebral cortex.

## Developmental Synaptic Maturation and Pruning Hypothesis

The lack of FMRP leads to a persistent abnormal dendritic spine structure in both humans and mice and to an elevated number of dendritic spines in humans. The neuronal structural abnormalities in FXS seem to be limited to dendritic spines, based on the results from in vivo studies, although the different in vitro study results may well provide important additional understanding of the role of FMRP in dendritic development. The results overall provide strong evidence for the association of FMRP with synaptic plasticity across brain regions and point to a cause of the behavioral deficits observed in both humans and mice lacking FMRP. The specific role played by FMRP in altering the structure of dendritic spines is not clear, although its possible role in regulating protein synthesis at the synapse certainly provides mechanisms through which such an effect could occur (see below). Several other genetic syndromes have been reported to be associated with neuronal structural abnormalities; however, the deficits associated with these syndromes have not been limited specifically to dendritic spines, nor have any of these syndromes been found to exhibit an increase in dendritic spine number. This suggests that FMRP may be specific to developmental maturation and pruning of dendritic spines (see Irwin et al. 2000a).

The in vivo increase in the density of dendritic spines on cortical cells of fragile X patients, combined with a clear tendency of spines to exhibit an immature morphology (Irwin et al. 2001), points to impaired activity-mediated synapse maturation during development, in which some synapses are eliminated while others are stabilized and strengthened (e.g., LeVay et al. 1980; Greenough and Chang 1985; Hwang and Greenough 1986; Schuz 1986; Galofre et al. 1987; Greenough and Chang 1988a; Horner 1993; Greenough et al. 1994).

A very recent finding supports the concept that fragile X KO mice are impaired in eliminating neuronal processes in development. Galvez et al. (2001) studied dendritic processes of spiny stellate neurons in barrels, the cylindrical arrangements of neuronal cell bodies that define the processing units in the somatosensory cortex for the large facial whiskers. In normal development, dendritic processes initially extend in all directions from the cell body; as development proceeds, branches directed toward the "hollow" or interior of the barrel continue to proliferate, while those directed away from it are withdrawn. In KO mice, the processes extending into the barrel hollow were identical to those of WT mice; those extending away from it, however, remained more extensive than in WT mice, suggesting a failure of dendritic process retraction, which could be associated with a failure to eliminate synapses.

An excess number of excitatory synapses could be involved in one of the occasionally observed features of clinical FXS, a tendency to exhibit seizures (chap. 1). A correlate of clinical and experimental seizures is sprouting of the mossy fiber axons arising from dentate gyrus granule cells, both within the den-

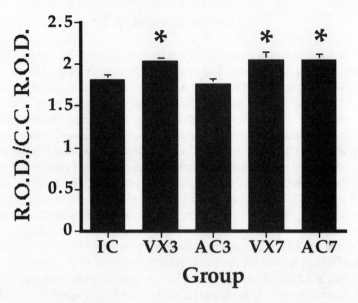

**Fig. 5.3.** Effects of individual laboratory cage housing (*IC*), voluntary exercise in an activity wheel attached to an individual laboratory cage (*VX*), or learning to traverse an elevated obstacle course (*AC*) for 3 or 7 days on the relative optical density (*R.O.D.*) of dentate gyrus molecular layer immunostained for FMRP. *Source:* Irwin et al. 2000b.

tate and in hippocampal subfield CA3 (Proper et al. 2000; Golarai and Sutula 1996). Ivanco and Greenough (2000) investigated mossy fiber sprouting in subfield CA3 in KO (FVB strain) and WT mice. They observed excess sprouting in the KO mice, suggesting that increased axonal branching and synaptogenesis might be either a cause or a consequence (or both) of the seizures.

The data reviewed thus far can be interpreted to suggest that synaptic pruning and maturation are impaired in cases of FXS and may imply a direct or indirect role in these processes for FMRP. Other findings support a potential role of FMRP in synaptic plasticity as well. For example, as figure 5.3 illustrates, a series of in vivo studies has demonstrated increased FMRP immunoreactivity in brain regions known to be undergoing active synaptogenesis in response to motor-skill learning or complex environment rearing, or increased activation in response to repetitive motor activity or sensory stimulation (Irwin et al. 2000b; Greenough et al. 2001). In related work, Todd and Mack (2000) similarly found that somatosensory stimulation increased FMRP levels in somatosensory cortex. It is possible that FMRP synthesis serves as an "activity detector," allowing initiation of synaptic protein synthesis, with other events related to learning, as opposed to activity, determining the final pattern of synaptic change.

## The Cellular Roles of FMRP

Clues to the function of FMRP may lie in its specific tissue localization and its association with rapidly dividing cells early in development (Abitbol et al. 1993; Hinds et al. 1993). FMRP and its closely related family members *FXR1* and *FXR2* have independent cellular distributions in fetal brain and testis (Tamanini et al. 1997), despite a high degree of sequence similarity and comparable RNA-binding properties. In adult testis, FMRP is strongly expressed in spermatogonia (Devys et al. 1993; Coy et al. 1995). In addition, FMRP is implicated in cellular remodeling by data demonstrating increased FMRP levels in quiescent mouse kidney cells when these cells were stimulated to resume proliferation (Khandjian et al. 1995). Devys et al. (1993) showed that dividing layers of epithelial tissues, as well as cells involved with wound healing and pathogenesis, such as heart myocytes during ischemic cardiomyopathy, exhibited strong FMRP expression. There are also high levels of FMRP in esophageal epithelium and thymus cortex of adult mice (Hinds et al. 1993). These data suggest that FMRP may be involved in cellular structural transformations outside of the central nervous system, such as those accompanying cellular proliferation, that may have mechanisms in common with neuronal structural transformations. Thus, unlike mature tissues such as muscle, where FMRP has not been observed, neurons, rapidly dividing tissues, and spermatogonia retain certain embryonic capacities and might require FMRP for regulated transport or translation of mRNAs needed for cell maturation.

Another clue to the cellular role of FMRP is its synthesis at synapses under the regulatory control of the neurotransmitter glutamate. An in vitro study has shown that FMRP is translated in a preparation of purified subcellular synapse-containing particles (termed *synaptoneurosomes*) in response to neurotransmitter stimulation. This result suggests that FMRP is made at synapses in response to synaptic activation (Weiler et al. 1997). Weiler and Greenough (1991, 1993) reported that protein synthesis in synaptoneurosomes is triggered by a class I metabotropic glutamate receptor that acts through phospholipase C production of diacylglycerol to activate protein kinase C.

Using the *fmr1* KO mice that, functionally resembling affected patients, are unable to produce a full-length FMRP protein (see chap. 4), we recently observed a deficit in synapse-associated protein translation. Synaptoneurosomes from rats and WT mice respond to stimulation by metabotropic glutamate agonists with rapid (1–2 min) increased polyribosome formation and transient accelerated protein translation (Weiler and Greenough 1993; Weiler et al. 1997). We observed that synaptoneurosomes from KO mice were unable to respond in this manner, although they were capable of basal levels of protein translation. Moreover, electron microscopic quantification showed that young (15 and 25 day) KO mice exhibited substantially fewer polyribosomal aggregates in dendritic spines than did WT mice of the same age (Weiler et al. 1999; Greenough et al. 2001). The absence, in KO mice, of neurotransmitter-stimulated protein synthesis in the isolated synapse preparation and the reduction in synapse-associated polyribosomes suggest that FMRP is necessary to support neuro-transmitter-actuated polyribosome assembly and dendritic protein synthesis. A deficit in some aspect of protein translation in dendritic processes of neurons might well underlie the deficiency in synaptic maturation observed in both KO mice and human patients.

There is also evidence suggesting a cellular transport role for FMRP. Bardoni et al. (1999) described a nuclear FMRP-interacting protein (NUFIP) that does not interact with the FXR homologs but does show RNA binding activity in vitro, suggesting a specific nuclear role for FMRP. Furthermore, leptomycin B, an antibiotic that inhibits the nuclear export of nuclear export signal (NES)–containing proteins, causes FMRP to accumulate in the nucleus (Tamanini et al. 1999), suggesting that FMRP shuttles between the nucleus and the cytoplasm. Indeed, FMRP has been observed in transit through nuclear pores by immunogold electron microscopy (Feng et al. 1997). However, the majority of FMRP has been reported to be located in the cytoplasm (Devys et al. 1993). In neurons, most FMRP is located in the cytoplasm of the cell body, but it is also detected in dendrites, at the origins of dendritic spine necks, in spine heads (Feng et al. 1997), and associated with polyribosomes in synaptoneurosomes (Weiler et al. 1997).

## Possible Mechanisms of Action of FMRP

Taking into account the association of FMRP with poly(A)+ mRNA in actively translating polyribosomes (Corbin et al. 1997), Khandjian (1999) suggested that FMRP might be a mRNA chaperone interacting with mRNP complexes. Thus, FMRP could act as a translational regulator at the synapse, where its function would be to selectively allow translation of a subset of mRNAs in response to cellular signals. In the absence of FMRP, translation would be unaffected by neurotransmitter stimuli; hence, the cells would appear normal but would not be able to achieve the normal degree of synaptic maturation or remodeling on demand (or other functions of synaptically regulated protein synthesis).

A translational regulator of relatively low abundance would most likely be specific to particular mRNAs. Several investigators have attempted to determine whether FMRP binds a subset of mRNAs. FMRP has been reported to bind to 4% of all brain mRNAs, including its own (Ashley et al. 1993). Several groups have identified some candidate mRNAs in this subset using a variety of in vitro methods (Sung et al. 2000; Brown et al. 1998), but as yet no common RNA sequence or putative RNA structure has emerged. There are other suggestions of specific proteins that differ, for example, in level of expression in *Fmr-1* knockout versus wild-type mice and in humans with fragile X syndrome. For example, using an RNA differential display assay, the mRNA for Ras-GTPase-activating protein SH3-domain-binding protein (G3PD) was found to be less abundant in lymphocytes derived from a fragile X patient compared to control cells (Zhong et al. 1999). Whether this transcript binds directly to FMRP is unknown, as is the significance of the observed difference in expression of the gene product. Preliminary tests of synaptic protein preparations revealed that, in young *Fmr-1* knockout mice, there are lowered levels of the glutamate receptor mGluR1 in cerebral cortex, although not in cerebellum or hippocampus (Weiler et al. 2000). Receptor binding studies and immunohistochemistry have also indicated a decrease in mGluR2 receptors in the granule cell layer of the cerebellum (Shi et al. 2000). If the balance of receptors at a synapse is not normal, due to disturbed translation regulation, the response of the synapse may be subtly altered. Such receptor alterations could also affect protein synthesis at the synapse.

Irwin et al. (2000b) and Greenough et al. (2001) proposed that FMRP may act as an "immediate early protein" in a manner similar to immediate early genes that are transcribed rapidly in response to neuronal activity (Sheng and Greenberg 1990; Clayton 2000). FMRP may be rapidly translated in response to neuronal activity in order to regulate the translation of other activity-dependent proteins at the synapse. It is widely recognized that activity drives nervous system organization in development and, given that proteins are synthesized at synapses in response to activity, it is plausible that these proteins might be involved in synaptic plasticity processes. Moreover, the fact that the absence of FMRP is associated with morphologic deficits of dendritic spines is compatible with this view. It is possible that FMRP is the "synaptic tag" proposed by Grey and Morris (1997). FMRP may set in motion a process at the synapse whereby new proteins are synthesized locally to interact with proteins that arrive via dendritic transport. Such interactions may be required for synaptic plasticity. This hypothesis reflects the finding that synaptic plasticity has a longer time course than would be expected if it depended on local processes alone; it also allows for synapse specificity and may require transcription, which has been shown to be important for some forms of synaptic plasticity (Huang and Kandel 1994; Kurotani et al. 1996).

## Acknowledgments

Supported by HD 37175, FRAXA Research Foundation, MH 11272, MH 35321, Illinois–Eastern Iowa District Kiwanis International Spastic Paralysis Research Foundation, NSF DBI 98-70821, and HD 07333.

## References

Abitbol, M., C. Menini, A. L. Delezoide, T. Rhyner, M. Vekemans, and J. Mallet. 1993. Nucleus basalis magnocellularis and hippocampus are the major sites of *FMR-1* expression in the human fetal brain. *Nat. Genet.* 4:147–153.

Ashley, C. T., K. D. Wilkinson, D. Reines, and S. T. Warren. 1993. *FMR1* protein: Conserved RNP family domains and selective RNA binding. *Science* 262:563–566.

Bailey, A., P. Luthert, A. Dean, B. Harding, I. Janota, M. Montgomery, M. Rutter, and P. Lantos. 1998. A clinicopathological study of autism. *Brain* 121:889–905.

Bakker, C. E., C. Verheij, R. Willemsen, R. van der Helm, et al. 1994. *Fmr1* knockout mice: A model to study fragile X mental retardation. *Cell* 78:23–33.

Bardoni, B., A. Schenck, and J. L. Mandel. 1999. A novel RNA-binding nuclear protein that interacts with the fragile X mental retardation (*FMR1*) protein. *Hum. Mol. Genet.* 8:2557–2566.

Bowes, C., T. Li, M. Danciger, L. C. Baxter, M. L. Applebury, and D. B. Farber. 1990. Retinal degeneration in the rd mouse is caused by a defect in the beta subunit of rod cGMP-phosphodiesterase. *Nature* 347:677–680

Braun, K., and M. Segal. 2000. FMRP involvement in formation of synapses among cultured hippocampal neurons. *Cereb. Cortex* 10:1045–1052.

Brown, V., K. Small, L. Lakkis, Y. Feng, C. Gunter, K. D. Wilkinson, and S. T. Warren. 1998. Purified recombinant FMRP exhibits selective RNA binding as an intrinsic property of the fragile X mental retardation protein. *J. Biol. Chem.* 273:15521–15527.

Brunjes, P. C., H. D. Schwark, and W. T. Greenough. 1982. Olfactory granule cell development in normal and hyperthyroid rats. *Brain Res.* 281:149–159.

Carper, R. A., and E. Courchesne. 2000. Inverse correlation between frontal lobe and cerebellum sizes in children with autism. *Brain* 123:836–844.

Clayton, D. F. 2000. The genomic action potential. *Neurobiol. Learn. Mem.* 74:185–216.

Comery, T. A., J. B. Harris, P. J. Willems, B. A. Oostra, S. A. Irwin, I. J. Weiler, and W. T. Greenough. 1997. Abnormal dendritic spines in fragile X knockout mice: Maturation and pruning deficits. *Proc. Natl. Acad. Sci. USA* 94:5401–5404.

Corbin F., M. Bouillon, A. Fortin, S. Morin, F. Rousseau, and E. W. Khandjian. 1997. The fragile X mental retardation protein is associated with poly(A)+ mRNA in actively translating polyribosomes. *Hum. Mol. Genet.* 6:1465–1472.

Coy, J. F., Z. Sedlacek, D. Bachner, H. Hameister, S. Joos, P. Lichter, H. Delius, and A. Poustka. 1995. Highly conserved 3′UTR and expression pattern of *FXR1* points to a divergent gene regulation of *FXR1* and *FMR1*. *Hum. Mol. Genet.* 4:2209–2218.

Devys, D., Y. Lutz, N. Rouyer, J. P. Bellocq, and J. L. Mandel. 1993. The *FMR-1* protein is cytoplasmic, most abundant in neurons and appears normal in carriers of a fragile X premutation. *Nat. Genet.* 4:335–340.

Falls, W., and S. Gobel. 1979. Golgi and EM studies of the formation of dendritic and axonal arbors: The interneurons of the substantia gelatinosa of Rolando in newborn kittens. *J. Comp. Neurol.* 187:1–18.

Feng, Y., C. A. Gutekunst, D. E. Eberhart, H. Yi, S. T. Warren, and S. M. Hersch. 1997.

Fragile X mental retardation protein: Nucleocytoplasmic shuttling and association with somatodendritic ribosomes. *J. Neurosci.* 17:1539–1547.

Galofre, E., I. Ferrer, I. Fabregues, and D. Lopez-Tejero. 1987. Effects of prenatal ethanol exposure on dendritic spines of layer V pyramidal neurons in the somatosensory cortex of the rat. *J. Neurol. Sci.* 81:185–195.

Galvez, R., A. R. Gopal, and W. T. Greenough. 2001. Dendritic abnormalities associated with a mouse model of the fragile X mental retardation syndrome. *Soc. Neurosci. Abstr.* In press.

Godfraind, J. M., E. Reyniers, K. De Boulle, R. D'Hooge, P. P. De Deyn, C. E. Bakker, B. A. Oostra, R. F. Kooy, and P. J. Willems. 1996. Long-term potentiation in the hippocampus of fragile X knockout mice. *Am. J. Med. Genet.* 64:246–251.

Golarai, G., and T. P. Sutula. 1996. Functional alterations in the dentate gyrus after induction of long-term potentiation, kindling, and mossy fiber sprouting. *J. Neurophysiol.* 75:343–353.

Greenough, W. T., and F-L. F. Chang. 1985. Synaptic structural correlates of information storage in mammalian nervous systems. In C. W. Cotman (ed.), *Synaptic plasticity.* New York: Guilford Press, pp. 335–371.

———. 1988a. Plasticity of synaptic structure in the cerebral cortex. In A. Peters and E. G. Jones (eds.), *Cerebral cortex.* New York: Plenum Press, 7:391–439.

———. 1988b. Dendritic pattern formation involves both oriented regression and oriented growth in the barrels of mouse somatosensory cortex. *Brain Res.* 471:148–152.

Greenough, W. T., K. E. Armstrong, T. A. Comery, N. Hawrylak, A. G. Humphreys, J. A. Kleim, R. A. Swain, and X. Wang. 1994. Plasticity related changes in synapse morphology. In A. I. Selverston and P. Ascher (eds.), *Cellular and molecular mechanisms underlying higher neural functions.* Chichester, England: Wiley, pp. 211–219.

Greenough, W. T., A. Y. Klintsova, S. A. Irwin, R. Galvez, K. E. Bates, and I. J. Weiler. 2001. Synaptic regulation of protein synthesis and the fragile X protein. *Proc. Natl. Acad. Sci. USA* 98:7101–7106.

Grey, U., and R. G. M. Morris. 1997. Synaptic tagging and long-term potentiation. *Nature* 385:533–536.

Hinds, H. L., C. T. Ashley, J. S. Sutcliffe, D. L. Nelson, S. T. Warren, D. E. Housman, and M. Schalling. 1993. Tissue specific expression of *FMR-1* provides evidence for a functional role in fragile X syndrome [see comments] [erratum in *Nat. Genet.* 5: 312]. *Nat. Genet.* 3:36–43.

Hinton, V. J., W. T. Brown, K. Wisniewski, and R. D. Rudelli. 1991. Analysis of neocortex in three males with the fragile X syndrome. *Am. J. Med. Genet.* 41:289–294.

Horner, C. H. 1993. Plasticity of the dendritic spine. *Prog. Neurobiol.* 41:281–321.

Huang, Y. Y., and E. R. Kandel. 1994. Recruitment of long-lasting and protein kinase A–dependent long-term potentiation in the CA1 region of hippocampus requires repeated tetanization. *Learn. Mem.* 1:74–82.

Hwang, H. M., and W. T. Greenough. 1986. Synaptic plasticity in adult rat occipital cortex following short-term, long term, and reversal of differential housing environment complexity. *Soc. Neurosci. Abstr.* 12:1284.

Irwin, S. A., M. Idupulapati, A. B. Mehta, R. A. Crisostomo, E. J. Rogers, B. P. Larsen, C. J. Alcantara, J. B. Harris, B. A. Patel, M. E. Gilbert, A. Chakravarti, R. A. Swain,

R. F. Kooy, P. B. Kozlowski, I. J. Weiler, and W. T. Greenough. 1999. Abnormal dendritic and dendritic spine characteristics in fragile-X patients and the mouse model of fragile-X syndrome. *Soc. Neurosci. Abstr.* 25:636;254.8.

Irwin, S. A., R. Galvez, and W. T. Greenough. 2000a. Dendritic spine structural anomalies in fragile-X mental retardation syndrome. *Cereb. Cortex* 10:1038–1044.

Irwin, S. A., R. A. Swain, C. A. Christmon, A. Chakravarti, I. J. Weiler, and W. T. Greenough. 2000b. Evidence for altered fragile-X mental retardation protein expression in response to behavioral stimulation. *Neurobiol. Learn. Mem.* 73:87–93.

Irwin, S. A., B. Patel, M. Idupulapati, J. B. Harris, R. A. Cristostomo, F. Kooy, P. J. Willems, P. Cras, P. B. Kozlowski, R. A. Swain, I. J. Weiler, and W. T. Greenough. 2001. Abnormal dendritic spine characteristics in the temporal cortex of patients with fragile-X syndrome: A quantitative examination. *Am. J. Med. Genet.* 98:161–167.

Ivanco, T. L., and W. T. Greenough. 2000. Fragile X knockout mice show an increase in mossy fiber sprouting in the hippocampus compared to wildtype mice. *Soc. Neurosci. Abstr.* 26:223;80.12.

Kates, W. R., M. T. Abrams, W. E. Kaufmann, S. N. Breiter, and A. L. Reiss. 1997. Reliability and validity of MRI measurement of the amygdala and hippocampus in children with fragile X syndrome. *Psychiatry Res.* 75:31–48.

Khandjian, E. W. 1999. Biology of the fragile X mental retardation protein, an RNA-binding protein. *Biochem. Cell Biol.* 77:331–342.

Khandjian, E. W., A. Fortin, A. Thibodeau, S. Tremblay, F. Cote, D. Devys, J. L. Mandel, and F. Rousseau. 1995. A heterogeneous set of *FMR1* proteins is widely distributed in mouse tissues and is modulated in cell culture. *Hum. Mol. Genet.* 4:783–789.

Kooy, R. F., R. D'Hooge, E. Reyniers, C. E. Bakker, G. Nagels, K. De Boulle, K. Storm, G. Clincke, P. P. De Deyn, B. A. Oostra, and P. J. Willems. 1996. Transgenic mouse model for the fragile X syndrome. *Am. J. Med. Genet.* 64:241–245.

Kooy, R. F., E. Reyniers, M. Verhoye, J. Sijbers, C. E. Bakker, B. A. Oostra, P. J. Willems, and A. Van Der Linden. 1999. Neuroanatomy of the fragile X knockout mouse brain studied using in vivo high resolution magnetic resonance imaging. *Eur. J. Hum. Genet.* 7:526–532.

Kurotani, T., S. Higashi, H. Inokawa, and K. Toyama. 1996. Protein and RNA synthesis-dependent and -independent LTPs in developing rat visual cortex. *Neuroreport* 8:35–39.

LeVay, S., T. N. Wiesel, and D. H. Hubel. 1980. The development of ocular dominance columns in normal and visually deprived monkeys. *J. Comp. Neurol.* 191:1–51.

Mostofsky, S. H., M. M. Mazzocco, G. Aakalu, I. S. Warsofsky, M. B. Denckla, and A. L. Reiss. 1998. Decreased cerebellar posterior vermis size in fragile X syndrome: Correlation with neurocognitive performance. *Neurology* 50:121–130.

Murphy, E. H., and R. Magness. 1984. Development of the rabbit visual cortex: A quantitative Golgi analysis. *Exp. Brain Res.* 53:304–314.

Nimchinsky, E. A., A. M. Oberlander, and K. Svoboda. 2000. Dendritic spine maturation and motility in *FMR1* knockout mice. *Soc. Neurosci. Abstr.* 26:357.

———. 2001. Abnormal development of dendritic spines in *FMR1* knock-out mice. *J. Neurosci.* 21:5139–5146.

Proper, E. A., A. B. Oestreicher, G. H. Jansen, C. W. M. von Veelen, P. C. van Rijen, W. H. Gispen, and P. N. E. de Graan. 2000. Immunohistochemical characterization of mossy fiber sprouting in the hippocampus of patients with pharmaco-resistant temporal lobe epilepsy. *Brain* 123 (pt. 1): 19–30.

Reiss, A. L., E. Aylward, L. S. Freund, P. K. Joshi, and R. N. Bryan. 1991. Neuroanatomy of fragile X syndrome: The posterior fossa. *Ann. Neurol.* 29:26–32.

Reiss, A. L., J. Lee, and L. Freund. 1994. Neuroanatomy of fragile X syndrome: The temporal lobe. *Neurology* 44:1317–1324.

Reiss, A. L., M. T. Abrams, R. Greenlaw, L. Freund, and M. B. Denckla. 1995. Neurodevelopmental effects of the *FMR-1* full mutation in humans. *Nat. Med.* 1:159–167.

Reyniers, E., J. J. Martin, P. Cras, E. Van Marck, I. Handig, H. Z. Jorens, B. A. Oostra, R. F. Kooy, and P. J. Willems. 1999. Postmortem examination of two fragile X brothers with an *FMR1* full mutation. *Am. J. Med. Genet.* 84:245–249.

Ritvo, E. R., B. J. Freeman, A. B. Scheibel, T. Duong, H. Robinson, D. Guthrie, and A. Ritvo. 1986. Lower Purkinje cell counts in the cerebella of four autistic subjects: Initial findings of the UCLA-NSAC Autopsy Research Report. *Am. J. Psychiatry* 143: 862–866.

Rudelli, R. D., W. T. Brown, K. Wisniewski, E. C. Jenkins, M. Laure-Kamionowska, F. Connell, and H. M. Wisniewski. 1985. Adult fragile X syndrome: Clinico-neuropathologic findings. *Acta Neuropathol. (Berl.)* 67:289–295.

Schuz, A. 1986. Comparison between the dimensions of dendritic spines in the cerebral cortex of newborn and adult guinea pigs. *J. Comp. Neurol.* 244:277–285.

Sheng, M., and M. E. Greenberg. 1990. The regulation and function of *c-fos* and other immediate early genes in the nervous system. *Neuron* 4:477–485.

Shi, G., J-H. Cha, L. A. Farrell, E. Torre, S. Warren, H. Yi, and S. M. Hersch. 2000. Altered mGluR2/3 receptor protein expression in the brains of fragile X knockout mice. *Soc. Neurosci. Abstr.* 26:1543.

Sung, Y. J., J. Conti, J. R. Currie, W. T. Brown, and R. B. Denman. 2000. RNAs that interact with the fragile X syndrome RNA binding protein FMRP. *Biochem. Biophys. Res. Commun.* 275:973–980.

Tamanini, F., R. Willemsen, L. Van Unen, C. Bontekoe, H. Galjaard, B. A. Oostra, and A. T. Hoogeveen. 1997. Differential expression of *FMR1, FXR1* and *FXR2* proteins in human brain and testis. *Hum. Mol. Genet.* 6:1315–1322.

Tamanini, F., L. Van Unen, C. Bakker, N. Sacchi, H. Galjaard, B. A. Oostra, and A. T. Hoogeveen. 1999. Oligomerization properties of fragile-X mental-retardation protein (FMRP) and the fragile-X-related proteins FXR1P and FXR2P. *Biochem. J.* 343 (pt. 3): 517–523.

Todd, P. K., and K. J. Mack. 2000. Sensory stimulation increases cortical expression of the fragile X mental retardation protein in vivo. *Brain Res. Mol. Brain Res.* 80:17–25.

Warren, S. T., and E. R. Torre. 2000. Dendritic spine maturation is delayed in cultured hippocampal neurons from the mouse model of fragile X syndrome. *Soc. Neurosci. Abstr.* 26:1543.

Weiler, I. J., and W. T. Greenough. 1991. Potassium ion stimulation triggers protein translation in synaptoneurosomal polyribosomes. *Mol. Cell. Neurosci.* 2:305–314.

————. 1993. Metabotropic glutamate receptors trigger postsynaptic protein synthesis. *Proc. Natl. Acad. Sci. USA* 90:7168–7171.

Weiler, I. J., S. A. Irwin, A. Y. Klintsova, C. M. Spencer, A. D. Brazelton, K. Miyashiro, T. A. Comery, B. Patel, J. Eberwine, and W. T. Greenough. 1997. Fragile X mental retardation protein is translated near synapses in response to neurotransmitter activation. *Proc. Natl. Acad. Sci. USA* 94:5395–5400.

Weiler, I. J., A. Y. Klintsova, C. C. Spangler, and W. T. Greenough. 1999. FMRP is necessary for rapid translational response to synaptic stimulation. Presented at the Ninth International Workshop on Fragile X Syndrome and X-linked Mental Retardation, Strasbourg, France.

Weiler, I. J., B. Belt, C. Spangler, A. Drew, and W. T. Greenough. 2000. Decreased levels of cortical mGluR1 in *FMR1*-KO mice. *Soc. Neurosci. Abstr.* 26:1540.

Wisniewski, K. E., S. M. Segan, C. M. Miezejeski, E. A. Sersen, and R. D. Rudelli. 1991. The Fra(X) syndrome: Neurological, electrophysiological, and neuropathological abnormalities. *Am. J. Med. Genet.* 38:476–480.

Zhong, N., W. Ju, D. Nelson, C. Dobkin, and W. T. Brown. 1999. Reduced mRNA for G3BP in fragile X cells: Evidence of *FMR1* gene regulation. *Am. J. Med. Genet.* 84:268–271.

# CHAPTER 6
# Neuropsychology

## Loisa Bennetto, Ph.D., and Bruce F. Pennington, Ph.D.

This chapter provides a comprehensive review of the neuropsychologic phenotype of fragile X syndrome in males and females. When the first edition of this volume was written, fragile X syndrome (FXS) was considered a relatively new genetic syndrome, and research on the neuropsychologic profile of affected individuals was still quite limited (Pennington et al. 1991). During the past 10 years, research on FXS has progressed significantly in several different areas, leading to a much more comprehensive understanding of this common genetic disorder.

The isolation and identification of the fragile X mental retardation 1 (*FMR1*) gene (Oberle et al. 1991; Verkerk et al. 1991, Yu et al. 1991), which is discussed in detail in chapter 2, has had important implications for neuropsychologic research. Researchers are now able to identify and classify subjects more accurately. Previously, subjects were classified according to the percentage of cells expressing the FXS mutation, which provided an incomplete picture of the subject's molecular makeup and may have obscured the relation between genotype and phenotype. Now, researchers can measure the size of the base pair insertion, the percentage of methylation, and, in females, the X activation ratio (i.e., percentage of cells with the normal *FMR1* allele on the active X chromosome). Recent studies have measured the amount of FMR1 protein (FMRP) expression and its relationship to physical and neurocognitive factors. With this additional information, researchers have begun to piece together the links from genetic and protein studies to neurologic phenotype to neuropsychologic and behavioral functioning. Ten years ago, we were working toward defining the neuropsychology of this disorder. Today, we are at the threshold of having an integrated understanding of the cognitive neuroscience of FXS.

Neuropsychologic research on FXS has also progressed in new directions during the past 10 years. Investigators have looked more specifically at the neu-

*Fragile X Syndrome: Diagnosis, Treatment, and Research,* third edition, ed. Randi Jenssen Hagerman and Paul J. Hagerman (Baltimore: Johns Hopkins University Press, 2002), © The Johns Hopkins University Press.

ropsychologic profile of affected individuals and are beginning to identify specific strengths and weaknesses *within* neuropsychologic domains. The developmental trajectory of IQ has been examined further in several longitudinal studies. High-functioning males with a full mutation are receiving more attention from researchers since, like women, their phenotypic profiles can increase understanding of the role of the *FMR1* gene in development.

In the following discourse, we address these and other neuropsychologic findings in more detail. Although information about both the neurologic and the psychiatric phenotypes in FXS is relevant to the neuropsychologic phenotype, this information is covered in chapter 1 and will not be repeated here. Before we begin, however, we will address some theoretical and methodologic issues germane to our review. These include important lessons learned from neuropsychologic studies of other genetic syndromes and issues that are specific to FXS.

## Theoretical and Methodologic Issues

The field of developmental neuropsychology provides a framework from which to examine the neurocognitive phenotype of FXS. Research on normal cognitive functioning suggests specific areas for further research, theoretical and empiric associations between cognitive domains, and an increasing number of well-validated measures for assessment. In addition, the relationship that exists between the phenotype definition of a syndrome like FXS and the field of developmental neuropsychology is reciprocal and dialectic (Pennington and Smith 1988). New syndromes may compel us to carve the domain of cognition somewhat differently, which may have important implications for phenotype definition in other syndromes and for studies of normal behavioral development. FXS is particularly exciting in this regard because it may provide insights about the intersection of neuropsychiatry and cognitive neuropsychology. For instance, FXS may illuminate disorders like autism, attention deficit hyperactivity disorder, and schizotypy, in which there are deficits both in purely cognitive functions and in social-emotional functions.

Conversely, research on the neuropsychology of related disorders and functions may provide us with theories and measures to better understand FXS. At this point, we have an increasingly well-described taxonomy of developmental learning disorders (Pennington 1991) and a beginning understanding of the neuropsychology of different retardation syndromes (Pennington and Bennetto 1998). We can ask whether the neuropsychologic phenotype in females and high-functioning males with FXS is similar to any of these better-understood developmental learning disorders and how the phenotype in full-mutation males with FXS compares and contrasts with that in other retardation syndromes. We can also ask whether the phenotypes in females and males with FXS are qualitatively similar despite varying considerably in overall level of function.

## Evaluation of Discriminant Validity, Specificity, Primacy, and Consistency

Finding that males or females with FXS are impaired on the same measures as individuals with a known type of retardation syndrome or learning disorder would be interesting but would not take us very far. We also need to evaluate whether they are relatively unimpaired in other neuropsychologic domains. If only areas of predicted deficit are tested, positive results are ambiguous because they may only be part of a more general pattern of impairment. This is the issue of *discriminant validity*.

The issue of *specificity* is closely related to the issue of discriminant validity. In attempting to understand the neuropsychologic phenotype in males and females with FXS, we would like to identify specific effects of the mutation on brain function, apart from nonspecific effects on overall developmental level. To control for this possible confound, one must use non-FXS control subjects with developmental disabilities (DD) who are similar in overall IQ to the subjects with FXS. Normally developing subjects who are matched on mental age obviously do not control for the nonspecific effects of a developmental disability. In considering the phenotypic characteristics of FXS, it is important to be able to decide which are attributable to developmental delay (nonspecific effects) and which are attributable to developmental deviance (specific effects). Over the past 10 years, more studies of FXS have used appropriate IQ-matched control groups with developmental disabilities.

Not all specific effects are *primary* because some specific effects may either be secondary to primary effects (e.g., gaze avoidance may be secondary to deficits in social understanding) or be correlated effects (e.g., stereotypies in males with FXS may be correlated rather than primary deficits). Evaluating whether observed deficits are primary, secondary, or correlated is difficult and is most definitively addressed by longitudinal studies.

If, in group studies of individuals with FXS, we find a neuropsychologic phenotype that has discriminant validity, specificity, and primacy, we still need to determine how *consistent* that phenotype is across individuals. Consistency is a continuous variable rather than a dichotomous one. At one extreme, there may be neuropsychologic effects of a disorder that are so variable across individuals as to make it meaningless to speak of *the* neuropsychologic phenotype. For example, neurocutaneous disorders may have a highly variable effect. If there is no consistency across affected individuals, then we will not find discriminant validity, specificity, or primacy. At the other, unlikely extreme, every affected individual will have the same phenotype. The actual situation in many genetic disorders probably falls somewhere between these two extremes; thus, we need to develop criteria for significant but less than complete consistency. These criteria must allow for the phenotypic variability usually found across affected individuals; this variability is caused by their genetic and environmental differences. It is easy to forget that individuals with a given genetic syndrome are different in the vast majority of both their genes and their specific environmental experiences. Consequently, the genetic defect must emit a strong signal for us to detect it in the noise caused by genetic and environmental differences. It would be very unusual for a neuropsychologic phenotype to be present in all affected individuals, and some phenotypes will not be present in the majority but will be detectable only as the central tendency of the group. It is thus unlikely that there will be a neuropsychologic profile that is diagnostic of a genetic syndrome at the individual level.

## Ascertainment Bias

In trying to arrive at the core set of neuropsychologic symptoms that are specific and primary in a genetic disorder, one must avoid ascertainment bias. Individuals referred for clinical services are more likely to have additional, unrelated diagnoses (Berkson 1946), which only add to our confusion in trying to sort out core symptoms. Prospective studies of infants with sex chromosome anomalies were initiated to avoid just this problem, and the phenotype results from such prospective samples did differ considerably from those reported for clinically ascertained cases (Robinson et al. 1979). In studies of females with FXS, an affected male is usually the proband who has come to clinical attention. His male and female relatives who also have the mutation would provide a less biased sample, although it would not be as unbiased as a sample identified through population screening.

## Issues Specific to FXS

Several aspects of this syndrome create special problems for research on the neuropsychologic phenotype. These include the late decline in IQ in males, comorbidity with psychiatric disorders, the extreme variation in penetrance observed in females and more recently in high-functioning males, and the challenge of identifying appropriate biologic variables to test putative links between genotype and phenotype. The first problem is a potential confound in studies with a wide age range of males with FXS. If the biologic changes responsible for this decline also affect the pattern of abilities, then group data across a broad age range will be misleading not only about the levels of IQ at different ages but also about developmental changes in the patterns of abilities at different ages. Other issues related to the IQ decline will be discussed later.

The frequency and variability of comorbid psychiatric symptoms found in samples of individuals with FXS (which can include attention deficit hyperactivity disorder, anxiety and social avoidance, depression, and autism) can also complicate neuropsychologic testing. Deciding which of these psychiatric symptoms are primary features of FXS is an important goal of phenotype analysis. Furthermore, since many of these disorders are characterized by distinct neuropsychologic profiles, a comparative approach can help in identifying the neuropsychologic strengths and weaknesses that are unique to FXS and may move us closer to understanding the pathways from the underlying neurocognitive phenotype to social and behavioral functioning.

Our understanding of the wide spectrum of clinical involvement in individuals with FXS has improved greatly since the identification of the *FMR1* gene and some of the mechanisms that control its expression. However, there is still much work to be done in specifying how these mechanisms lead to the cognitive and behavioral phenotype of FXS. As we will see below, new findings in genetic and protein studies of the syndrome provide the tools for more careful analyses of genotype-phenotype correlations. However, they also dictate a continual reevaluation of previous neuropsychologic findings. For example, we now know that there are considerable differences in the ability patterns of females with a premutation and females with a fully expanded mutation. Consequently, early studies that combined these two groups probably obscured distinctive ability profiles unique to each subgroup. Recent studies have highlighted the need to examine phenotypic variation based on even more specific biologic markers (e.g., degree of methylation, mosaicism, FMRP expression, and in women, X activation ratio).

Finally, although these biologic markers have greatly improved our ability to identify core phenotypic characteristics, the critical test for neuropsychology is how these mechanisms affect the developing central nervous system. Thus, we are primarily interested in the relationship between neuropsychologic functioning and FMRP expression in the brain. Most studies measure the *FMR1* gene, protein, and other molecular predictors from leukocytes or saliva-borne epithelial cells. These sources, however, may not be valid indictors of levels in brain tissue. Postmortem studies of males with FXS have been inconclusive, with some researchers finding no differences in *FMR1* variables across tissues (Tassone et al. 1999a) and others finding differences in both methylation and FMRP expression in different tissues, even across distinct regions of the brain (Taylor et al. 1999). Taylor et al. also found that FMRP was negatively related to degree of methylation, suggesting that, in males, methylation seems to predict FMRP expression, which in turn predicts cognitive functioning. Research on women has also identified tissue-specific heterogeneity in X activation ratio, but not repeat length, across leukocyte, lymphocyte, and fibroblast cell lines (Allingham-Hawkins et al. 1996). In this study, only X activation in fibroblast cell lines was related to IQ. Together, these studies caution against drawing strong conclusions about *FMR1* expression in brain tissues based on leukocyte and other cell lines. Moreover, they may help to explain the variability in phenotypic presentation, even within distinct subgroups of individuals with FXS.

## A Review of Studies of Males with FXS

### Cognitive Measures

Although the spectrum of involvement is quite variable, adult males with FXS function on average within the moderately to severely retarded range of intelligence (Herbst 1980; Hagerman and Smith 1983; Chudley et al. 1983). The range of functioning, however, can be much greater. Sutherland and Hecht (1985) reported findings from 21 studies in which the IQ for males with FXS ranged from normal intelligence to profound mental retardation. Recent studies of molecular correlates of IQ suggest that there may be a continuum of involvement in FXS, depending on the amount of FMRP produced. Below, we review the key studies of IQ in males with FXS. Studies with sufficient sample size and details that provide meaningful information about mean IQ in males are summarized in table 6.1.

### Overall IQ

A review of the cross-sectional studies indicates that the mean IQ of males with FXS ranges from a standardized score of 22 to 65. Several of these studies, however, used biased samples of males and thus provided unnaturally high or low estimates. Kemper et al. (1988) included only males with an IQ of 50 or greater; the sample in Dykens et al. (1988) was drawn from an institutional population. Considering the remaining studies, the mean IQs cluster roughly around two values—34 and 50. The two studies with the higher values used a younger age range, which is consistent with an age-related decline in IQ in males with FXS (discussed below). In general, the results of these studies are very consistent and indicate a mean IQ in the moderately to severely retarded range for males with FXS. However, these studies do not address variability in IQ based on molecular status.

The number of CGG repeats does not appear to be related to IQ in males with a full mutation (e.g., Fisch et al. 1996a; Merenstein et al. 1996; Steyaert et al. 1996). Other indices, such as degree of methylation and FMRP expression, seem to be better predictors of cognitive functioning, particularly in males with a standardized IQ score of 70 or higher.

Several studies focused on this group of high-functioning males (Goldfine

**Table 6.1**

**Cross-sectional Studies of IQ in Males with Fragile X Syndrome**

| Study | n | Age (yr) | Controls | Measures | FSIQ | VIQ | NVIQ |
|---|---|---|---|---|---|---|---|
| Chudley et al. 1983 | 37 | 6–65 | None | Wechsler, SB | 34.8 | ND | ND |
| Borghgraef et al. 1987 | 17 | 15–22 | DD males matched on age and IQ | Wechsler, SB | 34.5 | VIQ > PIQ for both groups | |
| Dykens et al. 1987 | 14 | 7–28 | None | K-ABC | 50.0 | Seq < Sim on K-ABC | |
| Veenema et al. 1987 | 14 | 26–74 | Normal relatives | WAIS | 22.0[a] | — | — |
| Dykens et al. 1988 | 12 | 23–62 | FXS-neg. autistic, MR | SB | MA = 3–2 | — | — |
| Kemper et al. 1988 | 20 | 4–12 | FXS-neg, DD | K-ABC | 65.0 | 62.0 (Seq) | 71.0 (Sim) |
| Prouty et al. 1988 | 93 | ? | None | Mixed | 33.0 | — | — |
| Freund and Reiss 1991 | 23 | 3–24 | None | SB | 50.0 | — | — |
| Hodapp et al. 1992 | 10 | 6–10 | DS, unknown MR (both CA, MA match) | K-ABC | | Seq < Sim for FXS and unknown MR | |
| Merenstein et al. 1996[b] | 35 | 3 mo–12 yr | None | Mixed | 51.3 | — | — |
| | 51 | 12–60 | None | Mixed | 41.2 | — | — |

*Note:* FSIQ, Full-Scale IQ; VIQ, Verbal IQ; PIQ, Performance IQ; NVIQ, Nonverbal IQ; SB, Stanford-Binet; ND, not done; K-ABC, Kaufman Assessment Battery for Children; WAIS, Wechsler Adult Intelligence Scale–Revised; DS, Down syndrome; DD, developmental delay; MR, mental retardation; CA, chronologic age; MA, mental age; Seq, Sequential IQ; Sim, Simultaneous IQ.
[a]Four at floor of test.
[b]Subjects reported in table had fully methylated full mutations.

et al. 1987; Hagerman 1991; Merenstein et al. 1994; Steyaert et al. 1996; Theobald et al. 1987). A report of prevalence rates in a clinic population of 250 males with FXS found that 13% of the expressing males were high functioning (Hagerman et al. 1994). In this sample, high-functioning males were more common among the young children with FXS (seven years or younger). This is consistent with a study of preschool-aged boys, which reported that 44% of a sample of 16–64-month-old boys with FXS had IQs in the normal or borderline range (Freund et al. 1995).

The Hagerman et al. (1994) study also examined the relation between IQ and molecular factors. On the whole, the higher-functioning group had a greater percentage of both mosaicism (i.e., both full-mutation and premutation cells) and incompletely methylated full mutations compared to mentally retarded males with FXS, who typically have fully methylated mutations and thus produce very limited amounts of FMRP. Merenstein et al. (1996) reported similar findings in a study of 218 males with FXS. Among postpubertal males, they found that subjects with a completely methylated full mutation had the lowest mean IQ (41.2) and the greatest physical involvement, compared to subjects with a mosaic pattern (mean IQ = 60.1). Significant differences in IQ were not observed between groups of prepubertal males, although the pattern of higher IQs in males with mosaic patterns was still evident. Steyaert et al. (1996) also found a significant negative correlation between IQ and the degree of methylation in a group of high-functioning males with full mutations but variable degrees of methylation. In contrast, neither de Vries et al. (1993) nor Rousseau et al. (1994) found phenotypic differences between males with mosaic patterns or full mutations, although Rousseau et al. reported significant correlations between clinical estimations of IQ and both CGG expansion length and methylation.

Recent studies of protein expression in subgroups of males may help to clarify these inconsistencies. FMRP seems to be a good predictor of IQ in mosaic or partially methylated full-mutation males, after adjusting for the averaged IQ of the proband's parents (Kaufmann et al. 1999). Kaufmann et al. also detected a limited amount of FMRP expression in all of their full-mutation males, suggesting that this group is not transcriptionally silent. Tassone et al. (1999b) found a similar relationship between IQ and FMRP expression in males with mosaicism and partially methylated full mutations. Moreover, FMRP expression was predictive of a nonretarded IQ in males with >50% of their leukocytes expressing the protein.

Several studies of high-functioning males with FXS examined the relation of age to IQ. Although declines in IQ seem to affect high-functioning individuals, approximately 30% maintained their nonretarded IQ into adolescence or adulthood (Hagerman et al. 1994). While the general cognitive abilities of high-functioning males are within the normal to low normal range, case studies suggest that they exhibit a neuropsychologic and psychiatric profile similar to that of women with the full mutation. This includes evidence of deficits in executive functioning, math, and attentional control, as well as mood lability and poor temper control (Hagerman et al. 1994; Merenstein et al. 1994).

Finally, there is a subgroup of males with an *FMR1* premutation. Although these males have traditionally been considered to be clinically unaffected, several reports indicate that they may have subtle deficits in cognitive performance (e.g., Hagerman et al. 1996; Hills et al. 2000; Murray et al. 1996; chaps. 1 and 12).

## The Developmental Trajectory of IQ

There is consistent evidence of a developmental decline in the IQ of males with FXS. Understanding more about the nature of the developmental trajectory of IQ is important for several reasons. First, it has direct implications for diagnosis and intervention. Second, uncovering the etiology of the IQ decline may lead to a better understanding of the neuropathology and neurophysiology of this disorder. Finally, differential developmental patterns are important for the issue of discriminant validity in mental retardation syndromes. In general, IQ scores among children with mental retardation have been reported to be relatively stable (Silverstein et al. 1982). However, an examination of different syndromes that cause mental retardation suggests distinct patterns of cognitive development (Pennington and Bennetto 1998). The cognitive ability of most children with autism, for example, is relatively stable across the life-span (Waterhouse and Fein 1984). In Down syndrome, there is a progressive decline in IQ beginning in about the first year of life and continuing across childhood (Hodapp et al. 1990a).

The decline in the intellectual performance of males with FXS was first observed in cross-sectional studies, which found that age was negatively correlated with IQ (e.g., Borghgraef et al. 1987, 1988; Chudley et al. 1983; Hagerman and Smith 1983; Prouty et al. 1988). Since then, the decline in IQ has been replicated in a series of more rigorous longitudinal studies, which we review below.

There are several methodologic issues to consider in evaluating these longitudinal studies (Hay 1994). Several of the longitudinal studies compare IQ data derived from different tests. This method has two inherent problems. First, it begs the question of whether the intelligence measured by two different tests is really the same construct. Even within a particular test, children of different ages often receive a different series of subtests (e.g., the Kaufman Assessment Battery for Children, or K-ABC). Second, the IQs used for comparison are based on population norms. Tests that are normed on different cohorts will yield significantly different scores for the same performance. Thus, the most reliable studies are based on IQ estimates using the same test at both time points.

A second general issue is the age levels at which the first and second testing are completed. Since the decline in IQ has been reported to occur at some time between the ages of 6 and 15 years, studies that do not effectively span this critical period may be less relevant. A third issue is related to ascertainment bias. Decreases or increases in IQ from studies based on unusually low- or high-functioning samples may be artifacts of regression to the mean. Finally, most of the longitudinal studies conducted have not included a control group. The use of an appropriately matched comparison sample can help to address some of the issues discussed above, as well as the issue of discriminant validity.

Table 6.2 summarizes the key longitudinal studies of IQ in males with FXS. In general, the results of these studies are remarkably consistent. All seven studies report declines in the mean IQ from the first to the second testing. This trajectory was observed in studies that used identical measures at both time points (Hagerman et al. 1989; Hodapp et al. 1990b; Wright-Talamante et al. 1996; Fisch et al. 1996b), suggesting that the decline is not an artifact of test differences. In the one study that employed a matched control group (Wright-Talamante et al. 1996), the mean IQ of boys with FXS declined significantly compared to controls, suggesting that the decline is not an artifact of sampling bias.

Although the average IQs in these studies declined with age, not all boys with FXS were affected. Fisch et al. (1992) further investigated this by examining the distribution of IQ scores from the Lachiewicz et al. (1987), Hagerman et al. (1989), and Fisch et al. (1992) studies. Their findings suggest that there may be two groups of males: one with relatively stable mental retardation and one with increasing levels of mental retardation related to decelerated cognitive development. Wright-Talamante et al. (1996) measured molecular status and methylation in a longitudinal study of IQ changes. They found no decline in the IQ of males with FXS who had a full mutation that was less than 50% methylated, compared to a significant decline for the remaining males with FXS. Those producing some FMRP seem to be protected from the IQ decline, whereas those with greater methylation and presumably less FMRP are more affected.

The results in table 6.2 also suggest that the IQs do not decline in a linear fashion. The Hagerman et al. (1989) and Lachiewicz et al. (1987) data suggest that IQs initially begin to decline in middle childhood and continue to decline through adolescence. Hagerman et al. hypothesized that this decline is related to changes in the tasks used to assess IQ. In early childhood, IQ tests stress single-word vocabulary and visual matching, which are relative strengths for many boys with FXS. By middle childhood, IQ tests require more abstract thinking and symbolic language skills, which are areas of specific weakness in this group. Other studies, however, suggest that the greatest decline in IQ occurs during the early pubertal years and may be related to regulatory factors involved in the onset of puberty (e.g., Dykens et al. 1989). Fisch et al. (1996b) also ar-

**Table 6.2**
**Longitudinal Studies of IQ Change in Males with Fragile X Syndrome**

| Study | n | Measures | Age | | | IQ | | |
|---|---|---|---|---|---|---|---|---|
| | | | *Time 1* | *Time 2* | *(Time 3)* | *Time 1* | *Time 2* | *(Time 3)* |
| Lachiewicz et al. 1987 | 21 | 11: same test at T1, T2 (primarily SB) | 5.6 (2.8–8.5) | 12.5 (5.0–19.7) | | 59.5 | 45.9 | |
| Dykens et al. 1989 | 10 | 8: SB at T1–T3; 1: WISC at T1–T3 | 5–10 | 10–15 | 15–20 | 53.8 | 47.2 | 40.6 |
| Hagerman et al. 1989 | 24 | All: SB at T1, T2 | 11.4 (4.5–29) | 16.3 (7.6–33.2) | | 54.9 | 48.4 | |
| Hodapp et al. 1990 (combined data from 3 studies above) | 66 | All: same test at T1, T2 (62 SB) | 9.2 (3–18) | 12.7 (5–20) | | 53.3 | 47.3 | |
| Fisch et al. 1991 | 60 | 46: SB at T1, T2; 13: Wechsler test at T1, T2 | 21.1 (2.6–53.7) | 27.0 (4.8–56.7) | | 40.1 | 35.8 | |
| Wright-Talamante et al. 1996 | 54 | K-ABC, SB, WISC | 8.9 | 13.9 (est.) | | 63.9 | 55.9 (est.) | |
| (similar tests only) | 35 | All: same test at T1, T2 | 9.9 | 13.5 (est.) | | 63.7 | 55.7 (est.) | |
| Fisch et al. 1996[a] | 17 | All: SB at T1, T2 | 7.8 | 10.2 | | 49.0 | 42.0 | |

*Note:* T1, time 1; T2, time 2; T3, time 3; SB, Stanford-Binet; WISC, Wechsler Intelligence Scale for Children; K-ABC, Kaufman Assessment Battery for Children.
[a]Subjects reported in table had fully methylated full mutations.

gued that the IQ decline observed in their sample did not seem to be due to changes in the testing instruments (e.g., increased abstraction) because the declines were present across all factors of Stanford-Binet, as well as all three areas of a parent-report adaptive behavior scale. This is supported by others' research on adaptive functioning profiles in males with FXS, as measured by both cross-sectional and longitudinal studies (Dykens et al. 1996; Fisch et al. 1999). In the Dykens et al. study, which reported both longitudinal and cross-sectional results, there were clear age-related increases in adaptive functioning until subjects were about 10 years old, after which the trajectory seemed to plateau. Similarly, in their cross-sectional study, adaptive functioning age equivalencies were no longer correlated with chronologic age for subjects older than 10 years. Both Dykens et al. and Fisch et al. reported variability in developmental trajectories across adaptive domains, with communication skills seeming to be most affected and to reach a developmental plateau earliest, while daily living skills seem to be a relative strength and reach a plateau later.

Hodapp et al. (1991) also examined changes in the pattern of cognitive strengths and weaknesses in boys with FXS over time. Using the K-ABC in a cross-sectional study of 21 males with FXS (aged 4 to 27 years), they found that subjects' chronologic age was related to performance on the Simultaneous Processing and Achievement components of this test. In contrast, subjects' age was not related to performance on Sequential Processing. These findings were confirmed with a smaller ($n = 10$) longitudinal study. These results suggest that the IQ decline may be related to a developmental plateau in the type of step-by-step processing required in the Sequential Processing tasks.

Finally, Bailey et al. (1998) examined developmental trajectories over several years in 46 young boys with FXS, ranging in age from 24 to 66 months. The authors assessed developmental skills every 6 months with the Battelle Developmental Inventory. Their results suggest that, even at this young age, the rate of development is significantly delayed—approximately half of what would be expected in normally developing peers. The slower rate of development was consistent across all areas measured by the Battelle, but the authors did note that, at every age tested, the participants showed a relative weakness in Communication and Cognitive scores compared to Motor and Adaptive Scores.

In summary, recent methodologic improvements in research have helped to resolve several issues regarding the developmental trajectory of IQ in males with FXS. New longitudinal studies have all replicated the IQ decline. More studies used only identical tests at both time points, demonstrating that the IQ decline is not an artifact of test differences. One study with a matched control group demonstrated that the IQ decline is not an artifact of sampling bias. The primary issue that remains unanswered, however, is the etiology of the IQ decline. Wright-Talamante et al. (1996) measured molecular variables in their subjects and obtained preliminary evidence that methylation status (and thus *FMR1* protein production) may have an effect on IQ decline.

## Neuropsychologic Profile

The initial evidence of a specific neuropsychologic profile in FXS came from studies that examined patterns of cognitive strengths and weaknesses on intelligence tests. At a preliminary level of analysis, there does not seem to be a significant discrepancy in the verbal and performance IQ scores of males with FXS on Wechsler tests. Although Borghgraef et al. (1988) found a significant verbal-performance difference in a sample of males with FXS, they also found a similar discrepancy in an age- and IQ-matched group of males with mental retardation and without FXS. At a more precise level of analysis, males with FXS have demonstrated a consistent pattern of cognitive strengths and weaknesses. On the K-ABC, males with FXS have consistently performed poorly on the Sequential Processing tasks, compared to the Simultaneous Processing and Achievement tasks (Dykens et al. 1987; Kemper et al. 1988; Hodapp et al. 1992). In particular, they show a pattern that includes relative weaknesses in several measures of short-term memory, including tasks of visual-motor memory (Hand Movements), visual-spatial memory (Spatial Memory), and Arithmetic. Relative strengths are typically observed on a task assessing long-term memory and perceptual closure (Gestalt Closure). These findings seem to have some specificity for FXS. For example, the Hodapp et al. study compared the performance of males with FXS to comparison groups of males with Down syndrome and unspecified mental retardation who were matched for chronologic age (CA) and mental age (MA). Unlike the males with FXS, males with Down syndrome showed almost identical levels of performance on Sequential and Simultaneous Processing. While the group with unspecified mental retardation showed a relative weakness in Sequential Processing, they also displayed a slightly different profile from the males with FXS, with no relative strengths on any tasks. In addition, it is possible that some subjects in this group may have actually carried the *FMR1* mutation.

Freund and Reiss (1991) examined the profiles of males with FXS on the Stanford-Binet Intelligence Scale, fourth edition. They found a distinct pattern that included weaknesses in visual-motor coordination, spatial memory, and arithmetic and strengths in verbal labeling and comprehension.

Finally, Maes et al. (1994) examined performance profiles on the McCarthy Scales of Mental Abilities in a sample of 43 mentally retarded men with FXS compared to MA- and CA-matched controls with nonspecific mental retardation. Compared to controls, the men with FXS did significantly worse on a visuospatial construction task. They also had significantly more difficulty remembering meaningless verbal information, such as strings of numbers. In

contrast, the men with FXS had a relative strength in remembering meaningful verbal information. This strength was also evident in their relatively strong
performance on measures of crystallized, or acquired, verbal knowledge (e.g.,
word meanings).

These studies point to consistent areas of weakness for males with FXS, including difficulties on tasks that tap short-term auditory memory, spatial skills,
and visual-motor skills. Furthermore, they demonstrate a consistent processing
style, in which they seem to have difficulty holding information on line as they
solve problems. In contrast, males with FXS seem to have a relative strength in
certain verbal abilities. The implications of this pattern are discussed below.

## Speech and Language

Abnormalities in both speech production and language competence have
consistently been noted in males with FXS. Sudhalter et al. (1991) argued that
language should be considered a combination of competencies, rather than a
unitary skill. We will follow this suggestion and discuss separately the different areas of linguistic functioning.

Speech Production. Speech production includes articulation, rate, and prosody (i.e., intonation, tone, and stress). Several studies of males with FXS have
revealed poor articulation (Paul et al. 1987; Prouty et al. 1988; Newell et al. 1983;
Hanson et al. 1986), including errors of substitution and omission. One question
is whether these errors are specific to FXS or a function of being mentally retarded. Several researchers examined the quality of these speech errors and concluded that they were not different from the types of errors produced by normally
developing children as they acquire language skills and were consistent with the
mental age of the subjects with FXS (Prouty et al. 1988; Newell et al. 1983). Paul
et al. (1987) compared articulation and other language characteristics in men with
FXS, matched on CA and MA to men with nonspecific mental retardation, and
men with autism. They found no significant differences in performance between
groups, with the exception of increased echolalia in subjects with autism. Prouty
et al. (1988) also examined articulatory structures in a group of males and females with FXS and found no abnormalities that could account for the articulation difficulties. Thus, these studies suggest that the articulatory errors of males
with FXS are an example of developmental delay, not deviance.

A second area in which males with FXS demonstrate impairments is in the
rate and prosody of their speech. The rate of their speech is often described as
rapid and dysrhythmic (Prouty et al. 1988; Borghgraef et al. 1987; Reiss and
Freund 1992). Hanson et al. (1986) described this as "cluttering," which they
viewed as a type of verbal clumsiness. Males with FXS also show an increase
in repetitions of parts of words or whole words (Newell et al. 1983; Vilkman et
al. 1988). Finally, the quality of their speech has been described as "jocular" or

"litany-like" (Turner et al. 1980) or as exhibiting a harsh or hoarse vocal quality (Prouty et al. 1988).

Several researchers have likened these difficulties with rate and prosody to those seen in verbal dyspraxia (e.g., Paul et al. 1984; Vilkman et al. 1988). Thus, some of the speech impairments in FXS may be caused by a high-level motor encoding or planning problem. Such a deficit is consistent with the impairments males show on the Hand Movements subtest of the K-ABC, which also involves the encoding and production of sequential motor plans.

**Language Competence.** Language competence can also be partitioned into several related skills. The most general level includes expressive and receptive language. Expressive language is the ability to produce meaningful words and sentences to convey one's ideas to the listener. Receptive language is the ability to understand correctly the meaning of others' language. These general categories can each be further divided into syntactic and pragmatic skills. *Syntax* refers to the grammatical arrangement of words to form structures such as sentences, phrases, questions, and negations. *Pragmatics* refers to the communicative level of language and includes such conversational skills as how to listen to others, initiate a conversation, take turns, and ask and answer questions appropriately.

These distinctions are important for understanding atypical language development and may shed light on the specificity of language deficits in FXS. Children with Down syndrome tend to show severe impairments in syntactic competence compared to other areas of language (e.g., Fowler 1990). Children with autism have striking difficulties with the pragmatic level of language (e.g., Prior 1977). Males with FXS tend to show varying degrees of impairment at both the syntactic and pragmatic levels of language. One important question is whether these impairments are simply delayed and consistent with mental age or whether they represent deviant development.

Males with FXS also seem to have delays in syntactic competence. Newell et al. (1983) examined speech and language skills in a group of 21 males with FXS who were 17 months to 21 years of age. They found that syntactic competence (as measured by mean length of utterance, or MLU) did not increase as IQ increased. This suggested that syntactic ability may reach an asymptote in males. More recently, Sudhalter et al. (1991) examined expressive language skills in a group of 19 males with FXS who were 5 to 36 years old. They used two variables to assess syntactic competence: MLU and a measure of syntactic complexity. The authors found that the relation between length and complexity was similar to that observed in normally developing children. Furthermore, syntactic scores were not correlated with measures of deviant pragmatic competence. The authors interpreted these results as suggesting that syntactic development is delayed, rather than deviant, in males with FXS.

Males with FXS also demonstrate impairments in pragmatic competence. An early study describing the conversational speech of males reported high levels of inappropriate or tangential responses, topic perseveration, rambling, and frequent use of repetitive phrases (Madison et al. 1986). Later studies began to examine the specificity of these deficits for males with FXS by comparing them to other groups of children with mental retardation. Wolf-Schein et al. (1987) compared males with FXS to a group of males with Down syndrome, matched on adaptive functioning. They found that the males with FXS were more likely than the Down syndrome comparison group to produce pragmatic abnormalities, including perseveration, stereotyped or repetitive statements, echolalia, and inappropriate or tangential remarks. They were also less likely than the males with Down syndrome to use appropriate nonverbal pragmatics, such as referential gestures and facial/head signals. Borghgraef et al. (1987) compared males with FXS to a matched group of males without FXS. In a sample of 7–11-year-old children, they found increased levels of perseverative speech in the group of males with FXS. In this study, however, 39% of the males with FXS had also received a diagnosis of autism. Thus, some of the language abnormalities may be a result of having autism rather than being specific to FXS.

Recently, two studies have compared the pragmatic competence of males with FXS, Down syndrome, and autism (Sudhalter et al. 1990; Ferrier et al. 1991). Sudhalter et al. measured the occurrence of "deviant repetitive language," which included behaviors such as perseverations on topics and phrases and echolalia. In maintaining a conversation topic, males with FXS produced significantly more deviant repetitive language than did males with Down syndrome but less than did those with autism. Furthermore, males with FXS tended to produce perseverative language, while males with autism exhibited more echolalia. Finally, the authors noted that males with FXS were able to do more appropriate conversational turn taking than were the subjects with autism.

Ferrier et al. (1991) also observed distinctions in the deviant language produced by males with FXS and autism. Those with FXS tended to produce more self-repetitions (palilalia), while those with autism exhibited more echolalia and multiply inappropriate responses (e.g., those including more than one example of pragmatic deviance). They also noted that males with FXS produced more utterances that required the listener to make a response, which suggested that they were aware of the social press of a conversation, even if they had trouble maintaining it.

In summary, males with FXS seem to display a consistent abnormality in the pragmatic level of language that consists of perseverations on words, phrases, and topics. The occurrence of these perseverations is greater than what would be expected based on mental age and apparently different from the deficits seen in other mental retardation groups. Hence, perseverative language in males with FXS is probably an example of developmental deviance. This raises the question of the etiology of this behavior, for which several theories have been proposed. As discussed above, Hanson et al. (1986) propose that perseverations on words and phrases may be a manifestation of higher-level motor encoding difficulties. Sudhalter examined both expressive syntactic (Sudhalter et al. 1991) and semantic (Sudhalter et al. 1992) deficits as possible explanations for perseverative speech in males with FXS. Their results suggest that syntactic delays are unrelated to pragmatic deviance. However, their results did suggest that difficulties related to expressive semantics (e.g., word retrieval problems) may be associated with the production of repetitive language. Ferrier et al. (1991) suggest that repetitions of words or parts of words may serve a place-holding function for males with FXS, which allows them to maintain and keep up with a conversation. We still do not know which, if any, of these theories is correct.

## Memory

Males with FXS show consistent weaknesses in certain aspects of memory on cognitive tests. On the memory subtests of the Stanford-Binet, they showed a consistent weakness on short-term memory for sentences and bead memory (a visual memory task) but did relatively well on object memory (Freund and Reiss 1991). These authors interpreted this finding as suggesting that the memory deficit in FXS is not pervasive but depends on the type of information to be remembered. Abstract visual information that is not easily labeled (e.g., Bead Memory) or information that requires sequencing ability (e.g., Sentence Memory) may be particularly difficult for males with FXS because these tasks require organizational or analytic skill. In addition, delays in syntactic skills may adversely affect their performance on more complex verbal memory tasks such as sentence memory. Maes et al. (1994) also found a dissociation between intact memory for meaningful verbal information but impaired memory for meaningless, rote information. Difficulties with remembering sequences or abstract visual information are also evident in the performance of males with FXS on the K-ABC (Dykens et al. 1987; Kemper et al. 1988; Hodapp et al. 1992). On this task, they tend to show deficits on Spatial Memory and Hand Movements (which measures memory for sequentially present visual-motor information). This pattern of memory deficits may be related to a deficit in executive functioning.

Recently, Munir, Cornish, and Wilding (2001) conducted a comprehensive evaluation of memory functioning in 25 young males with FXS (aged 8 to 15 years). The subjects were significantly worse than CA- and verbal mental age (VMA)-matched controls with Down syndrome on measures of meaningless verbal memory, which included nonword repetition and backward digit span. In contrast, there was no difference between the two groups on a forward digit span task or a more meaningful story memory task. Together, these studies suggest that the memory profile of males with FXS is largely determined by the degree of complexity and abstraction of the information to be remembered.

## Spatial Ability

An examination of cognitive profiles suggests that males with FXS may have some difficulties in spatial ability. Visuospatial tasks, such as Block Design on the Wechsler tests, are typically among the lowest IQ subtests for males with FXS (e.g., Kemper et al. 1986; Theobald et al. 1987).

Several neuropsychologic studies have examined spatial skills in males with FXS. Crowe and Hay (1990) compared eight adolescent and adult males with FXS to CA- and VMA-matched subjects with Down syndrome. The males with FXS performed significantly worse on tasks of visuospatial construction (e.g., block building, drawing), visuospatial perception (e.g., judgment of line orientation), and spatial memory. Although the authors hypothesized that FXS may be the result of right hemisphere dysfunction, they did not find evidence of lateralization of function on a pegboard task.

Cornish et al. (1999) examined spatial abilities in a sample of 15 boys with FXS, aged 7 to 14 years. In contrast to previous studies, the subjects with FXS were not impaired on any of the spatial tasks compared to CA- and MA-matched boys with Down syndrome. In fact, subjects with FXS performed significantly better than the Down syndrome group on a task of spatial memory, as well as two tasks that required some ability to either encode or use visuospatial gestalts to aid performance (Gestalt Closure, Object Assembly). These findings are similar to those reported for patterns of memory. Individuals with FXS may be able to use meaning or perceptual gestalts to improve their performance across a range of neuropsychologic domains.

## Executive Function

Executive functions (EF) refer to goal-directed, future-oriented behaviors that involve working memory, planning, flexible strategy employment, and inhibition. EF impairment is usually associated with patients with frontal lobe lesions. However, diffuse brain damage (Levin et al. 1994) or damage to subcortical structures connected to the frontal lobes (Cummings 1993) can also produce deficits in these skills. Although some studies have specifically tested EF in women with FXS, it has been examined in males only recently. These studies, however, suggest that males with FXS may have a specific deficit in EF.

Preliminary evidence for a deficit in EF came from the pattern of impairments that males with FXS show on the K-ABC. As we discussed above, performance on the Sequential Processing score is typically worse than performance on the Simultaneous Processing score. Tasks of sequential processing, such as imitating sequential hand movements, often rely on an individual's ability to hold a sequence of actions on line in working memory and formulate a motor plan to execute a response. Other tasks of motor sequencing have been shown to be sensitive to frontal lobe deficits (Kolb and Whishaw 1996).

Munir et al. (2000) examined inhibition in a group of 25 boys with FXS compared to CA- and VMA-matched boys with Down syndrome. The subjects with FXS had significantly more difficulty inhibiting a simple, practiced motor response but were relatively better than subjects with Down syndrome on an inhibition task that required shifting from one response strategy to another. The authors also administered several measures of attention. On a task of selective attention, in which subjects had to search for specific targets in a field of distractors, the boys with FXS found fewer correct targets than subjects with Down syndrome. They also made more false alarms, which suggests difficulty in inhibition. On a task of divided attention, both groups found a similar number of targets. Further analysis, however, revealed that the FXS group employed less efficient search strategies. Finally, on a task of sustained attention, FXS subjects again found as many correct targets as did subjects with Down syndrome but made significantly more false alarms. These results suggest that males with FXS have clear impairments in neuropsychologic measures of attention and inhibition relative to control subjects with developmental delays. In addition, they suggest a specific profile of attentional abilities within the FXS sample, which seems to be characterized by difficulties with inhibition across a range of tasks.

Cornish et al. (2001) examined EF and attentional processes in a group of 15 adult males with FXS, compared to CA- and VMA-matched males with Down syndrome and normally developing control subjects matched on VMA. On a shortened version of the Wisconsin Card Sorting Test, which measures cognitive set shifting and concept formation, the subjects with FXS made significantly more perseverative errors than did both the Down syndrome and normal control group. In contrast, subjects with FXS found more targets on a measure of sustained attention than did subjects with Down syndrome, which is consistent with the results of Munir et al. (2000). This second study did not measure false alarms.

Recent studies of carrier males have begun to examine specificity within their neurocognitive profile. A study by Hills et al. (2000) suggests that these deficits in EF may be present in a more titrated form in males with a premutation. The authors compared three groups of premutation males: 6 boys, 15 adults, and 5 elderly men. The first two groups were matched on CA and Verbal IQ with groups of control subjects. The authors found that, overall, the males with FXS made more perseverative errors than did controls on a standard measure of EF (Wisconsin Card Sorting Test). Moreover, there seemed to be a developmental trend in their EF skills. The younger group demonstrated only borderline weaker performance than their controls, but by adulthood, the males with FXS were showing significant impairments. The authors compared the performance of the elderly group to published norms for subjects of their age and found that their performance was significantly lower than one would predict based on their age and IQ.

A deficit in EF is consistent with some of the behavioral problems often observed in males with FXS. These problems include difficulty with attentional control, impulsivity, and difficulty with transitions or shifting from one activity to another, as discussed in chapter 1. A deficit in EF would also help to explain some of the deviant performance in language and memory. For example, perseverative thinking, difficulty with topic maintenance, and tangential conversational style are all common manifestations of an EF deficit. Finally, difficulties with the organizational aspects of memory may also be related to frontal lobe functioning (Moscovitch 1992).

In summary, existing studies of males with FXS indicate some specificity for their neuropsychologic phenotype, with regard to both domains of function and other developmentally delayed groups. Specifically, in the cognitive area, there is evidence for specific deficits in short-term auditory memory, sequential motor planning, spatial skills, and arithmetic. There is also clear evidence of a late decline in IQ that is unlike that observed in other mental retardation syndromes, but the mechanisms responsible for this decline are still unclear. Because of relative strengths in language and long-term memory, males with FXS can seem less affected during the preschool years than other individuals with mental retardation.

In the areas of speech and language, males seem to have a developmental delay in speech production and specific deviance in pragmatic and conversational skills. In contrast, other language processing, such as syntax, seems to be at an expected level for the level of mental retardation.

Preliminary evidence suggests that males with FXS have a specific deficit in certain aspects of EF, particularly those that require inhibiting prepotent responses and holding information or sequences on line in working memory. These EF deficits may be responsible, in part, for some of their difficulties in motor planning, memory, pragmatics, and behavioral control. Males with FXS also seem to have a distinct pattern of abilities within both memory and visuospatial skills. For example, they typically demonstrate preserved memory for meaningful information, such as stories, but have difficulty remembering abstract, meaningless, or sequential stimuli. This ability to use meaning effectively is also evident in their pattern of spatial abilities. Preliminary evidence suggests that males with FXS can encode and use perceptual gestalts to improve performance on visuospatial tasks involving meaningful stimuli. In contrast, abstract tasks, such as Block Design or Judgment of Line Orientation, seem to be consistent areas of weakness.

## A Review of Studies of Females with FXS

### Cognitive Studies

Our understanding of the cognitive and neuropsychologic profiles of females with FXS has increased dramatically in the past 10 years. Molecular discoveries have led to better definitions of affected and carrier women. Previously, women with FXS were categorized according to the percentage of fragility in tested cells, which may have obscured the boundary between the two groups. Women who were previously labeled as cytogenetically positive typically have a full, or expanded, mutation. Women who were cytogenetically negative, or obligate carriers, typically have a premutation. Studies have begun to look directly at the relationships of various phenotypic variables to size of amplification, percentage of methylation, and X activation ratio (e.g., de Vries et al. 1996; Loesch et al. 1993; Reiss et al. 1995; Sobesky et al. 1996; Taylor et al. 1994), as well as FMRP expression (Kaufmann et al. 1999; Tassone et al. 1999b). The findings from these studies help to elucidate the variability in the cognitive profiles of women with FXS.

Researchers have also made considerable progress in describing the neuropsychologic phenotype of women with FXS. They represent an ideal group for examining the neuropsychologic phenotype of the *FMR1* mutation. Their relatively higher IQ allows the use of a greater range of tests, as well as easier interpretation of results.

Many studies of IQ functioning in females with FXS were reviewed. Of these, 18 had sufficient sample sizes, clearly defined samples, and detail about measures and methods to permit a summary. These studies are presented in table 6.3. Results on premutation or carrier females are presented separately from results of samples that mainly or exclusively consisted of cytogenetically positive, full-mutation females. The results across studies are surprisingly consistent and warrant several conclusions.

### Overall IQ

Females with a full mutation (or cytogenetically positive) have mean IQs that consistently fall in the low average range (74.4–90.8). The sole exception is the very low mean reported by Prouty et al. (1988); however, the women who received IQ testing were only a subset of their total sample, and one suspects that more severely affected women were more likely to receive IQ testing. However, this low average mean IQ across studies is somewhat misleading, in that a significant number of women with a full mutation are mentally retarded. Cronister et al. (1991) examined IQs of 43 cytogenetically positive daughters of known carrier women. They found that 23% were mentally retarded (IQ < 70),

33% had IQs in the borderline range (70–84), and 44% had normal IQs (≥85). Of those with IQs in the normal range, almost half were diagnosed as learning disabled and received special education services. Another study compared cognitive abilities in 32 cytogenetically positive girls and their cytogenetically negative sisters in order to control for other genetic and environmental influences on IQ (Hagerman et al. 1992). This study reported similar findings, with a total of 25% of the cytogenetically positive girls and none of the sisters falling in the mentally retarded range. Other studies have reported similar proportions of cognitively affected women (e.g., Rousseau et al. 1991; Staley et al. 1993).

Researchers can now measure molecular variables to determine their relationship to neurocognitive functioning. As with males, studies of full-mutation women have generally not found a relationship between CGG repeat length and neurocognitive variables (Bennetto et al. 2001; de Vries et al. 1996; Reiss et al. 1995; Sobesky et al. 1996; Taylor et al. 1994), with a few exceptions (Abrams et al. 1994; Sobesky et al. 1994). In contrast, most studies of full-mutation women and girls have found a relationship between X activation ratios and IQ (Abrams et al. 1994; Bennetto et al. 2001; de Vries et al. 1996; Kaufmann et al. 1999; Reiss et al. 1995), but some have failed to find this correlation (Taylor et al. 1994). Several studies have also identified more specific neurocognitive variables or patterns that seem to be related to activation status. For example, studies have found significant correlations between EF and activation status (Bennetto et al. 2001; Sobesky et al. 1996) and between activation ratio and Performance IQ but not Verbal IQ (Bennetto et al. 2001; Reiss et al. 1995). Finally, protein expression studies have found strong correlations between FMRP and IQ in full-mutation females (Kaufmann et al. 1999; Tassone et al. 1999b).

Compared to women with the full mutation, those with a premutation seem to be unaffected cognitively. Their mean IQ in 10 separate studies was consistently at or above the population mean (range: 98.1–116.5). Of these studies, the most rigorous are those that employed control groups, either for age or for growing up with developmentally disabled individuals. In the six studies that used control groups, mean IQs ranged from 98.1 to 108.1 and were not significantly different from those of the controls. These results argue against a negative ascertainment bias in the selection of these families, at least for IQ; if such a bias were operating, we would expect lower mean IQs in the premutation women.

## The Developmental Trajectory of IQ

Several studies have examined the possibility of an IQ decline in females with FXS. Prouty et al. (1988) conducted a cross-sectional study of 33 girls with FXS and reported a significant negative correlation between age and IQ. Hagerman

**Table 6.3**
**IQ Results in Females with Fragile X Syndrome**

| Study | n | Age (yr) | Controls | Measures | FSIQ | VIQ | NVIQ |
|---|---|---|---|---|---|---|---|
| | | | *Full mutation/cytogenetically positive* | | | | |
| Chudley et al. 1983[a] | 32 | 10–88 | None | Mixed | 87.9 | ND | ND |
| Veenema et al. 1987 | 11 | Adults | Normal relatives | WAIS-R | 86.8 | VIQ = PIQ | |
| Loesch and Hay 1988 | 80 | Adults | None | PPVT, Block Design | — | 82.9 | 62.3 |
| | 19 | Children | | | — | 83.6 | 69.5 |
| Prouty et al. 1988 | 33 | N/A | None | Mixed, mostly SB | 54.5 | ND | ND |
| Brainard et al. 1991 | 21 | Adults | None | WAIS-R | 85.6 | 84.9 | 87.6 |
| Cronister et al. 1991 | 43 | Children | None | Mixed | 81.0 | ND | ND |
| Freund and Reiss 1991 | 11 | 6–20 | None | SB, 4th ed. | 84.0 | — | — |
| Hagerman et al. 1992 | 32 | 1–18 | Sisters without FXS | Mixed, mostly Wechsler | 80.4 | — | — |
| Mazzocco et al. 1993[b] | 22 | Adults | Relatives without FXS or mothers of DD children | WAIS-R | 90.8 | 92.2 | 91.6 |
| Abrams et al. 1994 | 31 | 4–27 | None | SB, 4th ed. or WISC-R | 82 | — | — |
| Sobesky et al. 1996[b] | 29 | Adults | Relatives without FXS or mothers of DD children | WAIS-R | 82.6 | 82.6 | 85.2 |
| de Vries et al. 1996[c] | 27 | Adults | Relatives without FXS | WAIS | 74.4 | 72.3 | 81.9 |
| Bennetto et al. 2001[b] | 32 | Adults | Relatives without FXS | WAIS-R | 82.7 | 82.6 | 85.3 |

*Premutation/cytogenetically negative carriers*

| Study | n | Age | Group | Test | FSIQ | VIQ | PIQ |
|---|---|---|---|---|---|---|---|
| Prouty et al. 1988 | 10 | Adults | None | WAIS-R | 102.3 | 103.6 | 100.8 |
| Wolff et al. 1988 | 9 | Adults | Relatives of DS males | WAIS-R | 105.2 | 104.2 | 106.1 |
| Brainard et al. 1991 | 38 | Adults | None | WAIS-R | 106.0 | 106.0 | 107.5 |
| de von Flindt et al. 1991 | 13 | Adults | CA-match | WAIS-R | 98.1 | 90.3 | 101.5 |
| Seyaert et al. 1992 | 11 | Adults | None | WAIS-R | 116.5 | 111.6 | 120.0 |
| Mazzocco et al. 1993[b] | 35 | Adults | Relatives without FXS or mothers of DD children | WAIS-R | 100.6 | 101.9 | 100.9 |
| Reiss et al. 1993 | 34 | Adults | Mothers of DD children | WAIS-R | 108.1 | 106.1 | 109.1 |
| Allingham-Hawkins et al. 1996 | 14 | Adults | None | WAIS-R | 105.8 | 107.1 | 103.0 |
| Sobesky et al. 1996[b] | 92 | Adults | Relatives without FXS or mothers of DD children | WAIS-R | 105.0 | 102.3 | 107.3 |
| Bennetto et al. 2001[b] | 96 | Adults | Relatives without FXS | WAIS-R | 105.1 | 102.5 | 107.4 |

*Note:* FSIQ, Full-Scale IQ; VIQ, Verbal IQ; PIQ, Performance IQ; NVIQ, Nonverbal IQ; ND, not done; SB, Stanford-Binet; PPVT, Peabody Picture Vocabulary Test; WAIS-R, Wechsler Adult Intelligence Scale–Revised; WISC-R, Wechsler Intelligence Scale for Children–Revised; N/A, not available; DD, developmentally delayed; CA, chronologic age.

[a]Included a few cytogenetically negative females.
[b]Included only women without mental retardation (IQ ≥ 70).
[c]Subjects reported in table had full mutations only.

et al. (1992) conducted a longitudinal follow-up study of 12 females with FXS. They did not find a significant decline in IQ; in fact, the IQs of 9 of the 12 girls increased with age (perhaps due to regression to the mean). Fisch et al. (1994) examined IQ changes in a multicenter study of 11 females with FXS. They found a significant IQ decline in 44% of their sample and an overall mean decline of approximately 6 points. However, the majority of these females were mentally retarded (mean IQ at first testing was approximately 64) and may have been more severely affected than the majority of females with FXS. Brun et al. (1995) conducted a longitudinal follow-up of 21 girls with FXS, who were initially matched with a control sample of 18 girls without FXS of similar age and IQ. The initial distribution of IQ scores was comparable to those in other studies, with 24% falling in the mentally retarded range. The mean age was 11 years at the first testing and 16 years at the final testing. The authors found a significant IQ decline in 29% of the sample with FXS and 22% of the control sample, suggesting that a decline in IQ is not a specific feature of the phenotype in women. This study, however, included some subjects who had received different tests at the initial and final testings. Wright-Talamante et al. (1996) examined a subgroup of 16 girls, who were given similar tests at both time points. The authors found no significant changes in these subjects' IQs, when compared to matched controls.

In summary, there is no consistent evidence of IQ decline in females with a full mutation. As seems to be the case for males, variations in *FMR1* expression (as measured by X activation) and amount of FMRP may mediate the developmental trajectory of IQ. Thus, it would be useful to examine larger longitudinal samples to see whether these molecular variables predict which females with FXS, if any, have IQ declines.

## Neuropsychologic Profile

As was the case for males, preliminary evidence about neuropsychologic strengths and weaknesses comes from examinations of profiles on standard cognitive tests. The data on Wechsler Verbal IQ (VIQ) versus Performance IQ (PIQ) differences are much better than those available for males with FXS, and the results provide no evidence for a specific cognitive phenotype at the level of VIQ-PIQ differences. The only exception is the Steyaert et al. (1992) study of carrier women. In this study, the authors did find a significantly higher Performance than Verbal IQ. However, the mean IQs of their sample are significantly higher than those reported in all of the other studies of premutation women, which suggests that this study may be compromised by sampling bias.

At the level of specific IQ subtests, there is consistent evidence for specificity. Many investigators have found particular weaknesses on several Wechsler subtests in full-mutation females. These subtests include Block Design, Arithmetic, and Digit Span. In contrast, women with a premutation typically do not show a specific profile on cognitive tests (e.g., de von Flindt et al. 1991; Mazzocco et al. 1993; Reiss et al. 1993), although two studies did find a specific weakness in verbal short-term memory (Wolff et al. 1988; Brainard et al. 1991). Below, we review several studies of the cognitive patterns of full-mutation women on Wechsler tests. We have limited our discussion to those that have well-defined samples and/or appropriate control groups.

Kemper et al. (1986) explored Wechsler profiles of 22 females with FXS, children and adults, with varying levels of fragility. A control group of 20 learning-disabled females was included to evaluate their subtest patterns. The group with FXS demonstrated weaknesses on the Arithmetic, Digit Span, and Block Design subtests that were not seen in the comparison groups. The Full-Scale IQ of the subjects with FXS was in the average range. Kemper et al. (1986) identified a correlation between percentage of fragility and both Verbal and Full-Scale IQ.

Grigsby et al. (1987) studied a subset of 20 of the cytogenetically positive women later studied by Brainard et al. (1991) for signs of Gerstmann syndrome. One control group consisted of cytogenetically negative relatives of the experimental group; the other consisted of a mixed group of females with head injuries and learning disabilities. The cytogenetically positive group did significantly worse than both control groups on measures of spatial dyscalculia, dysgraphia, finger agnosia, right-left disorientation (the four symptoms of Gerstmann syndrome), and constructional dyspraxia but not on measures of visual agnosia or ideomotor apraxia or on a screening test for aphasic symptoms. They also performed worse on the three Wechsler subtests found to be deficient in other studies—Digit Span, Arithmetic, and Block Design. However, less than half of the cytogenetically positive sample had all of the signs of full Gerstmann syndrome, which does not support the consistency of this putative phenotype at the individual level. Moreover, the range of discriminant measures was limited, and all seem to have been subject to floor effects. Finally and most importantly, both control groups had considerably higher Full-Scale IQs than those of the females with FXS (between 10 and 19 points higher), so we do not know if the Gerstmann deficits found in the group with FXS are an effect of lower overall neuropsychologic functioning or a specific effect of FXS.

Freund and Reiss (1991) described the performance of 11 cytogenetically positive females on the Stanford-Binet, 4th edition. The IQs of their subject group were consistent with previous studies (mean IQ = 84). They discussed a particular pattern of performance suggestive of strengths in inductive reasoning and semantic memory function. They postulated that the females compensated for short-term memory weaknesses to some degree with their stronger verbal processing skills. Particular weaknesses were identified in short-term memory, quantitative skills, and visual motor tasks, similar to those identified in studies using the Wechsler Scale.

Finally, Bennetto et al. (2001) examined cognitive profiles in 32 women with a FXS full mutation, compared to women with a premutation, and non-FXS controls raised in FXS families. The full-mutation women had a significantly lower Full-Scale IQ than the other groups, so the authors conducted ipsative analyses of Wechsler Adult Intelligence Scale–Revised (WAIS-R) subtest profiles to examine relative strengths and weaknesses separate from overall IQ. Compared to the profiles of the other groups, women with a full mutation showed a relative weakness on Arithmetic and strength on Picture Completion. These findings were confirmed in a second study, in which the full-mutation women were compared to an age- and IQ-matched control group of women with mild learning disabilities. Thus, this study did not support previous findings of impaired performance on Block Design or short-term memory, after accounting for overall IQ via ipsative analyses or an IQ-matched control group.

In summary, studies of cognitive functioning indicate that females with FXS have specific weaknesses in arithmetic and may demonstrate impairments on tasks of short-term auditory memory and some visual-spatial tasks. Further research that controls for overall impairment in cognitive functioning is needed to clarify these patterns.

### Speech and Language

In contrast to males, little research has specifically examined speech and language in women with FXS. Madison et al. (1986) examined the speech and language functioning of five adult females with FXS, ranging from moderate mental retardation to low average intelligence. They found that the articulation of the women was clear and intelligible. No oral or speech apraxia was noted in the women, but they did have hypernasal voices and were one standard deviation slower than normal on timed polysyllabic repetition tasks. The pitch, loudness, rate, and fluency (with the exception of frequent revisions, or self-corrections) of the women were within average limits. In terms of language, the three lowest-functioning women were described as occasionally inappropriate in speech content, and all women tended to use conditionalized, or automatic, phrases. Although Madison et al. used standardized measures, they did not include a control group, so we cannot determine whether this sample's behavior is consistent with or different from developmental levels.

A second study examined pragmatic competence in a sample of five adult women with FXS, with IQs in the nonretarded range (Canales and Thompson 1995). Subjects were matched individually with control subjects on age, IQ, socioeconomic status, ethnicity, and education. The authors scored communication skills from subjects' responses to projective pictures. The authors found that, compared to controls, women with FXS displayed more communicative deviance, which included contorted and peculiar language, a "flighty" attention style (e.g., interrupting, jumping from topic to topic), perceptual distortions, difficulties with story closure, and faulty overintellectualization and overpersonalization of the story. In addition, the overall communicative deviance score was positively associated with the number of CGG repeats in subjects with FXS. Although it has a small sample, this study provides preliminary evidence of an impairment in pragmatics similar to that found in males with FXS.

### Memory

As with males, females with FXS seem to have a pattern of memory deficits that reflects intact performance in some areas and clear deficits in others. Initial evidence for a specific deficit in memory came from consistently poor digit span scores on Wechsler intelligence tests. In a study of Stanford-Binet profiles in FXS, Freund and Reiss (1991) reported a dissociation between abstract and meaningful visual memory in females, with abstract visual memory the lowest point on the profile and meaningful (or easily labeled) visual memory the highest.

Several studies of females with FXS have explicitly examined memory performance. Grigsby et al. (1992) administered several measures of short-term memory and learning efficiency to a sample of 20 females with FXS (aged 8 to 42 years), matched on CA with carrier mothers and sisters and with females with head injuries and learning disabilities. The mean IQ of the group with FXS was significantly lower (10–15 points) than those of the other two groups. Nonetheless, the women with FXS showed no significant differences from either group on two tasks of paired-associate learning (verbal-verbal and verbal-visual) or on delayed recall for word learning. Compared to both control groups, the women with FXS did show significantly worse performance on a digit span task and a measure of verbal learning efficiency (trials to criterion on a list learning task). The authors suggested that the women with FXS may have specific trouble in the memory encoding process. Cues given in the paired associate task may facilitate learning and retrieval.

Mazzocco et al. (1993) examined neuropsychologic functioning in a group of 22 women with FXS (without mental retardation), 35 carrier women, and 60 controls (mother and sisters from families with FXS or developmentally delayed children). Memory was assessed with the story and figural memory subtests of the Wechsler Memory Scale–Revised (WMS-R), which includes both immediate and delayed recall. After covarying out the effects of IQ, there were no group differences on either immediate or delayed figural memory. On both the immediate and delayed trials of story memory, however, women with FXS scored *better* than controls.

These findings are further supported by Hinton et al. (1995), who found that full-mutation women were not different from age-matched controls on the WMS-R verbal memory tasks, even after controlling for overall differences in IQ. Bennetto et al. (2001) also found that full-mutation women were not different on the WMS-R verbal memory scale compared to a more rigorous control sample matched on both age and IQ.

Together, these studies suggest that women with FXS do well on verbal memory tasks that impose some external structure (e.g., the story narrative or encoding/retrieval cues) on the information to be remembered. Memory for abstract or rote auditory information is an area of weakness, which may be the result of poor encoding.

### Spatial Ability

The fact that Block Design is consistently among the lowest IQ subtests in the cognitive profiles of women with FXS could suggest that spatial ability is an area of weakness for them. Other evidence comes from deficits in spatial short-term memory (Kemper et al. 1986) and weaker performance on figural memory compared to verbal memory (Mazzocco et al. 1993). Recent studies, however, suggest that visuospatial abilities are not a uniform weakness; rather, women with FXS seem to have a distinct pattern of impaired and intact functioning within this domain.

Hinton et al. (1995) examined a group of nine nonretarded women with a FXS full mutation, compared to women with a premutation and controls, with a comprehensive battery of neuropsychologic tests including several measures of spatial skills. After covarying age and Full-Scale IQ, the full-mutation women performed significantly worse than the other groups on the Benton Visual Reminding Test and the visual index of the WMS-R but not on other spatial tasks that did not involve attention or memory.

Cornish et al. (1998) examined patterns of spatial ability in a group of 17 full-mutation girls, aged 7 to 14 years. Compared to MA-matched controls, the girls with FXS showed a clear pattern of abilities within the spatial domain. They were significantly impaired on tasks involving abstract visuospatial construction, including the Wechsler Block Design subtest and the Triangles task from the K-ABC. In contrast, they were not different from MA-matched controls on constructional tasks involving more meaningful material, including Draw-a-person and the Wechsler Object Assembly. The girls with FXS were also relatively unimpaired in other visuospatial domains including perception, motor skills, and memory. Finally, the authors also examined X activation ratio and found no evidence of a relationship to spatial abilities.

Bennetto et al. (2001) examined neuropsychologic functioning in their sample of women with full mutations, premutations, and control subjects. As described above, they found a relative strength for Picture Completion in the WAIS-R profiles of full-mutation women, which is consistent with previous findings of intact abilities for tasks involving meaningful content. On neuropsychologic tests, women with full mutations performed worse than the other groups, after covarying age and IQ, on spatial ability (measured by a visual rotation task) and WMS-R visual memory, as well as several tasks of EF. Correlations with molecular variables showed that X activation ratio was related to all three domains. The authors then conducted partial correlations to examine the relationship of activation ratio with either visuospatial or executive abilities while controlling for the other. They found that activation ratio remained significantly related to EF, even after controlling for its shared relationship with spatial ability or visual memory, but was no longer related to the visuospatial variables after accounting for EF. Thus, EF deficits seemed more primary in this sample of women with FXS. This was confirmed in a second study in which the full-mutation women were compared to age and IQ-matched controls; in this study, they showed deficits on EF but not spatial measures.

Additional support for a more general processing impairment comes from a study by Cianchetti et al. (1991), who administered the Raven's Progressive Matrices to a mixed group of cytogenetically positive and carrier women (IQ > 80) and an age- and IQ-matched control group. Compared to controls, the women with FXS performed significantly worse on the Raven's Matrices. The authors argued that these women may have a specific deficit in spatial ability because this task is a visuospatial test of logical thinking. However, the Raven's is also typically considered a test of fluid intelligence. Poor performance on this task, relative to a group matched on a less purely fluid measure of IQ (i.e., WAIS-R), may reflect a deficit in fluid intelligence rather than spatial cognition.

### Executive Function

One of the most consistent neuropsychologic findings in studies of females with FXS is a specific deficit in EF (e.g., Bennetto et al. 2001; Mazzocco et al. 1992a, 1992b, 1993; Sobesky et al. 1994, 1996; Thompson et al. 1994). Unlike studies of affected males with FXS, studies of high-functioning females (IQ > 70) are able to use standard clinical tasks that are sensitive to frontal lobe functioning.

In their study of the neuropsychologic performance of women with FXS, Mazzocco et al. (1993) reported their most consistent and strongest group differences on tasks of EF. Compared to both carrier women and controls, and after covarying IQ, expressing women were significantly impaired on relevant variables from the Wisconsin Card Sorting Test (which measures conceptual problem solving and flexibility in thinking), the Contingency Naming Test (which measures set shifting and inhibition), and the Visual-Verbal Test (which measures concept formation and flexible thinking).

Hinton et al. (1995) also examined EF skills in their neuropsychologic study of nonretarded women with a FXS full mutation, a premutation, and non-FXS controls. They used a version of the Continuous Performance Test, which taps both attention and inhibition. A series of four-digit numbers appear briefly on a computer screen, and subjects are instructed to press a key whenever a number is repeated immediately after its presentation. After covarying age and Full-Scale IQ, the full-mutation women were significantly more likely to miss the targets, which is thought to reflect poor attentional skills. However, they did not make more false alarms (a measure of inhibition), which differs from the pattern reported in males with FXS, who seem to have more trouble with inhibition than attention (Munir et al. 2000).

Sobesky et al. (1996) examined EF in a sample of 29 women with a full mutation, compared to women with a premutation and non-FXS controls. They found that the full-mutation women showed significant deficits in EF, as measured by the Wisconsin Card Sorting Test and the Contingency Naming Test, even after covarying age and Full-Scale IQ. Analysis of molecular data found a significant relationship between X activation ratio and EF.

Finally, the Bennetto et al. (2001) studies discussed above found significant EF deficits (as measured by the Wisconsin Card Sorting Test and Contingency Naming Test) in a sample of full-mutation women, even after covarying age and Full-Scale IQ. The authors also provide the clearest evidence of the specificity of EF deficits in women with FXS by replicating their initial findings in a second study in which women with FXS were compared to age- and IQ-matched controls with mild learning disabilities. Their data suggest the primacy of EF rather than spatial deficits in women with FXS, in terms of both their overall neuropsychologic profile and the relationship of neuropsychologic variables to the underlying biology of the syndrome.

There is clear evidence that women with the full mutation have deficits in EF and that this area of functioning may be particularly sensitive to the effects of the *FMR1* mutation. Deficits in EF may help to explain some of the other areas of weakness observed in this group. For example, pragmatics, organizational aspects of memory, and behavioral problems such as hyperactivity or impulsivity may be manifestations of a more general deficit in EF.

In summary, existing studies of women with FXS indicate some specificity in their neuropsychologic functioning. In the cognitive area, there is clear evidence that the full mutation in females does have a major effect on IQ, producing on average a standard deviation depression in performance (mean IQ of 85). Approximately half of these women have IQs in the borderline or mentally retarded range. Unlike males, they do not seem to show a developmental decline in IQ. In contrast, the premutation does not seem to have an effect on general cognitive performance.

There also seems to be some specificity in the profiles of full-mutation women. In particular, they tend to show significant and consistent deficits on tasks of EF, which are not accounted for by their lower IQs. These women also seem to have some deficits in spatial or nonverbal abilities. However, recent research suggests that these deficits may not be central to the phenotype, but rather effects of generally poor cognitive processing.

In terms of verbal abilities, preliminary evidence suggests that women with FXS have specific deficits in pragmatics similar to those found in males. These women also seem to have deficits in verbal memory for rote or abstract information. In contrast, several studies have found a relative strength in certain types of verbal memory that impose a clear structure on the information to be remembered (e.g., story memory, cued recall).

During the past five years, considerable progress has been made in understanding the neuropsychologic phenotype of women with FXS. Many studies have examined specific deficits with appropriate neuropsychologic tests, rather than relying exclusively on IQ measures. Now that several areas of impairment have been identified, further research is needed to determine which of these deficits are primary to the neuropsychologic phenotype. In addition, most of the research with women has employed normally developing control groups. Comparing the performances of full-mutation women to those of subjects with developmental disabilities will help to address the issue of discriminant validity. This is a particularly important task, since several other groups (e.g., autism, attention deficit hyperactivity disorder) also show deficits on EF tasks.

## Implications for Future Research

We will discuss two research implications of the work reviewed here, one synthetic and one analytic. On the synthetic side, we would like to know how many of the behavioral features of FXS can be explained by the neuropsychologic profile we have identified; we will focus on the relation between EF and intelligence. On the analytic side, more work is needed to characterize more precisely the executive deficit in FXS and to compare it to the executive deficit found in other developmental disorders. We will discuss the synthetic issue first.

An unresolved issue in the neuropsychology of females with FXS is the specificity of their neuropsychologic deficit and how this deficit relates to their lower IQ. On the one hand, it has been demonstrated that their neuropsychologic profile is not "flat" but instead is characterized by a relative peak in verbal memory and a pronounced valley in EF. Moreover, their deficit in EF is greater than that predicted by their IQ. On the other hand, they seem to have a deficit in fluid intelligence that is also greater than that predicted by their IQ (Cianchetti et al. 1991). So, do they have a specific deficit in EF that is independent of IQ, or are the deficits in EF and fluid intelligence related? This is a critical question because its answer has important implications for how we can conceptualize the neuropsychology of intelligence and mental retardation. Recent work in cognitive neuropsychology suggests an answer to this question, but determining whether this answer applies to individuals with FXS requires further study.

Although EF tasks are quite heterogeneous in their surface characteristics, they all require goal-directed behavior, usually in novel contexts with competing but erroneous response alternatives. Despite understanding the goal of the task, patients with frontal lesions fail to accomplish it because of perseveration, lack of persistence, intrusions of task-irrelevant behavior, or lack of initiative. It is this dysregulation of goal-directed behavior that cannot be attributed to a more basic deficit in perception, memory, or language comprehension and that occurs across tasks varying in content and surface characteristics, which has led to the current view in neuropsychology that the frontal lobes are important for the "executive" or "supervisory" aspect of task performance. Thus, the historical controversy over whether the frontal lobes play a special role in higher cognition has been partly resolved. At the same time, Hebb's (1945) view that psychometric intelligence tests are particularly insensitive to the effects of frontal lesions continues to be accepted in contemporary neuropsychology. As Duncan et al. (1995, 262) aptly pointed out, "The paradox has been accepted that frontal patients have impaired 'planning,' 'problem solving,' etc., but preserved 'intelligence.'"

A resolution to this paradox is that the frontal lobes may be particularly important for what is called "fluid" intelligence but much less important for the maintenance of accumulated information, which is mainly tapped by measures of "crystallized" intelligence (Duncan 1995; Pennington 1994). Hence, a patient with a frontal lesion would perform much worse on a fluid IQ measure, like the Raven's Progressive Matrices or the Culture Fair IQ test, than on a measure like the Wechsler, many subtests of which tap accumulated information. To test this hypothesis, Duncan et al. (1995) administered both the Wechsler and the Culture Fair IQ tests to patients with either frontal or posterior lesions and to controls. Only in patients with frontal lesions was there a marked disparity between the scores on the two IQ tests; in that group, the score on the fluid measure was about 1.5 to 3 standard deviations lower than the Wechsler score. In separate experiments, Duncan and colleagues found that goal neglect on an experimental task was closely related to fluid intelligence in both patients with frontal lesions and normal adults (Duncan 1995).

So, it may also be the case that the executive and fluid intelligence deficits in females with FXS are closely related. The reason that scores in both domains are worse than predicted by Wechsler IQ scores may be that the subjects' strength in verbal memory contributes to relatively higher crystallized intelligence, which is also tapped by the Wechsler. If this is the case, then FXS in females (and perhaps high-functioning and premutation males) may allow us to study the cognitive mechanisms underlying mental retardation in a titrated form.

We turn now to a second unresolved issue in the neuropsychology of FXS that requires further analysis. EF deficits have been identified in a broad range of other neuropsychiatric and developmental disorders, including autism, attention deficit hyperactivity disorder (ADHD), schizophrenia, obsessive-compulsive disorder, and Tourette syndrome (for reviews, see Pennington and Ozonoff, 1996; Ozonoff, 1997). To understand what makes the FXS phenotype unique, we must now focus our research on the specificity of the neuropsychologic phenotype among different developmental disorders.

Recent empiric and theoretical work points to several distinct functions within the executive domain, which may help to address this problem. Historically, EF has been used as an umbrella term to describe a range of cognitive processes involved in the planning and execution of complex behavior, without necessarily specifying the precise nature of the processes. The tasks traditionally used to assess EF are often quite complex, and poor performance on them may be affected by one or more distinct cognitive processes (Pennington et al. 1996). The imprecise definition and measurement of EF is a critical problem in research on FXS. Most of our evidence for an EF deficit in FXS comes from complex tasks such as the Wisconsin Card Sorting Task or from indirect analyses of strengths and weaknesses in cognitive profiles.

One solution to this problem can be found by examining components of EF. Recent studies that employ more precise tasks suggest that EF may instead be composed of a set of unique and dissociable components, including cognitive flexibility, planning, working memory, and inhibition (e.g., Burgess 1997; Duncan et al. 1995; Robbins 1998). Individuals with different disorders may demonstrate similar impairments on global tasks, yet show very different patterns on component processes. For example, Bennetto and Pennington (1999) compared EF performance across three disorders: autism, women with FXS, and ADHD. Each group was matched to its own control group on age and IQ. All three groups showed impairments on the Wisconsin Card Sorting Task, although subjects with autism showed the greatest impairment relative to their controls. When the authors examined components of EF, subjects with autism and FXS were significantly impaired on a task of verbal working memory, while subjects with ADHD were not. In contrast, subjects with ADHD were impaired on measures of inhibition, while the other groups were not. Thus, a component approach to EF may help explain why individuals who show impairments on traditional EF tasks can demonstrate such different behavior patterns and respond to different remediation strategies.

In the last decade, there have been exciting new developments in our understanding of FXS. Continued research on the neuropsychologic phenotype will play an important role in our achievement of an integrated understanding of the cognitive neuroscience of FXS. By identifying the primary neuropsychologic deficits in FXS, we can complete the bridge from molecular and neurologic levels, to neuropsychologic functioning, to some of the behavioral and psychiatric difficulties experienced by individuals with FXS.

## Acknowledgments

This work was supported in part by NIMH grant R01 MH45916 and NIH grant 5M01 RR00069. In addition, the second author was supported by NICHD grants P50 HD27802 and P30 HD04024 and NIMH grants 5 K02 MH00419 (RSA) and 5 R37 MH38820 (MERIT). Correspondence concerning this chapter should be addressed to Loisa Bennetto, Ph.D., University of Rochester, Clinical and Social Sciences in Psychology, Meliora Hall, RC 270266, Rochester, NY 14627.

## References

Abrams, M. T., L. Reiss, L. S. Freund, T. L. Baumgardner, G. A. Chase, and M. B. Denckla. 1994. Molecular-neurobehavioral associations in females with the fragile X full mutation. *Am. J. Med. Genet.* 51:317–327.

Allingham-Hawkins, D. J., C. A. Brown, R. Babul, D. Chitayat, K. Krekewich, T. Humphries, P. N. Ray, and I. E. Teshima. 1996. Tissue-specific methylation differences and cognitive function in fragile X premutation females. *Am. J. Med. Genet.* 64:329–333.

Bailey, D. B., D. Hatton, and M. Skinner. 1998. Early developmental trajectories of males with fragile X syndrome. *Am. J. Ment. Retard.* 103:23–39.

Bennetto, L., and B. F. Pennington. 1999. Dissociating components of executive functioning across developmental disorders. Presented at the Biennial Meeting of the Society for Research in Child Development, Albuquerque, April 15–18.

Bennetto, L., B. F. Pennington, D. Porter, A. K. Taylor, and R. J. Hagerman. 2001. Profile of cognitive functioning in women with the fragile X mutation. *Neuropsychology* 15:290–299.

Berkson, J. 1946. Limitations of the application of fourfold table analysis to hospital data. *Biometrics* 2:47–51.

Borghgraef, M., J. P. Fryns, A. Dielkens, K. Dyck, and H. Van den Berghe. 1987. Fragile (X) syndrome: A study of the psychological profile in 23 prepubertal patients. *Clin. Genet.* 32:179–186.

Borghgraef, M., J. P. Fryns, K. Dyck, and H. Van den Berghe. 1988. Fragile X syndrome: A study of the psychological profile of 40 pre- and postpubertal patients. Presented at the Eighth World Congress of the International Association for the Scientific Study of Mental Deficiency, Dublin, August 21–25.

Brainard, S. S., R. A. Schreiner, and R. J. Hagerman. 1991. Cognitive profiles of the adult carrier fra(X) female. *Am. J. Med. Genet.* 38:505–508.

Brun, C., J. E. Obiols, A. Cheema, R. O'Connor, J. Riddle, M. DiMaria, C. Wright-Talamante, and R. Hagerman. 1995. Longitudinal IQ changes in fragile X females. *Dev. Brain Dysfunct.* 8:230–241.

Burgess, P. W. 1997. Theory and methodology in executive function research. In P. Rabbitt (ed.), *Methodology of frontal and executive function.* Hove, U.K.: Psychology Press, pp. 81–111.

Canales, D. N., and N. M. Thompson. 1995. Communication deviance in females with fragile X syndrome. Presented at the 23rd Annual Meeting of the International Neuropsychological Society, Seattle, February 8–11.

Chudley, A. E., J. Knoll, J. W. Gerrard, L. Shepel, E. McGahey, and J. Anderson. 1983. Fragile (X) X-linked mental retardation. I: Relationship between age and intelligence and the frequency of expression of fragile (X) (q28). *Am. J. Med. Genet.* 14:699–712.

Cianchetti, C., G. Sannio-Fancello, A. L. Fratta, F. Manconi, A. Orano, M. P. Pischedda, D. Pruna, G. Spinicci, N. Archidiacono, and G. Filippi. 1991. Neuropsychological, psychiatric, and physical manifestations in 149 members from 18 fragile X families. *Am. J. Med. Genet.* 40:234–243.

Cornish, K. M., F. Munir, and G. Cross. 1998. The nature of the spatial deficit in young females with fragile-X syndrome: A neuropsychological and molecular perspective. *Neuropsychologia* 36:1239–1246.

———. 1999. Spatial cognition in males with fragile-X syndrome: Evidence for a neuropsychological phenotype. *Cortex* 35:263–271.

———. 2001. Differential impact of the FMR-1 full mutation on memory and attention functioning: A neuropsychological perspective. *J. Cog. Neurosci.* 13:144–150.

Cronister, A., R. J. Hagerman, M. Wittenberger, and K. Amiri. 1991. Mental impairment in cytogenetically positive fragile X females. *Am. J. Med. Genet.* 38:503–504.

Crowe, S. F., and D. A. Hay. 1990. Neuropsychological dimensions of the fragile X syndrome: Support for a non-dominant hemisphere dysfunction hypothesis. *Neuropsychologia* 28:9–16.

Cummings, J. L. 1993. Frontal-subcortical circuits and human behavior. *Arch. Neurol.* 50:873–880.

de von Flindt, R., B. Bybel, A. E. Chudley, and F. Lopes. 1991. Short-term memory and cognitive variability in adult fragile X females. *Am. J. Med. Genet.* 38:488–492.

de Vries, B. B. A., A. M. Wiegers, E. de Graaff, A. J. M. H. Verkerk, J. O. Van Hemel, D. J. J. Halley, J-P. Fryns, L. M. G. Curfs, M. F. Niermeijer, and B. A. Oostra. 1993. Mental status and fragile X expression in relation to *FMR-1* gene mutation. *Eur. J. Hum. Genet.* 1:72–79.

de Vries, B. B. A., A. M. Wiegers, A. P. T. Smits, S. Mohkamsing, H. J. Duivenvoorden, J-P. Fryns, L. N. G. Curfs, D. J. J. Halley, B. A. Oostra, A. M. W. van den Ouweland, and M. F. Niermeijer. 1996. Mental status of females with an *FMR1* gene full mutation. *Am. J. Hum. Genet.* 58:1025–1032.

Duncan, J. 1995. Attention, intelligence, and the frontal lobes. In M. S. Gazzaniga (ed.), *The cognitive neurosciences.* Cambridge: MIT Press, pp. 721–733.

Duncan, J., P. Burgess, and H. Emslie. 1995. Fluid intelligence after frontal lobe lesions. *Neuropsychologia* 3:261–268.

Dykens, E. M., R. M. Hodapp, and J. F. Leckman. 1987. Strengths and weaknesses in the intellectual functioning of males with fragile X syndrome. *Am. J. Med. Genet.* 28:13–15.

Dykens, E. M., J. F. Leckman, R. Paul, and M. Watson. 1988. Cognitive, behavioral, and adaptive functioning in fragile X and non-fragile X retarded men. *J. Autism Dev. Disord.* 18:41–52.

Dykens, E. M., R. Hodapp, S. Ort, B. Finucane, L. Shapiro, and J. Leckman. 1989. The trajectory of cognitive development in males with fragile X syndrome. *J. Am. Acad. Child Adolesc. Psychiatry* 28:422–426.

Dykens, E., S. Ort, I. Cohen, B. Finucane, G. Spiridigliozzi, A. Lachiewicz, A. Reiss, L. Freund, R. Hagerman, and R. O'Connor. 1996. Trajectories and profiles of adaptive behavior in males with fragile X syndrome: Multicenter studies. *J. Autism Dev. Disord.* 26:287–301.

Ferrier, L. J., A. S. Gashir, D. L. Meryash, J. Johnston, and P. Wolff. 1991. Conversational skills of individuals with fragile X syndrome: A comparison with autism and Down syndrome. *Dev. Med. Child Neurol.* 33:776–788.

Fisch, G. S., T. Arinami, U. Froster-Iskenius, J. P. Fryns, L. M. Curfs, M. Borghgraef, P. N. Howard-Peebles, C. E. Schwartz, R. J. Simensen, and L. R. Shapiro. 1991. Relationship between age and IQ among fragile X males: A multicenter study. *Am. J. Med. Genet.* 38:481–487.

Fisch, G. S., L. R. Shapiro, R. Simensen, C. E. Schwartz, J. P. Fryns, M. Borghgraef, L. M. Curfs, P. N. Howard-Peebles, T. Arinami, and A. Mavrou. 1992. Longitudinal changes in IQ among fragile X males: Clinical evidence of more than one mutation? *Am. J. Med Genet.* 43:28–34.

Fisch, G. S., R. Simensen, T. Arinami, M. Borghgraef, and J. P. Fryns. 1994. Longitudinal changes in IQ among fragile X females: A preliminary multicenter analysis. *Am. J. Med. Genet.* 51:353–357.

Fisch, G. S., N. Carpenter, P. N. Howard-Peebles, A. Maddalena, R. Simensen, J. Tarleton, C. Julien-Inalsingh, M. Chalifoux, and J. J. A. Holden. 1996a. Lack of association between mutation size and cognitive/behavior deficits in fragile X males: A brief report. *Am. J. Med. Genet.* 64:362–364.

Fisch, G. S., R. Simensen, J. Tarleton, M. Chalifoux, J. J. A. Holden, N. Carpenter, P. N. Howard-Peebles, and A. Maddalena. 1996b. Longitudinal study of cognitive abilities and adaptive behavior levels in fragile X males: A prospective multicenter analysis. *Am. J. Med. Genet.* 64:356–361.

Fisch, G. S., N. J. Carpenter, J. J. A. Holden, R. Simensen, P. N. Howard-Peebles, A. Maddalena, A. Pandya, and W. Nance. 1999. Longitudinal assessment of adaptive and maladaptive behaviors in fragile X males: Growth, development, and profiles. *Am. J. Med. Genet.* 83:257–263.

Fowler, A. 1990. The development of language structure in children with Down syndrome: Evidence for a specific syntactic delay. In D. Cicchetti and M. Beeghly (eds.), *Children with Down syndrome: A developmental approach.* New York: Cambridge Univ. Press, pp. 302–328.

Freund, L., and A. L. Reiss. 1991. Cognitive profiles associated with the FraX syndrome in males and females. *Am. J. Med. Genet.* 38:542–547.

Freund, L., C. A. Peebles, E. Aylward, and A. L. Reiss. 1995. Preliminary report on cognitive and adaptive behaviors of preschool-aged males with fragile X. *Dev. Brain Dysfunct.* 8:242–261.

Goldfine, P. E., P. M. McPherson, V. A. Hardesty, G. A. Heath, L. J. Beauregard, and A. A. Baker. 1987. Fragile-X chromosome associated with primary learning disability. *J. Am. Acad. Child Adolesc. Psychiatry* 26:589–592.

Goldman-Rakic, P. S. 1987. Circuitry of primate prefrontal cortex and regulation of behavior by representational memory. In F. Plum (ed.), *Handbook of physiology: Section I. The nervous system:* Vol. 5, *Higher functions of the brain.* Bethesda, Md.: American Physiology Association, pp. 373–417.

Grigsby, J., M. B. Kemper, and R. J. Hagerman. 1987. Developmental Gerstmann syndrome without aphasia in fragile X syndrome. *Neuropsychologia* 25:881–891.

———. 1992. Verbal learning and memory among heterozygous fragile X females. *Am. J. Med. Genet.* 43:111–115.

Hagerman, R. J. 1991. Physical and behavioral phenotype. In R. J. Hagerman and A. Cronister-Silverman (eds.), *Fragile X syndrome: Diagnosis, treatment, and research.* Baltimore: Johns Hopkins Univ. Press, pp. 3–68.

Hagerman, R. J., and A. C. M. Smith. 1983. The heterozygous female. In R. J. Hagerman and P. M. McBogg (eds.), *The fragile X syndrome: Diagnosis, biochemistry, and intervention.* Dillon, Colo.: Spectra Publishing, pp. 83–94.

Hagerman, R. J., R. A. Schreiner, M. B. Kemper, M. D. Wittenberger, B. Zahn, and K. Habicht. 1989. Longitudinal IQ changes in fragile X males. *Am. J. Med. Genet.* 33: 513–518.

Hagerman, R. J., C. Jackson, C. Amiri, A. Cronister-Silverman, R. O'Connor, and W. Sobesky. 1992. Girls with fragile X syndrome: Physical and neurocognitive status and outcome. *Pediatrics* 89:395–400.

Hagerman, R. J., C. E. Hull, J. F. Safanda, I. Carpenter, L. W. Staley, R. A. O'Conner, C. Seydel, M. M. M. Mazzocco, K. Snow, S. N. Thibodeau, D. Kuhl, D. L. Nelson, C. T. Caskey, and A. K. Taylor. 1994. High functioning fragile X males: Demonstration of an unmethylated fully expanded *FMR-1* mutation associated with protein expression. *Am. J. Med. Genet.* 51:298–308.

Hagerman, R. J., L. W. Staley, R. O'Connor, K. Lugenbeel, D. Nelson, S. D. McLean, and A. Taylor. 1996. Learning-disabled males with a fragile X CGG expansion in the upper premutation size range. *Pediatrics* 97:122–126.

Hanson, D. M., A. W. Jackson III, and R. J. Hagerman. 1986. Speech disturbances (cluttering) in mildly impaired males with the Martin-Bell/fragile X syndrome. *Am. J. Med. Genet.* 7:471–489.

Hay, D. A. 1994. Does IQ decline with age in fragile X? A methodological critique. *Am. J. Med. Genet.* 51:358–363.

Hebb, D. O. 1945. Man's frontal lobes: A critical review. *Arch. Neurol. Psychology* 54:10–24.

Herbst, D. S. 1980. Nonspecific X-linked mental retardation: I. A review with information from 24 families. *Am. J. Med. Genet.* 7:443–460.

Hills, J. L., R. Wilson, W. Sobesky, S. W. Harris, J. Grigsby, E. Butler, D. Loesch, R. Huggins, and R. J. Hagerman. 2000. Executive functioning deficits in adult males with the fragile X premutation: An emerging phenotype. Presented at the Seventh International Fragile X Foundation Conference, Los Angeles, July 19–22.

Hinton, V. J., J. M. Halperin, C. S. Dobkin, X. H. Ding, W. T. Brown, and C. M. Miezejeski. 1995. Cognitive and molecular aspects of fragile X. *J. Clin. Exp. Neuropsychol.* 17:518–528.

Hodapp, R. M., J. A. Burack, and E. Zigler. 1990a. *Issues in the developmental approach to mental retardation.* New York: Cambridge Univ. Press.

Hodapp, R. M., E. M. Dykens, R. J. Hagerman, R. A. Schreiner, A. M. Lachiewicz, and J. F. Leckman. 1990b. Developmental implications of changing trajectories of IQ in males with fragile X syndrome. *J. Am. Acad. Child Adolesc. Psychiatry* 29:214–219.

Hodapp, R. M., E. M. Dykens, S. I. Ort, D. G. Zelinsky, and J. F. Leckman. 1991. Changing patterns of intellectual strengths and weaknesses in males with fragile X syndrome. *J. Autism Dev. Disord.* 21:503–516.

Hodapp, R. M., J. F. Leckman, E. M. Dykens, S. Sparrow, D. Zelinsky, and S. Ort. 1992. K-ABC profiles in children with fragile X syndrome, Down syndrome, and nonspecific mental retardation. *Am. J. Ment. Retard.* 97:39–46.

Kaufmann, W. E., M. T. Abrams, W. Chen, and A. L. Reiss. 1999. Genotype, molecular phenotype, and cognitive phenotype: Correlations in fragile X syndrome. *Am. J. Med. Genet.* 83:286–295.

Kemper, M. B., R. J. Hagerman, R. S. Ahmad, and R. Mariner. 1986. Cognitive profiles and the spectrum of clinical manifestations in heterozygous fragile (X) females. *Am. J. Med. Genet.* 23:139–156.

Kemper, M. B., R. J. Hagerman, and D. Altshul-Stark. 1988. Cognitive profiles of boys with the fragile X syndrome. *Am. J. Med. Genet.* 30:191–200.

Kolb, B., and I. Q. Whishaw. 1996. *Fundamentals of human neuropsychology,* 4th ed. New York: W. H. Freeman.

Lachiewicz, A. M., C. M. Guillion, G. A. Spiridigliozzi, and A. S. Aylsworth. 1987. Declining IQs of young males with the fragile X syndrome. *Am. J. Ment. Retard.* 92: 272–278.

Levin, H. S., D. Mendelsohn, M. A. Lilly, J. M. Fletcher, K. A. Culhane, S. B. Chapman, H. Harward, L. Kusnerik, D. Bruce, and H. M. Eisenberg. 1994. Tower of London performance in relation to magnetic resonance imaging following closed head injury in children. *Neuropsychologia* 8:171–179.

Loesch, D. Z., and D. A. Hay. 1988. Clinical features and reproductive patterns in fragile X female heterozygotes. *J. Med. Genet.* 25:407–414.

Loesch, D. Z., R. Huggins, D. A. Hay, A. K. Gedeon, J. C. Mulley, and G. R. Sutherland. 1993. Genotype-phenotype relationships in fragile X syndrome: A family study. *Am. J. Hum. Genet.* 53:1064–1073.

Madison, L. S., C. George, and J. B. Moeschler. 1986. Cognitive functioning in the fragile-X syndrome: A study of intellectual, memory and communication skills. *J. Ment. Defic. Res.* 30:129–148.

Maes, B., J-P. Fryns, M. Van Walleghem, and H. Van den Berghe. 1994. Cognitive functioning and information processing of adult mentally retarded men with fragile-X syndrome. *Am. J. Med. Genet.* 50:190–200.

Mazzocco, M. M. M., R. J. Hagerman, A. Cronister-Silverman, and B. F. Pennington.

1992a. Specific frontal lobe deficits among women with the fragile X gene. *J. Am. Acad. Child Adolesc. Psychiatry* 31:1141–1148.

Mazzocco, M. M. M., R. J. Hagerman, and B. F. Pennington. 1992b. Problem solving limitations among cytogenetically expressing fragile X women. *Am. J. Med. Genet.* 43:78–86.

Mazzocco, M. M. M., B. F. Pennington, and R. J. Hagerman. 1993. The neurocognitive phenotype of female carriers of fragile X: Additional evidence for specificity. *Dev. Behav. Pediatr.* 14:328–335.

Mazzocco, M. M. M., B. F. Pennington, and R. J. Hagerman. 1994. Social cognition skills among females with fragile X. *J. Autism Dev. Disord.* 24:473–485.

Merenstein, S. A., V. Shyu, W. E. Sobesky, L. Staley, E. Berry-Kravis, D. L. Nelson, K. A. Lugenbeel, A. K. Taylor, B. F. Pennington, and R. J. Hagerman. 1994. Fragile X syndrome in a normal IQ male with learning and emotional problems. *J. Am. Acad. Child Adolesc. Psychiatry* 33:1316–1321.

Merenstein, S. A., W. E. Sobesky, A. K. Taylor, J. E. Riddle, H. X. Tran, and R. J. Hagerman. 1996. Molecular-clinical correlations in males with an expanded *FMR1* mutation. *Am. J. Med. Genet.* 64:388–394.

Moscovitch, M. 1992. Memory and working-with-memory: A component process model based on modules and central system. *J. Cogn. Neurosci.* 4:257–267.

Munir, F., K. M. Cornish, and J. Wilding. 2000. A neuropsychological profile of attention deficits in young males with fragile X syndrome. *Neuropsychologia* 38:1261–1270.

———. 2001. Nature of the working memory deficit in fragile X syndrome. *Brain Cogn.* 44:387–401.

Murray, A., S. Youings, N. Dennis, L. Latsky, P. Linehan, N. McKechnie, J. Macpherson, M. Pound, and P. Jacobs. 1996. Population screening at the FRAXA and FRAXE loci: Molecular analyses of boys with learning difficulties and their mothers. *Hum. Mol. Genet.* 5:727–735.

Newell, K., B. Sanborn, and R. J. Hagerman. 1983. Speech and language dysfunction in the fragile X syndrome. In R. J. Hagerman and P. M. McBogg (eds.), *The fragile X syndrome: Diagnosis, biochemistry, and intervention.* Dillon, Colo.: Spectra Publishing, pp. 175–200.

Oberle, I., F. Rousseau, D. Heitz, C. Kretz, D. Devys, A. Hanauer, J. Boue, M. F. Bertheas, and J. L. Mandel. 1991. Instability of a 550-base pair DNA segment and abnormal methylation in fragile X syndrome. *Science* 252:1097–1110.

Ozonoff, S. 1997. Components of executive function in autism and other disorders. In J. Russell (ed.), *Autism as an executive disorder.* New York: Oxford Univ. Press, pp. 179–211.

Paul, R. E., D. Cohen, R. Greg, M. Watson, and S. Herman. 1984. Fragile X syndrome: Its relation to speech and language disorders. *J. Speech Hear. Disord.* 49:328–332.

Paul, R., E. Dykens, J. F. Leckman, M. Watson, W. R. Breg, and D. J. Cohen. 1987. A comparison of language characteristics of mentally retarded adults with fragile X syndrome and those with nonspecific mental retardation and autism. *J. Autism Dev. Disord.* 17:457–468.

Pennington, B. F. 1991. *Diagnosing learning disorders: A neuropsychological framework.* New York: Guilford Press.

Pennington, B. F. 1994. The working memory function of the prefrontal cortices: Implications for developmental and individual differences in cognition. In M. M. Haith, J. Benson, R. Roberts, and B. F. Pennington (eds.), *Future oriented processes in development.* Chicago: Univ. of Chicago Press, pp. 243–289.

Pennington, B. F., and L. Bennetto. 1998. Toward a neuropsychology of mental retardation. In J. A. Burack, R. M. Hodapp, and E. Zigler (eds.), *Handbook of mental retardation and development.* Cambridge: Cambridge Univ. Press, 80–114.

Pennington, B. F., and S. Ozonoff. 1996. Executive functions and developmental psychopathology. *J. Child Psychol. Psychiatry* 37:51–87.

Pennington, B. F., and S. D. Smith. 1988. Genetic influences on learning disabilities: An update. *J. Consult. Clin. Psychol.* 36:817–823.

Pennington, B. F., R. A. O'Connor, and V. Sudhalter. 1991. Toward a neuropsychology of fragile(X) syndrome. In R. J. Hagerman and A. Cronister (eds.), *Fragile X syndrome: Diagnosis, treatment, and research.* Baltimore: Johns Hopkins Univ. Press, pp. 173–201.

Pennington, B. F., L. Bennetto, O. McAleer, and R. J. Roberts. 1996. Executive functions and working memory: Theoretical and measurement issues. In G. R. Lyon and N. A. Krasnegor (eds.), *Attention, memory, and executive function.* Baltimore: Paul H. Brookes, pp. 327–348.

Prior, M. 1977. Psycholinguistic disabilities of autistic and retarded children. *J. Ment. Defic. Res.* 21:37–45.

Prouty, L. A., R. C. Rogers, R. E. Stevenson, J. H. Dean, K. K. Palmer, R. J. Simensen, G. N. Coston, and C. E. Schwartz. 1988. Fragile X syndrome: Growth, development, and intellectual function. *Am. J. Med. Genet.* 30:123–142.

Reiss, A. L., and L. Freund. 1992. Behavioral phenotype of fragile X syndrome: DSM-III-R autistic behavior in male children. *Am. J. Med. Genet.* 43:35–46.

Reiss, A. L., L. Freund, M. T. Abrams, C. Boehm, and H. Kazazian. 1993. Neurobehavioral effects of the fragile X premutation in adult women: A controlled study. *Am. J. Hum. Genet.* 52:884–894.

Reiss, A. L., L. S. Freund, T. L. Baumgardner, M. T. Abrams, and M. B. Denckla. 1995. Contribution of the *FMR1* gene mutation to human intellectual dysfunction. *Nat. Genet.* 11:331–334.

Robbins, T. W. 1998. Dissociating executive functions of the prefrontal cortex. In A. C. Roberts, T. W. Robbins, and L. Weiskrantz (eds.), *The prefrontal cortex: Executive and cognitive functions.* Oxford: Oxford Univ. Press, pp. 117–130.

Robinson, A., H. A. Lubs, and D. Bergson. 1979. *Sex chromosomes aneuploidy: Prospective studies on children.* New York: Alan R. Liss.

Rousseau, F., D. Heitz, V. Biancalana, S. Blumenfeld, C. Kretz, J. Boue, N. Tommerup, C. Van Der Hagen, C. DeLozier-Blanchet, M-F. Croquette, S. Gilgenkrantz, P. Jalbert, M. A. Voelckel, I. Oberle, and J. L. Mandel. 1991. Direct diagnosis by DNA analysis of the fragile X syndrome of mental retardation. *N. Engl. J. Med.* 325:1673–1681.

Rousseau, F., D. Heitz, J. Tarleton, J. MacPherson, H. Malmgren, N. Dahl, A. Barnicoat, C. Mathew, E. Mornet, I. Tejada, A. Maddalena, R. Spiegel, A. Schinzel, J. A. G. Marcos, D. F. Schorderet, T. Schaap, L. Maccioni, S. Russo, P. A. Jacobs, C.

Schwartz, and J. L. Mandel. 1994. A multicenter study on genotype-phenotype correlations in the fragile X syndrome, using direct diagnosis with probe StB 12.3: The first 2,253 cases. *Am. J. Hum. Genet.* 55:225–237.

Sherman, A. C. 1991. Genetic counseling. In R. J. Hagerman and A. Cronister (eds.), *Fragile X syndrome: Diagnosis, treatment, and research.* Baltimore: Johns Hopkins Univ. Press, pp. 69–97.

Silverstein, A. B., G. Legutki, S. L. Friedman, and D. L. Takayama. 1982. Performance of Down syndrome individuals on the Stanford-Binet Intelligence Scale. *Am. J. Ment. Defic.* 86:548–551.

Sobesky, W. E., B. F. Pennington, D. Porter, C. E. Hull, and R. J. Hagerman. 1994. Emotional and neurocognitive deficits in fragile X. *Am. J. Med. Genet.* 51:378–385.

Sobesky, W. E., A. K. Taylor, B. F. Pennington, J. Riddle, and R. J. Hagerman. 1996. Molecular/clinical correlations in females with fragile X. *Am. J. Med. Genet.* 64: 340–345.

Staley, L., C. Hull, M. Mazzocco, S. Thibodeau, K. Snow, V. Wilson, A. Taylor, L. McGavran, J. Riddle, R. O'Connor, and R. Hagerman. 1993. Molecular-clinical correlations in fragile X children and adults. *Am. J. Dis. Child.* 147:724–726.

Steyaert, J., M. Borghgraef, C. Gaulthier, J. P. Fryns, and H. Van Den Berghe. 1992. Cognitive profile in adult, normal intelligent female fragile X carriers. *Am. J. Med. Genet.* 43:116–119.

Steyaert, J., M. Borghgraef, E. Legius, and J-P. Fryns. 1996. Molecular-intelligence correlations in young fragile X males with a mild CGG repeat expansion in the *FMR1* gene. *Am. J. Med. Genet.* 64:274–277.

Sudhalter, V., I. L. Cohen, W. P. Silverman, and E. G. Wolf-Schein. 1990. Conversational analyses of males with fragile X, Down syndrome and autism: A comparison of the emergence of deviant language. *Am. J. Ment. Retard.* 94:431–441.

Sudhalter, V., H. S. Scarborough, and I. C. Cohen. 1991. Syntactic delay and pragmatic deviance in the language of fragile X males. *Am. J. Med. Genet.* 38:493–497.

Sudhalter, V., M. Maranion, and P. Brooks. 1992. Expressive semantic deficit in the productive language of males with fragile X syndrome. *Am. J. Med. Genet.* 43:65–71.

Sutherland, G. R., and Hecht, F. 1985. *Fragile sites on human chromosomes.* New York: Oxford Univ. Press.

Tassone, F., R. J. Hagerman, L. W. Gane, and A. K. Taylor. 1999a. Strong similarities of the *FMR1* mutation in multiple tissues: Postmortem studies of a male with a full mutation and a male carrier with a premutation. *Am. J. Med. Genet.* 84:240–244.

Tassone, F., R. J. Hagerman, D. N. Ikle, P. N. Dyer, M. Lampe, R. Willemsen, B. A. Oostra, and A. K. Taylor. 1999b. FMRP expression as a potential prognostic indicator in fragile X syndrome. *Am. J. Med. Genet.* 84:250–261.

Taylor, A. K., J. F. Safanda, M. Z. Fall, C. Quince, K. A. Lang, C. E. Hull, I. Carpenter, L. W. Staley, and R. J. Hagerman. 1994. Molecular predictors of cognitive involvement in female carriers of fragile X syndrome. *JAMA* 27:507–514.

Taylor, A. K., F. Tassone, P. N. Dyer, S. M. Hersch, J. B. Harris, W. T. Greenough, and R. J. Hagerman. 1999. Tissue heterogeneity of the *FMR1* mutation in a high-functioning male with fragile X syndrome. *Am. J. Med. Genet.* 84:233–239.

Theobald, T. M., D. A. Hay, and C. Judge. 1987. Individual variation and specific cognitive deficits in the fra(X) syndrome. *Am. J. Med. Genet.* 28:1–11.

Thompson, N. M., M. L. Gulley, G. A. Rogeness, R. J. Clayton, C. Johnson, B. Hazelton, C. G. Cho, and V. T. Zellmer. 1994. Neurobehavioral characteristics of CGG amplification status in fragile X females. *Am. J. Med. Genet.* 54:378–383.

Turner, G., A. Daniel, and M. Frost. 1980. X-linked mental retardation, macroorchidism and the Xq27 fragile site. *J. Pediatr.* 96:837–841.

Veenema, H., T. Veenema, and J. P. Geraedts. 1987. The fragile X syndrome in a large family: II. Psychological investigations. *J. Med. Genet.* 24:32–38.

Verkerk, A. J., M. Pieretti, J. S. Sutcliffe, Y. H. Fu, D. P. Kuhl, A. Pizzuti, O. Reiner, S. Richards, M. F. Victoria, F. Zhang, B. E. Eussen, G. J. van Ommen, L. A. J. Blonden, G. J. Riggins, J. L. Chastain, C. B. Kunst, H. Galjaard, C. T. Caskey, D. L. Nelson, B. A. Oostra, and S. T. Warren. 1991. Identification of a gene (*FMR-1*) containing a CGG repeat coincident with a breakpoint cluster region exhibiting length variation in fragile X syndrome. *Cell* 65:905–914.

Vilkman, E., J. Niemi, and U. Ikonen. 1988. Fragile X speech phonology in Finnish. *Brain Lang.* 34:203–221.

Waterhouse, L., and D. Fein. 1984. Developmental trends in cognitive skills for children diagnosed as autistic and schizophrenic. *Child Dev.* 55:312–326.

Wolff, P. H., J. Gardner, J. Lappen, J. Paccia, and D. Meryash. 1988. Variable expression of the fragile X syndrome in heterozygous females of normal intelligence. *Am. J. Med. Genet.* 30:213–225.

Wolf-Schein, E. G., V. Sudhalter, I. L. Cohen, G. S. Fisch, D. Hanson, A. G. Pfadt, R. Hagerman, E. Jenkins, and W. T. Brown. 1987. Speech-language and the fragile X syndrome: Initial findings. *ASHA* 29:35–38.

Wright-Talamante, C., A. Cheema, J. E. Riddle, D. W. Luckey, A. K. Taylor, and R. J. Hagerman. 1996. A controlled study of longitudinal IQ changes in females and males with fragile X syndrome. *Am. J. Med. Genet.* 64:350–355.

Yu, S., M. Pritchard, E. Kremer, M. Lynch, J. Nancarrow, E. Baker, K. Holman, J. C. Mulley, S. T. Warren, D. Schlessinger, G. R. Sutherland, and I. R. Richards. 1991. Fragile X genotype characterized by an unstable region of DNA. *Science* 252:1179–1181.

# PART II
## Treatment and Intervention

# CHAPTER 7

# Genetic Counseling

## Louise W. Gane, M.S., and Amy Cronister, M.S.

Many families find relief in finally knowing the cause of their child's problems. At last there is a diagnosis, possible treatment, and, most importantly, answers. As with all inherited conditions, parents must face the difficult and emotionally charged issue that one of them may have passed this altered *FMR1* gene to their children. Explaining the molecular and hereditary aspects of fragile X syndrome (FXS) and helping families cope with and resolve feelings of guilt, anger, denial, and grief are primary goals of genetic counseling. When appropriate, available testing and family planning options should be discussed and a plan for approaching extended family members considered.

Since the discovery of the *FMR1* gene, many questions have been answered, but there remain many challenges for the genetic professional. These challenges include the variable expressivity seen in males and females with the full mutation or the premutation, recurrence risks, and prenatal testing. Genetic counselors should realize that most parents are overwhelmed by the vast amount of information given to them at the initial evaluation. Taking time to help families grasp all aspects of the diagnosis is essential, since it enables families to appreciate how the *FMR1* mutation affects their particular family.

Families dealing with the diagnosis of FXS have counseling needs beyond understanding the genetic aspects of the condition. With little information available to families and with many physicians, health care providers, and educators unfamiliar with this diagnosis and the spectrum of involvement, parents turn to the genetic counselor for information about medical management, educational options and recommendations as well as long-term prognostic implications. Many parents also need someone who will validate the varying emotions they experience and who will acknowledge the psychological stressors they feel are being placed upon personal relationships as a result of having a child with special needs. To address these and other aspects of the diagnosis,

*Fragile X Syndrome: Diagnosis, Treatment, and Research,* third edition, ed. Randi Jenssen Hagerman and Paul J. Hagerman (Baltimore: Johns Hopkins University Press, 2002), © The Johns Hopkins University Press.

the genetic counseling process cannot be hurried. Long-term contact and support are necessary. It is an enormous challenge, but with the help of other professionals on the team, including psychologists, social workers, and educational specialists, the needs of families can be met.

## Appropriate Referrals to Genetic Counseling Services

The vast majority of families with a member diagnosed with FXS and who receive genetic counseling services find them helpful (Turner et al. 1992; Roy et al. 1995). For this reason every individual receiving a diagnosis of FXS or every person considering FXS as a possible diagnosis for their child or relative should be offered genetic counseling. Health care providers, therapists, social workers, and educators, to name a few, may refer families. For many people self-referrals are also appropriate. To locate a genetic counselor in your area, please contact the National Society of Genetic Counselors, 233 Canterbury Drive, Wallingford, PA 19086-6617 or call 1-610-872-7608.

## Genetic Aspects of FXS

### A Dynamic Mutation

The gene associated with FXS, fragile X mental retardation 1 (*FMR1*) (Kremer et al. 1991; Oberle et al. 1991; Verkerk et al. 1991; Yu et al. 1991), is located on the X chromosome, as reviewed in chapter 2. The underlying mutation is caused by the addition of new genetic material. It is this mutation, termed a *dynamic mutation* or *trinucleotide repeat expansion,* which explains the common finding of mental retardation or learning disabilities (Turner et al. 1980; Sherman et al. 1984, 1985; Kemper et al. 1986; Miezejeski et al. 1986; Wolff et al. 1988; chap. 2). It also clarifies why Sherman et al. (1985) found that a woman's intellectual abilities in some way influence penetrance in her offspring. Expansion of the trinucleotide repeat has also resolved the issue of phenotypically normal male carriers (Martin and Bell 1943; Jacobs et al. 1980; Brøndum-Nielsen et al. 1981; Fryns and Van den Berghe 1982; Camerino et al. 1983; Sherman et al. 1985; Froster-Iskenius et al. 1986; Brown et al. 1987a; Sved and Laird 1990). The expansion also provides a molecular explanation for the Sherman paradox (Opitz 1986), the observation that daughters of nonpenetrant men are more likely to have affected offspring than are the mothers of nonpenetrant males.

## The *FMR1* Gene

The *FMR1* gene is polymorphic in the general population (Fu et al. 1991; Brown et al. 1993) and contains approximately 6 to 40 copies of the trinucleotide sequence, CGG. The trinucleotide CGG repeat sequence containing 41 to 54 copies is designated the *gray zone,* referring to the increased risk for repeat instability in this repeat range. A premutation, found in approximately 80% of normal IQ carrier females and the majority of nonpenetrant males, contains approximately 55 to 200 CGG repeats. The premutation is prone to expansion when passed from parent to child (Nolin et al. 1996). Decreases in size of a premutation, when transmission occurs through either a male or a female, have also been observed in subsequent generations (Oberle et al. 1991; Heitz et al. 1992; Vaisanen et al. 1994; Nolin et al. 1994, 1996; Fisch et al. 1995).

Individuals affected by FXS and approximately 20% of female carriers with a normal IQ will demonstrate a full mutation. A full mutation consists of an expansion greater than 200 CGG repeats and is susceptible to abnormal methylation (Rousseau et al. 1991). Methylation, as described in chapter 2, chemically modifies the gene so that it may no longer function correctly (Verkerk et al. 1991). Most males with the full mutation are mentally retarded. There is, however, no linear correlation between the number of CGG repeats greater than 200 and clinical severity. CGG repeat size does not explain the variability of cognitive involvement among males with the full mutation. Incompletely methylated full mutations have been observed in males with normal IQs (McConkie-Rosell et al. 1993; Hagerman et al. 1994; Rousseau et al. 1994a; chap. 1). These reports and other published studies (Taylor et al. 1994a; Tassone et al. 1999) suggested that methylation status is an important variable affecting clinical outcome in males with the full mutation. Later reports have established that it is the level of protein produced by the *FMR1* gene that is most likely related to the variability of cognitive involvement in males with the full mutation (see chap. 1) (Tassone et al. 1999; Kaufmann et al. 1999).

The protein produced by the *FMR1* gene is called the fragile X mental retardation protein (FMRP). In males with the full mutation, there is a decrease or complete lack of production of FMRP due to a translational block or error (see chaps. 2 and 12). It has been suggested that FMRP expression may be a prognostic indicator for males with FXS (Tassone et al. 1999). In addition, Tassone et al. (2000a, 2000b) and Hanauer and Hagerman (2000) reported that messenger RNA (mRNA) level is increased in males and females with the premutation and in some males and females with the full mutation. Recognition and understanding of increased mRNA levels in these patients are leading the way to further clarification of the molecular underpinnings of the phenotype in carriers, as described in chapters 1 and 12.

Approximately 53–71% of females with the full mutation have IQs in the borderline or mentally retarded range (Rousseau et al. 1991; Taylor et al. 1994b; de Vries et al. 1996). Those with a normal IQ may have learning disabilities or emotional problems (Mazzocco et al. 1993; Loesch et al. 1994; Sobesky et al. 1994; Franke et al. 1998). The variable expression in females with a full mutation is not fully understood. Some studies have found a correlation between IQ and X chromosome activation ratios (Abrams et al. 1994; Sobesky et al. 1996; Riddle et al. 1998; chap. 1). Regardless, researchers caution against using activation ratios in lymphocytes to accurately and reliably predict cognitive outcome in a female with the full mutation (Rousseau et al. 1991; Abrams et al. 1994; Taylor et al. 1994b).

An estimated 12% of males and 6% of females with the full mutation are mosaics, meaning that some of their cells contain a methylated full mutation whereas other cells contain an unmethylated premutation (Rousseau et al. 1994b). Mental retardation is not uncommon among mosaic males (de Vries et al. 1993; Rousseau et al. 1994b). Mosaic males with IQs in the normal range have also been reported. The mean IQ score for these males has been shown to be higher than for those males who carry only the full mutation (Merenstein et al. 1996). For a more thorough discussion of molecular clinical correlations, X activation studies, and clinical findings in individuals with the *FMR1* premutation and full mutation, see chapter 1.

## Other Causes of FXS

Although the majority of people diagnosed with FXS have the CGG expansion, several individuals have been shown to have different mutations in the *FMR1* gene. Specifically, point mutations (De Boulle et al. 1993) and deletions (Gedeon et al. 1992; Wöhrle et al. 1992; Tarleton et al. 1993; Gu et al. 1994; Hirst et al. 1995; Quan et al. 1995) have been reported. People with these rarer types of mutations tend to be physically, behaviorally, and intellectually similar to individuals with an expanded CGG repeat pattern. However, some have presented with an atypical FXS phenotype (De Boulle et al. 1993; Quan et al. 1995). Confirming the underlying mutation in individuals with clinical findings suggestive of FXS ensures the provision of accurate recurrence risks and is important when other family members are considering testing.

## Inheritance and Recurrence Risks

After identifying FXS in a family, relatives will seek genetic counseling for many different reasons. Often family members are uncertain of their risk of having a child with FXS. Each person will have a differing perception of his or her risk. One person may view the risk figure as very high. Yet another may view the same risk figure as being much lower (Pearn 1973). In any case, be-

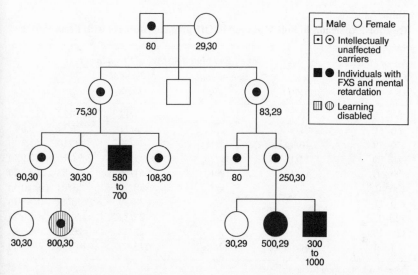

**Fig. 7.1.** A family with fragile X syndrome: the numbers represent repeats at *FMR1* in each X chromosome.

cause of the hereditary nature of FXS, all at-risk relatives or concerned family members should receive genetic counseling to review the inheritance pattern and discuss specific recurrence risks (McIntosh et al. 2000). Several examples of how the *FMR1* mutation is transmitted within a family are shown in figure 7.1.

### Females

A woman who carries the *FMR1* premutation on one of her X chromosomes has a 50% risk of passing the mutation to future offspring. A premutation is unstable and can expand to a full mutation or remain a premutation when passed from mother to child. Children who inherit the premutation are usually unaffected cognitively, whereas children with the full mutation are at risk for mental impairment.

Women who have a full mutation have a 50% risk with each pregnancy to pass the mutation to their offspring. Any male who inherits the full mutation is predicted to be mentally retarded. Any daughter who inherits the full mutation is at a 30% risk to have a normal IQ, but executive function deficits are common (Sobesky et al. 1996). A daughter with the full mutation is also at a 60% risk to have learning disabilities (particularly in math) or emotional difficulties and at a 70% risk to have an IQ in the borderline or mentally retarded range (deVries et al. 1996). Decreases in the size of the CGG expansion have

**Table 7.1**

**Risk for Expansion to Full Mutation in Offspring of Mothers with Premutation**

| No. of Maternal CGG Repeats | No. of Full Mutations/No. of Pregnancies | | | | |
|---|---|---|---|---|---|
| | Fu et al. (1991) | Snow et al. (1993) | Nolin et al. (1996) | Total | |
| 56–59 | 0/7 | 0/3 | 3/12 | 3/22 | (13.4%) |
| 60–69 | 1/6 | 2/7 | 4/21 | 7/34 | (20.6%) |
| 70–79 | 10/14 | 5/18 | 44/70 | 59/102 | (57.8%) |
| 80–89 | 14/17 | 19/24 | 45/66 | 78/107 | (72.9%) |
| 90–99 | 12/12 | 10/10 | 61/66 | 83/88 | (94.3%) |
| 100–109 | 7/7 | 4/4 | 70/70 | 81/81 | (100.0%) |
| 110–119 | . . . | 8/8 | 38/39 | 46/47 | (97.8%) |
| 120–129 | . . . | 2/2 | 22/22 | 24/24 | (100.0%) |
| 130–199 | . . . | . . . | 26/27 | 26/27 | (96.3%) |
| Total | 44/63 | 50/76 | 313/393 | 407/532 | (76.5%) |

*Source:* Adapted from Nolin et al. 1996.

also been documented in offspring of women who have a full mutation (Nolin et al. 1996). Loesch et al. (1995) also reported that, among 19 full mutation mothers, five daughters and one son had CGG repeat expansions in the premutation range.

Recurrence risks for premutation females vary. One factor that is known to influence a woman's risk is the length of the CGG repeat (Fu et al. 1991; Yu et al. 1991; Heitz et al. 1992; Snow et al. 1993; Turner et al. 1994; Fisch et al. 1995; Nolin et al. 1996; Kallinen et al. 2000; Pesso et al. 2000). In general, the larger the size of the CGG repeat the greater the chance a premutation will expand to a full mutation in subsequent generations (table 7.1).

Repeat length, though important, is not the only condition leading to instability (Reiss et al. 1994). CGG repeats of the same length have been shown to be stable in some people and prone to expansion in others. Eichler et al. (1994), Snow et al. (1994), and Zhong et al. (1995) suggest that the absence of interspersed AGG triplet repeats destabilizes the CGG region. By determining the actual number of AGGs in males with the pre- and full mutation and in male controls, Zhong et al. (1995) have shown that the threshold of instability is approximately 40 pure CGG repeats. Developing methods to analyze the AGG interspersion pattern in females should lead to more accurate genetic counseling for women, especially those with *FMR1* alleles in the gray zone range (see chap. 2).

Characterizing the trinucleotide repeat expansion mechanism is also under investigation and should contribute further to our understanding of recurrence risks. Ashley and Sherman (1995), in their meiotic/mitotic mutational model, hypothesize that the parental origin of a woman's premutation influences a woman's risk to have an affected child. That is, women who inherit a premutation from their father have a higher risk to have a child with a full mutation than women who inherit the premutation from their mother.

Work by Loesch et al. (1995) and Rousseau et al. (1994c) suggests that expansion of the CGG repeat depends on the sex of the offspring. Both studies found that sons had a higher risk of transforming their mother's premutation to a full mutation than did daughters. Testing these and other hypotheses, collecting and analyzing additional data, and exploring other mutational models should contribute to our understanding of the fragile X mutation and enable the genetic counselor to more accurately assess recurrence risks for women who have the premutation.

### Males

If a male carries the *FMR1* mutation (either a premutation or full mutation), he will pass the premutation to all of his daughters (100% risk) but none of his sons (0% risk). A premutation remains relatively stable in size when passed through a male, increasing or decreasing in size by only a few CGG repeats (Heitz et al. 1992; Vaisanen et al. 1994). Though previously thought to be rare events, Fisch et al. (1995) found that one-third of the daughters of nonpenetrant males demonstrated intergenerational decreases compared to 2% of the daughters of premutation carrier females. Expansion to a full mutation from a premutation male has never been documented.

Affected males with the full mutation usually do not reproduce (Sherman et al. 1984). Brown et al. (1987b) suggested that perhaps 1% will father children. As higher functioning individuals with the full mutation are identified, as the emphasis on inclusion grows, and as attitudes toward marriage of people with mental retardation change, this percentage will most likely increase. Reports suggest that males with FXS father intellectually normal daughters (reviewed by Willems et al. 1992). An intellectually normal male with the full mutation and an incomplete methylation pattern on Southern blot has been confirmed as having an intellectually normal daughter who carried a premutation (Rousseau et al. 1994a). The fact that the *FMR1* gene in the sperm of males with the full mutation contains a premutation explains this finding (Reyniers et al. 1993). As with any couple, accurate recurrence risks are based on both parents' clinical and family histories. Should a male with a full mutation father a child with a woman who is mentally impaired due to biologic or genetic reasons unrelated to FXS, offspring may still be at risk to have intellectual impairment.

### Isolated Cases

To date no laboratory has demonstrated a new mutation in a proband shown to have FXS caused by expansion of the CGG trinucleotide repeat. Nor has the change from a normal allele to a premutation allele been reported. These findings and studies of founder effects in FXS have led some authors to suggest that the transition from a normal-size *FMR1* allele to a premutation is a multistep process that occurs over an as yet undetermined number of generations (Smits et al. 1993; Montagnon et al. 1993; Ashley and Sherman 1995). Regardless of the mutational model, DNA analysis of families with apparently isolated cases of FXS (Smits et al. 1993; Holden 1995) indicates that even distant relatives are at risk to be carriers. For this reason, it is imperative that members of these families be offered *FMR1* DNA studies.

### The Gray Zone

A person who has 40 to 55 CGG repeats within the *FMR1* gene falls into the *gray zone*. Some alleles in this range have been shown to be unstable and to expand in subsequent generations, whereas others appear stable when transmitted to offspring. At this time the only way to distinguish stable from unstable alleles is with follow-up family studies (Brown et al. 1993; Reiss et al. 1994). To date no female with fewer than 55 CGG repeats on *FMR1* analysis has had a child with a full mutation (see chap. 2).

### Information Is Changing

Specific information about a person's risk may change as our understanding of the *FMR1* mutation increases. To receive the most accurate genetic counseling, families should be encouraged to recontact the genetic counseling clinic periodically to see whether additional testing or counseling is indicated.

## Working Up the Family

### Pedigree Analysis

Once an individual in a family is diagnosed with FXS, the next step involves the evaluation and molecular assessment of other family members (McIntosh et al. 2000). If the diagnosis is confirmed in a child, the primary focus is the mother's side of the family. Outlining the family history is the most efficient way to identify relatives at risk. Although a simple task in theory, gathering accurate and pertinent family information requires skill, experience, and persistence.

Frequently parents are so focused on their own child that they overlook other family members who have more variable or minimal expression of the *FMR1* mutation. Broader, more open-ended questions can help families explore the wide spectrum of features associated with the condition. For example, specifically asking how each relative did in school, whether anyone was slow in speaking or walking, what level of education was completed, and what jobs family members hold is more useful than simply asking who in a family is mentally retarded or learning disabled. It is important not to ignore the more subtle features noted among intellectually normal carriers, including difficulty in math and some of the emotional and behavioral problems discussed in chapters 1 and 9. Open-ended questions such as "How is your health?" will usually lead to more descriptive responses than "Are you healthy?" which usually elicits only a yes or no.

Having asked more general questions regarding the medical history, one can ask more specific questions related to FXS, such as "Has anyone ever had seizures, vision problems, heart murmurs, or multiple ear infections? Is anyone taking medication on a regular basis? If so, which medication and for what purpose? Is or has anyone regularly been seen by a psychiatrist or psychologist?" Sometimes asking the same question in multiple ways is more effective. For example, to determine whether any relatives have any of the physical features common among individuals with FXS, one can ask, "Does anyone resemble your son? Does anyone have the features you now know are common among people with FXS? Do you have any photographs of your family?"

While asking these questions about the family history, it is important to be sensitive to how the family is feeling. Some parents may be in denial and not feel their child is different in any way. Other parents may not have had the opportunity to gauge their child's development against a child who has had normal cognitive development. If asking specific questions, avoid medical or technical terms such as prominent ears, hyperextensible joints, otitis media, and strabismus, since these may distance you from the patient. Normalizing unusual characteristics can make parents feel more at ease and more trusting of you as a professional. It is also important to include a discussion of the strengths noted among individuals with FXS, such as sociability, sense of humor, ability to mimic or copy, and ability to use the computer to enhance learning.

It is not unusual to be counseling a mentally impaired parent or relative. These clients may be confused by questions that are too general. For these counseling situations, yes/no questions and either/or questions are recommended (Raeburn 1989). In some instances, with consent of the patient, it may be appropriate to invite a normally functioning relative to the genetic counseling session. If this is not possible, other relatives may be contacted for a more complete family history.

In addition to identifying other affected relatives, the pedigree can also help to identify potential carriers. Phenotypic expression in intellectually normal female carriers has been suggested by several authors (Fryns 1986; Loesch and Hay 1988; Cronister et al. 1991). Hull and Hagerman (1993) and Schwartz et al. (1994) suggest that a long face, prominent ears, shyness, anxiety, and ovarian problems are frequent findings in premutation females. Further investiga-

**Exhibit 7.1**
**Symptoms to Be Questioned When Taking the Family History**

| | |
|---|---|
| Long face | Strabismus |
| Long or prominent ears | Seizures |
| Hyperextensible joints | Hyperactivity |
| Joint dislocation | Attention deficit hyperactivity disorder |
| Hypotonia | Obsessive-compulsive behavior |
| Cerebral palsy | Motor or vocal tics |
| Poor eye contact | Premature menopause |
| Autism | Depression |
| Hernias | Sleep problems |
| Developmental delay | Shyness |
| Special education | Mood swings |
| Difficulty in math | Panic attacks/anxiety |
| Speech/language delay | Violent outbursts |
| Recurrent ear infections | Heart murmur, mitral valve prolapse |

tion of phenotypic expression in males within the premutation population is also warranted (Dorn et al. 1994; Loesch et al. 1994). Although an explanation for penetrance in premutation carriers is unclear (Feng et al. 1995), subtle clinical features suggestive of FXS observed among normally functioning relatives should alert the clinician (see chap. 1). Exhibit 7.1 lists symptoms that should be included when taking the family history.

## Diagnostic Testing

### *FMR1* DNA Analysis

After targeting affected individuals and potential carriers by pedigree analysis or clinical assessment, the genetic counselor should offer available diagnostic testing to appropriate family members. Individuals to consider for testing include all siblings of the person diagnosed with FXS and relatives who either present with any of the clinical or behavioral features of the condition or are women of reproductive age. Because the implications for grandchildren can be burdensome, carrier testing for phenotypically normal male relatives should also be suggested to men of reproductive age.

Carrier testing for children should be approached thoughtfully. The medical and psychosocial benefits to the child must be weighed against any harm to the child. Potential benefits include reduction of uncertainty and anxiety and early treatment of problems associated with carrier status. Potential risks of genetic testing include loss of a child's self-esteem, stigmatization, distortion of the parents' perception of the child, or inappropriate discrimination if he or she is shown to be a carrier. To determine whether testing is appropriate, one should have an open discussion that fully explores the potential benefits and harms of testing with the family. The child may be included in the decision-making process, if possible and if appropriate. To promote the interest of the child and family, information about the test should be presented in an understandable and usable form. Attitudes about carrier testing for children among carrier women were preliminarily investigated by McConkie-Rosell et al. (1995a, 1997). Of 28 obligate carrier women surveyed (23 to 72 years), 60% felt information about carrier status would have been helpful by the age of 12 to 15 years and 92.9% by high school. These attitudes seemed to influence when women felt their children should be tested, with most mothers encouraging testing in childhood as opposed to learning this information as adults.

Direct DNA analysis of the *FMR1* gene is now the method of choice for diagnosing both affected individuals and unaffected carriers (Rousseau et al. 1994b; chap. 2). Direct DNA analysis is usually performed by analysis of the CGG repeat within the *FMR1* gene by polymerase chain reaction (PCR) (Brown et al. 1993) and double digest of genomic DNA and Southern blot analysis (Rousseau et al. 1991; see chap. 2). DNA can be isolated from peripheral blood, amniocytes, chorionic villi (see under "Family Planning," below), and other tissues, including buccal cells. Key advantages of PCR are that the testing is rapid, it is less expensive than Southern blot analysis, and it can accurately determine the specific number of CGG repeats in the normal and premutation range. Although some PCR methods allow visualization of full mutations (Brown et al. 1993), accurate size determination of a large premutation or full mutation is very difficult. PCR may also preferentially amplify smaller fragments. In the experience of Berliner et al. (1994), premutations and full mutations failed to amplify by PCR 5% of the time. Most laboratories have more difficulty getting full mutations to amplify using this technology.

Southern blot analysis, using a double digest, will measure the size of the CGG repeat and determine methylation status. The latter is not possible by PCR. In addition to being the preferred method for detecting full mutations, Southern blot is particularly useful when evaluating repeats in the upper end of the premutation range. If abnormal methylation is observed, this would indicate a full mutation rather than a premutation. This technology is also helpful in confirming PCR results when only one band is visualized in a female. Southern blot will confirm whether the female is a normal homozygote, normal heterozygote, or actually a carrier whose larger-sized allele failed to amplify by PCR analysis. Distinguishing females with a premutation from those with a

CGG repeat in the normal range is difficult by Southern blot. In these instances confirmation by PCR is recommended. For a more thorough discussion of DNA analysis, please refer to chapter 2.

### Previous Testing by Chromosome or DNA-Linkage Analysis

Cytogenetic studies prepared using specialized culture techniques were the standard diagnostic test for FXS until the early 1990s. Although this testing was considered fairly accurate in detecting children and adults with the condition, direct DNA analysis is diagnostically superior (Rousseau et al. 1994b). For this reason, individuals who had cytogenetic testing to confirm a suspected diagnosis of FXS require follow-up molecular testing (Brown 1996; Gringras and Barnicoat 1998). DNA mutation analysis of individuals previously shown to be fragile X cytogenetically negative will detect false negatives. If the diagnosis of FXS in a family is based on a positive cytogenetic result, at least one affected relative should have DNA studies to confirm the *FMR1* mutation before further family studies are pursued (Policy Statement: American College of Medical Genetics 1994). In rare instances, molecular analysis of fragile X cytogenetically positive individuals will lead to an actual diagnosis of FRAXE or FRAXF (Nakahori et al. 1991; Sutherland and Baker 1992; Flynn et al. 1993; Knight et al. 1993; Jacky 1996).

The limitations of cytogenetic analysis when testing potential carriers have been realized for some time. Sherman et al. (1984), in their study of FXS pedigrees, found that 44% of all heterozygous females were both intellectually normal and fragile X negative, whereas 26% had normal IQs but were fragile X positive. These data suggest that approximately 60% of all normally functioning carrier females test negative cytogenetically. Nonpenetrant males frequently fail to express the fragile X site as well.

From the mid-1980s until the discovery of the *FMR1* gene, DNA linkage analysis was considered a reliable means of carrier detection for families found to be informative. Used in conjunction with clinical evaluation, cognitive assessment, and chromosome analysis, DNA linkage analysis might increase the accuracy of carrier detection to as high as 99%. Linkage testing, though a good option at the time, also had its limitations. Inherent limitations of restriction fragment length polymorphism (RFLP) analysis, including the possibility of recombination, made some results difficult to interpret and often inconclusive. As has been proven by follow-up direct DNA analysis, there was always concern that a person might be falsely predicted to be a carrier or vice versa (Curtis et al. 1994). Because of the limitations of both cytogenetic and DNA linkage analysis, any intellectually unaffected individual who was tested previously by fragile X cytogenetic and/or DNA linkage studies should be offered confirmatory studies using direct DNA methods.

## Family Planning

### Prenatal *FMR1* DNA Analysis

When the mother is a known carrier, prenatal diagnosis by direct DNA analysis is available. Prenatal diagnosis gives families options. Families who learn that the fetus is unaffected are relieved and, therefore, able to enjoy the remainder of the pregnancy. Families who learn their fetus has an increased chance to have FXS may choose to either discontinue or continue the pregnancy. Reliability for *FMR1* prenatal diagnosis is considered extremely high for both male and female fetuses (Brown et al. 1993; Berliner et al. 1994; Halley et al. 1994; Maddalena et al. 1994).

Until recently, the largest experience with prenatal detection of FXS had been with amniocentesis, a test offered to women during the second trimester, at 15 to 16 weeks gestation. Early amniocentesis, defined as earlier than 15 weeks, is not recommended for prenatal diagnosis of FXS, since the preferred amount of amniotic fluid (20–30 ml) cannot be obtained for DNA analysis. The risk for pregnancy loss associated with traditional amniocentesis may approach 0.5% (Tabor et al. 1986; reviewed by Elias and Simpson 1993). Amniocentesis can be performed at an outpatient facility. To perform this procedure, one inserts a spinal needle, no larger than 20 gauge, into the amniotic cavity. Ultrasound is used to visualize the needle. Once the needle is within the amniotic cavity, a syringe is attached and at 15 to 16 weeks gestation 20–30 ml of amniotic fluid can be withdrawn. This amount is sufficient for *FMR1* DNA analysis.

The mid- to late 1990s saw a shift to chorionic villus sampling (CVS) as the prenatal option of choice for women at risk to have a child with FXS. CVS is performed during the first trimester, usually at 10 to 11 weeks of gestation. This first trimester diagnosis offers families a result earlier in pregnancy, potentially reducing emotional and psychologic stress, and allows couples privacy, since the pregnancy at this stage is less obvious to others. A termination, if this is the woman's choice, can be performed earlier and is, therefore, considered safer. The safety of CVS is still under debate. Pregnancy loss associated with CVS has been reported as low as 1.2% and seems dependent on the experience of the center performing the procedure (reviewed by Rhoads et al. 1989). Similar to amniocentesis, CVS is an outpatient procedure. CVS involves the withdrawal of a small amount of the chorionic villus tissue from the placenta. The trimmed tissue is fetal in origin. To obtain the chorionic villus tissue, one inserts a thin catheter cervically or abdominally under ultrasound guidance. With gentle suction, chorionic villus tissue is removed and used for the genetic testing (see chap. 2).

The cells collected by CVS contain a random sample of the allele sizes present in the fetus. It is possible in a mosaic fetus (one with a premutation and a full mutation) that the CVS sample could contain predominantly DNA with the premutation. For this reason and because the mechanism that causes expansion from the premutation to the full mutation is still not understood, some molecular geneticists have recommended confirming CVS premutation results by amniocentesis or fetal blood sampling (Oostra et al. 1993; Maddalena et al. 1994). However, for most cases of CVS performed to rule out FXS, this is not necessary. *FMR1* DNA testing after delivery is always suggested to verify the prenatal testing result. In addition, it can be extremely helpful in clarifying the fetal result to obtain, before or at the time of prenatal diagnosis, peripheral blood samples from both parents to determine their *FMR1* repeat size.

It is still unclear when the methylation process is complete. Since it has been shown to be incomplete in the first trimester of pregnancy (Rousseau et al. 1991; Sutherland and Baker 1992; Brown et al. 1993), amniocentesis or fetal blood sampling may be required to confirm methylation status if CVS is performed and the band size visualized by DNA analysis falls in the upper end of the premutation range (Warren and Nelson 1994).

Fetal blood sampling is an outpatient procedure that can be safely performed starting at approximately 18 weeks of gestation. As described above, it may be considered for confirming certain CVS results. During this procedure ultrasound is used to guide a needle through a woman's abdomen into the umbilical cord. Sampling, usually from the umbilical vein, allows 3–4 ml of blood to be taken from the fetus. When performed by an experienced team, pregnancy loss rates following the procedure have been approximately 1% (reviewed by Ryan and Rodeck 1993).

A fetus shown to have a premutation on prenatal diagnosis is predicted to be a carrier who most likely will not be affected cognitively. Although there are reports of high-functioning males with IQs in the borderline or normal range (Hagerman et al. 1994; chap. 1), a male fetus with a completely methylated full mutation or a mosaic pattern is predicted to be affected by FXS and to have mental retardation. It is impossible to predict whether intellectual impairment will be mild, moderate, or severe. Predicting clinical outcomes for male fetuses with an incomplete methylation pattern is less certain. Some males with this pattern have mental retardation, whereas others have IQs in the borderline or normal range (McConkie-Rosell et al. 1993; Hagerman et al. 1994; Rousseau et al. 1994a). A female fetus with a full mutation is given approximately a 50–70% risk for cognitive deficits (borderline or mentally retarded IQ). The remaining 30–50% are at risk for learning disabilities or emotional problems. At this time, further studies on the fetus, mother, or any other family member are not helpful in more accurately predicting intellectual ability in a female fetus with a full mutation. The laboratory's inability to accurately predict clinical outcome or mental status must be clearly explained by the genetic counselor.

## Preimplantation Diagnosis

Another option families may wish to consider is preimplanation diagnosis. This procedure involves DNA testing of in vitro fertilized embryos and is therefore performed before pregnancy begins. Only embryos shown to be free of the *FMR1* mutation are implanted into the woman's womb. It is a highly technical procedure and has not met with much success when used for FXS. Numerous centers specializing in preimplantation diagnosis have reported difficulty in obtaining viable ova in sufficient numbers (thought to be related to the increased risk for premature ovarian failure in female carriers of the premutation) and in obtaining *FMR1* repeat size from the eight-cell embryo. Preimplantation diagnosis is available only through a few select centers in the United States, Europe, and Australia.

Another preimplantation diagnostic option that has recently become available to families at risk to have a child with FXS is polar body removal (Verlinsky et al. 1999; Strom et al. 2000). This procedure involves DNA analysis by PCR of the first polar body, which is produced from the division of the egg during meiosis, and of the second polar body, which is associated with cell division postfertilization. The polar bodies have no known function other than to assist in cell division and, as by-products of egg division, are available for analysis without harming the embryo. By testing the polar bodies for several dinucleotide polymorphic markers, one can determine the genetic composition of the egg and embryo. If the developing embryo is determined not to carry the *FMR1* gene mutation, embryo transfer will be performed. Prenatal diagnosis is recommended for all pregnancies that have undergone preimplantation diagnosis. Since the DNA analysis by PCR is dependent on each parent being informative for the *FMR1* dinucleotide polymorphic markers, not all families are candidates for this procedure.

## Preconceptional and Prenatal Counseling

Family planning is a common and serious concern for those with a family history of FXS (Curtis et al. 1994). The concerns for those at risk to have a child with FXS are similar whether the parent has the premutation or full mutation. However, if the parent at risk is a carrier of the full mutation and cognitively impaired, the genetic counselor may need to take a system-oriented approach and involve other relatives (de Vries et al. 1999). Couples contemplating pregnancies are best counseled before conception, and both partners should be encouraged to attend the counseling session. At this time, all factors that influence reproductive decisions can be discussed and a patient's particular decision acknowledged and validated. Meryash and Abuelo (1988) found that the majority of women at risk of having a child with FXS would consider pregnancy termination. Moreover, 81% of the women studied would opt for prenatal diagnosis during future pregnancies. Perception of burden has also been shown to influence reproductive decisions (Sorenson et al. 1981; Wertz et al. 1984). Meryash (1989) examined perception of burden among women at risk of having children with FXS. Although mothers who have a child with FXS seem to cope well with their child's special needs, they are more likely to consider pregnancy termination than are women without an affected child (Meryash and Abuelo 1988). This suggests that the apparent burden of having cared for and raised a child with FXS must in some way influence a woman's willingness to risk having another. When a family has one child with FXS, they will often voice their commitment to this child and state that to have a second child with FXS would diminish the time, attention, and therapeutic intervention they could provide to the first affected child. Thus, they feel that the possibility of the first affected child reaching his maximum potential would be reduced. Other variables, such as education, financial considerations, personal beliefs, and perceived social consequences should not be overlooked because they may also dramatically influence reproductive decisions (Lipperman-Hand and Fraser 1979; Wertz et al. 1984).

Exploration of these issues and family planning options, including prenatal diagnosis, preimplantation diagnosis, polar body retrieval, adoption, egg and sperm donor programs, and embryo transfer programs are critical in helping families make informed reproductive decisions (Curtis et al. 1994). If families decide to pursue a future pregnancy, prenatal genetic counseling is recommended. At this time, all prenatal procedures and available testing can be discussed in greater detail. Benefits and drawbacks of the testing should be outlined to help families decide whether they are willing to accept the limitations of the existing prenatal technology.

If a couple contacts the genetic counselor when the mother is already pregnant, which is frequently the case, all options may not be available. First, gestational age should be determined accurately by prenatal ultrasound. Depending on the gestational age, fetal sexing may also be possible. If a woman is in her first trimester, CVS and amniocentesis may be considered. Regardless of gestational age and regardless of whether a couple would consider prenatal diagnosis or pregnancy termination, all pregnant couples should be encouraged to have prenatal genetic counseling so that they more fully understand their risks and options and have a professional who can support them through this emotionally draining and extremely stressful time.

The psychosocial needs of families undergoing pregnancy should not be underestimated. Although couples may have made a rational decision to become pregnant, emotions may change when the pregnancy becomes reality. Couples may need support reevaluating their concerns about having a child with special needs and may need help exploring how a child affected by FXS will affect family life and their relationship with one another. At the same time couples may find themselves bonding to the pregnancy, hoping and believing that everything will be OK. They may also be uncertain whether they wish to pursue prenatal diagnosis. Exploring and acknowledging both the father's and the mother's choices throughout the decision-making process is important and will help strengthen the relationship between patient and professional. If a family chooses to continue a pregnancy without further testing, the genetic counselor should present possible plans for keeping in touch with them throughout the pregnancy. Some families may wish to be called frequently, while others may prefer only occasional contact. A mother may feel she needs more support. The suggestion that she be contacted by another mother who has had a similar experience may be well received.

Families who proceed with prenatal diagnosis will often need ongoing support throughout the pregnancy, especially from the time of the procedure to the time they receive a result. How the result will be given (i.e., what time of day they should call, where to call, and how soon the family can be seen in the clinic if the prenatal result shows the fetus is affected) is important to discuss, since it helps parents know what to expect. Should the fetus be affected, the couple should be given sufficient time to make a decision about the pregnancy. As long as 5 to 7 days may be required for some individuals. For couples deciding to continue the pregnancy, the genetic counselor must be available to support the family as they adjust emotionally and plan for the future. For couples deciding to terminate, ongoing contact and support are required. Some families will choose to treat the fetus as a child, and a name will be given, a burial service held or ashes scattered in a special place, or a memorial created in memory of the lost child. Others will mourn their loss in a different way. With the help of a social worker or other professionals, the genetic counselor can support the family. Supportive calls to the couple on any anniversary dates to comfort them about their loss are greatly appreciated.

## Other Prenatal Concerns

### Twinning

In 1986, Fryns was the first to report an increase in twins (1 in 35 live births) among women who were heterozygous for FXS. He suggested that this may have been due to a disturbed hypothalamic hypophyseal ovarian axis. Cronister et al. (1991) showed an increased rate of ovarian problems, including cysts, tumors, and premature menopause in heterozygous women compared to controls. Sherman et al. (1988), in a study of families affected by FXS in New South Wales, reported 17 twin births (both monozygotic and dizygotic) among 752 total births. This twinning rate of 1 in 44 was significantly different from that found in the general population (1 in 96). Sherman et al. (1988), however, questioned whether superovulation was related to the fragile X mutation or instead triggered by the advanced maternal age noted in the obligate carrier females studied. Turner et al. (1994) reported a threefold increase in the rate of twinning in females with the premutation compared to female controls and women with the full mutation. More recent data presented in chapter 3 and the authors' own clinical experience suggest that twinning may not be increased in carriers.

### Nondisjunction

There have been at least 10 reports in the literature of the concurrence of Klinefelter syndrome and the fragile X chromosome (Wilmot et al. 1980; Froster-Iskenius et al. 1982; O'Brien et al. 1982; Filippi et al. 1983; Fryns et al. 1983; Fryns et al. 1984; Schnur et al. 1986; Filippi et al. 1988; Fryns and Van den Berghe 1988; Kupke et al. 1991). Fryns and Van den Berghe (1988) in Belgium found that 3 of 465 fragile X–positive males also had Klinefelter syndrome (1 in 155). Importantly, several of these reports have suggested that nondisjunction was maternal in origin (Filippi et al. 1983; Fryns et al. 1984; Kupke et al. 1991). Down syndrome has also been shown to occur simultaneously with the fragile X mutation (reviewed by Turner et al. 1986), and Watson et al. (1988) reported that 6 of 931 children with FXS, from 236 carrier females, had trisomy 21. How the *FMR1* mutation might interfere with chromosomal separation at meiosis is unclear. Additional data are necessary, but clinicians should be aware that female carriers of the FXS may have an increased risk for meiotic nondisjunctional events over and above their age-dependent risks.

### Adoption

Some couples, when faced with the risk of having a child with a disability, choose not to have any biologic children or to limit the size of their existing family. For families who still have a strong desire to raise children, adoption may be an appropriate choice. Although fewer healthy babies are available for adoption now than in years past, the fact remains that thousands of couples still successfully adopt children every year. The possibility of adoption should be raised with any couple considering having a family.

Giving a child up for adoption is also an option to present to pregnant women at risk to have a child with FXS. An adoption agency can work with families to see if this is the appropriate choice for them. The trend currently is for open adoption with visitation rights for the biologic parents.

## Prenatal Diagnosis for Individuals with a Possible Family History of FXS

Taking a family history has become a routine aspect of obstetric health care. By asking about intellectual impairment in family members, the clinician may elicit a family history of mental retardation that would otherwise go undiscussed. Under other circumstances, a pregnant couple or a couple planning a future pregnancy may approach their physician concerned about a relative who is mentally impaired and their risks to have a similarly affected child. Brown et al. (1993) estimated that approximately 1 in 40 pregnant women with a family history of undiagnosed mental retardation may be a member of a FXS family. To rule out this and any other genetic cause for mental impairment, a comprehensive genetic evaluation of the mentally impaired relative is always indicated. Certain circumstances, however, such as death of the affected relative, can make this impossible.

How one counsels a couple with a possible family history of FXS will vary from case to case. Again, a thorough genetic evaluation of the individual with mental retardation is always the number one recommendation. *FMR1* DNA testing of any normal individual, however, can be pursued if there is a family history of mental retardation for which there is no known etiology (Policy Statement: American College of Medical Genetics 1994). The patient must understand that the testing is limited to the CGG expansion mutation and only rules out carrier status for FXS. As part of the pretest genetic counseling, the genetic counselor should review the limitations of FXS prenatal diagnosis, including the laboratories' inability to predict intellectual status, especially in a full mutation female. The patient should also understand that an inconclusive result is possible, and should the patient be shown to have a CGG repeat in the gray zone, follow-up family studies may be indicated. Prenatal diagnosis is not indicated for any woman found to have a CGG repeat of less than 50. Women found to have a CGG repeat between 50 and 59 should receive genetic counseling to review the most recent prenatal diagnostic recommendations. If a person is shown to have a pre- or full mutation, prenatal genetic counseling is indicated.

## Psychosocial Implications of the Fragile X Diagnosis

Having a child with a genetic disease has many social and psychologic ramifications. The level of burden and the number of psychologic dilemmas faced are dependent on a complex mixture of interpersonal skills, past experiences, philosophical beliefs, and perceived social consequences (Reif and Baitsch 1985). Only preliminary work has examined the psychosocial issues specific to FXS families (Roy et al. 1995). One must rely, at least for now, on information gathered from studying parents and families coping with a variety of genetic disorders.

Unquestionably, having a child with a genetic problem can have serious though often temporary effects on self-esteem. Feelings of blame, guilt, embarrassment, and stigmatization are commonly experienced (Shore 1975; Kiely et al. 1976; Falek 1984). A considerable amount has been written regarding the "stages" of the grief response noted in families who have a child born with mental retardation (Mercer 1974; Drotar et al. 1975; Kelly 1976; Emde and Brown 1978). When families are faced with the crisis of having a child with special needs, they initially experience shock, which is followed by denial. Then begins the more emotionally laden phase when feelings of grief, guilt, anger, disappointment, and low self-esteem prevail. Eventually, parents who have received information and ongoing support become focused on their child's needs and other concerns specific to the genetic diagnosis. The period of acceptance is considered the healthy outcome of parental coping and adjustment. Importantly, however, the past may never be totally forgotten. As a consequence, chronic sorrow (recalling past hardships, a deep sense of loss when expectations are not met, and grief) is a common characteristic among parents coping with genetic disease, especially during times of transition (Schild and Black 1984; Wikler et al. 1981).

The psychologic ramifications discussed above are not infrequent among parents of a child with FXS and should be discussed during the genetic counseling session. Additional psychosocial implications, however, may be more specific to the diagnosis of FXS. The study of parents of children with mental impairment (Drillien and Wilkenson 1964; Carr 1970; Watkins et al. 1989) showed that parents wish to be told about their child's diagnosis and prognosis as soon as possible. Many parents who recognized their child's disability early but were never given a diagnosis find initial relief in at last having an answer. However, the path from parental or professional recognition of the disability to the diagnosis is often one of difficulty involving not being listened to, being treated insensitively, and/or lack of support, which may continue even after receiving the diagnosis (Carmichael et al. 1999; Bailey et al. 2000). The grief response for the loss of a healthy child may be worsened when information is postponed (Schild 1981). Many children with FXS appear normal at birth and are undiagnosed until age 3 or later (Bailey et al. 2000). When the initial grief response is delayed, parents may experience intense and overwhelming feelings of loss and sorrow. Expectations parents had held for their child are shattered. As a consequence readjustment can be a slow and painful process.

Meryash's work (1989) suggests that mothers learn to cope and adjust to their child's special needs. The families reported in this study had an experienced and supportive FXS network available to them. For families in isolated communities where the professionals are unfamiliar with the diagnosis of FXS, issues such as appropriate medical treatment and educational intervention often remain problems and the perceived burden may be greater.

Financial considerations also affect the perceived burden for parents of handicapped children (Gath 1972; Nihira et al. 1980). Meryash (1989) found that, among at-risk women without children who had FXS, education level correlated with magnitude of perceived burden. Education, however, did not correlate with level of burden in mothers who had children with FXS, suggesting that more highly educated women, once faced with an affected son or daughter, are able to readjust and adapt to the problems and challenges inherent in raising a child with FXS. The mean number of years of education among the mothers studied was 12.7.

The coping and adjustment process and the perception of burden may differ for women who present with subtle emotional difficulties or neurocognitive deficits. Having a child with FXS is compounded by the fact that often these mothers themselves feel different. Shyness, social anxiety, paranoia, depression, and problems with mood lability are very real issues for some women (Sobesky et al. 1994; Franke et al. 1995, 1998). Understanding that these may actually be a subtle expression of clinical features associated with the female carrier phenotype can be comforting if presented appropriately. Another important counseling issue regarding mildly affected carrier females is patient compliance and willingness to participate in the genetic evaluation. The genetic counseling session is typically stressful for any individual. Fears about doctors, fears of being labeled, and fears of stigmatization may be exacerbated in a woman who has a poor self-concept as a result of learning difficulties (Watkins et al. 1989). Coming to the clinic for an evaluation or even genetic counseling may be too stressful. The genetic counselor must appreciate the special needs of these women. Usually, if the counselor is emotionally supportive and understanding, a lasting relationship will develop (see chap. 9).

## ZOE'S STORY

It is important to enjoy the optimistic elements of university, having good friends, interesting courses, etc. I've only really experienced those things you mentioned in the last few years and now. Previously, I was experiencing aspects of life that were—to sum up—negative and frustrating.

Living and dealing with fragile X personally could be compared to a plant which states on the label at the time of purchase that it has the capabilities to flower. In the meantime, the owner for some reason decides that this particular plant wouldn't flower so the owner relocates the plant to a corner of the garden where it is removed from view.

The plant does eventually flower. It took time. The plant suffered along the way, but it survived. Now, it finds itself in the best spot in the garden.

It is a welcomed change and one that members of the community are still coming to terms with—how could that plant possibly flower in the most un-viewed spot in the garden.

(Zoe in Australia, a woman with a full mutation, pers. comm.)

The same psychologic stress that affects personal feelings of self-worth can also influence interpersonal relationships. Meryash (1989) specifically examined marital relationships in families dealing with the diagnosis of FXS. He found that 81% of mothers were still married to the child's father. The experience of the Fragile X Treatment and Research Center in Denver, Colorado, is similar. McConkie-Rosell et al. (1995a) also found that the diagnosis had positive effects on the marital relationship. In this study, 13 of 17 obligate carrier women surveyed felt the diagnosis had positively changed their relationship with their husband by improving communication and understanding.

Having a child with a genetic condition may, however, disrupt marital relationships and family dynamics. An inherited condition that elicits feelings of blame or guilt is especially burdensome (Gath 1977; Schild 1981). Neglecting the spouse's and family's needs by focusing too much attention on the child with FXS can also negatively affect interpersonal relationships. Raising these issues and exploring each parent's perspective of their relationship with one another and with their other children is essential. Quality time spent as a family is important, but couples also need time alone. Arrangements for child or respite care that enable couples to spend time together, without interruption, should be encouraged. If possible, this should take place on a regular basis, ideally several hours each week.

Testing and physical evaluations may be threatening to individuals who are unwilling to consider that they or their children may be at risk for this disorder. McConkie-Rosell et al. (2000), in a longitudinal study of 42 women (20 carriers and 22 noncarriers) at risk to inherit the *FMR1* gene mutation, reported how upsetting these women found their carrier information, their perceptions of the seriousness of fragile X syndrome, and their descriptions of the carrier testing process, in addition to the coping behaviors employed during this process. In addition, parents may feel the need to protect their learning-disabled child from an evaluation that may be stressful to the child's self-esteem. Others, in denial, may refuse to acknowledge that their child's problems relate in any way to the relative already diagnosed with FXS. When some family members are resistant to coming in for an evaluation or counseling, information sharing facilitated by the genetic counselor is most useful (McConkie-Rosell et al. 1995b). Often relatives are unfamiliar with the medical intervention and treatment options available to them or their children. Families are often comforted by learning that FXS is a common disorder that may cause only minimal problems in one individual but more serious problems in another. Letters may sensitively address these and other issues. Literature written by families as well as other lay literature can be sent to those at risk. Providing telephone numbers and addresses of family support groups or informal contacts outside the family is also helpful.

Contacting relatives by telephone may also provide a less threatening environment in which initial questions can be answered and specific concerns raised. Sometimes a home visit is required. To avoid anyone feeling singled out, one can use large family gatherings to share information about the diagnosis. It is important to remember that each person is different. It is critical to acknowledge that one person in a family may be ready for information about FXS when another is not. Respecting each person's emotional needs is essential, and families should not be rushed into genetic counseling if they are not ready. Ideally, through education and understanding, a trusting relationship can be built between the professional and extended family members.

Another significant observation is the reaction of grandparents to the diagnosis of FXS. Grandparents may be intimidated by the word *genetics,* since this may carry more negative connotations and cause feelings of social stigmatization in grandparents raised during a time when people with special needs were sheltered from the rest of society. For these reasons and others, the idea that one grandparent may have passed the *FMR1* mutation to the grandchild is an especially sensitive issue. Overwhelming depression, sadness, and guilt in grandparents coping with the news that they are carriers are not uncommon. It is not infrequent, moreover, that a carrier parent is protective of her own parents' feelings, concerned that they will be unable to cope if they hear this news. Genetic counselors must be sensitive to these issues and respond accordingly.

## Counseling Needs of Families with FXS

Helping families adjust to and cope with the stresses of having a child with FXS is an important role of the genetic counselor. This can be accomplished in a variety of ways and includes presenting pertinent medical information about diagnosis and prognosis, reviewing the inheritance and recurrence risks, discussing available testing and family planning options, and, as already discussed, assisting families in identifying and addressing the underlying psychosocial issues. Combining education with emotional support ideally helps prepare families to make informed decisions regarding treatment, management, and testing (Fraser 1974; Kessler 1979; Sorensen et al. 1981; Reif and Baitsch 1985).

Attaining these goals when counseling families affected by FXS is a challenge. As already discussed, the inheritance pattern is still unclear and recurrence risks are not straightforward. The uncertainties and limitations in testing can lead to further confusion and in fact may raise anxiety. The challenge is to untangle all the facts and figures and simplify the information so that the families can truly understand their options. Care must be taken to create an environment that is relaxed, nurturing, and supportive. Time must simply be spent making families feel comfortable. Feelings of isolation, sadness, and depression can be normalized by acknowledging how common these emotions are among people who have children with special needs. The genetic counseling sessions should not focus always on the negative. If parents point out something special their child has accomplished or mention a particular strength they have noted in their child, one should respond empathetically and provide positive feedback. At the same time, the genetic counselor must remember that parents are continually dealing with feelings of loss. At times of transition, such as the end of the school year, changes in the school setting, or on birthdays, families may be overwhelmed by grief. For some, the pain may be cyclical but equally intense each time it occurs. For others, the coping process involves constant readjustment.

Appreciating a patient's prior knowledge, experiences, expectations, and apprehensions about FXS can provide insight into how to approach the counseling session (Staley-Gane et al. 1996). The most commonly asked question concerns treatment for the affected child and how to optimize his potential. Families are seeking information that will help them explore what life in the future will be like for their child with FXS, what they can expect for their child, and what they can hope for (Lipperman-Hand and Fraser 1979; Curtis et al. 1994). The role of the genetic counselor, therefore, moves beyond providing recurrence risks and available testing (Beeson and Golbus 1985; Staley-Gane et al. 1996). Genetic counselors must educate themselves about medical management and educational intervention available to families. As an example, when counseling families affected by FXS, genetic counselors should have a general understanding of sensory integration therapy, be aware of the speech/language needs of children with FXS, have an appreciation for available medical interventions, and understand the benefits and drawbacks of mainstreaming and inclusion. Certainly, genetic counselors are not expected to be experts in all of these areas. However, with few health care providers and educators experienced in FXS, genetic counselors must be prepared to answer general questions regarding long-term management and, importantly, must know where to refer families. With a solid knowledge base, the genetic counselor can also play an important role in educating other health care professionals and special educators about FXS. And, finally, a genetic counselor can play an important role in supporting the family in their advocacy efforts by providing expertise and validation. Ultimately, it is the family members themselves who become the best educators and advocates for their child.

## ALLISON AND JOSH'S STORY

We've gone into the classroom and talked about fragile X every year. In the earlier years, it was with our kids out of the class, but in the last couple of years
they've been in the class and even raised their hands and asked questions. Last
year, my daughter asked (in front of the whole class) "Is there a cure?" After
Arlene's heart skipped a couple of beats, she just said, "There's really nothing
to cure, honey. You're perfect just the way you are." In our son's class, we had
everyone, including Josh, come up with ways to be nice and help others and
took all their ideas and put them into a "kindness contract" that each kid got a
copy of and signed. Then, this year (sixth grade), our daughter did her science
current event on fragile X by herself, but with Arlene in the class for moral support. Allison had a poster board that showed our family tree and had a list of
characteristics of fragile X that she read to the class. The last one that she read
to the class was "When you have fragile X, it doesn't mean that you can't learn.
It just means you have to try harder." . . . We are very proud of her.
(Jeffrey Cohen, parent)

Because so few people are knowledgeable about FXS, parents will find
themselves advocating time and time again for their child and FXS in general.
Many parents become actively involved in formal advocacy groups and other
organizations that promote awareness about the condition. A number of news-
letters (see appendix 1), including the newsletter published by the National
Fragile X Foundation, are strongly supported by parents who are willing to de-
vote endless time. This work can be very fulfilling and provides a support network of compassionate families and professionals.

There are a variety of support groups for families with a disabled child.
Putting parents in touch with other families is important. Families benefit enor-
mously from contact with other parents who share similar experiences and who
may be better suited to provide emotional support. The National Fragile X
Foundation is an international organization whose purpose is education and research regarding FXS. Genetic counselors and other health care providers are
encouraged to refer all families affected by FXS and concerned professionals
to this organization for support, ongoing information, resource centers in their
area, and family contacts. Their address is PO Box 190488, San Francisco, California 94119-0488, and their telephone number is 1-800-688-8765 or 1-925-
938-9300.

Concerns and issues for families will change and fluctuate with time. To best
understand the specific needs of a particular family, the genetic counseling process cannot be hurried and long-term contact is often necessary. A lasting bond
based on trust and understanding must be made between the family and the genetic counselor. To specifically evaluate the counseling process and determine

whether a patient's needs were met, a satisfaction survey may be helpful. With time and commitment, the genetic counselor can successfully provide families with the information and support they need to adjust and to cope with the challenges and decisions that lie ahead.

## Conclusion

The genetic counselor plays a crucial role in the multidisciplinary approach to the family dealing with the diagnosis of FXS. Assessing and addressing the counseling needs of each family are paramount. Explaining complex medical and genetic information in a manageable and meaningful way is a challenge that demands time, consideration, and practice. Each family will bring into the counseling session their own unique set of experiences, personal attitudes, and philosophical beliefs. It is the goal of the genetic counselor to help families adjust to and cope with unexpected circumstances. Families grappling to understand are sometimes confused by feelings of anger, guilt, or disappointment and may be helped by the information shared by the genetic counselor. Through emotional support and understanding, moreover, families can once again feel in control and regain hope in the future.

## Acknowledgments

This work was supported in part by National Institutes of Child Health and Development grant HD36071, the Kenneth Kendal King Foundation of Denver, Colorado, and the Schramm Foundation of Denver, Colorado. It is with gratitude that the past and ongoing support of the entire staff from the Fragile X Treatment and Research Center at the Child Development Unit of the Children's Hospital in Denver is acknowledged. We thank Sandy Morrison and Melissa Brown of the Children's Hospital Foundation for their untiring efforts in identifying and obtaining support for our work. We would also like to thank all our patients who have fragile X syndrome, their parents, and family members. It is because of them that we learn, change, and grow as people and professionals.

## References

Abrams, M. T., A. L. Reiss, L. S. Freund, T. L. Baumgardner, G. A. Chase, and M. B. Denckla. 1994. Molecular-neurobehavioral associations in females with the fragile X full mutation. *Am. J. Med. Genet.* 51:317–327.

Ashley, A. E., and S. L. Sherman. 1995. Population dynamics of a meiotic/mitotic expansion model for fragile X syndrome. *Am. J. Hum. Genet.* 57:1414–1425.

Bailey, D. B., Jr., D. Skinner, D. Hatton, and J. Roberts. 2000. Family experiences and factors associated with the diagnosis of fragile X syndrome. *Dev. Behav. Pediatr.* 21(5):315–321.

Beeson, D., and M. S. Golbus. 1985. Decision making: Whether or not to have prenatal diagnosis and abortion for X-linked conditions. *Am. J. Med. Genet.* 20:107–114.

Berliner, J. L., F. N. Shapiro, S. L. Nolin, G. E. Houck Jr., X. Ding, C. Dobkin, S. S. Brooks, and W. T. Brown. 1994. Molecular carrier testing for the fragile X syndrome: Issues for genetic counselors. *J. Genet. Counsel.* 3:233–244.

Brøndum-Nielsen, K., N. Tommerup, H. Poulsen, P. Jacobsen, and M. Mikkelsen. 1981. A pedigree showing transmission by apparently unaffected males and partial expression in female carriers. *Hum. Genet.* 59:23–25.

Brown, W. T. 1996. The molecular biology of the fragile X mutation. In R. J. Hagerman and A. Cronister (eds.), *Fragile X syndrome: Diagnosis, treatment, and research,* 2d ed. Baltimore: Johns Hopkins Univ. Press, pp. 88–113.

Brown, W. T., E. C. Jenkins, A. C. Gross, C. B. Chan, M. S. Krawczun, M. L. Alonso, E. S. Cantú, J. G. Davis, R. J. Hagerman, R. Laxova, M. Liebowitz, V. B. Penchaszadeh, S. Thibodeau. A. M. Willey, M. K. Williams, J. P. Willner, and N. J. Zellers. 1987a. Clinical use of DNA markers in the fragile(X) syndrome for carrier detection and prenatal diagnosis. In A. M. Willey (ed.), *Nucleic acid probes in diagnosis of human genetic diseases.* New York: Alan R. Liss, pp. 11–34.

Brown, W. T., E. C. Jenkins, A. C. Gross, C. B. Chan, K. Wisniewski, I. L. Cohen, and C. M. Miezejeski. 1987b. Genetics and expression of the fragile X syndrome. *Ups. J. Med. Sci. Suppl.* 44:137–154.

Brown, W. T., G. E. Houck, A. Jeziorowska, F. N. Levinson, X. Ding, C. Dobkin, N. Zhong, J. Henderson, S. S. Sklower, and E. D. Jenkins. 1993. Rapid fragile X carrier screening and prenatal diagnosis using a nonradioactive PCR test. *JAMA* 270:1569–1575.

Camerino, G., M. G. Mattei, J. F. Mattei, M. Jaye, and J. L. Mandel. 1983. Close linkage of fragile X-mental retardation syndrome to haemophilia B and transmission through a normal male. *Nature* 306:701–704.

Carmichael, B., M. Pembrey, G. Turner, and A. Barnicoat. 1999. Diagnosis of fragile-X syndrome: The experiences of parents. *J. Intell. Dis. Res.* 43(1):47–53.

Carr, J. 1970. Mongolism: Telling the parents. *Dev. Med. Child Neurol.* 12:213–221.

Cronister, A., S. N. Thibodeau, J. Jirikowic, and R. J. Hagerman. 1990. The usefulness of cytogenetic and DNA linkage analysis in counseling families with fragile X syndrome. *Birth Defects* 26:238–253.

Cronister, A., R. Schreiner, M. Wittenberger, K. Amiri, K. Harris, and R. J. Hagerman. 1991. The heterozygous fragile X female: Historical, physical, cognitive, and cytogenetic features. *Am. J. Med. Genet.* 38:269–274.

Curtis, G., N. Dennis, and J. MacPherson. 1994. The impact of genetic counselling on females in fragile X families. *J. Med. Genet.* 31:950–952.

De Boulle, K., A. J. M. H. Verkerk, E. Reyniers, L. Vits, J. Hendrickx, B. Van Roy, F. Van Den Bos, E. de Graaff, B. A. Oostra, and P. J. Willems. 1993. A point mutation in the *FMR-1* gene associated with fragile X mental retardation. *Nat. Genet.* 3:31–35.

deVries, B. B. A., A. M. Wiegers, E. de Graaff, A. J. M. H. Verkerk, J. O. Van Hemel, D. J. J. Halley, J. P. Fryns, L. M. G. Curfs, M. F. Niemeijer, and B. A. Oostra. 1993. Mental status and fragile X expression in relation to *FMR-1* gene mutation. *Eur. J. Hum. Genet.* 1:72–79.

deVries, B. B. A., A. M. Wiegers, A. P. T. Smits, S. Mohkamsing, H. J. Duivenvoorden, J. P. Fryns, L. M. G. Curfs, D. J. J. Halley, B. A. Oostra, A. M. W. van der Ouweland, and M. F. Niermeijer. 1996. Mental status of females with an *FMR1* gene full mutation. *Am. J. Hum. Genet.* 58:1025–1032.

deVries, B. A., H. M. A. van den Boer-van den Berg, M. F. Niermeijer, and A. Tibben. 1999. Dilemmas in counselling females with the fragile X syndrome. *J. Med. Genet.* 36:167–170.

Dorn, M., M. Mazzocco, and R. J. Hagerman. 1994. Behavioral and psychiatric disorders in adult fragile X carrier males. *J. Am. Acad. Child Adolesc. Psychiatry* 33:256–264.

Drillien, C. M., and E. M. Wilkenson. 1964. Mongolism: When should be parents be told? *Br. Med. Bull.* 5420:1306–1307.

Drotar, D., A. Baskiewicz, N. Irvin, J. H. Kennell, and M. H. Klaus. 1975. The adaptation of parents to the birth of an infant with a congenital malformation: A hypothetical model. *Pediatrics* 56:710–717.

Eichler, E. E., J. J. A. Holden, B. W. Popovich, A. L. Reiss, K. Snow, S. N. Thibodeau, C. S. Richards, P. A. Ward, and D. L. Nelson. 1994. Length of uninterrupted CGG repeats determines instability in the *FMR1* gene. *Nat. Genet.* 8:88–94.

Elias, S., and J. L. Simpson. 1993. Amniocentesis. In J. L. Simpson and S. Elias (eds.), *Essentials of prenatal diagnosis.* New York: Churchill Livingston, pp. 27–44.

Emde, R. N., and C. Brown. 1978. Adaptation to the birth of a Down syndrome infant. *J. Am. Acad. Child Psychiatry* 17:299–323.

Falek, A. 1984. Sequential aspects of coping and other issues in decision making in genetic counseling. In A. E. H. Emery and I. Pellen (eds.), *Psychological aspects of genetic counseling.* London: Academic Press, pp. 23–36.

Feng, Y., L. Lakkis, D. Devys, and S. T. Warren. 1995. Quantitative comparison of *FMR1* gene expression in normal and premutation alleles. *Am. J. Hum. Genet.* 56:106–113.

Filippi, G., A. Rinaldi, N. Archidiacono, M. Rocchi, I. Balazs, and M. Siniscalco. 1983. Linkage between G6PD and fragile-X syndrome. *Am. J. Med. Genet.* 15:113–119.

Filippi, G., V. Pecile, A. Rinaldi, and M. Siniscalo. 1988. Fragile-X mutation and Klinefelter syndrome: A reappraisal. *Am. J. Med. Genet.* 30:99–107.

Fisch, G. S., K. Snow, S. N. Thibodeau, M. Chalifaux, J. J. A. Holden, D. L. Nelson, P. N. Howard-Peebles, and A. Maddalena. 1995. The fragile X premutation in carriers and its effect on mutation size in offspring. *Am. J. Hum. Genet.* 56:1147–1155.

Flynn, G. A., M. C. Hirst, S. J. L. Knight, J. N. MacPherson, J. C. K. Barber, A. V. Flannery, K. E. Davis, and V. J. Buckle. 1993. Identification of the FRAXE fragile site in two families ascertained for X-linked mental retardation. *J. Med. Genet.* 30:97–103.

Franke, P., W. Maier, B. Iwers, M. Hautzinger, and U. G. Froster. 1995. Fragile X carrier females: Evidence for a distinct psychopathologic phenotype? Presented at the

Seventh International Workshop on the Fragile X and X-Linked Mental Retardation, Tromso, Norway, August 2–5.

Franke, P., M. Leboyer, M. Gansicke, O. Weiffenbach, V. Biancalana, P. Cornillet-Lefebre, M. F. Croquette, U. Froster, S. G. Schwab, F. Poustka, M. Hautzinger, and W. Maier. 1998. Genotype-phenotype relationship in female carriers of the premutation and full mutation of *FMR-1*. *Psychiatry Res.* 80:113–127.

Fraser, F. C. 1974. Genetic counseling. *Am. J. Med. Genet.* 26:636–659.

Friedman, J. M., and P. N. Howard-Peebles. 1986. Inheritance of fragile-X syndrome: An hypothesis. *Am. J. Med. Genet.* 23:701–713.

Froster-Iskenius, U., E. Schwinger, M. Weigert, and C. Fonatsch. 1982. Replication pattern in XXY cells with fra(X). *Hum. Genet.* 60:278–280.

Froster-Iskenius, U., B. C. McGillivray, F. J. Dill, J. G. Hall, and D. S. Herbst. 1986. Normal male carriers in the fragile(X) form of X-linked mental retardation (Martin-Bell syndrome). *Am. J. Med. Genet.* 23:619–631.

Fryns, J. P. 1986. The female and the fragile X: A study of 144 obligate female carriers. *Am. J. Med. Genet.* 23:157–169.

Fryns, J. P., and H. Van den Berghe. 1982. Transmission of fragile (X)(q27) from normal male(s). *Hum. Genet.* 61:262–263.

———. 1988. The concurrence of Klinefelter's syndrome and fragile X syndrome. *Am. J. Med. Genet.* 30:109–113.

Fryns, J. P., A. Kleczkowska, E. Kubien, P. Petit, M. Haspeslagh, I. Lindemans, and H. Van den Berghe. 1983. XY/XXY mosaicism and fragile X syndrome. *Am. Genet.* 26:251–253.

Fryns, J. P., A. Klexzkowska, I. Wolfs, and H. Van den Berghe. 1984. Klinefelter syndrome and two fragile X chromosomes. *Clin. Genet.* 26:445–447.

Fu, Y., D. P. A. Kuhl, A. Pizzuti, M. Pieretti, J. S. Sutcliffe, S. Richards, A. J. M. H. Verkerk, J. J. A. Holden, R. G. Fenwick Jr., S. T. Warren, B. A. Oostra, D. L. Nelson, and C. T. Caskey. 1991. Variation of the CGG repeat at the fragile site results in genetic instability: Resolution of the Sherman paradox. *Cell* 67:1047–1058.

Gath, A. 1972. The effect of mental subnormality on the family. *Br. J. Hosp. Med.* 8:147–150.

———. 1977. The impact of an abnormal child upon the parents. *Br. J. Psychiatry* 130:405–410.

Gedeon, A. K., E. Baker, H. Robinson, M. W. Partington, B. Gross, A. Manca, B. Korn, A. Ppoustka, S. Yu, G. R. Sutherland, and J. C. Mulley. 1992. Fragile X syndrome without CCG amplification has an *FMR-1* deletion. *Nat. Genet.* 1:341–344.

Gringas, P., and A. Barnicoat. 1998. Retesting for fragile X syndrome in cytogenetically normal males. *Dev. Med. Child Neurol.* 40:62–64.

Gu, Y., K. A. Lugenbeel, J. G. Vockley, W. W. Grody, and D. L. Nelson. 1994. A de novo deletion in *FMR-1* in a patient with developmental delay. *Hum. Mol. Genet.* 3:1705–1706.

Hagerman, R. J., and W. E. Sobesky. 1989. Psychopathology in fragile X syndrome. *Am. J. Orthopsychiatry* 59:142–152.

Hagerman, R. J., C. E. Hull, J. F. Safanda, I. Carpenter, L. W. Staley, R. A. O'Connor, C. Seydel, M. M. M. Mazzocco, K. Snow, S. N. Thibodeau, D. Kuhl, D. L. Nelson,

C. T. Caskey, and A. K. Taylor. 1994. High functioning fragile X males: Demonstration of an unmethylated full mutation associated with protein expression. *Am. J. Med. Genet.* 51:298–308.

Halley, D., A. Van Den Ouweland, W. Deelen, I. Verma, and B. Oostra. 1994. Strategy for reliable prenatal detection of normal male carriers of the fragile X syndrome. *Am. J. Med. Genet.* 51:471–473.

Hanauer, A., and P. Hagerman. 2000. Conference report: Ninth International Workshop on Fragile X Syndrome and X-linked Mental Retardation. Molecular basis of fragile X syndrome: Part 2. *Am. J. Med. Genet.* 94:345–360.

Heitz, D., D. Devys, G. Imbert, C. Kretz, and J. Mandel. 1992. Inheritance of the fragile X syndrome: Size of the fragile X premutation is a major determinant of the transition to full mutation. *J. Med. Genet.* 29:794–801.

Hirst, M., P. Grewal, A. Flannery, R. Slatter, E. Maher, D. Barton, J. Fryns, and K. Davies. 1995. Two new cases of *FMR1* deletion associated with mental impairment. *Am. J. Hum. Genet.* 56:67–74.

Holden, J. J. A. 1995. Workshop for families and friends. *Dev. Brain Dysfunct.* 278:380–389.

Hull, C. E., and R. J. Hagerman. 1993. The physical and medical phenotype of fragile X females. *Am. J. Dis. Child* 147:1236–1241.

Jacky, P. 1996. Cytogenetics. In R. J. Hagerman and A. Cronister (eds.), *Fragile X syndrome: Diagnosis, treatment, and research,* 2d ed. Baltimore: Johns Hopkins Univ. Press.

Jacobs, P. A., T. W. Glover, M. Mayer, P. Fox, J. W. Gerrard, H. G. Dunn, and D. S. Herbst. 1980. X-linked mental retardation: A study of 7 families. *Am. J. Med. Genet.* 7:471–489.

Kallinen, J., S. Heinonen, A. Mannermaa, and M. Ryynanen. 2000. Prenatal diagnosis of fragile X syndrome and the risk of expansion of a premutation. *Clin. Genet.* 58(2): 111–115.

Kaufmann, W. E., M. T. Abrams, W. Chen, and A. L. Reiss. 1999. Genotype, molecular phenotype, and cognitive phenotype: Correlations in fragile X syndrome. *Am. J. Med. Genet.* 83:286–295.

Kelly, T. E. 1976. *Clinical genetics and genetic counseling.* Chicago: Yearbook Medical Publishers, pp. 343–364.

Kemper, M. B., R. J. Hagerman, R. S. Ahmad, and R. Mariner. 1986. Cognitive profiles and the spectrum of clinical manifestations in heterozygous fra(X) females. *Am. J. Med. Genet.* 23:139–156.

Kessler, S. 1979. The psychological foundations of genetic counseling. In S. Kessler (ed.), *Genetic counseling: Psychological dimensions.* New York: Academic Press, pp. 17–33.

Kiely, L., R. Sterne, and C. J. Witkop. 1976. Psychological factors in low-incidence genetic disease: The case of osteogenesis imperfecta. *Soc. Work Health Care* 1:409–420.

Knight, S. J. L., A. V. Flannery, M. C. Hirst, L. Campbell, Z. Christodoulou, S. R. Phelps, J. Pointon, H. R. Middleton-Price, A. Barnicoat, M. E. Pembrey, J. Holland, B. A. Oostra, M. Bobrow, and K. E. Davies. 1993. Trinucleotide repeat amplification and hypermethylation of a CpG island in FRAXE mental retardation. *Cell* 74:127–134.

Kremer, E., M. Pritchard, M. Lynch, S. Yu, K. Holman, E. Baker, S. T. Warren, D. Schlessinger, G. R. Sutherland, and R. I. Richards. 1991. Mapping of DNA instability at the fragile X to a trinucleotide repeat sequence p(CCG)n. *Science* 252:1711–1714.

Kupke, K. G., A. L. Soreng, and U. Müller. 1991. Origin of the supernumerary X chromosome in a patient with fragile X and Klinefelter syndrome. *Am. J. Med. Genet.* 38:440–446.

Lipperman-Hand, A., and F. C. Fraser. 1979. Genetic counseling: Parent's responses to uncertainty. *Birth Defects* 15:325–339.

Loesch, D. Z., and D. A. Hay. 1988. Clinical features and reproductive patterns in fragile X female heterozygotes. *J. Med. Genet.* 25:407–414.

Loesch, D. Z., D. A. Hay, and J. Mulley. 1994. Transmitting males and carrier females in fragile X—revisited. *Am. J. Med. Genet.* 51:392–399.

Loesch, D. Z., R. Huggins, V. Petrovic, and H. Slater. 1995. Expansion of the CGG repeat in fragile X in the *FMR1* gene depends on the sex of the offspring. *Am. J. Hum. Genet.* 57:1408–1413.

Maddalena, A., B. D. Hicks, W. C. Spence, G. Levinson, and P. N. Howard-Peebles. 1994. Prenatal diagnosis in known fragile X carriers. *Am. J. Med. Genet.* 51:490–496.

Martin, J. P., and J. Bell. 1943. A pedigree of mental defect showing sex-linkage. *J. Neurol. Neurosurg. Psychiatry* 6:154–157.

Mazzocco, M. M. M., B. Pennington, and R. J. Hagerman. 1993. The neurocognitive phenotype of female carriers of fragile X: Further evidence for specificity. *J. Dev. Behav. Pediatr.* 14:328–335.

McConkie-Rosell, A., A. M. Lachiewicz, G. A. Spiridigliozzi, J. Tarleton, S. Schoenwald, M. C. Phelan, P. Goonewardena, X. Ding, and W. T. Brown. 1993. Evidence that methylation of the *FMR-1* locus is responsible for variable phenotypic expression of the fragile X syndrome. *Am. J. Hum. Genet.* 53:800–809.

McConkie-Rosell, A., G. Spiridigliozzi, T. Iafolla, J. Tarleton, and A. Lachiewicz. 1995a. Attitudes regarding carrier testing in fragile X syndrome. Presented at the Seventh International Workshop on the Fragile X and X-Linked Mental Retardation, Tromso, Norway, August 2–5.

McConkie-Rosell, A., H. Robinson, S. Wake, L. Staley, K. Heller, and A. Cronister. 1995b. The dissemination of genetic risk information to relatives in the fragile X syndrome: Guidelines for genetic counselors. *Am. J. Med. Genet.* 59:426–430.

McConkie-Rosell, A., G. A. Spiridigliozzi, T. Iafolla, J. Tarleton, and A. M. Lachiewicz. 1997. Carrier testing in the fragile X syndrome. *Am. J. Med. Genet.* 68:62–69.

McConkie-Rosell, A., G. A. Spiridigliozzi, J. A. Sullivan, D. V. Dawson, and A. M. Lachiewicz. 2000. Longitudinal study of the carrier testing process for fragile X syndrome: Perceptions and coping. *Am. J. Med. Genet.* 98:37–45

McIntosh, N., L. W. Gane, A. McConkie-Rosell, and R. L. Bennett. 2000. Genetic counseling for fragile X syndrome: Recommendations of the National Society of Genetic Counselors. *J. Genet. Counsel.* 9:303–325.

Mercer, R. T. 1974. Mothers' response to their infants with defects. *Nurs. Res.* 23:133–137.

Merenstein, S. A., W. E. Sobesky, A. K. Taylor, J. E. Riddle, H. X. Tran, and R. J. Hagerman. 1996. Fragile X syndrome in normal IQ males with learning and behavioral problems: Molecular-clinical correlations in males with an expanded *FMR1* mutation. *Am. J. Med. Genet.* 64:388–394.

Meryash, D. L. 1989. Perception of burden among at risk women of raising a child with fragile X syndrome. *Clin. Genet.* 36:15–24.

Meryash, D. L., and D. Abuelo. 1988. Counseling needs and attitudes toward prenatal diagnosis and abortion in fragile-X families. *Clin. Genet.* 33:349–355.

Miezejeski, C. M., E. C. Jenkins, A. L. Hill, K. Wisniewski, J. H. French, and W. T. Brown. 1986. A profile of cognitive deficit in females from fragile X families. *Neuropsychologia* 24:405–409.

Montagnon, M., A. Bogyo, C. Deluchat, M. Jokic, C. Chateau, A. Taillandier, F. Thomas, B. Simon-Bouy, J. Boue, J. L. Serre, A. Boue, and E. Mornet. 1993. Transition from normal to premutated alleles in fragile X syndrome results from a multistep process. *Eur. J. Hum. Genet.* 2:125–131.

Nakahori, Y., S. J. L. Knight, J. Holland, C. Schwartz, A. Roche, J. Tarleton, S. Wong, T. J. Flint, U. Froster-Iskenius, D. Bentley, K. E. Davies, and M. C. Hirst. 1991. Molecular heterogeneity of the fragile X syndrome. *Nucleic Acids Res.* 19:4355–4359.

Nihira, K., C. E. Meyers, and I. T. Mink. 1980. Home environment, family adjustment and the development of mentally retarded children. *Appl. Res. Ment. Retard.* 1:5–24.

Nolin, S. L., F. A. Lewis, A. Glicksman, G. E. Houck Jr., and W. T. Brown. 1994. *FMR-1* CGG transitions in fragile X families. Presented at the Fourth International Fragile X Conference, Albuquerque, June 8–12.

Nolin, S. L., F. A. Lewis III, L. L. Ye, G. E. Houck Jr., A. E. Glicksman, P. Limprasert, S. Y. Li, N. Zhong, A. E. Ashley, E. Feingold, S. L. Sherman, and W. T. Brown. 1996. Familial transmission of the *FMR1* CGG repeat. *Am. J. Hum. Genet.* 59:1252–1261.

Oberle, I., F. Rousseau, D. Heitz, C. Kretz, D. Devys, A. Hanauer, J. Bour, M. F. Berteas, and J. L. Mandel. 1991. Instability of a 550-base pair DNA segment and abnormal methylation in fragile X syndrome. *Science* 252:1097–1102.

O'Brien, M. M., T. Padre-Mendoza, and S. M. Pueschel. 1982. Maternal nondysjunction of fragile X chromosome resulting in Klinefelter syndrome. *Am. J. Hum. Genet.* 35:146A.

Oostra, B. A., P. B. Jacky, W. T. Brown, and F. Rousseau. 1993. Guidelines for the diagnosis of fragile X syndrome. *J. Med. Genet.* 30:410–413.

Opitz, J. M. 1986. On the gates of hell and a most unusual gene: Editorial comment. *Am. J. Med. Genet.* 23:1–10.

Pearn, J. H. 1973. Patients' subjective interpretation of risks offered in genetic counseling. *J. Med. Genet.* 10:129–134.

Pesso, R., M. Berkenstadt, H. Cuckle, E. Gak, L. Peleg, M. Frydman, and G. Barkai. 2000. Screening for fragile X syndrome in women of reproductive age. *Prenat. Diagn.* 20:611–614.

Policy Statement: American College of Medical Genetics. 1994. Fragile X syndrome: Diagnostic and carrier testing. *Am. J. Med. Genet.* 53:380–381.

Quan, F., J. Zonana, K. Gunter, K. L. Peterson, R. E. Magenis, and B. W. Popovich. 1995. An atypical case of fragile X syndrome caused by a deletion that includes the *FMR-1* gene. *Am. J. Hum. Genet.* 56:1042–1051.

Raeburn, J. A. 1989. Mental handicap. In A. E. H. Emery and I. Pullen (eds.), *Psychological aspects of genetic counseling.* London: Academic Press, pp. 95–105.

Reif, M., and H. Baitsch. 1985. Psychological issues in genetic counseling. *Hum. Genet.* 70:193–199.

Reiss, A. L., H. H. Kazazian, C. M. Krebs, A. McAughan, C. D. Boehm, M. T. Abrams, and D. L. Nelson. 1994. Frequency and stability of the fragile X premutation. *Hum. Mol. Genet.* 3:393–398.

Reyniers, E., I. Vits, K. De Boulle, B. Van Roy, D. Van Velzen, E. de Graaff, A. J. M. H. Verkerk, H. Z. J. Jorens, J. K. Darby, B. A. Oostra, and P. Willems. 1993. The full mutation in the *FMR-1* gene of male fragile X patients is absent in their sperm. *Nat. Genet.* 4:143–146.

Rhoads, G. G., L. G. Jackson, S. E. Schlesselman, F. F. de la Cruz, R. J. Desnick, M. S. Golbus, D. H. Ledbetter, H. A. Lubs, M. J. Mahoney, E. Pergament, J. L. Simpson, N. J. Carpenter, S. Elias, N. A. Ginsberg, J. D. Goldberg, J. C. Hobbins, L. Lynch, P. Shiono, R. J. Wapner, and J. M. Zachary. 1989. The safety and efficacy of chorionic villus sampling for early prenatal diagnosis of cytogenetic abnormalities. *N. Engl. J. Med.* 320:609–616.

Riddle, J. E., A. Cheema, W. E. Sobesky, S. C. Gardner, A. K. Taylor, B. F. Pennington, and R. J. Hagerman. 1998. Phenotypic involvement in females with the *FMR1* gene mutation. *Am. J. Ment. Retard.* 102:590–601.

Rousseau, F., D. Heitz, V. Biancalana, S. Blumenfeld, C. Kretc, J. Boue, N. Tommerup, C. Van der Hagen, C. DeLozier-Blanchet, M. Croquette, S. Gilgenkrantz, P. Jalbert, M. Voelckel, I. Oberle, and J. L. Mandel. 1991. Direct diagnosis by DNA analysis of the fragile X syndrome of mental retardation. *N. Engl. J. Med.* 325:1673–1681.

Rousseau, F., L. J. Robb, P. Rouillard, and V. M. Der Kaloustian. 1994a. No mental retardation in a man with 40% abnormal methylation at the *FMR-1* locus and transmission of sperm cell mutations as premutation. *Hum. Mol. Genet.* 3:927–930.

Rousseau, F., D. Heitz, J. Tarleton, J. MacPherson, H. Malmgren, N. Dahl, A. Barnicoat, C. Mathew, E. Mornet, I. Tejada, A. Maddalena, R. Spiegel, A. Schinzel, J. A. G. Marcos, C. Schwartz, and J. L. Mandel. 1994b. A multicenter study on genotype-phenotype correlation in the fragile X syndrome, using direct diagnosis with the probe StB 12.3: The first 2,253 cases. *Am. J. Hum. Genet.* 55:225–237.

Rousseau, F., D. Heitz, J. Tarleton, J. MacPherson, H. Malmgren, N. Dahl, A. Barnicoat, et al. 1994c. Higher rate of transition from fragile X premutations into full mutations in males than in females suggest post-conceptional expansion of the CGG repeats. *Am. J. Hum. Genet. (Suppl.)* 55:A240.

Roy, J. C., J. Johnsen, K. Breese, and R. Hagerman. 1995. Fragile X syndrome: What is the impact of diagnosis on families? *Dev. Brain Dysfunct.* 8:327–335.

Ryan, G., and C. H. Rodeck. 1993. Fetal blood sampling. In J. L. Simpson and S. Elias (eds.), *Essentials of prenatal diagnosis.* New York: Churchill Livingston, pp. 63–75.

Schild, S. 1981. Social and psychological issues in genetic counseling. In S. R. Applewhite, D. C. Busbie, and D. H. Gorgaonkar (eds.), *Genetic screening and counseling: A multidisciplinary perspective.* Springfield, Ill.: Charles C. Thomas, pp. 104–133.

Schild, S., and R. B. Black. 1984. *Social work and genetics: A guide for practice.* New York: Haworth Press, pp. 49–70.

Schnur, R. E., D. H. Ledbetter, and R. L. Nussbaum. 1986. A family with a 47,XXY plus fragile X at Xq27.3 due to paternal nondisjunction. *Am. J. Hum. Genet. (Suppl.)* 39: A100.

Schwartz, C. E., J. Dean, P. N. Howard-Peebles, M. Brigge, M. Mikkelsen, N. Tommerup, C. Hull, R. J. Hagerman, J. J. A. Holden, and R. E. Stevensen. 1994. Obstetrical and gynecological complications in fragile X carriers: A multicenter study. *Am. J. Med. Genet.* 51:400–402.

Sherman, S. L., N. E. Morton, P. A. Jacobs, and G. Turner. 1984. The marker (X) syndrome: A cytogenetic and genetic analysis. *Ann. Hum. Genet.* 48:21–37.

Sherman, S. L., P. A. Jacobs, N. E. Morton, U. Froster-Iskenius, P. N. Howard-Peebles, K. B. Nielsen, M. W. Partington, G. R. Sutherland, G. Turner, and M. Watson. 1985. Further segregation analysis of the fragile X syndrome with special reference to transmitting males. *Hum. Genet.* 69:289–299.

Sherman, S. L., G. Turner, L. Sheffield, S. Laing, and H. Robinson. 1988. Investigation of the twinning rate in families with the fragile X syndrome. *Am. J. Med. Genet.* 30:625–631.

Shore, M. F. 1975. Psychological issues in counseling the genetically handicapped. In C. Birch and P. Albrecht (eds.), *Genetics and the quality of life.* New York: Pergamon Press.

Smits, A. P. T., J. C. F. M. Dreesen, J. G. Post, D. F. C. M. Smeets, C. de Die-Smulders, T. Spaans-van der Bijl, L. C. P. Govaerts, S. T. Warren, B. A. Oostra, and B. A. van Oost. 1993. The fragile X syndrome: No evidence for any recent mutations. *J. Med. Genet.* 30:94–96.

Snow, K., L. K. Doud, R. Hagerman, R. G. Pergolizzi, S. H. Erster, and S. N. Thibodeau. 1993. Analysis of a CGG sequence at the *FMR-1* locus in fragile X families and in the general population. *Am. J. Hum. Genet.* 53:1217–1228.

Snow, K., D. J. Tester, K. E. Kruckberg, D. J. Schaid, and S. N. Thibodeau. 1994. Sequence analysis of the fragile X trinucleotide repeat: Implications for the origin of the fragile X mutation. *Hum. Mol. Genet.* 3:1543–1551.

Sobesky, W. E., B. F. Pennington, D. Porter, C. E. Hull, and R. J. Hagerman. 1994. Emotional and neurocognitive deficits in fragile X. *Am. J. Med. Genet.* 51:378–385.

Sobesky, W. E., A. K. Taylor, B. F. Pennington, J. E. Riddle, and R. J. Hagerman. 1995. Molecular/clinical correlations in females with fragile X. Presented at the Seventh International Workshop on the Fragile X and X-Linked Mental Retardation, Tromso, Norway, August 2–5.

Sobesky, W. E., A. K. Taylor, B. F. Pennington, L. Bennetto, D. Porter, J. Riddle, and R. J. Hagerman. 1996. Molecular/clinical correlations in females with fragile X. *Am. J. Med. Genet.* 54:340–345.

Sorenson, J. R., J. P. Swazey, and N. A. Scotch. 1981. *Reproductive pasts, reproductive futures: Genetic counseling and its effectiveness.* New York: Alan R. Liss.

Staley-Gane, L. W., L. Flynn, A. Cronister-Silverman, and R. J. Hagerman. 1996. Expanding the role of the genetic counselor. *Am. J. Med. Genet.* In press.

Strom, C. M., R. Levin, S. Strom, C. Masciangelo, A. Kuliev, and Y. Verlinsky. 2000. Neonatal outcome of preimplantation genetic diagnosis by polar body removal: The first 109 infants. *Pediatrics* 106:650–653.

Sutherland, G. R., and E. Baker. 1992. Characterisation of a new rare fragile site easily confused with fragile X. *Hum. Mol. Genet.* 1:111–113.

Sutherland, G. R., A. Gedeon, L. Kornman, A. Donnelly, R. W. Byard, J. C. Mulley, E. Kremer, M. Lynch, M. Pritchard, S. Yu, and R. Richards. 1991. Prenatal diagnosis of fragile X syndrome by direct detection of the unstable DNA sequence. *N. Engl. J. Med.* 325:1720–1722.

Sved, J. A., and C. D. Laird. 1990. Population genetic consequences of the fragile-X syndrome based on the X-inactivation imprinting model. *Am. J. Hum. Genet.* 46: 443–451.

Tabor, A., J. Philip, M. Madsen, J. Bang, E. D. Obel, and B. Norgaard-Pederson. 1986. Randomised control trial of genetic amniocentesis in 4604 low-risk women. *Lancet* 2:1287–1293.

Tarleton, J., R. Richie, C. Schwartz, K. Roa, A. S. Aylsworth, and A. Lachiewicz. 1993. An extensive de novo deletion removing *FMR1* in a patient with mental retardation and the fragile X phenotype. *Hum. Mol. Genet.* 2:1973–1974.

Tassone, F., R. J. Hagerman, D. N. Inkle, P. N. Dyer, M. Lampe, R. Willemsen, B. A. Oostra, and A. K. Taylor. 1999. FMRP expression as a potential prognostic indicator in fragile X syndrome. *Am. J. Med. Genet.* 84:250–261.

Tassone, F., R. J. Hagerman, W. D. Chamberlain, and P. J. Hagerman. 2000a. Transcription of the *FMR1* gene in individuals with fragile X syndrome. *Semin. Med. Genet.* 97:195–203.

Tassone, F., R. J. Hagerman, A. K. Taylor, L. W. Gane, T. E. Godfrey, and P. J. Hagerman. 2000b. Elevated levels of *FMR1* mRNA in carrier males: A new mechanism of involvement in fragile X syndrome. *Am. J. Hum. Genet.* 66:6–15.

Taylor, A. K., J. F. Safanda, K. A. Lugenbeel, D. L. Nelson, and R. J. Hagerman. 1994a. Molecular and phenotypic studies of the fragile X males with variant methylation of the *FMR1* gene reveal that the degree of methylation influences clinical severity. *Am. J. Hum. Genet.* 55:A18;85.

Taylor, A. K., J. F. Safanda, M. Z. Fall, C. Quince, K. A. Lang, C. E. Hull, I. Carpenter, L. Staley, and R. J. Hagerman. 1994b. Molecular predictors of cognitive involvement in fragile X females. *JAMA* 271:507–514.

Turner, G., A. Daniel, and M. Frost. 1980. X-linked mental retardation macroorchidism, and the Xq27 fragile site. *J. Pediatr.* 96:837–841.

Turner, G., J. M. Opitz, W. T. Brown, K. E. Davies, P. A. Jacobs, E. C. Jenkins, M. Mikkelsen, M. W. Partington, and G. R. Sutherland. 1986. Conference report: Second International Workshop on the Fragile X and on X-linked Mental Retardation. *Am. J. Med. Genet.* 23:11–67.

Turner, G., and M. W. Partington. 1988. Fragile X expression, age and the degree of mental handicap in the male. *Am. J. Med. Genet.* 30:423–428.

Turner, G., H. Robinson, S. Laing, M. Van den Berk, A. Colley, A. Goddard, S. Sherman, and M. Partington. 1992. Population screening for fragile X. *Lancet* 339:1210–1213.

Turner, G., H. Robinson, S. Wake, and N. Martin. 1994. Dizygous twinning and premature menopause in fragile X syndrome. *Lancet* 344:1500.

Vaisanen, M., M. Kähkönen, and J. Leisti. 1994. Diagnosis of fragile X syndrome by direct mutation analysis. *Hum. Genet.* 93:143–147.

Verkerk, A. J. M. H., M. Pieretti, J. S. Sutcliffe, Y. Fu, D. P. A. Kuhl, A. Puzzuti, O. Reiner, S. Richards, M. F. Victoria, F. Zhang, B. E. Eussen, G. J. B. Van Ommen, L. A. J. Blonden, G. L. Riggins, J. L. Chastain, C. B. Kunst, H. Galjaard, C. T. Caskey, D. L. Nelson, B. A. Oostra, and S. T. Warren. 1991. Identification of a gene (*FMR-1*) containing a CGG repeat coincident with a breakpoint cluster exhibiting length variation in fragile X syndrome. *Cell* 65:905–914.

Verlinsky, Y., S. Rechitsky, O. Verlinsky, V. Ivachnenko, A. Lifchez, B. Kaplan, J. Moise, J. Valle, A. Borkowski, J. Nefedova, E. Goltsman, C. Strom, and A. Kuliev. 1999. Prepregnancy testing for single-gene disorders by polar body analysis. *Genet. Test.* 3(2):185–190.

Warren, S. T., and D. L. Nelson. 1994. Advances in molecular analysis of fragile X syndrome. *JAMA* 271:536–542.

Watkins, C., A. Lazzarini, M. K. McCormack, and C. S. Reis. 1989. Genetic counseling for the mildly mentally retarded client. In N. J. Zellers (ed.), *Strategies in genetic counseling*. New York: Human Sciences Press, pp. 219–234.

Watson, M. S., W. W. Breg, D. Pauls, W. T. Brown, A. J. Carroll, P. N. Howard-Peebles, D. Meryash, and L. R. Shapiro. 1988. Aneuploidy and fragile X syndrome. *Am. J. Med. Genet.* 30:115–121.

Wertz, D. C., J. R. Sorenson, and T. C. Heeren. 1984. Genetic counseling and reproductive uncertainty. *Am. J. Med. Genet.* 18:79–88.

Wikler, L., M. Wasow, and E. Hatfield. 1981. Chronic sorrow revisited: Parent vs. professional depiction of the adjustment of parents of mentally retarded children. *Am. J. Orthopsychiatry* 51:63–70.

Willems, P. J., B. Van Roy, K. De Boulle, L. Vits, E. Reyniers, O. Beck, J. E. Dumon, A. J. Verkerk, and B. Oostra. 1992. Segregation of the fragile X mutation from an affected male to his normal daughter. *Hum. Mol. Genet.* 1:511–515.

Wilmot, P. L., L. R. Shapiro, and P. A. Duncan. 1980. The Xq27 fragile site and 47,XXY. *Am. J. Hum. Genet.* 32:94A.

Wöhrle, D., D. Kotzot, M. C. Hirst, A. Manca, B. Korn, A. Schmidt, G. Barbi, H. Rott, A. Poustka, K. E. Davies, and P. Steinbach. 1992. A microdeletion of less than 250 kb, including the proximal part of the *FMR-1* gene and the fragile-X site, in a male with the clinical phenotype of fragile-X syndrome. *Am. J. Hum. Genet.* 51:299–306.

Wolff, P. H., J. Gardner, J. Lappen, J. Paccia, and D. Meryash. 1988. Variable expression of the fragile X syndrome in heterozygous females of normal intelligence. *Am. J. Med. Genet.* 30:213–225.

Yu, S., M. Pritchard, E. Kremer, M. Lynch, J. Nancarrow, E. Baker, K. Holman, J. C. Mulley, S. T. Warren, D. Schlessinger, G. R. Sutherland, and R. I. Richards. 1991. Fragile X genotype characterized by an unstable region of DNA. *Science* 252:1179–1181.

Zhong, N., W. Yang, C. Dobkin, and W. T. Brown. 1995. Fragile X gene instability: Anchoring AGGs and linked microsatellites. *Am. J. Hum. Genet.* 57:351–361.

# CHAPTER 8

# Medical Follow-up and Pharmacotherapy

Randi Jenssen Hagerman, M.D.

The physician who follows children and adults with fragile X syndrome (FXS) must be familiar with the physical and behavioral problems associated with this disorder to provide optimal treatment and intervention. Although a cure does not presently exist, a variety of effective interventions are available. In the future, gene therapy or protein replacement therapy will be a reality. The difficulties that must be overcome before this type of therapy can be utilized in patients are discussed in chapter 12. At present, optimal intervention is a multiprofessional approach that includes academic and behavioral interventions (chaps. 9–11), individual motor and language therapy (chap. 10), and the physician's input in health maintenance and, when necessary, pharmacotherapy for behavior problems. The physician's perspective regarding treatment and follow-up are described in this chapter. Usually special education, individual therapy, and medication work synergistically to allow children with FXS to achieve their highest potential. Although significant behavior and attention problems are present in the majority of males with FXS and in significantly affected females, treatment must be individualized because the severity of the problems varies.

The first section of this chapter focuses on medical complications and their treatment. This section is divided into age groups, with an emphasis on what the physician should assess at each stage of development. The second section concerns the pharmacotherapy of behavior problems and medical problems, including seizures.

*Fragile X Syndrome: Diagnosis, Treatment, and Research,* third edition, ed. Randi Jenssen Hagerman and Paul J. Hagerman (Baltimore: Johns Hopkins University Press, 2002), © The Johns Hopkins University Press.

## Medical Follow-up

### Infancy

Infants with FXS are usually identified after an older relative, such as a brother or cousin, is identified with FXS. Genetic counseling for extended family members should begin at the time of diagnosis and may also involve prenatal diagnosis for future pregnancies (chap. 7).

The newly diagnosed infant should be examined with a close look for possible connective tissue abnormalities (chap. 1). Infants with FXS are at increased risk for cleft palate, clubfoot, congenital hip dislocation, and hernias, perhaps all related to loose connective tissue. Fryns et al. (1988) also reported an increased incidence of sudden infant death syndrome (SIDS), so episodes of apnea, obstructed breathing, or possible seizures require a detailed workup and subsequent careful monitoring. Tirosh and Borochowitz (1992) reported obstructive sleep apnea in four boys with FXS, but this was recognized later in childhood. A subsequent sleep study of seven children with FXS (six boys and one girl, mean age 12.9 years) did not demonstrate evidence of obstructive sleep apnea (Musumeci et al. 1996). The authors suggest that children with FXS usually do not have problems with sleep apnea unless risk factors such as enlarged adenoids or tonsils or hypotonic oropharyngeal muscles are present. Sometimes severe snoring can be associated with obstructive sleep apnea, and a tonsillectomy and adenoidectomy may improve these symptoms. If obstructive sleep apnea persists after surgery, treatment with continuous positive airway pressure (CPAP) has been shown to be efficacious in children with neurodevelopmental disorders (Tirosh et al. 1995). CPAP delivered by nasal prongs at night improved sleep quality, daily arousal, frequency of seizures, and episodes of pneumonia in four boys with neurodevelopmental disorders, including one patient with FXS.

Although many babies with FXS do well in the newborn period, others have been described as stiff, unable to cuddle, irritable, and unable to feed well. Recurrent vomiting with feeding is not uncommon. Gastroesophageal reflux (GER) has been diagnosed in several infants with FXS, and it may be related to the connective tissue abnormalities, hypotonia, dysfunction of the gastroesophageal sphincter, or a hypersensitive gag reflex (Goldson and Hagerman 1993). The vomiting in patients with GER usually resolves with positioning upright after meals or with thickening of the feedings (Sondheimer 1994). Occasionally medication is needed to decrease reflux and improve gastric emptying time. The medications commonly used in GER include metoclopromide (Reglan), which is related to neuroleptic medication, and bethanacol, a cholinergic drug that stimulates intestinal smooth muscle contraction. Both medications will enhance the lower esophageal sphincter pressure, and metoclopromide will improve gastric emptying time. Both, however, can cause side effects in the central nervous system (CNS), including irritability, and metoclopromide can cause dystonic reactions. Cisapride (Propulsid), a prokinetic agent, has been used to treat reflux, but a recent association with arrhythmias has discouraged its use in young children.

Recurrent GER can cause significant esophagitis and pain. These problems can be treated with an $H_2$ blocker, such as ranitidine (Zantac), or a proton-pump inhibitor, omeprazole (Prilosec), if ranitidine is not effective (Karjoo and Kane 1995). Rarely surgery is needed to tighten the sphincter area with a Nissen or Thal fundoplication procedure and only after medical intervention has failed.

Some children with FXS will have habitual vomiting when they are upset, overwhelmed, or frustrated. Behavioral intervention to decrease vomiting and replace it with a more acceptable behavior can be helpful. We have noted several cases of failure to thrive related to difficulties in sucking, GER, tactile defensiveness, or aversion to food textures (Goldson and Hagerman 1993). If feeding difficulties are a problem, particularly sucking or intolerance of certain food textures, consultation with an occupational therapist and/or a speech and language therapist and subsequent work on oral desensitization, oral stimulation, and oral motor coordination can be helpful (chap. 10).

Significant hypotonia or motor delays require therapy from an occupational therapist (OT) and/or physical therapist (PT) during the first year. This can be obtained through an infant stimulation program, which should also include a language therapist. Such programs work with the child and the parents to teach them how to stimulate the baby optimally at home. If the mother herself is severely learning disabled or retarded because of FXS, intervention is essential to teach appropriate parenting skills and to provide ongoing guidance.

Beginning in the first year of life, frequent otitis media (middle ear infections) are a problem for approximately 60% of boys with FXS (Hagerman et al. 1987). As discussed in chapter 1, this problem requires vigorous therapy to avoid a fluctuating hearing loss that may further compromise language development. If a conductive hearing loss persists after acute antibiotic treatment, the physician should consider the insertion of polyethylene (PE) tubes through the tympanic membrane to normalize hearing. A recent intriguing study evaluated the use of xylitol, a commonly used sweetener that is effective in preventing dental cavities and inhibiting the growth of pneumococci, in the prevention of acute otitis media (Uhari et al. 1998). In 857 normal, healthy children recruited from day care centers, xylitol syrup or xylitol chewing gum significantly decreased the incidence of acute otitis media by 30–40% compared to controls.

Recurrent sinusitis is also a frequent problem in FXS, and it may be related to the facial changes or the connective tissue problems that lead to recurrent otitis in FXS. Prophylactic antibiotics may be helpful to decrease the incidence of recurrent otitis media and/or recurrent sinusitis. Rarely ENT surgery may be necessary to improve drainage of the sinuses.

## The Toddler Period

Language development is almost always delayed in boys with FXS. Normal language milestones include approximately six words by 16 months, two-word phrases by 18 months, and three-word phrases by 24 months (Hagerman 1995). In general, young boys with FXS are not talking by 2 years of age, and this is often the first sign of developmental problems. Because otitis media infections are so common in FXS, the language delay is often blamed on recurrent otitis media and associated conductive hearing loss. If language delays, articulation problems, or unusual characteristics such as cluttering, echolalia, stuttering, or perseveration develop, referral to a speech and language pathologist for a thorough evaluation and individual therapy is appropriate (chap. 10). The therapist can also develop a home program to enhance language stimulation.

Formal developmental testing allows the physician to monitor progress and focus on areas of delay. Overall development in FXS progresses at approximately half the rate expected for typically developing children (Bailey et al. 1998). Motor problems, sensory integration deficits, and hypotonia are common among children with FXS and can be addressed by the OT (chap. 10).

Behavioral difficulties often noted in the second and third years include excessive tantrums, eating problems, and sleeping difficulties. Maintaining consistency in routines, facilitating transitions, avoiding circumstances that are overwhelming in sensory input, and helping a child with calming routines are therapy techniques outlined in chapters 9 and 10. Basic principles of child rearing and discipline, such as reinforcing good behavior and ignoring or timing out negative behavior, can be discussed in detail with parents. Negative behavior cycles can develop at home, which involve negative attention for bad behavior and no reinforcement for appropriate behavior, both of which are counterproductive. If problems develop, early referral to a psychologist who can teach appropriate behavior modification techniques to the parents is essential.

Usually eye contact is good during the first year of life in infants with FXS. However, an increase in sensitivity to eye contact gradually develops by the second to the third year, and it is often associated with initial shyness and social anxiety. Although most boys with FXS warm up to social interaction and are considered friendly, approximately 15–38% will maintain more severe social deficits and will be diagnosed with autism (see chap. 1 for detailed discussion). For these individuals a more intensive preschool program with a focus on treating deficits related to autism is appropriate (Rogers and Lewis 1989; Rogers et al. 2000).

Pharmacotherapy, such as methylphenidate, is typically most helpful for the school-aged child, and it is used for impulsivity and attentional problems and not primarily for behavioral control. However, when episodes of outburst behavior, tantrums, or aggression are severe, clonidine can be cautiously used for the child who is at least three years old, as described below. Dextroamphetamine or methylphenidate in low doses has also been helpful for preschool children with severe symptoms of attention deficit hyperactivity disorder (ADHD). Many families have associated folic acid therapy with improvement in attention, language development, and mood lability during early childhood, as reviewed below. Folic acid therapy may be started during infancy or early childhood, unlike stimulants.

## The Preschool Period

Sensorimotor integration therapy by an OT can improve motor planning, motor coordination, joint stability, and coordination of visual, auditory, and tactile information into a motor output. The OT can be particularly helpful in teaching calming techniques to the parents, which may control tantrums (chap. 10). Continued language therapy to improve pragmatics, attention, and problem-solving skills in addition to other language deficits is beneficial for boys and girls affected by FXS. Regular preschool experience with normal children is helpful in providing normal role models for the child with FXS.

The physician must be vigilant about taking a history for possible seizures, which occur in approximately 15–20% of children with FXS. The type of seizure may include absence episodes, partial motor, generalized (grand mal), or partial complex seizures, as described in chapter 1. If such a history is obtained, an electroencephalogram (EEG) that includes both waking and sleeping states should be done. Pharmacotherapy for seizures is described below.

An ophthalmologic examination is recommended by four years of age or earlier because strabismus or other difficulties including ptosis, nystagmus, myopia, or hyperopia may occur in children with FXS (chap. 1). An obvious visual defect requires referral to an ophthalmologist as soon as it is noticeable.

Delays in toilet training are common in young children with FXS. The attention deficits and the sensorimotor integration problems add to toileting difficulties. An approach to toilet training is presented in appendix 4, and Luxem and Christopherson (1994) provide an excellent review of behavioral approaches to toilet training. Consistent use of positive behavior reinforcement and the use of a music video like the one developed by Duke University (1-800-23POTTY) are usually helpful. The average age for successful toilet training in males with FXS is between five and six years and for females it is by four years (Fragile X Society 1995).

## The School-Age Period

The physician can ensure that appropriate special education is provided for the school-aged child, including speech and language therapy and OT. As described in chapters 10 and 11, such support continues to be essential for sensory integration and motor and language development. If this therapy is not provided through the school, the family may need guidance in finding private therapy. Inclusion or mainstreaming into the regular classroom is recommended whenever possible so that the child will have models of normal behavior in the classroom and will learn appropriate social skills. The regular classroom assignments can be modified by an educational aide or special education teacher, so that the child with FXS can complete an appropriate amount of work without excessive frustration (Spiridigliozzi et al. 1994; chap. 11). Although inclusion is beneficial for the child with FXS, it should take place in addition to individual therapy in language and motor areas and support from the special education teacher. Often an aide is needed in a regular classroom for the child with FXS to modify work and support good behavior. Creativity, flexibility, and innovation are the key features for creating an educational environment that enhances the learning strengths and remediates the disabilities of the child with FXS (Schopmeyer and Lowe 1992; Braden 2000a, 2000b; chap. 11).

The assessment and treatment of attentional problems and hyperactivity are important components of the educational program for the young school-aged child. Successful treatment is multimodal, including behavior management, structure in the classroom, and individual therapy (Dykens et al. 1994; Keogh 1992; Wilson et al. 1994; chap. 9). In addition, medication to improve attention and reduce impulsivity and hyperactivity is often helpful in patients with ADHD, with or without FXS (MTA 1999a, 1999b; Hagerman et al. 1988). For evaluation of possible ADHD, a detailed history should be taken and questionnaires, such as the Conners (Conners 1973), can be given to the parent and teacher (Murphy and Hagerman 1992). For a thorough list and a review of a variety of ADHD behavior checklists, see Barkley (1995, 1997, 1998). In the clinical assessment of the child, behavior can be monitored during play and during tasks that require concentration (Hagerman 1984).

Further signs of connective tissue dysplasia may be evident at this age, including scoliosis, flat feet, hernias, and a cardiac murmur. Mitral valve prolapse (MVP) may be manifested by a click or an early systolic murmur and occurs in approximately 50% of adult males with FXS. On rare occasions, the MVP may be severe and a holosystolic murmur secondary to mitral regurgitation is heard. If evidence of MVP is detected on physical examination (a click or a murmur), further evaluation by a cardiologist, including an echocardiogram, is necessary. If the MVP is confirmed, prophylaxis for subacute bacterial endocarditis (SBE) is recommended for dental procedures or surgery that may be contaminated by endogenous bacteria (Durack 1995). If scoliosis is present, baseline films of the total spine should be performed with careful follow-up. Referral to an orthopedist is important because progression of the scoliosis may require treatment such as bracing well before puberty.

Enuresis (bedwetting) is a common problem in FXS. Although medication, particularly imipramine, can be helpful, as described below, other interventions should be tried first (Schmitt 1995; Moffatt 1997; von Gontard 1998). Decreasing fluids after dinner, urination at bedtime, waking the child to urinate again when the parents go to bed, building bladder musculature and size by intermittently stopping urine flow, and reinforcing the urination of larger and larger volumes can be helpful. However, further intervention is often necessary, and a trial of an alarm may be successful. Alarms are available and they include (1) the Potty Pager, a vibrating alarm from Ideas for Living in Boulder, Colorado, 1-800-497-6573; (2) Nytone alarm, a clip-on wet alarm from Nytone Medical Products, Salt Lake City, Utah, 1-801-973-4090; and (3) Wet-stop alarm with Velcro fasteners from Palco Labs in Santa Cruz, California, 1-800-346-4488. Most of these devices are $50 to $60. An alternative medication is desmopressin (DDAVP), a synthetic vasopressin analog, which is used nasally at bedtime. Although this has not been studied in FXS specifically, the response rate in enuretic children is 30–40% (Thompson and Rey 1995).

In our clinical experience we have seen 4 cases of significant and persistent ureteral reflux in approximately 350 children with FXS. In 3 cases this has led to nephrectomy because of renal complications, including hypertension. Perhaps the connective tissue dysplasia in FXS facilitates the ureteral dilation secondary to reflux. Severe reflux subsequently causes renal damage. Children with recurrent urinary infections and reflux should therefore be followed closely radiographically and treated aggressively to avoid kidney damage. Further studies regarding connective tissue abnormalities in the urinary system are needed in FXS.

Families who have ongoing difficulties with behavior in their child should be referred to a child psychologist with expertise in treating children with developmental disabilities. This therapist can provide ongoing support for the family and child with behavior modification programs and counseling (chap. 9).

## Early Adolescence

Often hyperactivity decreases before or during puberty, but attention problems usually persist into adulthood in boys with FXS (Einfeld et al. 1999). Aggressive behavior may be a problem for some boys, and episodic violent outbursts are particularly common during and after puberty, perhaps related to the increase in testosterone during puberty (Constantino 1995; Einfeld et al. 1999). Aggression can be associated with CNS dysfunction in the hypothalamus, orbital prefrontal cortex, and amygdaloid complex (Weiger and Bear 1988; Habib et al. 2000), and all of these brain areas are affected by the absence of the *FMR1* protein (FMRP) (Binstock 1995; Reiss et al. 1995; chap. 1). Treatment involves many of the same interventions mentioned at earlier ages, including calming techniques and individual counseling, as well as behavior management and perhaps use of visual imagery to calm behavior (Brown et al. 1991; Brown 1995; chap. 9). Bregman (1991) summarized the goals of counseling in individuals with developmental disabilities. The goals and treatment issues include increasing self-esteem, helping with emancipation from parents or caregivers, finding adaptive ways to cope with anger or social stigmatization, understanding one's cognitive limitations, and planning for independent or semi-independent living when possible. Monitoring the environment to avoid overwhelming stimuli and facilitating transitions are also helpful (chap. 10). Medical intervention with pharmacotherapy (as described below) may work synergistically with these other interventions (chap. 9).

Females with FXS usually have less severe hyperactivity compared to the males, but other ADHD symptoms including impulsivity and a short attention span are a problem for many (chaps. 1 and 9). Increasing problems with mood lability are noticeable as girls move into puberty. Frequent crying spells for no reason, verbal outbursts, or tantrums may occur around the menstrual period and may be labeled as premenstrual syndrome (PMS). When these problems are severe, use of a serotonin agent that helps to stabilize the mood during hormonal changes is often helpful, as described below (Steiner et al. 1995).

Testicular volume normally increases during the early stages of puberty, but in boys with FXS this increase is usually quite dramatic, leading to macroorchidism (enlarged testicles). During and after puberty, macroorchidism is represented by a testicular volume of >30 ml bilaterally. These changes are typical for FXS, and they do not require intervention. Lachiewicz and Dawson (1994) reported that the testicular volume begins to increase significantly in boys with FXS by 8 or 9 years of age, which is before pubic hair develops. Fryns (1994) reported 3 cases of massive hydrocele in 3 males with FXS ages 15, 16, and 19 years. The author postulated that males with FXS may be predisposed to hydrocele formation because of the large volume increase of the testicle during puberty. This problem could also be related to a connective tissue dysplasia, as are hernias.

The physician may be consulted by a teacher or psychologist concerning an IQ decrease in the early adolescent boy with FXS. A decrease in IQ is common in the majority of boys and girls with FXS (Wright-Talamante et al. 1996; chap. 6). Since it is commonly seen, a more detailed neurologic workup is usually not indicated. Problems that may interfere with learning, however, such as subtle seizures or absence episodes, significant attentional problems, and emotional or behavioral difficulties, must be identified and treated to optimize the cognitive development of children with FXS.

## Late Adolescence

The problems at this stage are an extension of many issues discussed in the previous sections. The transition to adulthood is difficult for all individuals but particularly so for individuals with severe learning disabilities or with mental retardation. Usually an adult program for individuals with developmental disabilities provides minimal to more extensive supervision so that the adult with FXS can live in an apartment setting and perform a job each day. Daily living skills are taught in school and in most adult programs. Some adult males learn how to drive, but the majority learn to use public transportation to travel to jobs or visit family and friends. Vocational training is important for utilizing cognitive abilities most optimally at work, and this training should be started in high school (Bodine et al. 2001; chap. 10). Wiegers et al. (1993) demonstrated that adaptive behaviors in FXS continue to improve even into adulthood, with particular strengths in daily-living skills. The physician can provide ongoing support for programming in the vocational area. Behavior problems in the workplace should be discussed with the patient's physician and therapist.

The stress of the transition from childhood to adulthood often intensifies emotional or behavioral problems in males or females with FXS. Individual counseling can be very helpful to the adolescent or young adult, particularly regarding sexuality issues and problems associated with separation from family (Brown et al. 1991; chap. 11).

Aggressive behavior is a common problem in adolescence and adulthood, and it requires a thorough medical and environmental assessment. Medical problems, such as psychomotor seizures, may precipitate aggressive behavior, and anticonvulsant therapy is often helpful, as described below. Various environmental stressors may also precipitate an outburst, including overstimulating situations, crowding, transitions, physical discomfort, staff changes, moves, death of a family member, and family conflict. Possible problems must be assessed and changes made to create an appropriate environment. Often a workplace without excessive stimuli and distractions or a living situation without disruptive roommates makes a significant difference in the frequency of aggressive outbursts. Additionally, a program of behavior management may include tokens for good behavior and calming techniques (chaps. 9 and 11). Outbursts may also occur when a male with FXS is around a female staff member or client in whom he is interested sexually, but the feelings may not be mutual. The issue of sexual frustration is probably more common than we realize, and it is treated most effectively in counseling. Medications, particularly serotonin agents as described in the next section, may work synergistically with behavior and environmental management to help some patients control aggressive behavior (Stewart et al. 1990). Serotonin agents probably work to improve aggression by decreasing anxiety and irritability. Often, however, a mood stabilizer or an atypical antipsychotic is needed to treat severe aggression if other medications are not helpful (Ruedrich et al. 1999; Hellings 1999; Hagerman 1999b). Medical studies outside the fragile X field suggest that aggression associated with sexual obsessions, deviant sexual behavior, or severe paraphilia usually responds to a long-acting analog of gonadotropin-releasing hormone, such as triptorelin, if serotonin agents or other interventions described below are not successful (Rosler and Witztum 1998). However, there are no controlled studies regarding the treatment of aggression in FXS; actually very little controlled work has been done regarding treatment of any behavioral problem in FXS. Therefore, the information regarding medications described in the following segment includes studies that have been done in the normal population or in children or adults with developmental disabilities.

Periodic physical examinations to monitor cardiovascular parameters including blood pressure, growth parameters, weight changes, and neurologic findings that may be influenced by medication are recommended. Health maintenance also includes an ongoing vigilance for connective tissue problems such as hernias, joint dislocations, scoliosis, and MVP besides behavior and developmental problems (American Academy of Pediatrics 1996; Hagerman 1997).

## Pharmacotherapy

### The Treatment of Seizures and Mood Instability

Approximately 15–20% of males with FXS have seizures; therefore, the medical history should always include questions concerning possible seizures (Musumeci et al. 1999). Although many seizures are grand mal or generalized tonic-clonic events, other episodes may be partial complex or partial motor seizures with subtle jerking of the face or hand associated with staring, sensory sensations, or guttural sounds. These episodes may be difficult to recognize as seizures, and careful questioning is necessary. Abruptly violent episodes that are not precipitated by environmental stimuli may be temporal lobe or partial complex seizures. If there are clinical questions about the possibility of seizures, an EEG is warranted (chap. 1).

The majority of males with FXS and seizures have a benign variety with rolandic spikes, and these patients usually respond well to anticonvulsants (Wisniewski et al. 1991; Musumeci et al. 1999). Carbamazepine (Tegretol) is the most commonly used anticonvulsant in FXS, perhaps because it has a beneficial behavioral effect in addition to the anticonvulsant effect. Carbamazepine is an iminostilbine with a tricyclic structure unique among anticonvulsants. It is the drug of choice for partial motor, partial complex, and secondary generalized tonic-clonic seizures. It is usually well tolerated, but up to 30% of individuals may experience sedation, which is usually transient. The dosage is gradually increased from a starting dosage of 10 mg/kg/day to a maintenance dosage of 20–40 mg/kg/day. Carbamazepine is usually given two or three times a day, and side effects may rarely include a rash, hyponatremia, hematopoietic alterations, and liver toxicity. A benign transient neutropenia occurs in up to 20%, but it rarely requires discontinuation of the medication (Dodson 1989). Serious severe hematologic problems such as agranulocytosis are very rare (Pellock 1987). An occasional patient will develop behavioral problems such as hyperactivity. Concurrent treatment with macrolide antibiotics (including erythromycin), cimetidine, propoxyphene, isoniazid, fluoxetine, and paroxetine can interfere with the metabolism of carbamazepine, causing an increase in the serum levels and possible development of symptoms of toxicity, including nausea, vomiting, ataxia, lethargy, and diplopia (Pippenger 1987).

In approximately 3% of patients treated with carbamazepine, a hypersensitivity reaction may be seen within 2 to 4 weeks of initiation of the medication. This presents with fever and a cutaneous eruption, sometimes like erythema multiforme (Bellman et al. 1995). Patients who are started on carbamazepine should be told to discontinue the medication if a rash develops. Some patients may require treatment with steroids if the hypersensitivity syndrome does not disappear after carbamazepine is discontinued.

Carbamazepine is helpful for behavioral and psychiatric disorders in both retarded and nonretarded patients (Berkheimer et al. 1985; Evans and Gualtieri 1985). Problems including episodic dyscontrol, violent outbursts, hyperactivity, and self-injurious behavior may respond to carbamazepine in those with or without EEG abnormalities or seizures (Reid et al. 1981; Langee 1989). Although some patients may respond to the anticonvulsant effect (i.e., the EEG abnormalities that may have precipitated the outburst are improved), there is also a direct effect on behavior, which includes stabilization of the mood (Ryan et al. 1999; Kowatch et al. 2000).

No controlled studies of the effect of carbamazepine on behavior problems in FXS have been carried out. Gualtieri (1992) reported anecdotally that carbamazepine was helpful for behavior problems resulting from mood instability in 8 or 9 patients with FXS. Carbamazepine may also be used with a variety of other medications, including stimulants and antidepressants described below. A study by Langee (1989) showed improvement in 39% of 76 mentally retarded institutionalized males with behavior problems (usually aggression or episodic dyscontrol) when treated with carbamazepine. This is a medication, therefore, that should be considered in violent or significantly aggressive males with FXS, particularly those with EEG findings of spike wave discharges or those with significant mood instability.

Valproic acid or divalproex (Depakote) is an effective anticonvulsant for absence episodes and major motor seizures, and it is probably effective for partial motor seizures. It may be particularly effective when bilateral and multifocal spikes are present in the EEG. Its mechanism of action includes the propensity to increase levels of gamma-aminobutyric acid (GABA) and decrease dopamine turnover and $N$-methyl-D-aspartate-mediated depolarization (Hellings 1999; Keck et al. 1998). Valproate is also an excellent mood stabilizer and is superior to lithium for mixed, chronic, or atypical forms of bipolar disorder, even in children (Kowatch et al. 2000; Hellings 1999; Bowden et al. 1994; Swann et al. 1997). It has also been successfully used to treat aggression in patients with FXS and in patients with autism (Hagerman 1999a, 1999b; Davis et al. 2000; Kastner et al. 1993). Although Hellings (1999) reported that blood levels of 75–100 micrograms/dl produce greater behavioral improvement than levels of less than 75 in children with autism or pervasive development disorder (PDD), the dose should be started at 10 mg/kg/day and gradually increased to 20–30 mg/kg/day (McElroy and Weller 1997). The side effects of valproic acid include appetite changes, usually weight gain, thrombocytopenia, neutropenia, sedation, ataxia, fine tremor and hair thinning. Stomachaches can be avoided by taking valproic acid after meals. The most serious side effects are hepatic toxicity, pancreatitis, and cholecystitis (Buzan et al. 1995). Hepatic failure can occur, with the greatest risk (1 in 500) in young patients treated with multiple drugs (Dreifuss and Langer 1987).

Monitoring of valproate therapy includes complete blood count, platelet level, hepatic enzymes, electrolytes, and blood level of valproate. Occasionally, blood levels may need to be cautiously increased to 125 micrograms/dl to control behavior or seizures, but side effects must be carefully monitored (McElroy and Weller 1997). A report links the development of polycystic ovarian disease with long-term use of valproate in women (Isojarvi et al. 1993). This association requires further study and cautious use of valproate in girls with careful follow-up, particularly regarding the menstrual history.

In the treatment of mood instability, a second mood stabilizer is often necessary (Kowatch et al. 2000). Often an atypical antipsychotic is utilized as described below. Lithium carbonate has a long history of use in treatment of bipolar disorder (Kafantaris 1995), aggression in children with conduct disorder (Campbell et al. 1995), or behavior problems in those with mental retardation (Dale 1980; Gadow and Poling 1988). Although anecdotal evidence suggests that it is also effective in patients with FXS (Hagerman 1996), there are no controlled studies using lithium for this syndrome. It is not the first drug of choice for stabilizing mood because of the need for careful monitoring of kidney function and blood levels and the risk of diabetes insipidus with long-term use. However, it is a useful medication that is often effective when other medications do not control aggression or mood instability.

A group of new anticonvulsants can be helpful for adjunctive seizure control and for mood stabilization (Bowley and Kerr 2000). Gabapentin (Neurontin) can be used to augment seizure control, and it works well with valproate or carbamazepine. It has also shown efficacy in augmenting treatment for bipolar disorder and schizoaffective disorder (Bennett et al. 1997; Hellings 1999), so it was considered likely to be helpful in treatment of mood instability in FXS. However, we have not seen beneficial effects in either children or adults with FXS, with only 1 exception in 10 patients treated with gabapentin. Typically, patients have become more irritable, with an increase in outburst behavior at relatively low doses (100–500 mg/day).

Lamotrigine (Lamictal) has been approved to treat partial and secondary generalized seizures, and it inhibits the release of excitatory neurotransmitters such as glutamate and aspartate (Post et al. 1998). Efficacy has been demonstrated in treating bipolar disorder, but 5–10% of patients may experience a maculopapular rash, which can progress to a Stevens-Johnson syndrome (Hellings 1999). Use with valproate can exacerbate this side effect. Dosing in children is 0.5 mg/kg/day for two weeks with a gradual increase to 2–5 mg/kg/day with twice-daily dosing and a careful look at side effects (McElroy and Weller 1997). The adult dosing is 25 mg daily for two weeks, then 25 mg twice a day for two weeks, with a gradual increase if needed to a maximum of 500 mg/day (Hellings 1999).

Topiramate (Topamax), tiagabine (Gabitril), and vigabatrin (Sabril) are three additional new anticonvulsants that also seem to have mood-stabilizing effects and have shown efficacy in seizure control in patients with mental retardation (Bowley and Kerr 2000; Alvarez et al. 1998). However, experience in patients with FXS is limited to the rare patient whose seizures are not well controlled with valproate or carbamazepine.

Although phenobarbital is effective for controlling seizures, it commonly increases hyperactivity and it is therefore not recommended for use in patients with FXS or other developmental disabilities. Primidone (Mysoline) may also exacerbate hyperactivity because it is metabolized to phenobarbital.

Phenytoin (Dilantin) is effective for all types of partial seizures, generalized tonic clonic seizures, and status epilepticus. Side effects include gingival hyperplasia, hirsutism, acute cerebellar ataxia, and idiosyncratic allergic reactions. It can also lower serum folic acid levels, which is of concern in patients with FXS because behavioral improvements can be seen with high serum folic acid levels (Hagerman et al. 1986; Turk 1992). There is animal evidence that long-term use of phenytoin is associated with cerebellar atrophy, and phenytoin has the most significant cognitive effects, including memory and performance deficits, of the commonly used anticonvulsants (Trimble 1987). It is, therefore, not the drug of choice for seizures, but it is certainly an effective alternative drug if carbamazepine or valproic acid are not beneficial. If possible, serum folic acid levels should be brought to the normal range in individuals treated with phenytoin to avoid possible deleterious long-term effects of a lowered folic acid level in FXS.

The use of medications in children with FXS often poses a problem if the child cannot swallow a capsule or pill. Although some medications come in liquid form, most do not. Typical pill-taking training programs were reviewed by Pelco et al. (1987); they include modeling or demonstration and contingent reinforcers. Babbitt et al. (1991) described a behavioral training program for swallowing capsules designed for children with developmental delays that begins with swallowing oblong cake decorations (sprinkles) and then moves to Tic Tacs and on to increasing sizes of gelatin capsules.

## The Treatment of Attention Deficit Hyperactivity Disorder

Attention deficits with or without hyperactivity are significant problems for almost all young males with FXS and for many females who are intellectually affected by FXS (chap. 1). Treatment for these problems includes behavioral approaches, structure in the environment with positive reinforcement, as well as individual therapies, such as language therapy, occupational therapy, and cognitive behavior therapy (see chaps. 9, 10, and 11). Medication can also significantly improve attention, concentration, impulsivity, and hyperactivity. A variety of medications improve ADHD symptoms, but the first-line medications for attentional problems are the CNS stimulants.

## CNS Stimulants

Stimulants have been used to treat ADHD symptoms since Bradley's report of benzedrine's effectiveness in 1937. A dramatic increase in the use of stimulants occurred in the 1950s associated with the development of other psychotropic medications, including antipsychotics and antidepressants. Although stimulant medication is commonly used for intellectually normal children with ADHD, stimulant use in children with cognitive deficits has emerged over the last decade as well-designed studies demonstrating efficacy have been published (Handen et al. 1990, 1992, 1994, 1996, 2000; Mayes et al. 1994; Aman et al. 1991a, 1991b; Gillberg et al. 1997). Although children with mild and moderate mental retardation and ADHD were included in these studies, there is evidence that children with severe mental retardation do not usually respond to stimulants (Aman 1982). Aman et al. (1991b) found that IQ correlated significantly with response to methylphenidate and that an IQ below 45 was associated with a poor response.

Although methylphenidate has demonstrated efficacy (Barkley et al. 1991; MTA 1999a, 1999b), there is evidence that children with mental retardation have an increased number of side effects with methylphenidate, compared to normal-IQ children with ADHD. These side effects are worse at higher doses, and they include an increase in irritability, a decrease in verbalizations, social withdrawal, or an increase in stereotypic behavior, such as finger picking (Gadow and Pomeroy 1990; Handen et al. 1991; Arnold 1993; Gadow et al. 1992; Handen et al. 2000).

The two stimulants that are most commonly used are methylphenidate (Ritalin) and dextroamphetamine (Dexedrine; Adderall). Adderall is a mixture of four different dextro- and levoamphetamine salts that have a longer half-life than methylphenidate and less of a rebound when the medication wears off (Swanson et al. 1998; Pelham et al. 1999). Controlled studies have demonstrated efficacy in treatment of ADHD, and once-a-day dosing with Adderall is comparable to twice-a-day dosing with short-acting methylphenidate (Manos et al. 1999; Pliszka et al. 1996).

Experience in FXS is limited and includes a double-blind crossover trial of methylphenidate and dextroamphetamine compared to placebo in 15 prepubertal boys with FXS (Hagerman et al. 1988). Ten were clinical responders to stimulants with improvements in attention span and socialization skills. Seven were improved on methylphenidate, and two were improved on dextroamphetamine. A subsequent trial of Adderall in children with FXS demonstrated only a 50% response rate because of side effects, including irritability and an increase in anxiety (Riley et al. 2000). Pemoline (Cylert) is an alternative long-acting stimulant medication (fig. 8.1) and has been associated with less irritability and rebound than has methylphenidate or dextroamphetamine in anecdotal experience with FXS (Hagerman 1996), but reports of rare liver failure, which appears to be an autoimmune process, have curtailed its use (Rosh et al. 1998).

Recently, a new long-acting methylphenidate preparation, Concerta, available in 18-mg, 36-mg, and 54-mg tablets, has been released. It is typically taken once per day in the morning with a unique slow-release system. In our experience, Concerta has been effective for children with FXS and ADHD with fewer side effects, such as irritability or rebound in the late afternoon, compared to short-acting methylphenidate. All stimulants work by stimulating dopaminergic and norepinephrine pathways (Raskin et al. 1984). They seem to stimulate inhibitory systems, allowing children to inhibit their responses to extraneous stimuli and stay focused on the tasks at hand (Barkley 1997; Solanto 1998; Hagerman et al. 2001). Improved inhibition can also decrease impulsivity and

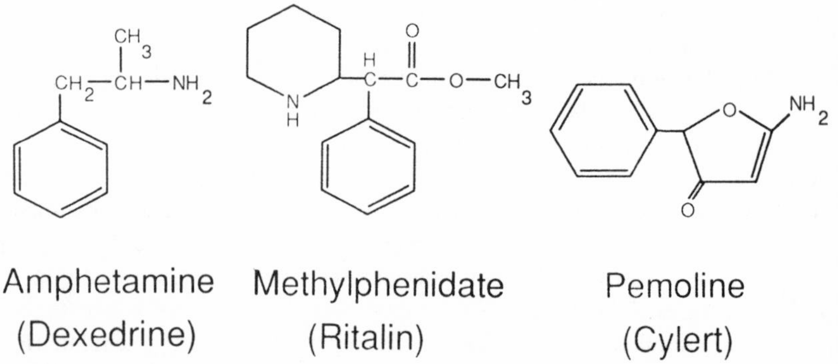

Amphetamine    Methylphenidate         Pemoline
(Dexedrine)        (Ritalin)                (Cylert)

**Fig. 8.1.** Stimulant medications commonly used to treat ADHD. Brand names are in parentheses.

hyperactivity. The overall effect is a child who is in better control of attention, impulsivity, and hyperactivity. Auditory processing, reaction time, and even sensory integration and visual motor coordination are improved (DuPaul and Barkley 1990; Jerome 1995; Barkley 1997). Douglas et al. (1986) also showed academic improvements, particularly in the accuracy and efficiency of academic tests in children with a normal IQ and ADHD who are treated with stimulants.

The side effects of stimulant medication include appetite suppression with possible weight loss, which, when excessive, can decrease height growth. The cardiovascular system is also stimulated, including heart rate and blood pressure. Children on stimulant medication should be seen by their physicians at least every four to six months to monitor height, weight, and cardiovascular parameters. If weight is maintained at the pretreatment percentile and has a steady normal increase with time, height growth does not decline. In approximately 10% of ADHD cases, stimulants may exacerbate an underlying tic disorder because of dopaminergic stimulation (Lipkin et al. 1994).

Stimulants are commonly used in boys with FXS even before the diagnosis is made. In general, children with FXS are sensitive to stimulants, and their mood often becomes brittle, with an increase in outbursts at higher doses. For children up to five years old, a starting dose would be 2.5 mg of methylphenidate or dextroamphetamine twice a day. For children older than five years, a methylphenidate dose of 0.2–0.3 mg/kg/dose is usually sufficient. Higher doses of stimulants may cause a decrease in verbalizations (Gadow et al. 1995) or an increase in perseverations (Dyme et al. 1982), both of which are counterproductive in children with FXS. An occasional male with FXS may develop motor tics on stimulants, and then an alternative medication such as clonidine should be considered.

Since ADHD symptoms in children with FXS usually begin in the preschool period, families are often ready to start medication treatment before the child is five years of age. Although stimulants can be efficacious under five years in children with ADHD (Rappley et al. 1999), our experience in preschoolers with FXS has shown that the majority can become irritable with exacerbation of behavioral problems so it is suggested that other medications, such as clonidine or guanfacine (described below), be tried first. In a recent survey of medication use in 177 children between 5 and 18 years with FXS, 39% of boys and 19% of girls were treated with methylphenidate; 22% of boys and girls were treated with Adderall; 2% of boys and 3% of girls were treated with Dexedrine (Amaria et al. 2001). Similar percentages were reported for more than 100 children with FXS treated in Chicago (Berry-Kravis 2000).

A novel treatment for ADHD in FXS, the use of L-acetylcarnitine, was reported by Torrioli et al. (1999) in Italy, where stimulants are difficult to obtain. They treated 20 boys with FXS between the ages of 6 and 13 years with either 50 mg of L-acetylcarnitine or placebo twice a day and found a significant improvement in ADHD behavior by parent rating, but not by teacher rating, in those treated with L-acetylcarnitine. There was no change in IQ or in other neurocognitive testing. This medication is an acetyl derivative of carnitine, and in vitro it will inhibit the cytogenetic expression of the fragile site. This preliminary work deserves further study in a larger number of patients with FXS.

Alternative treatments for ADHD include the use of mixed noradrenergic-serotonin reuptake inhibitors such as venlafaxine (Effexor) and nefazodone (Serzone). These medications hold promise for treatment of ADHD in children and adolescents with FXS. Although controlled studies are not available, anecdotal experience suggests that venlafaxine is often helpful for ADHD in patients with FXS. Venlafaxine has been efficacious in child and adult studies for treatment of ADHD and for autism combined with ADHD (Olvera et al. 1996; Findling et al. 1996b; Findling and Dogin 1998; Hollander et al. 2000). As with most medication regimens described here, the combined use of these agents and psychotherapy, together, leads to improved outcome compared to medication alone (Keller et al. 2000).

Other alternative treatments of ADHD in children with FXS include the use of amantadine. Amantadine (Symmetrel), an antiviral agent, is also a dopaminergic agent. It can be helpful for aggressive behavior and agitation in some individuals with developmental disabilities. Formal studies have been performed only on head-injured patients (Gualtieri et al. 1989) and in persons with hyperactivity and mental retardation, with a response rate of approximately 40% (Gualtieri 1990). Anecdotal reports and our experience suggest that amantadine

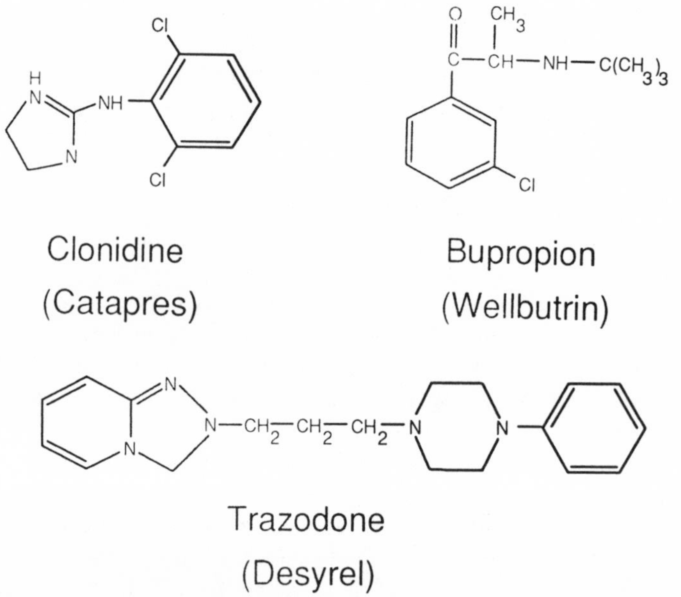

Clonidine
(Catapres)

Bupropion
(Wellbutrin)

Trazodone
(Desyrel)

**Fig. 8.2.** Clonidine and bupropion have been used to treat ADHD, and trazodone has been used to treat sleep disturbances. Brand names are in parentheses.

can be helpful for the treatment of ADHD in children with FXS (Gualtieri 1992).

Bupropion (Wellbutrin) (fig. 8.2) is an antidepressant that has shown efficacy in treatment of ADHD in young patients in controlled trials (Barrickman et al. 1995; Conners et al. 1996), but it carries a significant risk of seizures, particularly for patients with FXS who are predisposed to seizures (chap. 1). This medication is therefore not a drug of choice for patients with FXS (Tranfaglia 2000).

Tricyclics are antidepressant medications with known efficacy in the treatment of ADHD primarily because the reuptake of norepinephrine is blocked (Pliszka et al. 1996). Among patients with tics and ADHD, desipramine is more effective than clonidine for treatment of both problems (Singer et al. 1995). There has been one published report of the use of a tricyclic, imipramine, in a patient with FXS (Hilton et al. 1991). This patient was a six-year-old boy who had a negative response to methylphenidate, but imipramine improved his hyperactivity, insomnia, and enuresis. Berry-Kravis (2000) found that approximately 50% of children with FXS have improved ADHD symptoms with a tricyclic, usually imipramine, but it is typically tried only after failure on a stimulant.

The cardiovascular side effects, specifically prolongation of conduction, are the main impediment to use, and several cases of unexplained sudden death have been reported with desipramine (Riddle et al. 1993). Cardiovascular monitoring with electrocardiograms (EKGs) is necessary with tricyclics, as outlined by Gutgesell et al. (1999). A report by Mezzacappa et al. (1998) showed that tricyclics decrease vagal tone, which is already reduced in children with FXS compared to controls (Boccia and Roberts 2000).

Last, buspirone (Buspar), an anxiolytic agent that is a partial agonist at 5HT1A serotonin receptors in addition to stimulating dopamine and alpha-adrenergic systems, has been shown to be helpful in an open trial for treatment of ADHD (Malhotra and Santosh 1998). It has also been shown to be effective in treatment of anxiety and irritability in children with PDD or autism (reviewed by Buitelaar et al. 1998). We have not seen efficacy in treatment of ADHD in children with FXS, but buspirone can be helpful in treatment of anxiety, although it does not seem to be as effective as selective serotonin reuptake inhibitors (SSRIs), described below, in our experience.

## Clonidine

Clonidine (Catapres) is an antihypertensive drug (Manheim et al. 1982) that is effective in the treatment of ADHD (Hunt et al. 1985; Steingard et al. 1993). It has also been used to treat Tourette syndrome by reducing tics, improving hyperactivity, and decreasing obsessive-compulsive symptoms (Leckman et al. 1985, 1991; Hewlett et al. 1992). Clonidine is an alpha-adrenergic stimulating agent that acts on presynaptic neurons to inhibit norepinephrine activity (fig. 8.2). Hunt et al. (1985) suggested that clonidine may be most beneficial in children with ADHD, who are easily emotionally overwhelmed, are anxious, and have a low frustration tolerance. Clonidine also stimulates growth hormone release (Leckman et al. 1984), and it causes sedation, so it may be helpful in treating the ADHD of children with FXS who have sleep disturbances, motor tics, or hyperarousal (chap. 1).

Leckman (1987) reported improved ADHD symptoms in three males with FXS treated with clonidine. Hagerman et al. (1995) reported a survey of 35 children with FXS who were treated with clonidine. Overall, 63% of the parents said clonidine was very beneficial for their child, 20% said clonidine helped their child a little, 6% said clonidine had no effect, and 11% said their child's behavior was worse on clonidine. Although 89% of the children were taking clonidine for hyperactivity, other problems, including aggression, tantrums, anxiety, and sleep disturbances, were common and were somewhat improved on clonidine. Most of the patients (69%) were also on other medications, including methylphenidate. For instance, in a young boy with FXS, clonidine was used successfully in the afternoon and evening, with methylphenidate in the morning and at lunchtime. Clonidine helped to alleviate the irritability in the late afternoon exacerbated by stimulants, the sleeping problems at bedtime, and the ADHD symptoms at home. Methylphenidate was better at school because a greater degree of concentration was demanded at school compared to home. The use of combined pharmacotherapy is an emerging trend in pediatric psychopharmacology because of the frequency of comorbid disorders and the benefit of a synergistic effect from two medications (Wilens et al. 1995, 1998, 1999).

There have been four sudden deaths reported in children taking clonidine and methylphenidate together (Swanson et al. 1995; Cantwell et al. 1997; Fenichel 1995). Review of the case details demonstrated other causes of death, including an anomalous coronary artery, postnatal cardiac damage, and a grand mal seizure (Wilens et al. 1999; Hagerman 1996; Dech 1999). However, these reports led to the recommendation of cardiac monitoring with an EKG when clonidine or guanfacine is used, particularly in patients with FXS, because rare cases of sudden death have been reported even when no medication has been used (chap. 1). Clonidine can prolong conduction through the atrioventricular (AV) node, and rare dysarrhythmias have been reported (Dawson et al. 1989; Chandran 1994). The use of clonidine both with and without a stimulant has grown considerably over the last decade, and Wilens et al. (1999) reported that more than 1,200 children have received clonidine and methylphenidate in their two clinics without adverse cardiovascular events. We have also had no cardiac problems in using clonidine and methylphenidate together in more than 50 children with FXS, except for two young children who ate their clonidine patch and were hospitalized (Amaria et al. 2001; Delahunty et al., unpublished manuscript). Kofoed et al. (1999) followed the EKG in 42 children treated with clonidine for ADHD and/or tic disorder, and 30 were also on stimulants. Significant EKG abnormalities were not seen either with clonidine alone or when combined with stimulants.

The side effects of clonidine include sleepiness, which is dose-dependent and usually subsides within two to three weeks after the medication is begun. The dose should be started low at 0.05 mg twice a day to avoid excessive sedation and gradually increased as tolerated over two to three weeks to clinical effectiveness (approximately 4–5 micrograms/kg/day for school-aged children). The sleepiness with clonidine can often be helpful in treating bedtime wakefulness or sleep disturbances in children with ADHD (Wilens et al. 1994; Prince et al. 1996). Clonidine is also marketed in a patch form (Catapres TTS), which comes in three strengths and is effective for treatment of ADHD and tics (Comings et al. 1990). It provides a steady level for five to seven days and can be placed in the mid-back area so the child may not easily remove it. Sedation is less in the patch form compared to the tablet form. However, the patch may be irritating to the skin in approximately 30% of patients. Vancenase AQ double strength nasal spray may be sprayed on the back and allowed to dry before placing the patch to decrease skin irritation (Hagerman et al. 1996). In young children, four to six years of age, the Catapres TTS1 patch may be cut in half or smaller to decrease the dosage (Hagerman et al. 1995). The patch should be avoided in the child under four years, who may eat it and thereby cause a significant overdose, which requires hospitalization. When clonidine is discontinued, the dose should be tapered gradually to avoid a significant increase in blood pressure and severe headaches, which may occur with abrupt withdrawal. When the patch is removed, there is a gradual natural taper of the medication from skin stores.

Guanfacine (Tenex) is chemically related to clonidine, but it has a lower half-life (18 hours vs. 6 hours) and it is less sedating. Hunt et al. (1995) recently reported that guanfacine significantly improved hyperactivity and inattention in 13 children with ADHD. They also mentioned that several patients responded better to a combination of guanfacine and methylphenidate than to either medication alone. Many children with FXS have been successfully treated with guanfacine when the side effects from clonidine, particularly sedation, have been intolerable (Amaria et al. 2001). Guanfacine can also be substituted for clonidine when the child wakes up at 1:00 or 2:00 A.M. after a bedtime dose of clonidine. The longer half-life of guanfacine facilitates a full night of sleep.

## Folic Acid

Folic acid was the first medication reported to be beneficial for individuals with FXS (Lejeune 1982). When added to tissue culture media, folate will decrease cytogenetic expression of the fragile site (Jacky 1996). However, its mechanism of action in the central nervous system seems to be unrelated to its cytogenetic effect. In the CNS folate is involved with methylation and hydroxylation, and both reactions are important in neurotransmitter synthesis and metabolism (Greenblatt et al. 1994). Folate is concentrated in the synaptic regions of CNS neurons (McClain et al. 1975). Levine et al. (1981) speculated that exogenous folate may accelerate dopamine synthesis in nigrostriatal neurons through effects on tyrosine hydroxylase. Preliminary reports from Lejeune (1982) and others (Harpey 1982; Lacassie et al. 1984; Lejeune et al. 1984) anecdotally demonstrated improvement in behavior and development in males with FXS treated with folic acid. Subsequent controlled studies showed mixed results, with some reporting no benefit from folic acid (Rosenblatt et al. 1985; Brown et al. 1986; Froster-Iskenius et al. 1986; Madison et al. 1986; Fisch et al. 1988), whereas others demonstrated improvement with folic acid treatment (Carpenter et al. 1983; Brown et al. 1984; Gustavson et al. 1985; Gillberg et al. 1986; Hagerman et al. 1986; for review see Aman and Kern 1990; Turk 1992; and Greenblatt et al. 1994).

Clearly, not all patients with FXS respond to folic acid, but a significant number of prepubertal boys with FXS are reported by their families to be less hyperactive and to have a better attention span on folate. The cognitive improvements in young boys with FXS reported by Hagerman et al. (1986) seem to be the result of improvement in attention span and concentration, which is consistent with the hypothesized effect on dopamine synthesis (Levine et al. 1981). The effect of folic acid is similar to the response noted with stimulant medication, although the latter usually causes a more dramatic improvement in attention. A rare patient will become more hyperactive on folate, and an occasional adult with FXS will have more outbursts on folate. It is, therefore, not recommended for adult patients, who are less frequently plagued by hyperactivity.

Improvements in speech, language, and motor coordination are also occasionally reported by parents when their children are taking folic acid (Hagerman et al. 1986; Turk 1992). The effectiveness of folic acid has been difficult to document in controlled studies; if a child responds to folate, however, parents usually insist on using it. As many parents are adamant about its effectiveness, perhaps future studies should focus on identifying the subgroup of children with FXS who respond. There is no evidence for a metabolic defect in folate metabolism in FXS (Brøndum-Nielsen et al. 1983; Wang and Erbe 1984). There is one report of a child with FXS who deteriorated behaviorally and developmentally after treatment with trimethoprim, an antibiotic that interferes with the metabolism of folic acid (Hecht and Glover 1983). Therefore, caution should be used in treating patients with FXS with drugs that lower folate levels, including phenytoin.

Folate has been tolerated without significant side effects in dosages as high as 250 mg and 1,000 mg/day (Zettner et al. 1981; Brown et al. 1986). However, Hunter et al. (1970) reported malaise, sleep problems, irritability, and an increased activity level when folate was given to normal, healthy volunteers. Folate has been reported to exacerbate the frequency of seizures in epilepsy (Reynolds 1967), but we have not experienced this problem in patients with FXS and seizures. Folate treatment should be avoided, however, in patients with poorly controlled seizures. Folate may occasionally cause loose stools and can prolong diarrhea in children recovering from gastroenteritis. If diarrhea occurs, the dose of folate should be lowered or discontinued until the diarrhea resolves. We reported vitamin $B_6$ deficiency in males with FXS taking 10 mg of folic acid per day (Hagerman et al. 1986). To avoid this problem, patients should take daily a multiple vitamin with $B_6$ while on folic acid therapy. Folate can also interfere with zinc absorption in the intestine, and serum zinc levels should therefore be monitored at least once a year (Milne et al. 1984).

Folic acid is manufactured only in 1-mg tablets in the United States. A liquid preparation of 5 mg/ml is more convenient and less expensive than the tablet form. Most patients who respond will demonstrate improvement on a dose of 10–50 mg/day. Many pharmacies will prepare the liquid preparation after a special request. Pharmacies can obtain folic acid powder U.S.P. through Tanabe U.S.A., Inc., 7930 Conroy Ct., San Diego, California 92111 (1-619-571-8410) or Mike Jones at Gallipot (1-800-423-6967). The following formula can be used to mix the folic acid solution to a dilution of 5 mg/ml (provided by Rob Rodgers, Pharm.D., at The Children's Hospital in Denver, Colo.): 10 g folic acid, 2,000 ml $H_2O$ (sterile), 15 ml NaOH 20%—add by titration until mixture clarifies in solution. Folic acid solution is sensitive to heat and photodegradation, and it must be refrigerated and protected from light in a covered or brown bottle. A syringe can be used to measure a typical dose of 5 mg or 1 ml twice a day. As folic acid is relatively tasteless, it can be squirted directly in the mouth or added to juice. The dose is usually given twice a day to avoid stomach irritation or diarrhea, which occasionally occurs.

The medical follow-up of patients treated with high-dose folic acid includes a periodic physical and neurologic examination and at least annual blood work including a complete blood count (CBC): serum glutamic-oxaloacetic transaminase (SGOT); blood urea nitrogen (BUN); creatinine; urine analysis; and serum levels of zinc, vitamin $B_6$, and folate. A trial of folic acid therapy should last at least three months because improvements in behavior or attention may not begin until the second month. If folate is helpful, it should be continued, and it can be used together with stimulant medication. At least once every one to two years, the folic acid can be discontinued to assess whether it remains effective. There is some evidence to suggest a mild withdrawal effect in a limited number of patients, characterized by mood lability lasting one to two weeks. This is not uncommon in megavitamin therapy, and it has been described in pyridoxine and ascorbic acid therapy (American Psychiatric Association 1973; Gualtieri et al. 1987).

## Selected Serotonin Reuptake Inhibitors and Treatment of Aggression

Intermittent explosive disorder is common in adolescents and adults with FXS, as described in chapter 1. Episodic and unpredictable aggression was a common reason for institutionalization of men with FXS in the past. Sometimes aggression can be treated successfully with a stimulant if ADHD symptoms are a component of the clinical picture (Bukstein and Kolko 1998). Clonidine can also be helpful in calming down hyperarousal to sensory stimuli (Miller et al. 1999), which is a common problem in FXS and may be linked to aggression. If aggression is associated with an abnormal EEG that has spike-wave discharges, particularly in the temporal region, trial of an anticonvulsant such as carbamazepine or valproic acid is appropriate, as previously discussed. Most commonly, however, aggression is associated with anxiety, which can be treated with a selective serotonin reuptake inhibitor (SSRI) (fig. 8.3).

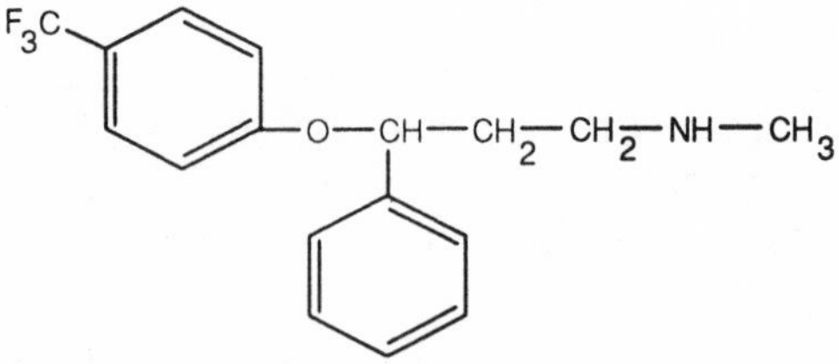

Fluoxetine
(Prozac)

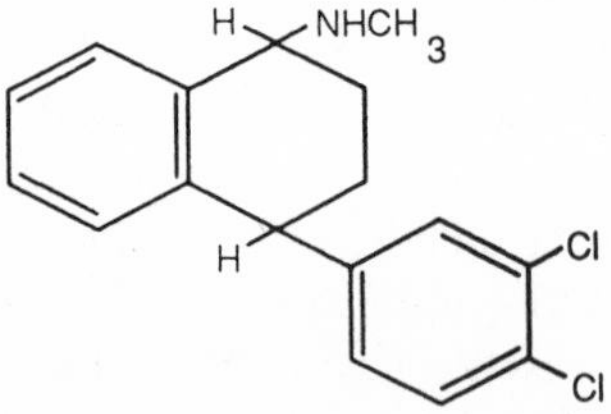

Sertraline
(Zoloft)

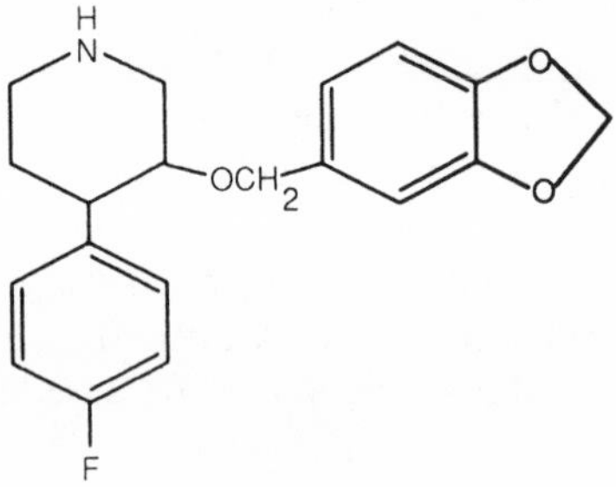

Paroxetine
(Paxil)

**Fig. 8.3.** Three commonly used SSRIs. Brand names are in parentheses.

The first SSRI, fluoxetine (Prozac), became available in the late 1980s. At the time of this writing, five SSRIs are available in the United States: fluoxetine (Prozac), sertraline (Zoloft), fluvoxamine (Luvox), paroxetine (Paxil), and citalopram (Celexa). In both adults and children with normal intellectual function, they effectively treat depression (Rey-Sanchez and Gutierrez-Casares 1997; DeVane and Sallee 1996; Mendels et al. 1999; Ambrosini et al. 1999), anxiety (Birmaher et al. 1994; March et al. 1998; Fairbanks et al. 1997; Lepola et al. 1994), obsessive-compulsive disorder (OCD) (Geller et al. 1995; Rosenberg et al. 1999, 2000; Thomsen 1997), panic disorder and school phobia (Lepola et al. 1996), ADHD (Barrickman et al. 1991), and irritable, difficult temperament (Garland and Weiss 1996). Because of their efficacy for a variety of problems and because of their relative safety compared to tricyclics, they are used by millions of patients worldwide (Kramer 1993).

In individuals with developmental disabilities, SSRIs have been helpful in decreasing obsessive-compulsive behavior (Dech and Budow 1991; Warnock and Kestenbaum 1992; Bodfish and Maddison 1993), self-injurious behavior (Markowitz 1992), autistic behavior (Cook et al. 1992; Hellings et al. 1996; Steingard et al. 1997), emotional lability (Sloan et al. 1992; Selinger et al. 1992), and aggression (Ghaziuddin and Tsai 1991).

In an open trial of fluoxetine in 37 children with autism between the ages of two and seven years, 22 (59%) had a positive response with improvements in behavior, cognition, and social abilities and marked increase in language acquisition (DeLong et al. 1998). The SSRIs block reuptake of serotonin, thereby enhancing levels in the synapse, particularly in the raphe nucleus and upper brain stem. The major ascending serotonin pathways go to the frontal cortex, cingulate cortex, and other limbic structures that are important for emotions.

The use of fluoxetine in FXS was surveyed by Hagerman et al. (1994). All males and females at our center who were affected by FXS and were prescribed fluoxetine for behavioral or emotional problems were surveyed with a questionnaire to evaluate the benefits and problems associated with the use of fluoxetine. The study of patients included 18 females (6 with the premutation and 10 with the full mutation) and 17 males with FXS (10 with the full mutation and 4 with a mosaic pattern). Overall fluoxetine was helpful in 83% of the females who were treated for depression, mood lability, anxiety, panic attacks, outburst behavior, or obsessive-compulsive symptoms. In the males fluoxetine was helpful in 71%, and it was usually prescribed for physical outbursts or severe verbal outbursts. Five males (29%) did not improve or had worse behavior on fluoxetine. Occasionally an increase in outburst behavior occurred in the males, probably related to the activation effect of fluoxetine. Other side effects included nausea in 12%, insomnia 6%, increased hyperactivity 6%, weight gain 6%, and weight loss in 6% of the males. In the females similar side effects were noted, in addition to one woman who developed hypomania and another woman who experienced suicidal ideation, which was a problem before starting fluoxetine. In general fluoxetine was a very helpful medication for the majority of males and females who were treated. In women with the premutation, fluoxetine decreased obsessive worries, anxiety, and/or depression, and in women with the full mutation fluoxetine improved mood lability and the occasional problem with outburst behavior. In males fluoxetine usually improved physical or verbal outbursts, which are a common problem for the adolescent or adult male with FXS. This study was not a controlled and blinded assessment of the efficacy of fluoxetine in FXS. Instead, this report suggests efficacy and the need for controlled studies.

Although fluoxetine was generally safe and well tolerated (Hagerman et al. 1994), the occasional occurrence of suicidal ideation or the development of hypomania reinforces the need for weekly counseling to monitor a patient's response to the SSRI and to treat emotional problems, such as depression, anxiety, or obsessive-compulsive behavior. Suicidal ideation with fluoxetine has been somewhat sensationalized in the lay press; however, controlled studies have shown suicidal ideation to be less in patients taking fluoxetine (1.2%) compared to tricyclic antidepressants (3.6%) or placebo (2.6%) (Beasley et al. 1991). Fluoxetine and other SSRIs are relatively safe in an overdose in contrast to tricyclics, which can cause fatal arrhythmias. In general SSRIs are relatively nontoxic. They do not cause cardiac or liver problems, and blood levels or EKGs do not need to be monitored. However, fluoxetine and paroxetine are inhibitors of the cytochrome P450 enzyme system, which metabolizes other medications, so that the blood level of other concurrent medications, particularly anticonvulsants, may increase significantly.

Sertraline interferes very little with the P450 system, and citalopram, which is the most recent addition to the SSRIs, has no effect on the P450 system. Citalopram is the most selective for blocking serotonin reuptake of all of the SSRIs, and it has very little effect on reuptake inhibition of norepinephrine (Thomsen 1997). A rare patient may experience extrapyramidal side effects, including an acute dystonic reaction, particularly when SSRIs are used in combination with other medications (Bouchard et al. 1989; Budman et al. 1995).

In adult patients treated with SSRIs, a decrease in libido is a frequent complaint. The use of a serotonin receptor blocker, such as cyproheptadine (Periactin), which is also an antihistamine with anticholinergic properties, can improve the libido when taken on appropriate occasions.

Another approach to the treatment of the sexual dysfunction is to increase dopamine levels either with stimulants on the day of sex or by using buproprion augmentation. Switching to a different antidepressant, such as Serzone or Rimeron, which is associated with less sexual dysfunction may be helpful. Last, use of Viagra in a dose of 50 to 100 mg approximately one hour before intercourse is perhaps the most effective intervention.

When excessive serotonin stimulation occurs, a serotonin syndrome can develop, which includes confusion, diaphoresis, hyperreflexia, ataxia, and myoclonus, and it often occurs when SSRI agents are used together with monoamine oxidase inhibitors (MAOIs) (Lappin and Auchincloss 1994). The combined use of MAOIs and SSRIs can lead to fatal outcomes.

Although SSRIs often help with mood lability, on occasion hypomania or mania may develop with longer term use, particularly if there is a genetic predisposition to bipolar disorder (Sovner and Pary 1993). In patients with FXS, hypomania, mania, or severe agitation develops in 25% who are treated with SSRIs. Although the makers of citalopram have reported the lowest risk for mania in the initial study population, it is unclear whether this medication will have the lowest risk of all SSRIs for these symptoms in patients with FXS. If agitation or an increase in aggressive behavior occurs, then the SSRI dose should be lowered or discontinued (Hagerman 1999a, 1999b). If mood lability or aggression persists, then a mood stabilizer such as valproate, carbamazepine, lithium, or an atypical antipsychotic can be added.

In the report by Hagerman et al. (1994), four males with FXS experienced a significant increase in verbalizations and less social withdrawal on fluoxetine. This may be related to the activation effect of fluoxetine or to a decrease in anxiety, which facilitates social interaction. Such an effect has also been reported in autism (Cook et al. 1992; DeLong et al. 1998). There may also be a direct beneficial effect on language. For example, Kramer (1993) reported a case with improved language skills in an intellectually normal female who was treated for depression. Fluoxetine or fluvoxamine have also been used to treat selective mutism (Black and Uhde 1994; Lafferty and Constantino 1998). This disorder is related to anxiety, and the improvement in language on fluoxetine or fluvoxamine may be related to the antianxiety effects of SSRIs. Anxiety is a significant problem in FXS; we have seen seven cases of selective mutism in girls with FXS, and fluoxetine improved language in one girl in whom it was tried (Hagerman et al. 1999). A novel treatment for selective mutism which may have a synergistic effect with SSRIs is the audio feedforward treatment reported by Blum et al. (1998).

## Antipsychotics

The use of antipsychotic medication has changed dramatically over the last five years with the introduction of atypical antipsychotics that have a lower risk of extrapyramidal symptoms (EPS) and tardive dyskinesias than classical antipsychotics (Findling et al. 1998). EPS include acute dystonic reactions, akathesia or involuntary motor restlessness, and a Parkinsonian syndrome of mask-like facial expression, rigidity in the extremities, and tremor. EPS typically occur in the first few weeks of antipsychotic treatment, whereas tardive dyskinesias (which are rhythmic, repetitive, stereotypic movements, such as lip smacking) occur later in treatment and may be irreversible. Typical antipsychotics block both dopamine-$D_2$ receptors and serotonin $5HT_2$ receptors, and it is the serotonin blockade that leads to protection from EPS, perhaps by increasing dopamine frontally and in the basal ganglia, most often when doses are kept low (Kapur and Remington 1996; Livingston 1994; Honey et al. 1999). The most commonly used atypical antipsychotic in pediatric practice is risperidone (Risperidal), which is not only helpful in treatment of schizophrenia (Quintana and Keshavan 1995; Honey et al. 1999) but also in treatment of tic disorder (Lombroso et al. 1995), bipolar disorder and aggression (Fras and Major 1995; Findling et al. 2000; Demb and Espiritu 1999), and treatment of behavior problems in children with mental retardation, autism, or PDD (Vanden Borre et al. 1993; Findling et al. 1997; Horrigan and Barnhill 1997; McDougle et al. 1997, 1998; Zuddas et al. 2000).

The wider utility of atypicals beyond schizophrenia, coupled with their superior safety profile, has led to their frequent use in the last few years. They should not be considered first-line treatments for aggression or mood stabilization, but they can be helpful when other medications previously described are not beneficial. In our experience, risperidone can be remarkably helpful in both children and adults with FXS who have significant aggression, mood instability, tantrums, or psychotic thinking, including paranoia (chap. 1). It is best to start at a low dose, 0.5 mg at bedtime, although increases to twice a day are often needed. Usually a dose of only 1 or 2 mg/day suffices (Demb and Espiritu 1999; Findling et al. 1998). Whenever possible, doses should be kept under 4 mg/day to avoid an increased risk of EPS (Kapur and Remington 1996).

Two newer atypical antipsychotics, olanzepine (Zyprexa) and quetiapine (Seroquel), have a similar safety profile to risperidone, but pediatric experience with their use is limited, particularly in developmental disabilities (Aman and Madrid 1999; Findling et al. 1998). Six of eight patients with autism or PDD responded clinically to olanzepine, with improvements in several behavioral areas, including socialization, in an open trial (Potenza et al. 1999). McConville et al. (2000) found that quetiapine was well tolerated and effective in an open trial in 10 adolescents with psychosis. However, in an open trial of 6 children and adolescents with autism, quetiapine was found to be helpful in only 2, and side effects such as sedation and behavioral activation were common (Martin et al. 1999). In our experience quetiapine has often been helpful in treating adolescents and adults with FXS who did not respond well to risperidone.

The most common side effect of risperidone and olanzapine is weight gain, which for many patients can lead to significant obesity. These medications cause a drug-induced satiety dysregulation (Findling et al. 1998), which may be less severe with quetiapine. The increase in weight can lead to a fatty liver or steatohepatitis (Kumra et al. 1997), so liver function studies should be followed in patients treated with atypicals, particularly if weight gain is seen. Sedation is common unless the atypical is given at bedtime. A slow increase in dose will reduce the chance of EPS, although they occasionally occur and necessitate lowering of the dose (Findling et al. 1998). Acute dystonic reactions are treated with diphenhydramine or benzotropine. Parkinsonism may respond to amantadine, and akathesia may improve with propranolol or clonazepam if benzotropine is not helpful (Findling et al. 1998). Another side effect of risperidone is prolactin elevation, which can cause breast tenderness, enlargement, and even galactorrhea in females and gynecomastia and sexual dysfunction in males (Findling et al. 1998). Olanzepine and quetiapine do not lead to substantial prolactin elevation, so they are good alternatives if these symptoms become significant. This seems to be a significant problem in less than 10% of the patients treated with risperidone (Findling et al. 1998). Cataracts have been reported occasionally in patients treated with quetiapine, so ophthalmoscopy is recommended at six-month intervals with quetiapine treatment (Findling et al. 1998).

## Sleep Disturbances

Sleep problems are common in young children with FXS (chap. 1). A variety of medications have been used to treat the sleeping difficulties, including clonidine, described previously, and trazodone, an antidepressant (fig. 8.2). Trazodone selectively blocks reuptake of serotonin, but it is also a potent antagonist of the 5-$HT_2$ receptor (Preskorn 1993). Trazodone has strong sedative effects, and it is often utilized at bedtime to counteract sleep disturbance. No published information is available concerning its efficacy in FXS. Carbamazepine or valproic acid may also improve sleep disturbances, particularly if spike-wave discharges or seizures are interfering with sleep.

Melatonin is a sleep hormone that is produced in the pineal gland from metabolism of serotonin. Melatonin's production is stimulated by darkness, and it is important for the induction and maintenance of sleep (Jan et al. 1994). Melatonin has been synthesized and is available in an oral form through health food stores in the United States. It has been shown to be effective for the treatment of chronic insomnia (MacFarlane et al. 1991), sleep problems related to jet lag (Arendt 1987), and delayed sleep phase syndrome (Dahlitz et al. 1991). Jan and O'Donnell (1996) and Jan et al. (1994) showed that melatonin given at bedtime, usually at a dose of 1 to 3 mg, can improve sleep disturbances in 82% of more than 100 children with developmental disabilities and sleep problems. No significant side effects were reported, even after continuous use for more than four years (Jan and O'Donnell 1996). Melatonin was nontoxic and without significant side effects, but it improved the mood and disposition of individuals who had improved sleep. Sadeh et al. (1995) suggested that melatonin might also improve aggressive behavior, as seen in their case study of a blind boy with severe mental retardation. Further studies are warranted in FXS concerning possible melatonin deficiency and the efficacy of melatonin for sleep disturbances.

## Combined Pharmacotherapy

There has been an emerging trend in psychopharmacology over the last decade to combine medications to more specifically cover multiple diagnoses in a child with comorbid conditions (Wilens et al. 1995; Jensen et al. 1999; Woolston 1999; Conner et al. 1997). The benefit of such a practice is that each specific diagnosis can be treated with the most effective medication, but the pitfalls include deleterious effects of medication combinations, which are not predictable from knowledge of the individual medications or their additive effect (Woolston 1999). There is a lack of controlled research on individual medications, much less combined pharmacologic effects, so it will take a while for research to document the benefits that an experienced clinician may discover in practice (Jensen et al. 1999).

In the fragile X field, we usually encounter comorbid diagnoses including ADHD, mood instability, and anxiety. As described here and in chapter 1, the use, therefore, of combined pharmacotherapy is common in both males and females with FXS, as illustrated in the survey described below. Importantly, however, combining psychopharmacologic treatment with counseling and therapies, as described in chapters 9, 10, and 11, is essential for an optimal treatment program.

We carried out a survey of the pharmacologic agents currently used by the children and adolescents with FXS seen in clinic between 1997 and 2000 (Amaria et al. 2001). There were 140 males and 37 females with FXS seen during this time. A summary of their medication use is found in figures 8.4 and 8.5. Among the males, only 9% were not taking any medication, 26% were taking a single medication that was usually a stimulant, and the rest were taking two or more medications. The most common combination was a stimulant, typically methylphenidate, combined with a SSRI, typically either fluoxetine (16%) or sertraline (18%) (Amaria et al. 2001). Risperidone was used in 13% of males and was often combined with a stimulant and/or a SSRI. Females with FXS (fig. 8.5) were more frequently taking either no medication (19%) or a single medication (35%). The single medication was often a stimulant or a SSRI agent. Anxiety is a frequent problem in females; 27% were treated with fluoxetine,

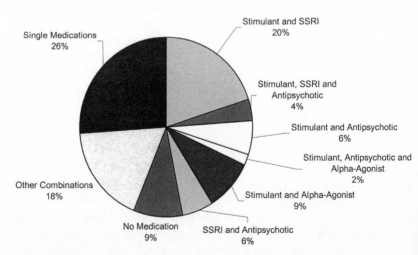

**Fig. 8.4.** Medication use in 140 males with FXS, ages 5 to 18 years, seen in clinic, 1997–2000. *Source:* Amaria et al. 2001. Reprinted with permission.

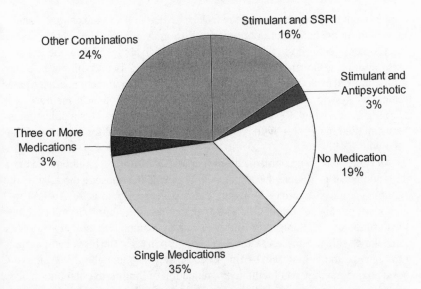

**Fig. 8.5.** Medication use in 37 girls with FXS, ages 5 to 18 years, seen in clinic, 1997–2000. *Source:* Amaria et al. 2001. Reprinted with permission.

and 16% were treated with sertraline. In general, such behavior problems as severe ADHD or aggression are less common in females with FXS, and this is reflected in their medication usage (Amaria et al. 2001).

## Future Prospects

Nootropics were introduced more than 20 years ago with piracetam as the prototype. The name is derived from *noos* (mind) and *tropin* (toward), and their pharmacologic effects are focused on improving higher cerebral functions, such as integration and memory (Ban 1995). Piracetam is a cyclic derivative of gama-aminobutyric acid (GABA), and several analogs have been synthesized, including oxiracetam, etiracetam, promiracetam, and aniracetam. These medications are used experimentally and have not been released for patient use in the United States. Extensive animal testing has shown positive effects on memory, object recognition, performance in radial mazes, and passive and active avoidance (reviewed by Mondadori 1994). Human studies have shown that a subgroup of patients with dementia (10–30%) have improved memory with nootropics, and this effect seems to be mediated by cholinergic systems (Mondadori 1993, 1994). In both Down syndrome and in dyslexia, there is evidence that the combined effects of piracetam and educational programs can enhance some types of learning compared to controls (Deberdt 1994). Since the cholinergic system may be affected by the lack of FMRP in FXS (see chap. 1), studies regarding the benefit of nootropics in FXS are warranted.

Another agent used in Alzheimer disease, which also works on the cholinergic system, is donepezil (Aricep). This medication is a cholinesterase inhibitor that enhances the effect of acetylcholine, which in turn enhances the glutamatergic system. The combined effect on both systems enhances memory and learning in aging rats. Results are similar in human studies. This medication is being studied in children with ADHD and has the potential for benefit in children with FXS.

An additional group of medications that may be helpful in children, and perhaps adults with FXS, are the ampakines. These medications are modulators of DL-alpha-amino-3-hydroxy-5-methyl-4-isoxazoleproprionic acid (AMPA) receptors of glutamate stimulation. They can increase the amplitude and prolong the duration of AMPA responses in slices of hippocampus (Staubli et al. 1994). Ampakines enhance fast excitatory synaptic responses in the hippocampus and rapidly cross the blood-brain barrier. Because they augment glutamatergic synaptic responses, they can facilitate the induction of long-term potentiation and perhaps enhance memory and cognitive function in those with developmental disabilities.

Studies in rats have shown that ampakine compounds improve olfactory learning, facilitate acquisition of a conditioned fear response, improve short-term memory, reverse age-associated memory impairment in middle-aged rats, reduce spontaneous unmotivated exploratory activity in familiar environments, increase speed at which rats collect rewards in a spatial maze, and improve methamphetamine-induced hyperactivity and stereotypic behavior (Granger et al. 1993, 1996; Hampson et al. 1998; Staubli et al. 1994; Larson et al. 1996). Many of the ampakine studies in rats and humans have utilized a benzamide compound, CX516 (1-quinoxalin-6-ylcarbonyl piperidine). Although this compound has a shorter half-life and lowered potency compared to newer ampakines, it has shown relative safety in human trials. In young adult men, CX516, in doses in the 600- to 1,200-mg range, helped delayed recall of nonsense words but not immediate recall, compared to controls (Lynch et al. 1996). There were no significant changes in mood or arousal as determined by self-report questionnaires after the use of CX516. A study by Ingvar et al. (1997) found improvement in visual associations, recognition of odors, and visuospatial information in a maze task in young adult males given 300 mg of CX516 per day. Improvement in a finger-tapping task and in a digit cancellation task was not seen, nor were changes in mood reported by the subjects who took CX516 (Ingvar et al. 1997). Improvements in delayed recall have been reported in elderly human subjects (65–76 years old) given CX516 (Lynch et al. 1997). With doses up to 900 mg of CX516 per day, a twofold improvement was seen 75 minutes posttreatment, but this seemed to diminish by 135 minutes after the dose.

Trials have also taken place in schizophrenic patients and have been initiated in adults with ADHD, but results are not yet available. There have been no studies of ampakines in patients with developmental disabilities, including patients with FXS. The ampakines hold significant potential for improving memory and cognition in adults and children with FXS, and controlled trials are warranted.

## Conclusions

The patient with FXS usually presents with an array of physical and behavioral problems that require monitoring and treatment. Medical complications associated with the syndrome require detection and early treatment. Although no cure is available, several medication possibilities have been presented and can be used to treat specific behavior problems. Although some patients with FXS have not required psychopharmacologic intervention, many have benefited from one or more of the medications discussed. If behavior problems exist, an appropriate medication trial can be considered in conjunction with additional intervention, discussed in chapters 9, 10, and 11. Further research involving controlled medication trials is necessary to clarify the most effective medication options in children and adults with FXS.

## Acknowledgments

I gratefully acknowledge grant support from NICHD (HD36071), the FRAXA Foundation, the National Fragile X Foundation, and the Lang Family Fund. I also thank Susan Harris and Andrew Wheeler for their wonderful expertise and support, which made this chapter possible.

## References

Aguglia E., M. Casacchia, G. B. Cassano, C. Faravelli, G. Ferrari, P. Giordano, P. Pancher, L. Ravizza, M. Trabucchi, F. Bolino, A. Carpato, D. Berardi, G. Provenzano, R. Brugnoli, and R. Rozzini. 1993. Double-blind study of the efficacy and safety of sertraline versus fluoxetine in major depression. *Int. Clin. Psychopharmacol.* 8:197–202.

Alvarez, N., R. A. Kern, N. N. Cain, D. L. Coulter, M. Iivanainen, and A. T. Plummer. 1998. Antiepileptics. In S. Reiss and M. G. Aman (eds.), *Psychotropic medication and developmental disabilities: The international consensus handbook.* Columbus: Ohio State Univ. Nisonger Center.

Aman, M. G. 1982. Stimulant drug effects in developmental disorders and hyperactivity: Toward a resolution of disparate findings. *J. Autism Dev. Disord.* 12:385–398.

Aman, M. G., and R. A. Kern. 1990. The efficacy of folic acid in the developmental disabilities. *J. Child Adolesc. Psychopharmacology* 1:285–295.

Aman, M. G., and A. Madrid. 1999. Atypical antipsychotics in persons with developmental disabilities. *Ment. Retard. Dev. Disabil. Res. Rev.* 5:253–263.

Aman, M. G., and A. J. White. 1988. Thioridazine dose effects with reference to stereotypic behavior in mentally retarded residents. *J. Autism Dev. Disord.* 18:355–366.

Aman, M. G., R. E. Marks, S. H. Turbott, C. P. Wilsher, and S. N. Merry. 1991a. Clinical effects of methylphenidate and thioridazine in intellectually subaverage children. *J. Am. Acad. Child Adolesc. Psychiatry* 30:246–256.

———. 1991b. Methylphenidate and thioridazine in the treatment of intellectually subaverage children: Effects on cognitive-motor performance. *J. Am. Acad. Child Adolesc. Psychiatry* 30:816–824.

Amaria, R. N., L. L. Billeisen, and R. J. Hagerman. 2001. Medication use in fragile X syndrome. *Ment. Health Aspects Dev. Disabil.* 4:143–147.

Ambrosini, P. J., K. D. Wagner, J. Biederman, I. Glick, C. Tan, J. Elia, J. R. Hebeler, H. Rabinovich, J. Lock, and D. Geller. 1999. Multicenter open-label sertraline study in adolescent outpatients with major depression. *J. Am. Acad. Child Adolesc. Psychiatry* 38:566–572.

American Academy of Pediatrics, Committee on Genetics. 1996. Health supervision for children with fragile X syndrome. *Pediatrics* 98:297–300.

American Psychiatric Association. 1973. *APA task force on vitamin therapy in psychiatry: Mega vitamin and ortho molecular therapy in psychiatry.* Washington, D.C.

Arendt, J., M. Aldhous, J. English, V. Marks, J. H. Arendt, M. Marks, and S. Folkard. 1987. Some effects of jet lag and their alleviation by melatonin. *Ergonomics* 30: 1379–1393.

Arnold, L. E. 1993. Clinical pharmacological issues in treating psychiatric disorders in patients with mental retardation. *Ann. Clin. Psychiatry* 5:189–197.

Arnold, E. L., K. Gadow, D. A. Pearson, and C. K. Varley. 1996. Stimulants in patients with mental retardation. In M. Aman and S. Reiss (eds.), *Handbook of psychopharmacology and mental retardation.* Washington, D.C.: American Association on Mental Retardation.

Babbitt, R. L., J. M. Parrish, P. E. Brierley, and M. A. Kohr. 1991. Teaching developmentally disabled children with chronic illness to swallow prescribed capsules. *J. Dev. Behav. Pediatr.* 12:229–235.

Bailey, D. B., D. D. Hatton, and M. Skinner. 1998. Early developmental trajectories of males with fragile X syndrome. *Am. J. Ment. Retard.* 103:29–39.

Ban, T. A. 1995. Psychopharmacology and successful cerebral aging. *Prog. Neuropsychopharmacol. Biol. Psychiatry* 19:1–9.

Barkley, R. A. 1995. *Taking charge of ADHD: The complete, authoritative guide for parents.* New York: Guilford Press.

———. 1997. *ADHD and the nature of self control.* New York: Guilford Press.

———. 1998. *Attention deficit hyperactivity disorder: A handbook for diagnosis and treatment,* 2d ed. New York: Guilford Press.

Barkley, R. A., G. J. DuPaul, and M. B. McMurray. 1991. Attention deficit disorder with and without hyperactivity: Clinical response to three dose levels of methylphenidate. *Pediatrics* 87:519–531.

Barrickman, L., R. Noyes, S. Kuperman, E. Schumacher, and M. Verda. 1991. Treatment of ADHD with fluoxetine: A preliminary trial. *J. Am. Acad. Child Adolesc. Psychiatry* 30:762–766.

Barrickman, L. L., P. J. Perry, A. J. Allen, S. Kuperman, S. V. Arndt, K. J. Herrmann, and E. Schumacher. 1995. Bupropion versus methylphenidate in the treatment of attention-deficit hyperactivity disorder. *J. Am. Acad. Child Adolesc. Psychiatry* 34: 649–657.

Beasley, C. M., B. E. Dornself, J. C. Bosomworth, M. E. Sayler, A. H. Rampsey, J. H. Heiligenstein, V. L. Thompson, and D. N. Mason. 1991. Fluoxetine and suicide: A meta analysis of controlled trials of treatment for depression. *Br. Med. J.* 303:685–692.

Bellman, B., L. A. Schachner, L. Pravder, S. McFalls, and B. Shapiro. 1995. Carbamazepine hypersensitivity. *J. Am. Acad. Child Adolesc. Psychiatry* 34:1405–1406.

Bennett, J., W. T. Goldman, and T. Suppes. 1997. Gabapentin for treatment of bipolar and schizoaffective disorders [letter]. *J. Clin. Psychopharmacol.* 17:141–142.

Berkheimer, J. L., J. L. Curtis, and M. W. Lann. 1985. Use of carbamazepine in psychiatric disorders. *Clin. Pharm.* 4:425–434.

Berry-Kravis, E. 2000. Medication use in fragile X. Presented at the Seventh International Fragile X Foundation Conference, Los Angeles, July 19–22.

Binstock, T. 1995. Fragile X and the amygdala: Cognitive, interpersonal, emotional, and neuroendocrine considerations. *Dev. Brain Dysfunct.* 8:199–217.

Birmaher, B., G. S. Waterman, N. Ryan, M. Cully, L. Balach, J. Ingram, and M. Brodsky. 1994. Fluoxetine for childhood anxiety disorders. *J. Am. Acad. Child Adolesc. Psychiatry* 33:993–999.

Black, B., and T. W. Uhde. 1994. Treatment of elective mutism with fluoxetine: A double-blind, placebo-controlled study. *J. Am. Acad. Child Adolesc. Psychiatry* 33:1000–1006.

Blacklidge, V., and R. L. Ekblad. 1971. The effectiveness of methylphenidate hydrochloride (Ritalin) on learning and behavior in public-school educable mentally retarded children. *Pediatrics* 47:923–926.

Blackwell, B., and J. Currah. 1973. The psychopharmacology of nocturnal enuresis. In I. Kalvin, R. C. MacKeith, and S. R. Meadow (eds.), *Bladder control and enuresis.* London: Heinemann, pp. 231–257.

Blum, N. J., R. S. Kell, H. L. Starr, W. L. Lender, K. L. Bradley-Klug, M. L. Osborne, and P. W. Dowrick. 1998. Case study: Audio feedforward treatment of selective mutism. *J. Am. Acad. Child Adolesc. Psychiatry* 37:40–43.

Boccia, M. L., and J. E. Roberts. 2000. Behavior and autonomic nervous system function assessed via heart period measures: The case of hyperarousal in boys with fragile X syndrome. *Behav. Res. Methods Instruments Computers* 32:5–10.

Bodfish, J. W., and J. T. Maddison. 1993. Diagnosis and fluoxetine treatment of compulsive behavior disorder of adults with mental retardation. *Am. J. Ment. Retard.* 98: 360–367.

Bodine, C., J. Sandstrum, J. L. Hills, K. Riley, L. Gane, and R. J. Hagerman. 2001. Vocational use of assistive technology for young adults with fragile X syndrome (submitted).

Borison, R. L., and J. M. Davis. 1983. Amantadine in Tourette syndrome. *Curr. Psychiatr. Ther.* 20:127–130.

Bouchard, R. H., E. Pourcher, and P. Vincent. 1989. Fluoxetine and extrapyramidal side effects [letter]. *Am. J. Psychiatry* 146:1352–1353.

Bowden, C. L., A. M. Brugger, A. C. Swann, J. R. Calabrese, P. G. Janicak, F. Petty, S. C. Dilsaver, J. M. Davis, A. J. Rish, J. G. Small, E. S. Garza-Trevino, S. C. Risch, P. J. Goodnick, and D. D. Morris. 1994. Efficacy of divalproex vs. lithium and placebo in the treatment of mania. *JAMA* 271:918–924.

Bowley, C., and M. Kerr. 2000. Epilepsy and intellectual disability. *J. Intellect. Disabil. Res.* 44:529–543.

Braden, M. L. 2000a. *Fragile X, handle with care: More about fragile X syndrome— adolescents and adults.* Dillon, Colo.: Spectra Publishing Co.

———. 2000b. Education. In J. Weber (ed.), *Children with fragile X syndrome: A parent's guide.* Bethesda, Md.: Woodbine House, pp. 243–305.

Bradley, C. 1937. The behavior of children receiving benzedrine. *Am. J. Psychiatry* 94: 557–585.

Bregman, J. D. 1991. Current developments in understanding mental retardation: Part II. Psychopathology. *J. Am. Acad. Child. Adolesc. Psychiatry* 30:861–872.

Brøndum-Nielsen, K., N. Tommerup, B. Frilis, K. Hjelt, and E. Hippe. 1983. Folic acid metabolism in a patient with fragile X. *Clin. Genet.* 24:153–155.

Brown, J., M. Braden, and W. Sobesky. 1991. The treatment of behavior and emotional problems. In R. J. Hagerman and A. C. Silverman (eds.), *Fragile X syndrome: Diagnosis, treatment, and research.* Baltimore: Johns Hopkins Univ. Press, pp. 311–326.

Brown, J. L. 1995. Imagination training: A tool with many uses. *Contemp. Pediatr.* 12: 22–36.

Brown, W. T., E. C. Jenkins, E. Friedman, J. Brooks, I. L. Cohen, C. Duncan, A. L. Hill, M. N. Malik, V. Morris, E. Wolf, K. Wisniewski, and J. H. French. 1984. Folic acid therapy in the fragile X syndrome. *Am. J. Med. Genet.* 17:289–297.

Brown, W. T., I. L. Cohen, G. S. Fisch, E. Wolf, V. A. Jenkins, M. N. Milik, and E. C. Jenkins. 1986. High dose folic acid treatment of fragile(X) males. *Am. J. Med. Genet.* 23:263–271.

Budman, C. L., M. Sherling, and R. D. Bruun. 1995. Combined pharmacotherapy risk [letter]. *J. Am. Acad. Child Adolesc. Psychiatry* 34:263–264.

Buitelaar, J. K., R. J. van der Gaag, and J. van der Hoeven. 1998. Buspirone in the management of anxiety and irritability in children with pervasive developmental disorders: Results of an open-label study. *J. Clin. Psychiatry* 59:56–59.

Bukstein, O. G., and D. J. Kolko. 1998. Effects of methylphenidate on aggressive urban children with attention deficit hyperactivity disorder. *J. Clin. Child Psychol.* 27:340–351.

Buzan, R. D., D. Firestone, M. Thomas, and S. L. Dubovsky. 1995. Valproate-associated pancreatitis and cholecystitis in six mentally retarded adults. *J. Clin. Psychiatry* 56: 529–532.

Campbell, M., and J. E. Cueva. 1995. Psychopharmacology in child and adolescent psychiatry: A review of the past seven years. Part I. *J. Am. Acad. Child Adolesc. Psychiatry* 34:1124–1132.

Campbell, M., P. B. Adams, A. M. Small, V. Kafantaris, R. R. Silva, J. Shell, R. Perry, and J. E. Overall. 1995. Lithium in hospitalized aggressive children with conduct disorder: A double-blind and placebo-controlled study. *J. Am. Acad. Child Adolesc. Psychiatry* 34:445–463.

Cantwell, D. P., J. Swanson, and D. F. Connor. 1997. Case study: Adverse response to clonidine. *J. Am. Acad. Child Adolesc. Psychiatry* 36:539–544.

Carpenter, N. J., D. H. Barber, M. Jones, W. Lindley, and C. Carr. 1983. Controlled six-month study of oral folic acid therapy in boys with fragile X-linked mental retardation [abstract 243]. *Am. J. Hum. Genet. (Suppl.)* 35:82A.

Chandran, K. S. K. 1994. ECG and clonidine. *J. Am. Acad. Child Adolesc. Psychiatry* 33:1351–1352.

Comings, D. E., B. F. Comings, T. Tacket, and S. Li. 1990. The clonidine patch and behavior problems. *J. Am. Acad. Child Adolesc. Psychiatry* 29:667–668.

Conners, C. K. 1973. Rating scales for use in drug studies with children. *Psychopharmacol. Bull.,* special issue, pp. 24–84, 219–222.

Conners, C. K., C. D. Casat, C. T. Gualtieri, E. Weller, M. Reader, A. Reiss, R. A. Weller, M. Khayrallah, and J. Ascher. 1996. Bupropion hydrochloride in attention deficit disorder with hyperactivity. *J. Am. Acad. Child Adolesc. Psychiatry* 35:1314–1321.

Connor, D. F., K. R. Ozbayrak, K. A. Kusiak, A. B. Caponi, and R. H. Melloni Jr. 1997. Combined pharmacotherapy in children and adolescents in a residential treatment center [see comments]. *J. Am. Acad. Child Adolesc. Psychiatry* 36:248–254.

Constantino, J. N. 1995. Testosterone and aggression [letter]. *J. Am. Acad. Child Adolesc. Psychiatry* 34:535.

Cook, E. H., Jr., R. Rowlett, C. Jaseiskis, and B. L. Leventhal. 1992. Fluoxetine treatment of children and adults with autistic disorder and mental retardation. *J. Am. Acad. Child Adolesc. Psychiatry* 31:739–750.

Dahlitz, M., B. Alvarez, J. Vignau, J. English, J. Arendt, and J. D. Parkes. 1991. Delayed sleep phase syndrome response to melatonin. *Lancet* 333:1121–1124.

Dale, P. G. 1980. Lithium therapy in aggressive mentally subnormal patients. *Br. J. Psychiatry* 137:469–474.

Dasgupta, K. 1990. Additional cases of suicidal ideation associated with fluoxetine. *Am. J. Psychiatry* 147:1570–1571.

Davis, L. L., W. Ryan, B. Adinoff, and F. Petty. 2000. Comprehensive review of the psychiatric uses of valproate. *J. Clin. Psychopharmacol.* 20 (suppl. 1): 1S–17S.

Dawson, P. M., J. A. VanderZanden, S. L. Werkman, R. L. Wahington, and T. A. Tyma. 1989. Cardiac dysrhythmia with the use of cloncine in explosive disorder. *DICP* 23: 465–466.

Deberdt, W. 1994. Interaction between psychological and pharmacological treatment in cognitive impairment. *Life Sci.* 55:2057–2066.

Dech, B. 1999. Clonidine and methylphenidate [letter; comment]. *J. Am. Acad. Child Adolesc. Psychiatry* 38:1469–1470.

Dech, B., and L. Budow. 1991 The use of fluoxetine in an adolescent with Prader-Willi syndrome. *J. Am. Acad. Child Adolesc. Psychiatry* 30:208–302.

DeLong, G. R., L. A. Teague, and M. McSwain Kamran. 1998. Effects of fluoxetine treatment in young children with idiopathic autism [see comments]. *Dev. Med. Child Neurol.* 40:551–562.

Demb, H. B., and C. R. G. Espiritu. 1999. The use of risperidone with children and adolescents with developmental disabilities: Effects on some common challenging behaviors. *Ment. Health Aspects Dev. Disabil.* 2:73–82.

DeVane, C. L., and F. R. Sallee. 1996. Serotonin selective reuptake inhibitors in child and adolescent psychopharmacology: A review of published experience. *J. Clin. Psychiatry* 57:55–66.

Dillon, D. C., I. J. Salzman, and D. A. Schulsinger. 1985. The use of imipramine in Tourette's syndrome and attention deficit disorder: Case report. *J. Clin. Psychiatry* 46:348–349.

Dodson, E. W. 1989. Medical treatment and pharmacology of antiepileptic drugs. *Pediatr. Clin. North Am.* 36:421–433.

Douglas, V. I., R. G. Barr, M. E. O'Neill, and B. G. Britton. 1986. Short-term effects of methylphenidate on the cognitive, learning and academic performance of children with attention deficit disorder in the laboratory and in the classroom. *J. Child Psychol. Psychiatry* 27:191–211.

Dreifuss, F. E., and D. H. Langer. 1987. Hepatic considerations in the use of antiepileptic drugs. *Epilepsia* 28 (suppl. 2): S23.

DuPaul, G. J., and R. A. Barkley. 1990. Medication therapy. In R. A. Barkley (ed.), *Attention deficit hyperactivity disorder.* New York: Guilford Press, pp. 573–612.

Durack, D. T. 1995. Prevention of infective endocarditis. *N. Engl. J. Med.* 332:38–44.

Dykens, E. M., R. M. Hodapp, and J. F. Leckman. 1994. *Behavior and development in fragile X syndrome.* London: Sage Publications.

Dyme, Z., B. J. Sahakian, B. E. Golinko, and E. F. Rabe. 1982. Perseveration induced by methylphenidate in children: Preliminary findings. *Prog. Neuropsychopharmacol. Biol. Psychiatry* 6:269–273.

Einfeld, S., B. Tonge, and G. Turner. 1999. Longitudinal course of behavioral and emotional problems in fragile X syndrome. *Am. J. Med. Genet.* 87:436–439.

Evans, R. W., and C. T. Gualtieri. 1985. Carbamazepine neurophysiological and psychiatric profile. *Clin. Neuropharmacol.* 8:221–241.

Fairbanks, J. M., D. S. Pine, N. K. Tancer, E. S. Dummit 3d, L. M. Kentgen, J. Martin, B. K. Asche, and R. G. Klein. 1997. Open fluoxetine treatment of mixed anxiety disorders in children and adolescents. *J. Child Adolesc. Psychopharmacol.* 7:17–29.

Fenichel, R. F. 1995. Combining methylphenidate and clonidine: The role of post-marketing surveillance. *J. Child Adolesc. Psychopharmacol.* 5:155–156.

Findling, R. L., and J. W. Dogin. 1998. Psychopharmacology of ADHD: Children and adolescents. *J. Clin. Psychiatry* 59:42–49.

Findling, R. L., S. J. Grcevich, I. Lopez, and S. C. Schulz. 1996a. Antipsychotic medications in children and adolescents. *J. Clin. Psychiatry* 57:19–23.

Findling, R. L., M. A. Schwartz, D. J. Flannery, and M. J. Manos. 1996b. Venlafaxine in adults with attention-deficit/hyperactivity disorder: An open clinical trial [see comments]. *J. Clin. Psychiatry* 57:184–189.

Findling, R. L., K. Maxwell, and M. Wiznitzer. 1997. An open clinical trial of risperidone monotherapy in young children with autistic disorder. *Psychopharmacol. Bull.* 33:155–159.

Findling, R. L., S. C. Schulz, M. D. Reed, and J. L. Blumer. 1998. The antipsychotics: A pediatric perspective. *Pediatr. Clin. North Am.* 45:1205–1232.

Findling, R. L., N. K. McNamara, L. A. Branicky, M. D. Schluchter, E. Lemon, and J. L. Blumer. 2000. A double-blind pilot study of risperidone in the treatment of conduct disorder. *J. Am. Acad. Child Adolesc. Psychiatry* 39:509–516.

Fisch, G. S., I. L. Cohen, A. C. Gross, V. Jenkins, E. C. Jenkins, and W. T. Brown. 1988. Folic acid treatment of fragile X males: A further study. *Am. J. Med. Genet.* 30:393–399.

Fragile X Society (England). 1995. Bowel control questionnaire. *Fragile X Society Newsletter* 11:11–12.

Fras, I., and L. F. Major. 1995. Clinical experience with risperidone [letter]. *J. Am. Acad. Child Adolesc. Psychiatry* 34:833.

Freeman, T. W., J. L. Clothier, P. Dazzaglia, M. D. Lesem, and A. C. Swann. 1992. A double-blind comparison of valproate and lithium in the treatment of acute mania. *Am. J. Psychiatry* 149:108–111.

Froster-Iskenius, U., K. Bodeker, T. Oepen, R. Matthes, U. Piper, and E. Schwinger. 1986. Folic acid treatment in males and females with fragile(X) syndrome. *Am. J. Med. Genet.* 23:273–289.

Fryns, J. P. 1994. Massive hydrocele in post pubertal fra (X) males [letter]. *Am. J. Med. Genet.* 49:259.

Fryns, J. P., P. Moerman, F. Gilis, L. d'Espallier, and H. Van den Berghe. 1988. Suggestively increased incidence of sudden death in children of fra(X) positive mothers. *Am. J. Med. Genet.* 30:73–75.

Gadow, K. D., and A. G. Poling. 1988. *Pharmacotherapy and mental retardation.* Boston: College Hill Press.

Gadow, K. D., and J. C. Pomeroy. 1990. A controlled case study of methylphenidate and fenfluramine in a young mentally retarded, hyperactive child. *Aus. N.Z. J. Dev. Disabilities* 16:323–334.

Gadow, K. D., J. C. Pomeroy, and E. E. Nolan. 1992. A procedure for monitoring stimulant medication in hyperactive mentally retarded school children. *J. Child Adolesc. Psychopharmacol.* 2:131–143.

Gadow, K. D., E. Nolan, J. Sprafkin, and J. S. Verd. 1995. School observations of children with attention deficit hyperactivity disorder and comorbid tic disorder: Effects of methylphenidate treatment. *J. Dev. Behav. Pediatr.* 16:167–176.

Garland, E. J., and M. Weiss. 1996. Case study: Obsessive difficult temperament and its response to serotonergic medication. *J. Am. Acad. Child Adolesc. Psychiatry* 35:916–920.

Geller, D. A., J. Biederman, E. D. Reed, T. Spencer, and T. E. Wilens. 1995. Similarities in response to fluoxetine in the treatment of children and adolescents with obsessive-compulsive disorder. *J. Am. Acad. Child Adolesc. Psychiatry* 34:36–44.

Ghaziuddin, M., and L. Tsai. 1991. Depression in autistic disorder. *Br. J. Psychiatry* 159:721–723.

Gillberg, C., J. Wahlstrom, R. Johansson, M. Tornblom, and K. Albertsson-Wikland.

1986. Folic acid as an adjunct in the treatment of children with the autism fragile X syndrome (A FRA X). *Dev. Med. Child Neurol.* 28:624–627.

Gillberg, C., H. Melander, A. L. von Knorring, L. O. Janols, G. Thernlund, B. Hagglof, L. Eidevall-Wallin, P. Gustafsson, and S. Kopp. 1997. Long-term stimulant treatment of children with attention-deficit hyperactivity disorder symptoms: A randomized, double-blind, placebo-controlled trial. *Arch. Gen. Psychiatry* 54:857–864.

Gittelman-Klein, R., and D. F. Klein. 1971. Controlled imipramine treatment of school phobia. *Arch. Gen. Psychiatry* 25:204–207.

Glazer, W. M. 1997. Olanzapine and the new generation of antipsychotic agents: Patterns of use. *J. Clin. Psychiatry* 58:18–21.

Goldson, E., and R. J. Hagerman. 1993. Fragile X syndrome and failure to thrive. *Am. J. Dis. Child.* 147:605–607.

Gordon, C. T., R. C. State, J. E. Nelson, S. D. Hamburger, and J. L. Rapoport. 1993. A double-blind comparison of clomipramine, desipramine, and placebo in the treatment of autistic disorder. *Arch. Gen. Psychiatry* 50:441–447.

Granger, R., U. Staubli, M. Davis, Y. Perez, L. Nilsson, G. Rogers, and G. Lynch. 1993. A drug that facilitates glutaminergic transmission reduces exploratory activity and improves performance in a learning-dependent task. *Synapse* 15:326–329.

Granger, R., S. Deadwyler, M. Davis, B. Moskovitz, M. Kessler, G. Rogers, and G. Lynch. 1996. Facilitation of glutamate receptors reverses an age associated memory impairment in rats. *Synapse* 22:332–337.

Greenblatt, J. M., L. C. Huffman, and A. L. Reiss. 1994. Folic acid in neurodevelopment and child psychiatry. *Prog. Neuropsychopharmacol. Biol. Psychiatry* 18:647–660.

Greendyke, R. M., and D. R. Kanter. 1986. Therapeutic effects of pindolol on behavioral disturbances associated with organic brain disease: A double blind study. *J. Clin. Psychiatry* 47:423–426.

Gualtieri, C. T. 1977. Imipramine and children: A review and some speculations about the mechanism of drug action. *Dis. Nerv. Syst.* 38:368–375.

———. 1990. *Neuropsychiatry and behavioral pharmacology.* Berlin: Springer Verlag.

———. 1992. Psychopharmacology and the fragile X syndrome. In R. J. Hagerman and P. McKenzie (eds.), *1992 International Fragile X Conference Proceedings.* Dillon, Colo.: National Fragile X Foundation and Spectra Publishing, pp. 167–178.

Gualtieri, C. T., R. W. Evans, and D. R. Patterson. 1987. The medical treatment of autistic people: Problems and side effects. In E. Shopler and G. Mesibov (eds.), *Neurobiological issues in autism.* New York: Plenum Publishing.

Gualtieri, C. T., M. Chandler, T. B. Coons, and L. T. Brown. 1989. Amantadine: A new clinical profile for traumatic brain injury. *Clin. Neuropharmacol.* 12:258–270.

Gustavson, K. H., K. Dahlblom, A. Flood, G. Holmgren, H. K. Blomquist, and G. Sanner. 1985. Effect of folic acid treatment in fragile X syndrome. *Clin. Genet.* 27:463–467.

Gutgesell, H., D. Atkins, R. Barst, M. Buck, W. Franklin, R. Humes, R. Ringel, R. Shaddy, and K. A. Taubert. 1999. AHA Scientific Statement: Cardiovascular monitoring of children and adolescents receiving psychotropic drugs. *J. Am. Acad. Child Adolesc. Psychiatry* 38:1047–1050.

Habib, K. E., K. P. Weld, K. C. Rice, J. Pushkas, M. Champoux, S. Listwak, E. L. Webster, A. J. Atkinson, J. Schulkin, C. Contoreggi, G. P. Chrousos, S. M. McCann, S. J. Suomi, J. D. Higley, and P. W. Gold. 2000. Oral administration of a corticotropin-releasing hormone receptor antagonist significantly attenuates behavioral, neuroendocrine, and autonomic responses to stress in primates. *Proc. Natl. Acad. Sci. USA* 97:6079–6084.

Hagerman, R. J. 1984. Pediatric assessment of the learning disabled child. *J. Dev. Behav. Pediatr.* 5:274–284.

———. 1987. Fragile X syndrome. *Curr. Probl. Pediatr.* 11:627–674.

———. 1995. Growth and development. In W. W. Hay, J. R. Groothuis, A. R. Hayward, and M. J. Levin (eds.), *Current pediatric diagnosis and treatment,* 12th ed. Hartford, Conn.: Appleton & Lange, pp. 65–84.

———. 1996. Medical follow-up and pharmacotherapy. In R. J. Hagerman and A. Cronister (eds.), *Fragile X syndrome: Diagnosis, treatment, and research,* 2d ed. Baltimore: Johns Hopkins Univ. Press, pp. 283–331.

———. 1997. Fragile X: Treatment of hyperactivity [letter]. *Pediatrics* 99:753.

———. 1999a. Fragile X syndrome. In: *Neurodevelopmental Disorders: Diagnosis and Treatment.* New York: Oxford University Press, pp. 61–132.

———. 1999b. Psychopharmacological interventions in fragile X syndrome, fetal alcohol syndrome, Prader-Willi syndrome, Angelman syndrome, Smith-Magenis syndrome, and velocardiofacial syndrome. *Ment. Retard. Dev. Disabil. Res. Rev.* 5:305–313.

Hagerman, R. J., A. W. Jackson, A. Levitas, B. Rimland, and M. Braden. 1986. Oral folic acid versus placebo in the treatment of males with the fragile X syndrome. *Am. J. Med. Genet.* 23:241–262.

Hagerman, R. J., D. Altshul-Stark, and P. McBogg. 1987. Recurrent otitis media in boys with the fragile X syndrome. *Am. J. Dis. Child.* 141:184–187.

Hagerman, R. J., M. Murphy, and M. Wittenberger. 1988. A controlled trial of stimulant medication in children with fragile X syndrome. *Am. J. Med. Genet.* 30:377–392.

Hagerman, R. J., M. J. Fulton, A. Leaman, J. Riddle, K. Hagerman, and W. Sobesky. 1994. A survey of fluoxetine therapy in fragile X syndrome. *Dev. Brain Dysfunct.* 7:155–164.

Hagerman, R. J., J. E. Riddle, L. S. Roberts, K. Brease, and M. Fulton. 1995. A survey of the efficacy of clonidine in fragile X syndrome. *Dev. Brain Dysfunct.* 8:336–344.

Hagerman, R. J., J. D. Bregman, and E. Tirosh. 1998. Clonidine. In S. Reiss and M. G. Aman (eds.), *Psychotropic medications and developmental disabilities: The international consensus handbook.* Columbus, Ohio: OSU Nisonger Center (distributed by the American Association on Mental Retardation), pp. 259–269.

Hagerman, R. J., J. Hills, S. Scharfenaker, and H. Lewis. 1999. Fragile X syndrome and selective mutism. *Am. J. Med. Genet.* 83:313–317.

Hagerman, R. J., L. J. Miller, J. McGrath-Clarke, K. Riley, E. Goldson, S. W. Harris, J. Simon, K. Church, J. Bonnell, and D. McIntosh. 2001. The influence of stimulants on electrodermal studies in fragile X syndrome. *Microsc. Res. Tech.* In press.

Hagino, O. R., E. B. Weller, R. A. Weller, D. Washing, M. A. Fristad, and S. A. Kontras. 1995. Untoward effects of lithium treatment in children aged four through six years. *J. Am. Acad. Child. Adolesc. Psychiatry* 34:1584–1590.

Hampson, R. E., G. Rogers, G. Lynch, and S. A. Deadwyler. 1998. Facilitative effects of the ampakine CX516 on short term memory in rats: Enhancement of delayed-nonmatch-to-sample performance. *J. Neurosci.* 18:2740–2747.

Handen, B. L., A. M. Breaux, A. Gosling, D. L. Ploof, and H. Feldman. 1990. Efficacy of methylphenidate among mentally retarded children with attention deficit hyperactivity disorder. *Pediatrics* 86:922–930.

Handen, B. L., H. Feldman, A. Gosling, A. M. Breaux, and S. McAuliffe. 1991. Adverse side effects of methylphenidate among mentally retarded children with ADHD. *J. Am. Acad. Child Adolesc. Psychiatry* 30:241–245.

Handen, B. L., A. M. Breaux, J. Janosky, S. McAuliffe, H. Feldman, and A. Gosling. 1992. Effects and noneffects of methylphenidate in children with mental retardation and ADHD. *J. Am. Acad. Child Adolesc. Psychiatry* 31:455–461.

Handen, B. L., J. Janosky, S. McAuliffe, A. M. Breaux, and H. Feldman. 1994. Prediction of response to methylphenidate among children with ADHD and mental retardation. *J. Am. Acad. Child Adolesc. Psychiatry* 33:1185–1193.

Handen, B. L., S. McAuliffe, and L. Caro-Martinez. 1996. Learning effects of methylphenidate in children with mental retardation. J. Dev. Phys. Disabil. 8:335–346.

Handen, B. L., C. R. Johnson, and M. Lubetsky. 2000. Efficacy of methylphenidate among children with autism and symptoms of attention-deficit hyperactivity disorder. *J. Autism Dev. Disord.* 30:245–255.

Harpey, J. P. 1982. Treatment of fragile X [letter]. *Pediatrics* 69:670.

Hartman, N., R. Kramer, W. T. Brown, and R. B. Devereux. 1982. Panic disorder in patients with mitral valve prolapse. *Am. J. Psychiatry* 139:669–670.

Hecht, F., and T. W. Glover. 1983. Antibiotics containing trimethoprim and the fragile X chromosome [letter]. *N. Engl. J. Med.* 308:285.

Hellings, J. A. 1999. Psychopharmacology of mood disorders in persons with mental retardation and autism. *Ment. Retard. Dev. Disabil. Res. Rev.* 5:270–278.

Hellings, J. A., L. A. Kelley, W. F. Gabrielli, E. Kilgore, and P. Shah. 1996. Sertraline response in adults with mental retardation and autistic disorder. *J. Clin. Psychiatry* 57:333–336.

Hewlett, W. A., S. Vinogradov, and W. S. Agras. 1992. Clomipramine, clonacepan and clonidine treatment of obsessive/compulsive disorder. *J. Clin. Psychopharmacol.* 12:420–426.

Hilton, D. K., C. A. Martin, W. M. Heffron, D. D. Hall, and G. L. Johnson. 1991. Imipramine treatment of ADHD in a fragile X child. *J. Am. Acad. Child Adolesc. Psychiatry* 30:831–834.

Hoge, S. K., and J. Biederman. 1986. A case of Tourette's syndrome with symptoms of attention deficit disorder treated with desipramine. *J. Clin. Psychiatry* 47:478–479.

Hollander, E., A. Kaplan, C. Cartwright, and D. Reichman. 2000. Venlafaxine in children, adolescents, and young adults with autism spectrum disorders: An open retrospective clinical report. *J. Child Neurol.* 15:132–135.

Honey, G. D., E. T. Bullmore, W. Soni, M. Varatheesan, S. C. Williams, and T. Sharma. 1999. Differences in frontal cortical activation by a working memory task after substitution of risperidone for typical antipsychotic drugs in patients with schizophrenia [see comments]. *Proc. Natl. Acad. Sci. USA* 96:13432–13437.

Horrigan, J. P., and L. J. Barnhill. 1997. Risperidone and explosive aggressive autism. *J. Autism Dev. Disord.* 27:313–323.

Hunt, R. D. 1987. Treatment effects of oral and transdermal clonidine in relation to methylphenidate: An open pilot study. *Psychopharmacol. Bull.* 23:111–114.

Hunt, R. D., R. B. Mindera, and D. J. Cohen. 1985. Clonidine benefits children with attentional deficit disorder and hyperactivity. *J. Am. Acad. Child Adolesc. Psychiatry* 24:617–629.

Hunt, R. D., A. F. T. Arnsten, and M. D. Asbell. 1995. An open trial of guanfacine in treatment of attention deficit hyperactivity disorder. *J. Am. Acad. Child Adolesc. Psychiatry* 34:50–54.

Hunter, R., J. Barnes, H. F. Oakeley, and D. M. Matthews. 1970. Toxicity of folic acid given in pharmacological doses to healthy volunteers. *Lancet* 1:61–63.

Ingvar, M., J. Ambros-Ingerson, M. Davis, R. Granger, M. Kessler, G. Rogers, R. S. Schehr, and G. Lynch. 1997. Enhancement by an ampakine of memory encoding in humans. *Exp. Neurol.* 146:553–559.

Isojarvi, J. I., T. J. Laatikainen, A. J. Pakarinen, K. T. Juntunen, and V. V. Myllyla. 1993. Polycystic ovaries and hyperandrogenism in women taking valproate for epilepsy. *N. Engl. J. Med.* 329:1383–1388.

Jacky, P. 1996. Cytogenetics. In R. J. Hagerman and A. Cronister (eds.), *Fragile X syndrome: Diagnosis, treatment, and research,* 2d ed. Baltimore: Johns Hopkins Univ. Press, pp. 114–164.

Jan, J. E., and M. E. O'Donnell. 1996. Use of melatonin in the treatment of paediatric sleep disorders. *J. Pineal Res.* 21:193–199.

Jan, J. E., H. Esperzel, and R. E. Appleton. 1994. The treatment of sleep disorders with melatonin. *Dev. Med. Child Neurol.* 36:97–107.

Jann, M. 1988. Buspirone: An update on a unique anxiolytic agent. *Pharmacotherapy* 8:100–116.

Jenkins, S. C., and T. Maruta. 1987. Therapeutic use of propranolol for intermittent explosive disorder. *Mayo Clin. Proc.* 62:204–214.

Jensen, P. S., V. S. Bhatara, B. Vitiello, K. Hoagwood, M. Feil, and L. B. Burke. 1999. Psychoactive medication prescribing practices for U.S. children: Gaps between research and clinical practice. *J. Am. Acad. Child Adolesc. Psychiatry* 38:557–565.

Jerome, L. 1995. Neurophysiological effects of stimulants. *J. Am. Acad. Child Adolesc. Psychiatry* 34:126–127.

Kafantaris, V. 1995. Treatment of bipolar disorder in children and adolescents. *J. Am. Acad. Child Adolesc. Psychiatry* 34:732–748.

Kapur, S., and G. Remington. 1996. Serotonin-dopamine interaction and its relevance to schizophrenia. *Am. J. Psychiatry* 153:466–476.

Karjoo, M., and R. Kane. 1995. Omeprazole treatment of children with peptic esophagitis refractory to ranitidine therapy. *Arch. Pediatr. Adolesc. Med.* 149:267–271.

Karrer, R., M. Nelson, and G. C. Galbraith. 1979. Psychophysiological research with the mentally retarded. In N. R. Ellis (ed.), *Handbook of mental deficiency, psychological theory, and research,* 2d ed. Hillsdale, N.J.: L. Erlbaum Associates, pp. 231–288.

Kastner, R., R. Finesmith, and K. Walsh. 1993. Long-term administration of valproic acid in the treatment of affective symptoms in people with mental retardation. *J. Clin. Psychopharmacol.* 13:448–451.

Keck, P. E., S. L. McElroy, and S. M. Strakowski. 1998. Anticonvulsants and antipsychotics in the treatment of bipolar disorder. *J. Clin. Psychiatry* 59:74–81.

Keller, M. B., J. P. McCullough, D. N. Klein, B. Arnow, D. L. Dunner, A. J. Gelenberg, J. C. Markowitz, C. B. Nemeroff, J. M. Russell, M. E. Thase, M. H. Trivedi, and J. Zajecka. 2000. A comparison of nefazodone, the cognitive behavioral-analysis system of psychotherapy, and their combination for the treatment of chronic depression [see comments]. *N. Engl. J. Med.* 342:1462–1470.

Keogh, M. J. 1992. Intervention to enhance attention skills in children with attention deficit hyperactivity disorder. In R. J. Hagerman and P. McKenzie (eds.), *1992 International Fragile X Conference proceedings.* Dillon, Colo.: National Fragile X Foundation and Spectra Publishing, pp. 251–259.

Klein, D. F. 1964. Delineation of two drug responsive anxiety syndromes. *Psychopharmacology (Berl.)* 5:397–408.

Kofoed, L., G. Tadepalli, J. R. Oesterheld, S. Awadallah, and R. Shapiro. 1999. Case series: Clonidine has no systematic effects on PR or QTc intervals in children. *J. Am. Acad. Child Adolesc. Psychiatry* 38:1193–1196.

Kowatch, R. A., T. Suppes, T. J. Carmody, J. P. Bucci, J. H. Hume, M. Kromelis, G. J. Emslie, W. A. Weinberg, and A. J. Rush. 2000. Effect size of lithium, divalproex sodium, and carbamazepine in children and adolescents with bipolar disorder. *J. Am. Acad. Child Adolesc. Psychiatry* 39:713–720.

Kramer, P. D. 1993. *Listening to Prozac.* New York: Viking/Penguin.

Kumra, S., D. Herion, L. K. Jacobsen, C. Briguglia, and D. Grothe. 1997. Case study: Risperidone-induced hepatotoxicity in pediatric patients [see comments]. *J. Am. Acad. Child Adolesc. Psychiatry* 36:701–705.

Lacassie, Y., B. Curotto, M. A. Alliende, I. de Andraca, and A. Zavala. 1984. Evaluacion preliminar del tratamiento con acido folico en dos pacientes con retraso mental ligado al sexo y macroorquidismo. *Rev. Med. Chil.* 112:469–473.

Lachiewicz, A. M., and D. V. Dawson. 1994. Do young boys with fragile X syndrome have macroorchidism? *Pediatrics* 93:992–995.

Lafferty, J. E., and J. N. Constantino. 1998. Fluvoxamine in selective mutism [letter]. *J. Am. Acad. Child Adolesc. Psychiatry* 37:12–13.

Langee, H. R. 1989. A retrospective study of mentally retarded patients with behavior disorders who were treated with carbamazepine. *Am. J. Ment. Retard.* 93:640–643.

Lappin, R. I., and E. L. Auchincloss. 1994. Treatment of the serotonin syndrome with cyproheptadine [letter]. *N. Engl. J. Med.* 331:1021–1022.

Larson, J., C. N. Quach, B. Q. LeDuc, A. Nguyen, G. A. Rogers, and G. Lynch. 1996. Effects of an AMPA receptor modulator on methamphetamine-induced hyperactivity in rats. *Brain Res.* 738:353–356.

Leboyer, M. 1990. A double blind study of naltrexone in infantile autism. Presented at the Consensus Conference on Biological Basis and Clinical Perspective in Autism, Troina, La Citta dell'Oasi, Sicilia, October 19.

Leckman, J. F. 1987. Medications in fragile X children. Presented at the First National Fragile X Conference, Denver, December 3–4.

Leckman, J. F., D. J. Cohen, J. M. Dertner, S. Ort, and D. F. Harcherik. 1984. Growth hormone response to clonidine in children age 4–17: Tourette's syndrome vs. children with short stature. *J. Am. Acad. Child Psychiatry* 23:174–181.

Leckman, J. F., J. Detlor, D. F. Harcherik, S. Ort, B. A. Shaywitz, and D. J. Cohen. 1985. Short and long-term treatment of Tourette's syndrome with clonidine: A clinical perspective. *Neurology* 35:343–351.

Leckman, J., M. Hardin, M. Riddle, J. Stevenson, S. Ort, and D. Cohen. 1991. Clonidine treatment of Gilles de la Tourette's syndrome. *Arch. Gen. Psychiatry* 48:324–328.

Lejeune, J. 1982. Is the fragile X syndrome amaenable to treatment? [letter]. *Lancet* 1:273–274.

Lejeune, J., M.-O. Rethore, M. C. de Blois, and A. Ravel. 1984. Assay of folic acid treatment in fragile-X syndrome. *Ann. Genet.* 27:230–232.

Lepola, U., E. Leinonen, and H. Koponen. 1994. Citalopram in anxiety disorder of childhood and adolescence [letter]. *Eur. Child Adolesc. Psychiatry* 3:277–279.

———. 1996. Citalopram in the treatment of early-onset panic disorder and school phobia. *Pharmacopsychiatry* 29:30–32.

Levine, R. A., L. P. Milles, and W. Lovenberg. 1981. Tetrahydrobiopterin in striatum: Localization in dopamine nerve terminals and role in catecholamine synthesis. *Science* 214:919–921.

Lipkin, P. H., I. J. Goldstein, and A. R. Adesman. 1994. Tics and dyskinesias associated with stimulant treatment in attention-deficit hyperactivity disorder. *Arch. Pediatr. Adolesc. Med.* 148:859–861.

Livingston, M. G. 1994. Risperidone. *Lancet* 343:457–460.

Lombroso, P. J., L. Scahill, R. A. King, K. A. Lynch, P. B. Chappell, B. S. Peterson, C. J. McDougle, and J. F. Leckman. 1995. Risperidone treatment of children and adolescents with chronic tic disorders: A preliminary report. *J. Am. Acad. Child Adolesc. Psychiatry* 34:1147–1152.

Luxem, M., and E. Christopherson. 1994. Behavioral toilet training in early childhood: Research practice and implications. *J. Dev. Behav. Pediatr.* 15:370–378.

Lynch, G., M. Kessler, G. Rogers, J. Ambros-Ingerson, R. Granger, and R. S. Schehr. 1996. Psychological effects of a drug that facilitates brain AMPA receptors. *Int. Clin. Psychopharmacol.* 11:13–19.

Lynch, G., R. Granger, J. Ambros-Ingerson, C. M. Davis, M. Kessler, and R. Schehr. 1997. Evidence that a positive modulator of AMPA-type glutamate receptors improves delayed recall in aged humans. *Exp. Neurol.* 145:89–92.

MacFarlane, J. G., J. M. Cleghorn, G. M. Brown, and D. L. Streiner. 1991. The effects of exogenous melatonin on the total sleep time and daytime alertness of chronic insomniacs: A preliminary study. *Biol. Psychiatry* 30:371–376.

Madison, L. S., T. E. Wells, T. E. Fristo, and C. G. Benesch. 1986. A controlled study of folic acid treatment in 3 fragile X syndrome males. *J. Dev. Behav. Pediatr.* 7:253–256.

Malhotra, S., and P. J. Santosh. 1998. An open clinical trial of buspirone in children with attention deficit/hyperactivity disorder. *J. Am. Acad. Child Adolesc. Psychiatry* 37:364–371.

Malone, R. P., R. Sheikh, and J. M. Zito. 1999. Novel antipsychotic medications in the treatment of children and adolescents. *Psychiatr. Services* 50:171–174.

Manheim, D., L. Paalzow, and B. Hokfelt. 1982. Plasma clonidine in relation to blood pressure, catecholamines, and renin activity during long-term treatment of hypertension. *Clin. Pharmacol. Ther.* 31:445–451.

Manos, M. J., E. J. Short, and R. L. Findling. 1999. Differential effectiveness of methylphenidate and Adderall in school-age youths with attention-deficit/hyperactivity disorder. *J. Am. Acad. Child Adolesc. Psychiatry* 38:813–819.

March, J. S., J. Biederman, R. Wolkow, A. Safferman, J. Mardekian, E. H. Cook, N. R. Cutler, R. Dominguez, J. Ferguson, B. Muller, R. Riesenberg, M. Rosenthal, F. R. Sallee, K. D. Wagner, and H. Steiner. 1998. Sertraline in children and adolescents with obsessive-compulsive disorder: A multicenter randomized controlled trial [see comments] [published erratum appears in *JAMA* 283:1293, 2000]. *JAMA* 280:1752–1756.

Markowitz, P. I. 1992. Effect of fluoxetine on self-injurious behavior in the developmentally disabled: A preliminary study. *J. Clin. Psychopharmacol.* 12:27–31.

Martin, A., K. Koenig, L. Scahill, and J. Bregman. 1999. Open-label quetiapine in the treatment of children and adolescents with autistic disorder. *J. Child Adolesc. Psychopharmacol.* 9:99–107.

Massand, P., S. Gupta, and M. Dewan. 1991. Suicidal ideation related to fluoxetine treatment [letter]. *N. Engl. J. Med.* 324:420.

Mayes, S. D., D. L. Crites, E. O. Bixler, F. J. Humphrey, and R. E. Mattison. 1994. Methylphenidate and ADHD: Influence of age, IQ and neurodevelopmental status. *Dev. Med. Child Neurol.* 36:1099–1107.

McClain, L. D., G. F. Carl, and W. F. Bridges. 1975. Distribution of folic acid coenzymes and folate dependent enzymes in mouse brain. *J. Neurochem.* 24:719–722.

McConville, B. J., L. A. Arvanitis, P. T. Thyrum, C. Yeh, L. A. Wilkinson, R. O. Chaney, K. D. Foster, M. T. Sorter, L. M. Friedman, K. L. Brown, and J. E. Heubi. 2000. Pharmacokinetics, tolerability, and clinical effectiveness of quetiapine fumarate: An open-label trial in adolescents with psychotic disorders. *J. Clin. Psychiatry* 61:252–260.

McDougle, C. J., J. P. Holmes, M. R. Bronson, G. M. Anderson, F. R. Volkmar, L. H. Price, and D. J. Cohen. 1997. Risperidone treatment of children and adolescents with pervasive developmental disorders: A prospective open-label study [see comments]. *J. Am. Acad. Child Adolesc. Psychiatry* 36:685–693.

McDougle, C. J., J. P. Holmes, D. C. Carlson, D. H. Pelton, D. J. Cohen, and L. H. Price. 1998. A double blind, placebo-controlled study of risperidone in adults with autistic disorder and other pervasive developmental disorders. *Arch. Gen. Psychiatry* 55:633–641.

McElroy, S. L., and E. Weller. 1997. Psychopharmacological treatment of bipolar disorder across the life span. In S. L. McElroy (ed.), *Psychopharmacology across the life span.* Washington, D.C.: American Psychiatric Press, pp. 31–85.

Mendels, J., A. Kiev, and L. F. Fabre. 1999. Double-blind comparison of citalopram and placebo in depressed outpatients with melancholia. *Depress. Anxiety* 9:54–60.

Mezzacappa, E., R. Steingard, D. Kindlon, J. P. Saul, and F. Earls. 1998. Tricyclic antidepressants and cardiac autonomic control in children and adolescents. *J. Am. Acad. Child Adolesc. Psychiatry* 37:52–59.

Miller, L. J., D. N. McIntosh, J. McGrath, V. Shyu, M. Lampe, A. K. Taylor, F. Tassone, K. Neitzel, T. Stackhouse, and R. J. Hagerman. 1999. Electrodermal responses to sensory stimuli in individuals with fragile X syndrome: A preliminary report. *Am. J. Med. Genet.* 83:268–279.

Milne, D. B., W. K. Canfield, J. R. Mahalko, and H. H. Sandstead. 1984. Effect of oral folic acid supplements on zinc, copper and iron absorption and excretion. *Am. J. Clin. Nutr.* 39:535–539.

Moffatt, M. E. 1997. Nocturnal enuresis: A review of the efficacy of treatments and practical advice for clinicians. *J. Dev. Behav. Pediatr.* 18:49–56.

Mondadori, C. 1993. The pharmacology of the nootropics: New insights and new questions. *Behav. Brain Res.* 59:1–9.

———. 1994. In search of the mechanism of action of the nootropics: New insights and potential clinical implications. *Life Sci.* 55:2171–2178.

MTA Cooperative Group. 1999a. A 14-month randomized clinical trial of treatment strategies for attention-deficit/hyperactivity disorder. Multimodal Treatment Study of Children with ADHD. *Arch. Gen. Psychiatry* 56:1073–1086.

———. 1999b. Moderators and mediators of treatment response for children with attention-deficit/hyperactivity disorder. *Arch. Gen. Psychiatry* 56:1088–1096.

Murphy, M. A., and R. J. Hagerman. 1992. Attention deficit hyperactivity disorder in children: Diagnosis, treatment and followup. *J. Pediatr. Health Care* 6:2–11.

Musumeci, S. A., R. Ferri, M. Elia, S. Del Gracco, C. Scuderi, and M. C. Stefanini. 1996. Normal respiratory pattern during sleep in young fragile X-syndrome patients [letter]. *J. Sleep Res.* 5:272.

Musumeci, S. A., R. J. Hagerman, R. Ferri, P. Bosco, K. Dalla Bernardina, C. A. Tassinari, G. B. DeSarro, and M. Elia. 1999. Epilepsy and EEG findings in males with fragile X syndrome. *Epilepsia* 40:1092–1099.

Naylor, G. T., J. M. Donald, D. Le Poidevin, and A. H. Reid. 1974. A double-blind trial of long-term lithium therapy in mental defectives. *Br. J. Psychiatry* 124:52–57.

O'Hare, J. P., I. A. D. O'Brian, J. Arendt, P. Astley, W. Ratcliffe, H. Andres, R. Walters, and R. S. M. Correll. 1986. Does melatonin deficiency cause the enlarged genitalia of the fragile X syndrome? *Clin. Endocrinol.* 24:327–333.

Olvera, R. L., S. R. Pliszka, J. Luh, and R. Tatum. 1996. An open trial of venlafaxine in the treatment of attention-deficit/hyperactivity disorder in children and adolescents. *J. Child Adolesc. Psychopharmacol.* 6:241–250.

Pascualvaca, D. 1995. Attention capacities in children with pervasive developmental disorders. *Int. Pediatr.* 10:166–170.

Pelco, L. E., R. C. Kissel, J. M. Parrish, and R. G. Miltenberger. 1987. Behavioral management of oral medication administration difficulties among children: A review of literature with case illustrations. *J. Dev. Behav. Pediatr.* 8:90–96.

Pelham, W. E., H. R. Aronoff, J. K. Midlam, C. J. Shapiro, E. M. Gnagy, A. M. Chronis, A. N. Onyango, G. Forehand, A. Nguyen, and J. Waxmonsky. 1999. A comparison of ritalin and Adderall: Efficacy and time-course in children with attention-deficit/hyperactivity disorder. *Pediatrics* 103:e43.

Pellock, J. M. 1987. Carbamazepine side effects in children and adults. *Epilepsia* 28 (suppl. 3): S64–S70.

Pippenger, C. E. 1987. Clinically significant carbamazepine drug interactions: An overview. *Epilepsia* 28 (suppl. 3): S71–S76.

Pliszka, S. R. 1987. Tricyclic antidepressants in the treatment of children with attention deficit disorder. *J. Am. Acad. Child Adolesc. Psychiatry* 26:127–132.

Pliszka, S. R., J. T. McCracken, and J. W. Maas. 1996. Catecholamines in attention deficit hyperactivity disorder: Current perspectives. *J. Am. Acad. Child Adolesc. Psychiatry* 35:264–272.

Polakoff, S. A., P. J. Sorgi, and J. J. Ratey. 1986. The treatment of impulsive and aggressive behavior with nadolol. *J. Clin. Psychopharmacol.* 6:125–126.

Post, R. M. 1989. Introduction: Emerging perspectives on valproate in affective disorders. *J. Clin. Psychiatry* 50 (suppl. 3): 3–9.

Post, R. M., M. A. Frye, and G. S. Leverich. 1998. The role of complex combination therapy in the treatment of refractory bipolar illness. *CNS Spectrums* 3:66–86.

Potenza, M. N., J. P. Holmes, S. J. Kanes, and C. J. McDougle. 1999. Olanzapine treatment of children, adolescents, and adults with pervasive developmental disorders: An open-label pilot study. *J. Clin. Psychopharmacol.* 19:37–44.

Preskorn, S. H. 1993. Recent pharmacologic advances in antidepressant therapy for the elderly. *Am. J. Med.* 94 (suppl. 5A): 2S–12S.

———. 1994. Antidepressant drug selection: Criteria and options. *J. Clin. Psychiatry* 55 (suppl. 9): 6–22.

Prince, J. B., T. E. Wilens, J. Biederman, T. J. Spencer, and J. R. Wozniak. 1996. Clonidine for sleep disturbances associated with attention-deficit hyperactivity disorder: A systematic chart review of 62 cases. *J. Am. Acad. Child Adolesc. Psychiatry* 35: 599–605.

Quintana, H., and M. Keshavan. 1995. Case study: Risperidone in children and adolescents with schizophrenia. *J. Am. Acad. Child. Adolesc. Psychiatry* 34:1292–1296.

Racusin, R., K. Kovner-Kline, and B. H. King. 1999. Selective serotonin reuptake inhibitors in intellectual disability. *Ment. Retard. Dev. Disabil. Res. Rev.* 5:264–269.

Rapoport, J. L. 1988. The neurobiology of obsessive-compulsive disorder. *JAMA* 260: 2888–2890.

Rapoport, J. L., D. O. Quinn, G. Bradbard, K. D. Riddle, and S. E. Brook. 1974. Imipramine and methylphenidate treatment of hyperactive boys. *Arch. Gen. Psychiatry* 30:789–793.

Rappley, M. D., P. B. Mullan, F. J. Alvarez, I. U. Eneli, J. Wang, and J. C. Gardiner. 1999. Diagnosis of attention-deficit/hyperactivity disorder and use of psychotropic medication in very young children [see comments]. *Arch. Pediatr. Adolesc. Med.* 153: 1039–1045.

Raskin, L. A., S. E. Shaywitz, B. A. Shaywitz, G. M. Anderson, and D. J. Cohen. 1984. Neurochemical correlates of attention deficit disorder. *Pediatr. Clin. North Am.* 31: 387–396.

Ratey, J. J., K. Sovner, E. Mikkelsen, and H. E. Chmielinski. 1989. Buspirone therapy for maladaptive behavior and anxiety in developmentally disabled persons. *J. Clin. Psychiatry* 50:382–384.

Reid, A. H., G. T. Naylor, and D. S. G. Kay. 1981. A double-blind placebo-controlled crossover trial of carbamazepine in overactive, severely mentally handicapped patients. *Psychol. Med.* 11:109–113.

Reiss, A. L., M. T. Abrams, R. Greenlaw, L. Freund, and M. B. Denckla. 1995. Neurodevelopmental effects of the *FMR-1* full mutation in humans. *Nat. Med.* 1:159–167.

Reynolds, E. H. 1967. Effects of folic acid on the mental state and fit frequency of drug treated epileptic patients. *Lancet* 1:1086–1088.

Rey-Sanchez, F., and J. R. Gutierrez-Casares. 1997. Paroxetine in children with major depressive disorder: An open trial. *J. Am. Acad. Child Adolesc. Psychiatry* 36:1443–1447.

Riddle, M. A., B. Geller, and N. Ryan. 1993. Another sudden death in a child treated with desipramine. *J. Am. Acad. Child Adolesc. Psychiatry* 32:792–796.

Riley, K., L. O. Ikle, and R. J. Hagerman. 2000. A randomized, double-blind comparative trial of Adderall in the treatment of attention deficit disorder in children with fragile X. Presented at the Seventh International Fragile X Conference, Los Angeles, July 19–23.

Ritvo, E. R., R. Ritvo, A. Yuwiler, and A. Brothers. 1993. Elevated daytime melatonin concentrations in autism: A pilot study. *Eur. Child Adolesc. Psychiatry* 2:75–78.

Rogers, S. J., and H. Lewis. 1989. An effective day treatment model for young children with pervasive developmental disorders. *J. Am. Acad. Child Adolesc. Psychiatry* 28:207–214.

Rosenberg, D. R., J. Holttum, and S. Gershon. 1994. *Textbook of pharmacotherapy for child and adolescent psychiatric disorders.* New York: Brunner/Mazel Publishers.

Rosenberg, D. R., C. M. Stewart, K. D. Fitzgerald, V. Tawile, and E. Carroll. 1999. Paroxetine open-label treatment of pediatric outpatients with obsessive-compulsive disorder. *J. Am. Acad. Child Adolesc. Psychiatry* 38:1180–1185.

Rosenberg, D. R., F. P. MacMaster, M. S. Keshavan, K. D. Fitzgerald, C. M. Stewart, and G. J. Moore. 2000. Decrease in caudate glutamatergic concentrations in pediatric obsessive-compulsive disorder patients taking paroxetine. *J. Am. Acad. Child Adolesc. Psychiatry* 39:1096–1103.

Rosenblatt, D. S., E. A. Duschenes, F. V. Hellstrom, M. S. Golick, M. J. Vekemans, S. F. Zeesman, and E. Andermann. 1985. Folic acid blinded trial in identical twins with fragile X syndrome. *Am. J. Hum. Genet.* 37:543–552.

Rosh, J. R., S. F. Dellert, M. Narkewicz, A. Birnbaum, and G. Whitington. 1998. Four cases of severe hepatotoxicity associated with pemoline: Possible autoimmune pathogenesis. *Pediatrics* 101:921–923.

Rosler, A., and E. Witztum. 1998. Treatment of men with paraphilia with a long-acting analogue of gonadotropin-releasing hormone [see comments]. *N. Engl. J. Med.* 338:416–422.

Ruedrich, S., T. P. Swales, C. Fossaceca, J. Toliver, and A. Rutkowski. 1999. Effect of divalproex sodium on aggression and self-injurious behaviour in adults with intellectual disability: A retrospective review. *J. Intellect. Disabil. Res.* 43:105–111.

Ryan, N. D., V. S. Bhatara, and J. M. Perel. 1999. Mood stabilizers in children and adolescents. *J. Am. Acad. Child Adolesc. Psychiatry* 38:529–536.

Sadeh, A., M. Klitzke, T. F. Anders, and C. Acebo. 1995. Case study: Sleep and aggressive behavior in a blind retarded adolescent. A concomitant schedule disorder? *J. Am. Acad. Child Adolesc. Psychiatry* 34:820–824.

Safer, D. J., and J. M. Krager. 1988. A survey of medication treatment for hyperactive/inattentive students. *JAMA* 260:2256–2258.

Schmitt, B. D. 1995. Nocturnal enuresis: Finding the treatment that fits the child. *Contemp. Pediatr.* 12:3–15.

Schopmeyer, B., and F. Lowe. 1992. *The fragile X child.* San Diego: Singular Publishing Group.

Selinger, G. M., A. Hornstein, J. Flax, J. Herbert, and K. Schroeder. 1992. Fluoxetine improves emotional incontinence. *Brain Inj.* 6:267–270.

Shapiro, A. K., E. S. Shapiro, J. G. Young, and T. E. Feinberg. 1988. *Gilles de la Tourette syndrome,* 2d ed. New York: Raven Press, pp. 405–410.

Scholomaskas, A. J. 1990. Mania in a panic disorder patient treated with fluoxetine. *Am. J. Psychiatry* 147:1090–1091.

Singer, H. S., J. Brown, S. Quaskey, L. A. Rosenberg, E. D. Mellits, and M. B. Denckla. 1995. The treatment of attention deficit hyperactivity disorder in Tourette's syndrome: A double-blind placebo-controlled study with clonidine and desipramine. *Pediatrics* 95:74–82.

Sloan, R. L., K. W. Brown, and B. Pentland. 1992. Fluoxetine as a treatment for emotional lability after brain injury. *Brain Inj.* 6:315–319.

Solanto, M. V. 1998. Neuropsychopharmacological mechanisms of stimulant drug action in attention-deficit hyperactivity disorder: A review and integration. *Behav. Brain Res.* 94:127–152.

Sondheimer, J. M. 1994. Gastroesophageal reflux in children: Clinical presentation and diagnostic evaluation. *Gastrointest. Endosc. Clin. N. Am.* 4:55–74.

Sovner, R., and R. J. Pary. 1993. Affective disorders in developmentally disabled persons. In J. L. Matson and R. P. Barrett (eds.), *Psychopathology in the mentally retarded.* Needham Heights, Mass.: Allyn & Bacon, pp. 87–147.

Spiridigliozzi, G. A., A. M. Lachiewicz, C. S. MacMurdo, A. D. Vizoso, C. M. O'Donnell, A. McConkie-Rosell, and D. J. Burges. 1994. *Educating boys with fragile X syndrome: A guide for parents and professionals.* Durham: Duke University Medical Center.

Staubli, U., G. Rogers, and G. Lynch. 1994. Facilitation of glutamate receptors enhances memory. *Proc. Natl. Acad. Sci. USA* 91:777–781.

Steiner, M., S. Steinberg, D. Stewart, D. Carter, C. Berger, R. Reid, D. Grover, and D. Streiner. 1995. Fluoxetine in the treatment of premenstrual dysphoria. *N. Engl. J. Med.* 332:1529–1534.

Steingard, R., J. Biederman, J. Spencer, T. Wilens, and A. Gonzalez. 1993. Comparison of clonidine response in treatment of attention deficit hyperactivity disorder with and without comorbid tic disorders. *J. Am. Acad. Child Adolesc. Psychiatry* 32:350–353.

Steingard, R. J., M. Goldberg, D. Lee, and D. R. Demaso. 1994. Adjunctive clonazepam treatment of tic symptoms in children with comorbid tic disorders and ADHD. *J. Am. Acad. Child Adolesc. Psychiatry* 33:394–398.

Steingard, R. J., B. Zimnitzky, D. R. DeMaso, M. L. Bauman, and J. P. Bucci. 1997. Sertraline treatment of transition-associated anxiety and agitation in children with autistic disorder. *J. Child Adolesc. Psychopharmacol.* 7:9–15.

Stewart, J. T., W. C. Myers, R. C. Burket, and W. B. Lyles. 1990. A review of the pharmacotherapy of aggression in children and adolescents. *J. Am. Acad. Child Adolesc. Psychiatry* 29:269–277.

Swann, A. C., C. L. Bowden, and D. Morris. 1997. Depression during mania: Treatment response to lithium and divalproex. *Arch. Gen. Psychiatry* 54:37–42.

Swanson, J., S. Wigal, L. Greenhill, R. Browne, B. Waslick, M. Lerner, L. Williams, D. Flynn, D. Agler, K. L. Crowley, E. Fineberg, R. Regino, M. Baren, and D. Cantwell. 1998. Objective and subjective measures of the pharmacodynamic effects of Adderall in the treatment of children with ADHD in a controlled laboratory classroom setting. *Psychopharmacol. Bull.* 34:55–60.

Swanson, J. M., D. Flockhart, D. Udrea, D. Cantwell, D. Connor, and L. Williams. 1995. Clonidine and the treatment of ADHD: Questions about safety and efficacy. *J. Child Adolesc. Psychopharmacol.* 5:301–304.

Thomaidis, L., E. Kaderoglou, M. Stefou, S. Damaniou, and C. Bakoula. 2000. Does early intervention work? A controlled trial. *Infant Young Child.* 12:17.

Thompson, S., and J. M. Rey. 1995. Functional enuresis: Is Desmopressin the answer? *J. Am. Acad. Child Adolesc. Psychiatry* 34:266–271.

Thomsen, P. H. 1997. Child and adolescent obsessive-compulsive disorder treated with citalopram: Findings from an open trial of 23 cases. *J. Child Adolesc. Psychopharmacol.* 7:157–166.

Tirosh, E., and Z. Borochowitz. 1992. Sleep apnea in fragile X syndrome. *Am. J. Med. Genet.* 43:124–127.

Tirosh, E., Y. Tal, and M. Jaffe. 1995. CPAP treatment of obstructive sleep apnoea and neurodevelopmental deficits. *Acta Paediatr.* 84:791–794.

Torrioli, M. G., S. Vernacotola, P. Mariotti, E. Bianchi, M. Calvani, A. De Gaetano, P. Chiurazzi, and G. Neri. 1999. Double-blind, placebo-controlled study of L-acetyl-carnitine for the treatment of hyperactive behavior in fragile X syndrome [letter]. *Am. J. Med. Genet.* 87:366–368.

Tranfaglia, M. R. 2000. A medication guide for fragile X syndrome, version 3.1. West Newbury, Mass.: FRAXA Research Foundation.

Trimble, M. R. 1987. Anticonvulsant drugs and cognitive function: A review of the literature. *Epilepsia* 28 (suppl. 3): S37–S45.

Turk, J. 1992. Fragile X syndrome and folic acid. In R. J. Hagerman and P. McKenzie (eds.), *1992 International Fragile X Conference proceedings.* Dillon, Colo.: National Fragile X Foundation and Spectra Publishing, pp. 195–200.

Uhari, M., T. Kontiokari, and M. Niemela. 1998. A novel use of xylitol sugar in preventing acute otitis media [see comments]. *Pediatrics* 102:879–884.

Vanden Borre, R., R. Vermote, M. Buttiëns, P. Thiry, G. Dierick, J. Geutjens, G. Sieben, and S. Heylen. 1993. Risperidone as an add-on therapy in behavioural disturbances in mental retardation: A double-blind placebo-controlled cross-over study. *Acta Psychiatr. Scand.* 83:167–171.

von Gontard, A. 1998. Annotation: Day and night wetting in children—a paediatric and child psychiatric perspective [see comments]. *J. Child Psychol. Psychiatry* 39:439–451.

Wang, J., and R. W. Erbe. 1984. Folate metabolism in cells from fragile X syndrome patients and carriers. *Am. J. Med. Genet.* 17:303–310.

Warnock, J. K., and T. Kestenbaum. 1992. Pharmacologic treatment of severe skin-picking behaviors in Prader-Willi syndrome. *Arch. Dermatol.* 128:1623–1625.

Weiger, W. A., and D. M. Bear. 1988. An approach to the neurology of aggression. *J. Psychiatr. Res.* 22:85–98.

Wilens, T. E. 1999. *Straight talk about psychiatric medications for kids.* New York: Guilford Press.

Wilens, T. E., J. Biederman, and T. Spencer. 1994. Clonidine for sleep disturbances associated with attention deficit hyperactivity disorder. *J. Am. Acad. Child Adolesc. Psychiatry* 33:424–426.

Wilens, T. E., T. Spencer, J. Biederman, J. Wozmak, and D. Connor. 1995. Combined pharmacotherapy: An emerging trend in pediatric psychopharmacology. *J. Am. Acad. Child Adolesc. Psychiatry* 34:110–112.

Wilens, T. E., D. Wyatt, and T. J. Spencer. 1998. Disentangling disinhibition. *J. Am. Acad. Child Adolesc. Psychiatry* 37:1225–1227.

Wilens, T. E., T. J. Spencer, J. M. Swanson, D. F. Connor, and D. Cantwell. 1999. Combining methylphenidate and clonidine: A clinically sound medication option [see comments]. *J. Am. Acad. Child Adolesc. Psychiatry* 38:614–619; discussion 619–622.

Wilson, P., T. Stackhouse, R. O'Connor, S. Scharfenaker, and R. Hagerman. 1994. *Issues and strategies for educating children with fragile X syndrome: A monograph.* Dillon, Colo.: Spectra Publishing Company.

Wisniewski, K. E., S. M. Segan, C. M. Miezejeski, E. A. Sersen, and R. D. Rudelli. 1991. The fragile X syndrome: Neurological, electrophysiological, and neuropathological abnormalities. *Am. J. Med. Genet.* 38:476–480.

Woolston, J. L. 1999. Combined pharmacotherapy: Pitfalls of treatment. *J. Am. Acad. Child Adolesc. Psychiatry* 38:1455–1457.

Wright-Talamante, C., A. Cheema, J. E. Riddle, D. W. Luckey, A. K. Taylor, and R. J. Hagerman. 1996. A controlled study of longitudinal IQ changes in females and males with fragile X syndrome. *Am. J. Med. Genet.* 64:350–355.

Zettner, A., G. Boss, and J. E. Seegmiller. 1981. A long-term study of the absorption of large doses of folic acid. *Ann. Clin. Lab. Sci.* 11:517–524.

Zuddas, A., A. Di Martino, P. Muglia, and C. Cianchetti. 2000. Long term risperidone for pervasive developmental disorder: Efficacy, tolerability, and discontinuation. *J. Child Adolesc. Psychopharmacol.* 10:79–90.

# CHAPTER 9

# The Treatment of Emotional and Behavioral Problems

## Jennifer L. Hills Epstein, Psy.D., Karen Riley, Ph.D., and William E. Sobesky, Ph.D.

In previous editions of this book, this chapter began with the observation that there was little empiric work regarding the effectiveness of different treatment strategies with individuals who display symptoms of fragile X syndrome (FXS) (Sobesky 1996; Brown et al. 1991). Unfortunately, this is still the case. Thus, the present chapter, like the previous ones, will be based on the authors' clinical experiences with clients with FXS and on anecdotal information from other clinicians. Although we are now more aware of some of the typical emotional and behavioral difficulties experienced by individuals with FXS (see chap. 1 of this volume), research in this area is still continuing.

To plan treatment interventions, one must know what problems are characteristic of FXS. Two difficulties arise in trying to describe characteristic problems connected with FXS. The first is that it can be difficult to determine when a problem is directly caused by the FXS mutation, when it is secondary to other difficulties in FXS, or when it is simply an emotional or behavioral problem that is not related to FXS at all. For example, there is now ample evidence to suggest that certain features of schizotypal personality disorder, such as social and interpersonal deficits related to odd thinking and speech patterns, suspiciousness or guardedness, and excessive social anxiety, are characteristic of FXS (Reiss et al. 1988, 1989; Sobesky et al. 1994a), whereas the evidence for depression as a characteristic of FXS is now more equivocal (Reiss et al. 1993; Sobesky et al. 1994b; Franke et al. 1998). It is possible that individuals with FXS may be at risk for depression secondary to other difficulties characteristic of FXS and not as a primary deficit. Finally, other problems, such as Tourette

*Fragile X Syndrome: Diagnosis, Treatment, and Research,* third edition, ed. Randi Jenssen Hagerman and Paul J. Hagerman (Baltimore: Johns Hopkins University Press, 2002), © The Johns Hopkins University Press.

syndrome, that occur in the population with FXS may be unrelated to the FXS gene or the result of a secondary gene effect acting independently or in concert with the fragile X mutation (Hagerman 1999).

The second issue has to do with the variability of the symptom picture among individuals with FXS. Physical symptoms such as outer ear prominence (Hull and Hagerman 1993), cognitive symptoms such as intellectual ability (Mazzocco et al. 1993), and emotional/behavioral symptoms (Sobesky et al. 1996) may all vary a great deal even within a specific genetic subgroup, such as individuals with a premutation or a full mutation. This may be related to background gene effects interacting with the variability within the *FMR1* gene. Perhaps after we are better able to understand the mechanisms that translate genotypic effects into phenotypic behaviors, we will be better able to define what constitutes characteristic problems for various subgroups of individuals with FXS. On the other hand, virtually no research on individuals with FXS has focused on factors other than genetic variables that may give rise to various emotional or behavioral difficulties. Preliminary data on this topic (Sobesky et al., unpublished) suggest that emotional/behavioral symptoms may be strongly influenced by stress, although stress does not typically influence physical or cognitive symptoms. Thus, as with individuals who do not display FXS, the population with FXS may exhibit a symptom pattern that is a function of the interaction of the FXS characteristics with environmental stresses over time.

In the first edition of this chapter, the majority of the treatment suggestions were focused on providing psychotherapeutic services to those who have mental retardation, particularly persons with the full mutation for FXS (Brown et al. 1991). In the second edition, treatment suggestions targeted higher-functioning males and females with FXS (Sobesky 1996). The present version of this chapter will propose a model for psychotherapy and behavioral interventions for the more common and, in some ways, the most severe problems experienced by persons with the full fragile X mutation and their families. The primary focus will be on full mutation males, although some case studies will also describe females. Characteristic strengths as well as difficulties will be addressed because it is crucial to build on strengths to help neutralize or compensate for difficulties. Possible intervention strategies based on the authors' clinical experiences will be outlined. Interventions to be discussed will focus on individual and family psychotherapy, as well as the specifics of developing a behavior plan. The reader is also encouraged to review material presented in the previous two editions of this chapter, as this information is still relevant but will not be repeated again here.

## Emotional Phenotype

The full fragile X mutation influences an individual on a variety of levels, resulting in a range of symptoms that vary in effect and intensity from person to person. FXS causes a broad range of cognitive disabilities ranging from mild to moderate learning disabilities to various ranges of mental retardation (see chap. 6). By adulthood, the majority of males with FXS function within the moderate range of mental retardation. Women with FXS have a greater diversity in cognitive profiles. By adulthood, approximately 70% of women have an IQ less than or equal to 85, many with weaknesses in math, visual spatial skills, auditory processing, and executive functioning (deVries et al. 1996). Approximately 30% of women with the full mutation have cognitive abilities in the average or greater range, but this is frequently accompanied by mild to moderate learning disabilities as well.

Regardless of level of cognitive ability, most individuals with FXS show deficits in executive functioning (see chap. 6; also Sobesky et al. 1996). Deficits in executive functioning result in problems with attention and concentration, working memory, and behavioral impulsivity and disinhibition. Many people with FXS also show hyperactivity and restlessness, which is more severe during childhood and improves somewhat in adulthood. These symptoms are all included in the diagnosis of attention deficit hyperactivity disorder, which is commonly assigned to individuals with FXS (Turk 1998; Munir et al. 2000).

Another set of emotional symptoms common for those with FXS includes anxiety problems. Across all individuals with FXS, anxiety issues are the most common underlying emotional feature and account for a variety of behavioral issues that require intervention (Franke et al. 1998; Mazzocco et al. 1998; Wisbeck et al. 2000). A continuum of the symptoms seen includes shyness (Sobesky 1995), generalized anxiety, fear or apprehension regarding novel or unfamiliar people or places, gaze avoidance, social anxiety resulting in social withdrawal, obsessive patterns of thinking, compulsive patterns of behavior, and panic attacks. Symptoms of anxiety are very common and can be quite severe.

Sometimes the symptoms become so severe that the individual does not want to leave home, resulting in agoraphobia. This severe picture seems to occur more often for men than women and frequently accompanies schizotypal features, including tangential thoughts, social withdrawal, and difficulty maintaining social relationships. Most people feel more comfortable at home than in the community. Sometimes, social anxiety becomes so severe that the person may restrict with whom they speak. They may have certain rules about with whom they can and cannot speak. At school, they may whisper answers to a close friend rather than talk in front of the whole class. This cautious communication pattern can develop into selective mutism, which seems to be more common in girls than boys (Hagerman et al. 1999).

Social skill deficits are a common symptom in FXS. Although many individuals with mental retardation syndromes show social deficits secondary to cognitive limitations, the social deficits seen in FXS seem to be more severe, regardless of cognitive ability. Women with FXS and average IQ often have difficulties sustaining friendships or understanding the nuances of social situations. There is also an overlap of autism spectrum disorders with FXS, and some individuals with FXS have autistic-like features including gaze avoidance, repetitive behaviors such as hand biting or rocking, and perseverative speech patterns, which may include practiced or rote phrases (Cohen et al. 1988; Kerby and Dawson 1994; Turk and Graham 1997; see chap. 1). Individuals with autistic-like features often withdraw from others and seem socially aloof or resistant. At present, the term *autism* is used descriptively, and the diagnosis of autism is made based on a pattern of behavior. Specifically, there are three main sets of symptoms, including impairments in communication and in socialization and repetitive behaviors or restricted interests. Some individuals with FXS have both disorders. The co-occurrence of autism and FXS seems greatest in early childhood (Bailey et al. 2000, 2001; Rogers et al. 2001), but in our experience, it may decrease as speech language skills of children with FXS improve (see chap. 1). A smaller subset of adults with FXS seem to meet diagnostic criteria for autistic disorder, while many adults with FXS may show features of pervasive developmental disorder, not otherwise specified.

The underlying anxiety seen in FXS seems to result in awkward social behavior, such as deficits in social initiation. People with FXS often use some appropriate gestures paired with incongruent gestures related to their social anxiety. For example, during a social introduction they may reach to shake someone's hand but simultaneously pull away with the rest of their body, while averting their gaze and turning their face away from the person. Their communication partner may be confused by the contradictory messages. People with FXS are most comfortable with people they know really well, such as immediate family members. Spontaneous eye contact is most commonly seen during interactions within the family or with very close friends. People with FXS may not feel comfortable making requests of other people and, as a result, may have difficulty in getting their needs met. This is frequently a target skill for intervention.

Mood swings are another area where problems in adjustment may be identified. People with FXS often experience rapidly changing moods. They may feel happy one moment and then feel overwhelmed with sadness or anger the next. They may be unable to describe their feelings to others. Those who have language impairments or a moderate level of mental retardation may not have learned the vocabulary with which to express feelings. Adolescents with FXS may feel anger about having the syndrome but may be afraid to discuss their feelings. They may experience strong feelings of sadness resulting in bouts of depression as they reach the age when many of their peers are marrying or leaving for college.

Many individuals with FXS experience mood instability. That is, their moods are unstable and they do not stay with a particular mood for a sustained period. This has a great influence on their family system, as those around the individual are frequently reacting to each mood change, resulting in everyone feeling a lack of control or stability. Mood instability also results in frequent, severe tantrum behavior. Tantrums and disruptive behavior patterns often begin in early childhood. These patterns of behavior often include aggressive behavior such as biting, scratching, kicking, or hitting and may also include destructive behavior. If the individual also has problems with hyperactivity, parents often find a time-out procedure more difficult to implement for their children with FXS than for their children who do not have FXS. Thus, behavior patterns can intensify and, left untreated, can lead to the development of very severe aggressive and disruptive behavior patterns in adulthood. In our experience, disruptive behavior, rather than degree of cognitive impairment, is the most common cause for the need for a segregated classroom placement and/or loss of participation in community-based activities.

## Interventions

Interventions for emotional and behavioral features of FXS are varied. Interventions may be designed by various qualified professionals and may also be implemented by families. Any specific intervention plan needs to be individualized and tailored to the specific behavior or symptom and the particular person in need of services. Treatment modalities include individual psychotherapy, family psychotherapy, behavioral therapy, group therapy, and specific social skills training programs that can be designed for specific settings. It is very important that the professional involved considers the symptoms from a transdisciplinary perspective (Linder 1983). This is integral for understanding the whole individual and for designing the best intervention. Without this perspective, some specific intervention strategies and the underlying etiology of some symptoms may be overlooked. For example, a young adult male with FXS may be showing aggression in the workshop setting when he is given a particularly difficult task. At first glance, the root of this problem may be viewed as related to poor tolerance for frustration. However, by gathering additional information, a professional may find that this task is always assigned at the end of the day. It may also become clear that this task is performed in a particularly busy and loud part of the room and that the person is a fairly nonverbal communicator. By gathering information from other perspectives such as occupational therapy and speech therapy, it is possible to highlight additional contributing factors in the behavior pattern. The individual may behave aggressively because he is tired, the room may be overstimulating, and/or he may not have communication skills to protest in a more appropriate manner. Each of these considerations may influence the direction of the intervention strategy. Close collateral contact with other disciplines is key to effective intervention for FXS.

## Developing a Behavior Plan

Attempting to change an individual's behavior can be a difficult undertaking. It requires a great deal of effort. The expenditure of energy, however, is somewhat like a scale. Change is initiated when the amount of effort required to modify the behavior is outweighed by the amount of energy expended by allowing the behavior to continue. The following approach has its roots in functional analysis (O'Neill et al. 1990) while combining elements of many other types of behavior management methods. The fundamentals of the ABC (Antecedent-Behavior-Consequence) model are also included in the plan. Both the ABC model and the Functional Analysis approach have been found to be effective in working with children with FXS (Braden 2000a, 2000b). This eclectic approach (outlined below) has been used successfully with many families who have children with FXS. Before initiating a behavior plan, however, there are several general considerations to review and to keep in mind throughout the process. The first and most important consideration is that behavior does not occur in isolation. The behavior of an individual is a result of complex interactions between the individual and the environment. The previous chapters within this book serve as a foundation for understanding the complex nature and unique profile of individuals with FXS. Although it is often understandable why individuals with FXS might react aggressively or inappropriately given their special needs and a stressful environment, inappropriate behavior should not be allowed (Moor 2000). Understanding and considering the individual as a whole is paramount. A mother of a child with fragile X syndrome expressed it well: "I guess that I had been so worried about trying to make him happy that I didn't concentrate on discipline."

**Step 1.** The first step is to identify one specific behavior to target. Examples of specific behaviors include hitting, screaming, rewinding a VCR tape, or watching too much television. After the target behavior has been identified, it is necessary to determine whether in fact this is a disruptive behavior. A disruptive behavior is one that interferes with the individual's ability to perform optimally at home, at school, or in social settings, it interferes with others' ability to perform optimally, or it presents a danger to self or others. If the target behavior meets the criteria, it is appropriate to move to the next step.

**Step 2.** To change or modify a behavior, one must understand when, where, and how often it occurs. All behavior occurs for a reason. To change a behavior, one must first understand the antecedent, the action that occurs directly before the behavior, and the consequence, what happens directly after the behavior. This ABC (Antecedent-Behavior-Consequence) model of behavior management can help address inappropriate behaviors. Modifying or eliminating the antecedent can change or cease to produce the ensuing behavior (Braden 2000a, 2000b) and is addressed in step 4. The consequence of the behavior is typically the key to understanding how to modify or change the behavior. It is the consequence that maintains the cycle of the behavior and provides the reinforcement that the individual is seeking. Keeping a log or a diary of when the behavior occurs can often reveal a pattern. The pattern may suggest that the behavior is related to a specific time of day or a specific event. Logging the occurrence of the behavior can also clarify the frequency of the behavior. This clarification may serve to reinforce the need for a behavior plan by exposing a greater than expected frequency. The converse may also hold true, bringing to light the fact that the behavior does not occur with sufficient frequency to warrant the initiation of the behavior plan.

Step 3. Physiologic causes can range from low blood sugar to a mild hearing impairment; from medication wearing off to environmental allergens. Attempting to change a behavior that is physiologically based will only serve to frustrate all involved. The eradication of a physiologic cause may eliminate the behavior entirely.

Step 4. Examine and modify the structure of the situation, when possible, to decrease the opportunity for the behavior to occur. Often it is easier to modify the environment or the structure of a routine than to change the resulting behavior of the individual. Changes in structure can be as simple as changing the routine of the day. For example, during the school day it may involve moving a challenging subject such as math to the morning from the afternoon. At home it may mean changing the morning routine so that getting dressed occurs after breakfast. If a child has difficulty getting ready for school because he or she is distracted by a favorite morning cartoon, then the television should probably be left off before school.

Step 5. Provide the individual with additional resources for dealing with the stressors associated with the behavior. An additional resource can be an intervention, such as a social skills group to deal with interpersonal issues, or it can be a physical aide, such as earphones to decrease the noise in the cafeteria. Commonly used resources include, but are not limited to, adding a sensory diet into the child's programming (e.g., heavy work activities, see chap. 10), using a picture schedule to help the child in sequencing and completing difficult tasks, and implementing a communication system so that he or she can communicate frustrations appropriately.

**Step 6.** Outline natural consequences for the behavior. This again requires some forethought. Determine what the response will be when the behavior occurs, and be specific. Learning through natural consequences is optimal. When this does not or cannot occur, the interventionist must manufacture consequences that are natural and logical for the situation (Braden 2000b). For example, if the child misuses a toy, then the natural consequence is the loss of that toy for a period of time. If an individual is unable to self-regulate the amount of television that he watches, then he loses the privilege of choosing how much he will watch.

**Step 7.** Be consistent. This is easier said than done and is undoubtedly the most difficult part of modifying behavior. Consistency is also the most crucial component to an effective behavior plan. Consistency and predictability of routine and expectations are calming and reassuring for all children, particularly those with FXS. Individuals with FXS are typically unable to differentiate between subtle variations that may change the appropriateness of a specific behavior. They also often have difficulty accurately reading a social situation. As a result it is imperative to provide clear limits for behavior. The consequence for the targeted behavior should also be applied in a consistent manner. If a natural consequence, such as not getting what has been asked for when throwing a temper tantrum, is employed inconsistently, what the individual has actually learned is that sometimes tantrumming is effective and sometimes it is not. This is called *intermittent reinforcement* and actually serves to strengthen a behavior pattern rather than to decrease it.

**Step 8.** Provide a substitute behavior. Identify what you want the person to do instead of what they are currently doing. A behavior should never be taken away without providing an alternate appropriate behavior. For example, instead of screaming when they are finished with something, have them indicate that they are done through signing, talking, or using the Picture Exchange Communication System (PECS) (Frost and Bondy 1994).

**Step 9.** Reinforce positive behavior. Identify reinforcers that work for the child. All children are different. The most effective reinforcers are those that are naturally occurring, such as positive attention, receiving an item when it is requested in the appropriate manner, or participating in a group game because they are abiding by the rules. Unlike typically developing children, children with mental retardation and autism spectrum disorders may not respond well to merely social reinforcement. Many children need external reinforcers such as stickers, small toys, or extra TV time. For older children, a token system can be very effective (Barkley 1995). Rotate reinforcers frequently, so that an individual does not become satiated on any one reinforcer. This helps to maintain the value of the reinforcers. It is important that children are able to immediately attain the reinforcer at the start of a positive behavior program. This allows them to clearly link the appropriate, desired behavior to the reinforcers. If the reinforcement regime does not seem to be effective, then return to step 2 and reassess the frequency of the target behavior, so that the reinforcement schedule can be redesigned. The use of reinforcement is not restricted to children with FXS but can also be used effectively for working with adults.

Step 10. Start in a controlled setting. The initiation of a behavior plan is very important, both for the individual whose behavior is being addressed and for the person who is addressing it. Initial feelings of success are important for the continuation of the program. It is easier for all involved to begin a plan at home or at school where there is more control over the environment. After all involved feel comfortable, it is time to take the plan on the road, so to speak. Using the plan in a variety of settings clearly conveys to the child that the same rules apply regardless of the setting.

Step 11. The final step is to provide opportunities for both success and failure. Initially it is important for the child to succeed and to be reinforced for the substitute behavior. For the child to succeed, the reinforceable behavior must be attainable for the individual. Setting unrealistic expectations is one of the most common reasons for ineffective behavior plans. After success, it is important to plan for failures. For example, if the targeted behavior involves begging for toys or treats at the store and throwing a temper tantrum when the child does not get what he or she wants, initiate consequences for the temper tantrums at home, and reinforce positive behavior. Finally, initiate a trip to the grocery store where this behavior is likely to occur. The key is to plan the trip as a function of the behavior plan, not out of need for items at the store. The focus of the trip or outing is to be ready and to have the time to follow through on the previously determined consequences when the target behavior occurs. This again reinforces the child's understanding that the consequences are real and that the person imposing the consequences will follow through in all settings.

As previously stated, changing behavior is not an easy task, but it can be done. Only one behavior should be targeted at a time. Several modifications to the environment can be employed at the same time; however, when more than one behavior is being targeted, the effectiveness decreases. Remember that the behavior will actually get worse before it gets better. This is referred to as an *extinction burst* and is actually a sign that the plan is working. Changing the rules for a child can cause frustration, which may lead to a temporary increase of inappropriate behavior until the individual learns the new routine. Any plan should be implemented for a sustained period before a decision is made about its efficacy. About two weeks is an optimal time to gather data regarding efficacy, and then modifications can be made. If adjustments are made too early or too frequently, it will be hard to determine which factors are leading to a change in behavior.

## Time-out

Time-out is a natural consequence for aggressive behaviors and for those situations in which the individual may harm others. Time-out, when used appropriately and as a component of a complete behavior plan, has been shown to be an effective means of significantly decreasing and often eliminating the targeted behavior (Barkley 1995). Time-out is not an appropriate consequence for avoidance behaviors (e.g., throwing a math book on the floor to get out of completing a difficult math assignment), as this serves only to reinforce the behavior because the individual is actually receiving the desired outcome for the behavior. Understanding and employing the time-out technique effectively is fundamental to its success.

What is time-out? Time-out does not need to be a specific place, location, or piece of furniture (i.e., a kitchen chair or a corner). Time-out is simply time away from your attention. The basis for the efficacy of time-out is that attention, be it positive or negative, is reinforcing. As a result, removal of attention as a consequence for a negative behavior requires complete removal of your attention. The effective use of time-out has been outlined by Barkley (1995) for use with children with ADHD but without developmental disabilities. The following modified approach builds on that sound foundation while incorporating adaptations, which are essential for individuals with special needs.

Time-out needs to be linked to one specific behavior. Particularly in dealing with a child with FXS, who has difficulty with abstract concepts, the consequence for the inappropriate behavior must be linked to something that is clear and easily understood. Time-out needs to be used in a consistent manner and should be imposed immediately after the targeted behavior. The longer the period between the behavior and the consequence, the more difficult it is for the child, especially the child with FXS, to make the connection between behavior and consequence, thus decreasing the potency of time-out. Do not engage in repartee. Talking, arguing, or discussing the issue with the individual defeats the purpose of time-out because all of those behaviors provide attention to the individual. Do not address the behaviors that occur on the way to time-out. Stopping and discussing comments or actions that occur during the process of initiating time-out delays the time between the behavior and the consequence and also allows the child to engage the attention of the person administering the consequence. For example, if he or she throws something on the way to time-out, ignore it. If the child gets out of time-out before the designated time has elapsed, put him back. Do this as many times as necessary. Decide what you are going to say before you start, and use a consistent phrase. When it is introduced, the length of time-out should be very brief. This ensures that the individual is able to comply with the consequence. As the individual becomes more compliant and learns the routine, the time can be extended, gradually. Time-out should not be longer, in minutes, than a child's age, for typically developing children. For children with FXS, we recommend using half this amount of time. Thus, a child with FXS who is six might receive a three-minute time-out.

Using a simple and concise predetermined phrase consistently is critical when using time-out with children who have FXS. Deciding what you are going to say ahead of time provides you with the luxury of time. Use this time to clearly choose your words so that you do not have to think in the heat of the moment. Previous chapters have outlined the language and processing delays associated with FXS. A consistent phrase such as "No hitting, time-out" is clear and easily understood. This phrase labels both the behavior and the consequence. It allows the individual to understand what she has done that was unacceptable and what the consequence is for that behavior. Additional discussion around the behavior or the consequences of that behavior only serves to prolong the time between the action and the consequence, thus decreasing the effect of the consequence. Using a consistent phrase also allows the interventionist, be it a professional or a parent, to change locations without disrupting the routine.

This following case study illustrates the use and effectiveness of a holistic approach to modifying aggressive behavior while employing time-out as a component of a complete behavior plan.

## CASE HISTORY

AB is a five-year-old boy with the full mutation. He presented with significant cognitive and speech and language delays. He had difficulty with impulse control, anxiety, transitions, and aggression. The aggression was particularly directed toward his mother. When he became frustrated or anxious, he lashed out at his mother, hitting, kicking, or throwing objects at her. When he was originally evaluated, he was about to enter into kindergarten. His mother was very concerned about his behavior.

AB underwent a complete evaluation. Interventions such as speech and language therapy, occupational therapy, and special education were recommended and initiated. Observation of the interaction between AB and his mother revealed that he would become frustrated with an object or bored with a situation and then lash out at his mother. She in turn would attempt to ameliorate the situation. Discussions with his mother allowed her to understand that her behavior was reinforcing his aggressive behavior. His treatment plan included modeling appropriate touching without hitting and providing him with short phrases to use to get his needs met. Techniques were instituted by his mother with the help of the speech therapist. Positive reinforcement was used for appropriate attempts at gaining her attention. Time-out using the simple phrase "No hitting, time-out" was a consequence for any type of hitting.

Two months after the initial contact and the implementation of the treatment plan, AB was observed in his kindergarten program. He appeared happy and content. When asked about his behavior, his teachers reported few problems and no current issues with aggression. His mother reported a significant decrease in hitting after the implementation of the plan. She reported some difficulty in being consistent but was able to execute the plan effectively most of the time.

The discussion of consequences would not be complete without addressing spanking. We are not going to discuss all of the cultural differences associated with spanking. Some issues specifically relate to individuals with FXS. Children with FXS are good imitators and have a relative strength in gestalt memory. As we have previously outlined, individuals with FXS often use physical means to express frustration and anger. As a result, we do not recommend spanking. Spanking or hitting as a consequence provides an undesirable model to imitate, and it does not significantly decrease the targeted behaviors.

Structure and predictability, as previously mentioned, are essential to an optimal home, school, social, or vocational environment for the individual with FXS. Even within an optimal environment, noncompliance issues are likely to arise. One of the most effective ways to deal with noncompliance is to provide choices within the structure. First, outline the main objective of the task and then provide the individual with acceptable choices for how that task can be completed. Writing tasks are often sources of contention, both at home and at school, because writing is usually difficult for individuals with FXS. Rather than engaging in a battle of wills around the writing, which needs to be completed, focus the child's attention on the aspects of the task over which they have control. These choices can include where they would like to do their work (e.g., in the kitchen or in the den) and what they would like to write with (e.g., a pen, a marker, or a pencil). The number of choices should be limited. Too many choices can actually be anxiety producing. The key to using this effectively is to minimize the focus of the main objective and increase discussion and attention onto the choices.

The following case study illustrates a combined intervention approach. Referrals were made for the family and a plan was outlined for one specific behavior. This behavior plan emphasizes the use of choices, a visual schedule, and consistency of reinforcement.

## CASE HISTORY

CD is a six-year-old girl with the full mutation. Her cognitive abilities are within the low normal range. Anxiety, language delays, and temper tantrums when she was denied her way were the primary concern for her family. Medication was prescribed to address her anxiety; however, taking the medication caused so much anxiety that she would vomit. The parents had tried several dif-

ferent types of behavioral intervention, but nothing had proven to be successful. CD's behavior was causing a great deal of disruption to her family. Her parents reported feeling powerless and hopeless.

The *Steps for Creating a Treatment Plan* were reviewed with CD's parents.
Taking the medication was determined to be the target behavior. A physical was
completed to rule out any physiologic causes for the vomiting. Some degree of
tactile defensiveness was present in the oral area. As a result, a sensory diet was
recommended (see chap. 10). A behavior plan was developed using choices as
a strategy to alleviate the power struggle concerning medication. Due to her severe anxiety, the medication was necessary. While she did not have a choice
about taking the medication, she could choose how she would take it. Did she
want it mixed in peanut butter or honey, applesauce or jelly? To involve her in
the process, CD and her parents went to the store together to buy the foods that
would be used to camouflage the taste of the medication. A primary reinforcer
(candy) was used after the successful ingestion of the medication. These reinforcers were not given at any other time during the day, which was a change
from what had happened previously. An enjoyable task (e.g., watching her favorite video or playing Nintendo) was also included as part of the plan after she
had successfully taken the medication. Again, these special tasks were reserved
only for reinforcement purposes and were not available during other parts of
the day. These enjoyable activities were used primarily to shift her attention
from the stressful and anxiety-producing act of taking the medication to a familiar and calming activity. A picture schedule outlining the events preceding
(sensory activity and choices) and following (primary reinforcers and familiar
activity) the ingestion of the medication was used whenever medications were
presented. Family counseling was also recommended for the family (Sobesky
1996).

CD was able to take her medication successfully using the plan. The combination of appropriate medication and a structured plan served to decrease her
anxiety. This decrease in anxiety, paired with the sensory diet, alleviated the
tantrums to some extent. The family continues to work with a therapist on setting appropriate limits and the consistent use of consequences.

## Psychotherapy

Many individuals with FXS benefit from individual psychotherapy. For the
FXS population, individual therapy seems to be most effective when it is a
structured approach designed to teach new skills. It can be helpful for males or
females and for a variety of ages, including children, adolescents, and adults.
Individual therapy may target a variety of symptoms, including reduction of
anxiety, anger management techniques, improved social skills, and help processing moods and feelings. For adolescent girls and women, there may be feel-

ings of grief regarding their carrier status. They may also experience social anxiety or anger about being "different." While males of this age may struggle with some similar concerns, often their families seek assistance in response to their sons' difficulties with anger management and outburst behavior.

Family therapy is helpful because it provides an opportunity for everyone to understand one another better while growing in their relationships to one another. Because FXS is a genetic disorder, parents often struggle with guilt and grief regarding the transmission of FXS to their children (Weber 2000). Parents also have concerns regarding how to balance the needs of all of their children fairly. Regardless of how many of the children are affected by FXS, everyone in the family is affected by the presence of FXS in any family members. Family therapy also provides an opportunity for family members to learn more about FXS and understand its impact. By gaining greater understanding of FXS, the family may learn different patterns of working together and strategies for helping everyone to adjust.

Group therapy and social skills therapy can be helpful in providing an opportunity for a child or adult with FXS to learn and practice social skills. Often, these groups can be conducted in the school setting or through the adult programs offered through state and federally subsidized developmental disabilities centers. The most effective groups are those that teach very specific skills. Role-playing and dramatic play can provide an opportunity to practice how to handle a specific situation. There should be a natural social component as part of the group. For example, the TEACCH program at the University of North Carolina, Chapel Hill (Mesibov 1992), developed a specific social group for adolescents and adults with autism. In this program, social interaction and social skills development are fostered during weekly group meetings. The routine of the group is very consistent. Each participant has an individual goal. The group meets weekly, and structured social activities (e.g., games, special interest night, parties) are planned. Food is always part of the group activity because eating is a social event and also provides a calming and reinforcing activity. Daily living skills such as food preparation can also be targeted through this format.

Pragmatic psychotherapy (exhibit 9.1) is a model that has been developed by one of the authors (J.L.H.E.) in her work with the FXS community in a private practice setting. It is presented to provide a foundation for intervention strategies for other mental health professionals who are working with families affected by FXS. Pragmatic psychotherapy is a model that emphasizes an eclectic theoretical approach while primarily emphasizing practical behavioral interventions. It is goal oriented, and energy is invested in developing a specific solution or set of solutions to specific problem areas. There is an assessment phase and an intervention phase of therapy. The behavior or treatment plan,

**Exhibit 9.1**
**Pragmatic Psychotherapy: A Model for Psychological Intervention in Fragile X Syndrome**

---

Holistic
Eclectic theoretical approach
Goal oriented
Emphasizes practical behavioral interventions
Two-phase approach
Specific solutions to specific problem areas
Builds on relative strengths

| *Assessment Phase* | *Intervention Phase* |
|---|---|
| Specific problem areas | Brainstorming |
| Maintaining variables | Collaboration with family, caregiver, and individual |
| Role of anxiety | Consistent routine within sessions |
| Other psychiatric conditions | Environmental modifications |
| Relative strengths and weaknesses | Visual representations |

---

**Exhibit 9.2**
**Steps for Developing a Treatment Plan**

---

1. Isolate one specific behavior.
2. Identify when, where, and how often the behavior occurs.
3. Rule out any physiologic causes.
4. Examine and modify the environment.
5. Provide the child with additional resources.
6. Outline natural consequences for the behavior.
7. Be consistent.
8. Provide a substitute behavior.
9. Reinforce positive behavior.
10. Start in a controlled and safe setting.
11. Provide opportunities for both success and failure.

---

which has been previously described, can be used within this framework (exhibit 9.2).

During the assessment phase, specific "problem areas" are identified. These "problems" are defined as carefully as possible, so that the clinician, family members, and client all understand the "target behavior." To gather enough information, the clinician adopts a transdisciplinary lens. This is accomplished primarily by meeting with the main people who are involved with the client.

Then it is important to determine the underlying sensory integration, communication impairments, and social skill deficits that may relate to or maintain inappropriate patterns of behavior. For example, the clinician may meet in person or interview by phone the family, the individual client, and any collateral agencies or professionals who are involved with the client (e.g., school personnel, a job coach, extended family members). The problem, including determination of the maintaining variables, is then clarified. It is also important to discuss with the individual and families what interventions have been unsuccessful. Otherwise, the clinician may suggest a strategy that has already failed. This can be very frustrating to the individual and/or family and may discourage them from engaging in the therapeutic process.

Regardless of the presenting problem, the clinician must pay attention to the role of anxiety. Anxiety is the underlying trigger of many of the most common behavioral problems seen in FXS. For this reason, its presence has to be identified in the chain of behaviors leading to the "problem area." In addition to anxiety, the individual may have symptoms related to other psychiatric conditions. The clinician should assess for a dual diagnosis, since it is common for individuals with FXS to have symptoms of other psychiatric conditions (see chap. 1).

Once the assessment process has been thoroughly completed, it is time to move to specific intervention strategies. The strategies should begin to emerge based on the information gained in a thorough assessment. During the intervention phase of therapy, all participants are involved in brainstorming ideas. The clinician should include the family and individual in the process. Without this collaboration, intervention is likely to fail, since the family and individual may not feel invested in the treatment process. Intervention strategies will include consideration of all issues that may contribute to the "problem area." Thus, the clinician and family should consider environmental modifications as a way of providing some immediate relief. Physiologic etiologies must be ruled out. It is also important to understand the role of routines within the context of the individual's life. Most individuals with FXS crave routines. If an intervention strategy unknowingly interrupts a routine, anxiety and subsequent anger are likely to emerge. In contrast, by building in a calming routine, some problems will abate.

The pragmatic psychotherapy model is tailored to common strengths and weaknesses seen in those who have FXS. For example, the session generally follows the same routine or flow. The therapist spends a few minutes with the care giver or parent first, following up on suggestions made by the therapist from the previous session. The therapist spends the majority of time with the individual who has the "problem." The session concludes with a discussion with the individual and care givers or parents, discussing any new findings, reinforcing positive changes in behavior, and making suggestions for the upcoming week.

Many individuals with FXS have difficulty when they are the focus of attention. They report that this is overwhelming and that it increases feelings of anxiety. For this reason, the therapist directs attention to the family and describes the therapeutic process as involving change in everyone. The therapist also minimizes time talking about the individual with the family and individual present simultaneously, as this often increases anxiety for the individual.

A key component to pragmatic psychotherapy is time spent with the individual client. It provides the therapist with time to build a relationship with the individual. It also allows for assessment of the individual's specific strengths and weaknesses. The individual may have a very different perspective from that of his or her family but may be too anxious to discuss his or her opinion in front of the family. The individual and therapist can use role-playing and practice how to handle specific anxiety-evoking situations. The therapist may also teach specific strategies such as breathing exercises or modified progressive muscle relaxation during this time.

In pragmatic psychotherapy, the therapist uses visual representations of specific ideas to provide enhanced understanding of the material. Individuals with FXS rely on visual cues, and this strength can be directly targeted in the therapy process. For example, the therapist may illustrate specific ideas while a discussion is occurring, using colored markers to diagram a social situation and possible roles and outcomes. The use of Social Stories or Comic Strips allows the clinician to highlight salient features of a common social event, thus improving the client's understanding (Gray 1994a, 1994b). Drawing also provides a direction for the focus of attention that does not require eye contact. If the clinician draws on paper, there is a final product that can be used later as a visual prompt, when the new strategy will be implemented.

The routine of the session may be enhanced and made more concrete for the participants by introducing a visual schedule (Braden 2000b; also see chaps. 10 and 11). This marks the sequence of events for that session, which may decrease anxiety. The visual schedule may be represented by line drawings, photographs, or other visual cues that represent key activities (e.g., clinician talks to parents, clinician talks to individual, clinician and individual practice role-play, clinician talks with parents and individual, time to go home). Visual schedules are commonly used when working with younger children but may be helpful for adults, especially men, who are more cognitively affected.

It is often difficult for families to seek help. Parents may be concerned that a therapist, especially a mental health professional, may negatively judge their parenting skills or the decisions they have made. The person with FXS may feel quite anxious about meeting a new person, especially if he or she perceives that they are going to therapy because of "bad" behavior. It is important to reduce anxiety for everyone involved by "demystifying" the process of therapy. An emphasis should be placed on open communication and on everyone working together as a team. This helps by reducing the pressure experienced by the individual with FXS. A healthy alliance can be nurtured.

Another helpful approach is to externalize the symptom from the individual by labeling it. Thus, the clinician encourages the family to confront "the anxiety," not the individual. Individuals with FXS generally respond well to humor. The clinician can use humor to an advantage, while externalizing the symptoms. Rather than directing frustration toward the person experiencing the symptoms of anxiety, the clinician directs the family and individual to be frustrated with "anxiety." For example, during a session the clinician would model, "Sounds like anxiety showed up at Thanksgiving and wasn't even invited," when a family reports frustration regarding the individual's behavior at a large family gathering.

The use of familiar routines helps everyone in the family to feel more comfortable about coming to the clinician's office. They know what to expect, and they understand the process. The use of strong positive reinforcers is essential in an effective intervention. The clinician, the family, and the individual must attend to what will be motivating to begin the process of behavior change.

Confidentiality must be protected in all psychotherapeutic processes, but to be most effective, the clinician must have permission to talk with a client's parents or care givers. This idea should be discussed early in the process so that a comfortable relationship can be developed. The clinician should not share all information with the care givers but should talk about themes that may relate to the maintaining variables or the design of appropriate intervention strategies.

The following case study is presented to highlight the use of pragmatic psychotherapy. It illustrates a combination of approaches including interventions based on physiology, the use of relaxation strategies, and an emphasis on collateral communication within the construct of individual therapy. The use of the Ticklebox provides an example of how the implementation of additional resources, in this case assistive technology, can modify behavior (Riley et al. 2001). This also demonstrates how a plan can be implemented at home first, to ensure its success, before its transition to a community setting.

## CASE HISTORY

EF is a woman who struggles with social anxiety, panic attacks, and attentional problems. EF has average intellectual functioning with specific learning disabilities in arithmetic and visual spatial reasoning. EF was struggling with career options. Her social anxiety and executive functioning deficits along with sensory integration issues affected her ability to sustain employment. Mood lability also led to extreme emotional outbursts, including tearfulness and anger.

EF received support through a vocational program. Job coaching provided someone who could sculpt an appropriate job situation. The coach could match EF's skills to particular job situations and target the acquisition of specific skills to help build necessary skills for prospective employment. Skill training focused on areas of her interest, such as computers. A stimulant medication was also tried for attentional problems; however, negative side effects, including increased anxiety, resulted in a cessation of this medication. An antidepressant was used to successfully treat symptoms of anxiety, depression, and general mood lability (see chap. 8). Individual therapy to address improved coping skills, to teach strategies to minimize symptoms of anxiety and panic, to target inattention, and to provide support regarding depression and grief regarding FXS was provided.

The Ticklebox system (Riley et al. 2001) was used to target issues related to poor attention in the workplace. The Ticklebox is a pager, a vibrating reminder system, which can send an alphanumeric reminder for certain tasks. For example, reminders were sent to cue times to leave the house for work, to leave for a break, to return from a break, and to clean her desk before the end of the workday. Medication cues were also programmed. Relaxation strategies including deep breathing exercises and progressive muscle relaxation were taught, to be used prophylactically, to prevent emotional outbursts and panic attacks. The combination of interventions allowed EF to obtain and sustain a job in an office setting, which included computer and clerical tasks.

Pragmatic psychotherapy can also be an effective approach for treating the severe symptoms of anxiety sometimes seen in men with FXS. The following case study illustrates the use of traditional methods of behavioral therapy, which have been modified to use with individuals with FXS. This case also presents the systematic use of primary and secondary reinforcers, implementation of a specific routine, and the role of ongoing collateral contact with family and other care givers as a means of ensuring success.

## CASE HISTORY

GH is a 35-year-old man with the full mutation for FXS and a secondary diagnosis of autism. He lives at home with his mother and sister. After many years working successfully in a workshop setting, he became increasingly unwilling to leave his house. His symptoms of anxiety worsened as he aged. Community outings were often triggers for extreme panic attacks, which included sweating, facial flushing, and difficulty breathing. Although he was able to speak, he was unable to engage in sustained conversations. He was unable to describe his experience of anxiety to others. The majority of his symptoms were inferred based on his behavior or based on parent report. At the beginning of the intervention, GH had been homebound for approximately two years.

Attempts were made to take GH to a physician to rule out any medical etiology for his intensifying anxiety. GH was unable to tolerate a trip from home
to the physician's office. His primary care doctor came to his home and completed an exam. No underlying etiology was identified except for FXS. Consultation with a psychiatrist led to a medication regimen that included buspirone,
sertraline, and olanzapine (see chap. 8 for more details regarding medication).
Psychologic intervention focused on a combination of individual and family interventions. Weekly sessions focused on identifying triggers of anxiety and developing interventions to decrease his experience of anxiety. A modified cognitive behavioral approach included gradual, in vivo systematic desensitization
(Wolpe 1958). It was modified from traditional systematic desensitization by
removing the verbal, cognitive component. GH could not verbally describe his
feelings during this process, and therefore it was not possible to construct an
anxiety hierarchy. Instead, his behavioral responses and his compliance with
the steps of the program served to provide information about his level of anxiety. The anxiety-provoking situation was first broken down into smaller units.
Primary reinforcers (potato chips) and high-interest materials (books with real
animal photographs) were paired with the early steps in treatment, such as sitting in the car, to provide activities that were incongruent with anxiety, thus interfering with the anxiety response. These activities served to distract his attention from feelings of anxiety. GH was also taught to verbalize, "All done"
and "Go home," when he began to demonstrate signs of anxiety while in the
car. In response to using these statements, the car activity would be discontinued. If he was in the community, the driver would take him home.

Desensitization to the trigger of anxiety (driving in the car) was introduced
in gradual increments by pairing each step with the above reinforcers. These
steps included walking from his home to the car, sitting in the car with the therapist and his mother with the car turned off, sitting in the car with the therapist
and his mother with the car turned on, driving up and down the driveway, driving out of the driveway and up and down the street, driving up and down familiar streets in the neighborhood, driving to a specific nearby location to receive reinforcers (to the mall, to get a snack), and driving to a sibling's house
to visit animals. As GH began to make progress, it became clear that he also
enjoyed identifying the make and model of cars. This routine was an additional activity that was antagonistic to anxiety. Thus, the need for the use of
primary reinforcers diminished as GH became more confident. The last step
of the program involved the introduction of a schedule to cue GH when an
outing would occur. A calendar was used to help prepare GH for transitions.
Once this routine was developed, GH began to look forward to weekly outings with his family.

Collateral contact with GH's family provided an opportunity to coordinate the intervention. The use of familiar routines within the intervention helped to decrease the family's secondary anxiety and increased the likelihood of compliance. Collaboration with the local community center board provided access to a job developer and community support.

Over time, the emphasis in intervention shifted to the generalization of skills. A service provider was hired to provide family respite in the form of two outings per week. The psychologist initially facilitated generalization of skills by spending time with GH and the new provider. GH successfully generalized his skills to the new provider and continues to leave his home two or three times per week, approximately three years after the initial intervention. Consultation with the treating psychologist is only necessary regarding setting new goals for outings and at times when symptoms have recurred. GH has become less verbal with medications; however, any reduction in medications resulted in a return of agoraphobia.

## Summary

Just as there are a variety of symptoms that may be associated with FXS, there are a variety of interventions that may prove helpful. At present, there are few empirically demonstrated treatments for specific symptoms associated with FXS (see chaps. 8 and 11). However, there are techniques that have proved helpful for problems similar to those experienced by individuals with FXS. It is essential for consumers to realize that they are active participants in any treatment process. They must feel comfortable with the people with whom they are working. It is important for them to ask questions and offer their own opinions and preferences regarding interventions, both initially and as the treatment proceeds. While medications may be quite helpful, they are often most helpful when combined with some type of therapy so that individuals can find ways to deal more actively with their symptoms or find ways to change their lifestyle so that their symptoms do not recur.

## Acknowledgments

A special thanks to all of the families who have shared a portion of their busy lives with us in the hopes of helping other families along the way. We have learned so much and continue to grow in our understanding of FXS each day. This work was made possible in part by funding from FRAXA, the Kenneth Kendal King Foundation, the Schramm Foundation, NICHD grant HD36071, and donations made to the Fragile X Treatment and Research Center.

## References

Bailey, D. B., Jr., D. D. Hatton, G. B. Mesibov, N. Ament, and M. Skinner. 2000. Early development, temperament and functional impairment in autism and fragile X syndrome. *J. Autism Dev. Disord.* 30:49–59.

Bailey, D. B., Jr., D. D. Hatton, M. Skinner, and G. B. Mesibov. 2001. Autistic behavior, FMRP, and developmental trajectories in young males with fragile X syndrome. *J. Autism Dev. Disord.* In press.

Barkley, R. A. 1995. *Taking charge of ADHD: A complete, authoritative guide for parents.* New York: Guilford Press.

Borghgraef, M., J. P. Fryns, and H. Van den Berge. 1990. The female and the fragile X syndrome: Data on clinical and psychological findings in fragile X carriers. *Clin. Genet.* 37:341–346.

Braden, M. 2000a. Education. In Weber, J. D. (ed.), *Children with fragile X syndrome: A parent's guide.* Bethesda, Md.: Woodbine House, pp. 243–306.

———. 2000b. *Fragile X; handle with care: More about fragile X syndrome—adolescents and adults.* Dillon, Colo.: Spectra Publishing.

Brown, J., M. Braden, and W. E. Sobesky. 1991. The treatment of emotional and behavioral problems. In R. J. Hagerman and A. C. Silverman (eds.), *Fragile X syndrome: Diagnosis, treatment, and intervention.* Baltimore: Johns Hopkins Univ. Press, pp. 311–326.

Cohen, I. L. 1995. A theoretical analysis of the role of hyperarousal in the learning and behavior of fragile X males. *Ment. Retard. Dev. Disabil. Res. Rev.* 1:286–291.

Cohen, I. L., G. S. Fisch, V. Sudhalter, E. G. Wolf-Schein, D. Hanson, R. Hagerman, E. C. Jenkins, and W. T. Brown. 1988. Social gaze avoidance, and repetitive behavior in fragile X males: A controlled study. *Am. J. Ment. Retard.* 92:436–446.

de Vries, B. B., A. M. Wiegers, A. P. Smits, S. Mohkamsing, H. J. Duivenvoorden, J. P. Fryns, L. M. Curfs, D. J. Halley, B. A. Oostra, A. M. van den Ouweland, and M. F. Niermeijer. 1996. Mental status of females with an *FMR1* gene full mutation. *Am. J. Med. Genet.* 58:1025–1032.

Dorn, M., M. Mazzocco, and R. J. Hagerman. 1994. Behavioral and psychiatric disorders in adult fragile X carrier males. *J. Am. Acad. Child Adolesc. Psychiatry* 33:256–264.

Franke, P., W. Maier, M. Hautzinger, O. Weiffernbach, M. Gansicke, B. Iwers, F. Poustka, S. G. Schwab, and U. Foster. 1996. Fragile-X carrier females: Evidence for a distinct psychopathological phenotype? *Am. J. Med. Genet.* 64:334–339.

Franke, P., M. Leboyer, M. Gansicke, O. Weiffenbach, V. Biancalana, P. Cornillet-Lefebre, M. F. Croquette, U. Froster, S. G. Schwab, F. Poustka, M. Hautzinger, and W. Maier. 1998. Genotype-phenotype relationship in female carriers of the premutation and full mutation of *FMR-1. Psychiatry Res.* 80:113–127.

Freund, L. S., C. D. Peebles, E. Aylward, and A. L. Reiss. 1993. Psychiatric disorders associated with fragile X in the young female. *Pediatrics* 91:321–329.

Frost, L., and A. Bondy. 1994. *The Picture Exchange Communication System training manual.* Cherry Hill, N.J.: Pyramid Educational Consultants.

Gray, C. 1994a. *The original social story book.* Arlington, Tex.: Future Education.

———. 1994b. *Comic strip conversation.* Arlington, Tex.: Future Education.

Hagerman, R. J. 1999. Tourette syndrome. In *Neurodevelopmental disorders: Diagnosis and treatment.* New York: Oxford Univ. Press, pp. 133–172.

Hagerman, R. J., J. Hills, S. Scharfenaker, and H. Lewis. 1999. Fragile X syndrome and selective mutism. *Am. J. Med. Genet.* 83:313–317.

Hagerman, R. J., C. E. Hull, J. F. SaLanda, I. Carpenter, L. W. Staley, R. O'Connor, C. Seydel, M. M. Mazzocco, K. Snow, S. Thibodeau, D. Kuhl, D. L. Nelson, C. T. Caskey, and A. Taylor. 1994. High functioning fragile X males: Demonstration of an unmethylated, fully expanded *FMR-1* mutation associated with protein expression. *Am. J. Med. Genet.* 51:298–308.

Hull, C. E., and R. J. Hagerman. 1993. A study of the physical, behavioral, and medical phenotype including anthropometric measures of females with fragile X syndrome. *Am. J. Dis. Child.* 147:1236–1241.

Kerby, D. S., and Dawson, B. L. 1994. Autistic features, personality, and adaptive behavior in males with the fragile X syndrome and no autism. *Am. J. Ment. Retard.* 98:455–462.

Lachiewicz, A. M., and D. V. Dawson. 1994. Behavioral problems of young girls with fragile X syndrome: Factor scores on the Connor's parent questionnaire. *Am. J. Med. Genet.* 15:364–369.

Linder, T. 1983. *Early childhood special education: Program development and administration.* Baltimore: Paul H. Brookes Publishing, pp. 21–43.

Mazzocco, M. M. M., B. F. Pennington, and R. J. Hagerman. 1993. The neurocognitive phenotype of female carriers of fragile X: Additional evidence for specificity. *J. Dev. Behav. Pediatr.* 14:328–335.

Mazzocco, M. M. M., T. Baumgardner, L. S. Freund, and A. L. Reiss. 1998. Social functioning among girls with fragile X or Turner syndrome and their sisters. *J. Autism Dev. Dis.* 28:509–517.

Merenstein, S. A., V. Shyu, W. E. Sobesky, L. W. Staley, A. K. Taylor, and R. J. Hagerman. 1994. Fragile X syndrome in a normal IQ male with learning and emotional problems. *J. Am. Acad. Child Adolesc. Psychiatry* 33:1316–1321.

Mesibov, G. 1992. Treatment issues with high-functioning adolescents and adults with autism. In E. Schopler and G. Mesibov (eds.), *High-functioning individuals with autism.* New York: Plenum Press, pp. 143–155.

Moor, D. Y. 2000. Daily care. In J. D. Weber (ed.), *Children with fragile X syndrome: A parent's guide.* Bethesda, Md.: Woodbine House, pp. 121–154.

Munir, F., Cornish, K. M., and Wilding, J. 2000. A neuropsychological profile of attention deficits in young males with fragile X syndrome. *Neuropsychologia* 28:1261–1270.

O'Neill, R., R. Horner, R. Albin, K. Storey, and J. Sprague. 1990. *Functional analysis of problem behavior: A practical assessment guide.* Sycamore, Ill.: Sycamore Publishing Co.

Reiss, A. L., R. J. Hagerman, S. Vinogradov, M. Abrams, and R. J. King. 1988. Psychiatric disability in female carriers of the fragile X chromosome. *Arch. Gen. Psychiatry* 45:25–30.

Reiss, A. L., L. Freund, S. Vinogradov, R. Hagerman, and A. Cronister. 1989. Parental inheritance and psychological disability in fragile X females. *Am. J. Hum. Genet.* 45:697–705.

Reiss, A. L., L. Freund, M. T. Abrams, C. Boehm, and H. Kazazian. 1993. Neurobe-havioral effects of the fragile X premutation in adult women: A controlled study. *Am. J. Hum. Genet.* 52:884–894.

Riley, K., C. Bodine, J. Hills, L. W. Gane, J. Sandstrum, and R. J. Hagerman. 2001. The Ticklebox assistive technology device: Piloted on a young woman with fragile X syndrome. *Ment. Health Aspects Dev. Disabil.* 4:138–142.

Rogers, S. J., E. A. Wehner, and R. Hagerman. 2001. The behavioral phenotype in fragile X syndrome: Symptoms of autism in very young children with fragile X syndrome, idiopathic autism, and other developmental disorders. *J. Dev. Behav. Pediatr.* In press.

Schopler, E., G. B. Mesibov, and K. Hearsey. 1995. Structured teaching in the TEACCH system. In E. Schopler and G. B. Mesibov (eds.), *Learning and cognition in autism.* New York: Plenum Press, pp. 243–268.

Sobesky, W. E. 1996. The treatment of emotional and behavioral problems. In R. J. Hagerman and A. Cronister (eds.), *Fragile X syndrome: Diagnosis, treatment, and research,* 2d ed. Baltimore: Johns Hopkins Univ. Press, pp. 332–348.

Sobesky, W. E., C. E. Hull, and R. J. Hagerman. 1994a. Symptoms of schizotypal personality disorder in fragile X females. *J. Am. Acad. Child Adolesc. Psychiatry* 33: 247–255.

Sobesky, W. E., B. F. Pennington, D. Porter, C. E. Hull, and R. J. Hagerman. 1994b. Emotional and neurocognitive deficits in fragile X. *Am. J. Med. Genet.* 51:378–384.

Sobesky, W. E., D. Porter, B. F. Pennington, and R. J. Hagerman. 1995. Dimensions of shyness in fragile X females. *Dev. Brain Dysfunct.* 8:280–292.

Sobesky, W. E., A. K. Taylor, B. F. Pennington, L. Bennetto, D. Porter, J. Riddle, and R. J. Hagerman. 1996. Molecular/clinical correlations in females with fragile X. *Am. J. Med. Genet.* 64:340–345.

Turk, J. 1998. Fragile X syndrome and attention deficits. *J. Appl. Res. Intellect. Disabil.* 11:175–191.

Turk, J., and P. Graham. 1997. Fragile X syndrome, autism, and autistic features. *Autism* 1:175–197.

Weber, J. D. 2000. *Children with fragile X syndrome: A parent's guide.* Bethesda, Md.: Woodbine House.

Wisbeck, J. M., L. C. Huffman, L. Freund, M. Gunnar, E. P. Davis, and A. L. Reiss. 2000. Cortisol and social stressors in children with fragile X: A pilot study. *J. Dev. Behav. Pediatr.* 21:278–282.

Wolpe, J. 1958. *Reciprocal inhibition therapy.* Stanford: Stanford Univ. Press.

# CHAPTER 10

# An Integrated Approach to Intervention

Sarah Scharfenaker, M.A., C.C.C.,
Rebecca O'Connor, M.A., Tracy Stackhouse, O.T.R.,
Marcia L. Braden, Ph.D., and Kristen Gray, M.S.

An integrated approach to intervention begins with knowledge of and sensitivity to the very special needs displayed by individuals with fragile X syndrome (FXS). In clinical interviews hundreds of families of children with FXS have reported that one of their greatest goals is to ensure they are providing their children with the most appropriate treatment, intervention, and educational services. Although there is no cure for FXS, there are many treatments for the challenging symptoms and behaviors displayed. Because of the multifaceted needs of these patients, an integrated approach to intervention and education that combines the expertise of the parents, speech and language pathologist, occupational therapist, physician, psychologists, special education teacher, and regular education teacher is most beneficial. The importance of medical management in conjunction with other supportive services must be stressed. Medical management of attentional and behavioral issues can begin as early as the toddler years. Because of the complex needs these children have, medical intervention is an essential component of integrated services.

In this chapter, we review the history and philosophy behind the concept of integrated services and discuss its implications for working with individuals with FXS. Specific strategies applicable within the academic, speech/language, and occupational therapy domains are presented for the infant-toddler, school-aged child, and late adolescent–adult. Although the emphasis of this chapter is on integrated services for the male with FXS, the information can be extrapolated for use with learning-disabled and mildly to moderately impaired females with FXS.

Many methods discussed in this chapter are based on the successes noted by

*Fragile X Syndrome: Diagnosis, Treatment, and Research,* third edition, ed. Randi Jenssen Hagerman and Paul J. Hagerman (Baltimore: Johns Hopkins University Press, 2002), © The Johns Hopkins University Press.

clinical observation and reported by parents, teachers, and therapists and in limited controlled research. Further research is necessary to improve our understanding of beneficial treatment techniques in all areas of education and intervention.

In this chapter applicable research using people with FXS or other populations whose features are similar to those of the population with FXS is cited, while we bear in mind the unique cognitive, speech/language, and sensory processing characteristics of individuals with FXS.

## Cognitive Foundations for Intervention

Most boys and some girls with FXS present with some degree of cognitive deficit, most often diagnosed as mental retardation. The American Association on Mental Retardation (AAMR) provides a new and very specific definition of mental retardation (2000):

—Mental retardation refers to substantial limitations in present functioning. It is characterized by: significantly subaverage intellectual functioning, existing concurrently with:

—Related limitations in two or more of the following applicable adaptive skill areas: Communication, self care, community use, functional academics, work, or play.

—Mental retardation manifests before age 18.

—Four critical assumptions must be considered when applying the definition of mental retardation:

- Valid assessment considers cultural and linguistic diversity, as well as differences in communications and behavioral factors.
- The existence of limitations in adaptive skills occurs within the context of community environments typical of the individual's age peers and is indexed to the person's individualized needs for supports.
- Specific adaptive limitations often coexist with strengths in other adaptive skills or other personal capabilities.
- With appropriate supports over a sustained period, the life functioning of the person with mental retardation will generally improve.

AAMR's newest definition of mental retardation describes four different levels of functional ability. The newest categories are based on IQ assessment, as well as the level of support a person requires to deal with everyday living situations: (1) intermittent, (2) limited, (3) extensive, and (4) pervasive. The majority of males with FXS and one-third of females present with mental retardation secondary to FXS. Males and females present with levels of functioning across the four categories, with most adult males requiring limited to extensive levels of support.

All individuals with FXS continue to learn new skills over time, though it takes them much longer to do so. A child with FXS may take a full year to learn a concept that may take another child six months to learn. The child with FXS can generally master many of the same kind of typical skills at a much older age. Children with FXS progress through the typical sequence of developmental milestones and build more complex skills from simpler ones.

Levels of function are determined by ranges of performance on standardized intellectual and adaptive behavior assessments. Usually a psychologist gathers information about the child through parent report, teacher report, observation, and standardized testing. The psychologist identifies strengths and needs and how to help children learn. By comparing cognitive and adaptive abilities, one can determine levels of function. This information will aid in treatment planning and educational intervention strategies. The psychologist works with the speech therapist, occupational therapist, and special education and regular education teacher. All intervention strategies are devised to be developmentally appropriate so that children experience success in what they are being taught. Sometimes the rate of learning seems very slow and inconsistent. This is often the case when academic material becomes more and more abstract.

Mental retardation generally affects all areas of development—language, motor, social, and cognitive. What is seen as fairly pervasive in most children with FXS are difficulties with attention, problem solving, abstract thinking, memory, and applying information they know in a new or different way. This last concept is often referred to as *generalization.* Generally, the greater the degree of retardation, the more difficult things are to do. Individuals with FXS need to have experiences and instruction on a level they can understand to promote feelings of positive self-worth. When the goals of intervention address the unique characteristics of those with FXS, successes are more easily achieved. Some general examples of such recommendations are modifications in curriculum that respect the simultaneous learning style, opportunities that promote appropriate engagement with peers, and preparation of the individual with the skills necessary to successfully manage independent living. Most individuals with FXS present with challenging characteristics that affect their learning ability. We know of cognitive deficits ranging from learning disabilities to severe mental retardation, communication difficulties, sensory integration disorder, anxiety, and attentional problems, including hyperactivity and impulsivity.

The majority of males with FXS function within the mild to moderate ranges on standardized assessments of intelligence and adaptive behavior. A characteristic pattern of performance has been documented on standardized intellectual tests that supports relative strengths in visual memory, simultaneous processing, and long-term memory for specific facts related to high-interest areas. Great difficulties are observed with auditory processing, sequential processing, abstract reasoning, and arithmetic skills. Generalization is very difficult in that many individuals cannot apply specific knowledge in a new or novel way and are limited in their ability to be mentally flexible (chaps. 1, 6, and 11).

Males present with a characteristic pattern of performance on several IQ tests (see chap. 6). Awareness of these patterns is helpful in educational planning and can support programs and curriculums that are designed for children who are relatively strong visual simultaneous learners and who benefit from experiential hands-on learning with materials of high interest. Boys with FXS also present with a characteristic pattern of performance (different from other learning-disabled or mentally retarded children) on the Kaufman Assessment Battery for Children (Kemper et al. 1988; Hodapp et al. 1992; chap. 11):

Mental Processing Composite < Achievement Standard Score

Sequential Processing < Simultaneous Processing Score

Arithmetic < Mean Achievement Standard Score

Spatial Memory < Matrix Analogy Subtest Score

On the Standard Binet Fourth Edition Intelligence Scale, significant strengths in comprehension and verbal labeling, as well as significant weaknesses in visual motor coordination, spatial memory, and arithmetic, are documented (Freund and Reiss 1991).

Males with FXS also demonstrate a decline in IQ score over time (Wright-Talamante et al. 1996). The decline in IQ does not reflect a regression in ability or loss of skill. This unusual trajectory, not observed in other mental retardation syndromes, is hypothesized to be related to the lack of ability to reason abstractly and apply knowledge and judgment (see chap. 6).

## An Overview of Integrated Services

The concept of integrated services emerged when special education legislation was passed at the federal level in the mid-1970s (U.S. Congress 1975). PL 94-142 posited that all handicapped children were entitled to a free and appropriate education within the "least restrictive environment." The term *least restrictive environment* implies that handicapped children are entitled to the same education as their nonhandicapped peers and that the school experience should not be restricted to the programs already established or available within school districts.

When PL 94-142 was passed, the new objective was to identify individuals with multiple needs in the cognitive, behavioral, speech/language, and occupational therapy areas as "multiply handicapped." The development of a trans-disciplinary team model evolved to accommodate the needs of these children within a public school setting (Hutchinson 1983). Within this model, each member of the team trains others, thus abandoning a traditional role and building competence in other disciplines to meet the complex needs of the student (Sternat et al. 1977).

In October 1986, another public law was passed, PL 99-457, which ensured that each infant and toddler with a handicap and their families receive a written individualized family service plan (IFSP) (U.S. Congress 1986). This act further served to acknowledge the multidisciplinary team concept by including the parent or guardian as a member of the team and thus an active participant in the educational process.

PL 94-142 and PL 99-457 significantly changed the public school system. With this legislation, more multiply handicapped children moved from private and public institutions into the public school system. As a consequence, the growing need for mainstreaming and providing the least restrictive environment was evident. These laws also caused changes in educational treatment, related services, and therapeutic intervention. It was no longer appropriate to educate a child in an isolated facility, with occupational therapy in a hospital and speech therapy in a rehabilitation center. Instead, there was a legal mandate to centralize services within the public school. Thus, the focus shifted from isolated delivery to a multidisciplinary approach. Input from speech pathologists, occupational and physical therapists, educators, psychologists, and other specialists provided an integrated framework within which a child's educational curriculum could evolve. The success of treatment was less contingent on the technique or philosophy of an individual therapist or educator and more dependent on the positive treatment effects of an integrated program. Only a few studies have evaluated the advantages of integrative therapy and the multidisciplinary model. Preliminary findings from several studies suggest that implementing therapy within a functional environment and context is more effective than teaching skills in isolated environments (Campbell et al. 1984; Giangreco 1986).

Views about curriculum for students with mental retardation (MR) are changing. Research demonstrates that individuals with MR learn more effectively and maintain more skills if education is provided in a functional setting (Brown et al. 1983). We know that boys with FXS demonstrate strengths in their ability to remember episodes and events that they participate in directly. Providing education in functional settings would promote opportunities to practice skills and provide generalizable knowledge. At times, practicing specific academic foundations in highly motivating, one-on-one or small-group settings and then moving into functional environments allows the student to expand and rehearse the use of these skills in more natural settings. Combinations of these approaches seem to work very well for individuals with FXS.

In 1997 the Handicapped Children's Act was changed to the Individuals with Disabilities in Education Act (IDEA). In addition to the name of the act, there were several changes related to inclusion. Inclusion simply brings a stronger emphasis to what was implied in the earlier act. In other words, more emphasis is to be placed on including the person with a disability in the regular mainstream of society. The emphasis includes infant through school-aged and community placements.

This federal law exists to ensure that individuals with disabilities receive appropriate education. Specific sections within the law relate to services for different age groups. The section relating to services for children under 3 years of age is usually referred to as part C. Individuals aged 3–21 receive services under part B. Individuals are eligible to receive the following services:

1. Multidisciplinary evaluation
2. Individual service plan
3. Service coordination assistance
4. Prior notice of change of service providers
5. Information provided in native language
6. Informed consent regarding decision making
7. Confidentiality regarding all information
8. Access to all records
9. Process to appeal decision regarding recommendations
10. Supports provided in natural environments
11. Assistance in finding funding for supports and services

Other changes include more emphasis on training specialized and nonspecialized personnel to adapt to the inclusionary emphasis. There is also more emphasis on technical assistance, instructional media, and transition from school to community.

The Americans with Disabilities Act (ADA) prohibits discrimination against children and adults with disabilities, including mental retardation. It operates in the same way as do other federal laws that outlaw discrimination. It applies to most private employees, public and private services, and public accommodations.

## Fragile X and Integrated Service Delivery

Application of intervention models from the related fields of autism, mental retardation, and learning disabilities, as well as clinical knowledge of the specific cognitive profiles in FXS, may be integrated to provide appropriate service delivery. In addition, observations from trained professionals can provide insight into the individual special educational needs of children with FXS.

The individual with FXS has complex needs that present the educator and therapist with a programming challenge (see chaps. 1, 6, 9, and 11). These complex needs include

—Hypersensitivity to visual, auditory, olfactory, and tactile stimuli as well as movement, gravity, and eye contact, collectively known as sensory defensiveness

—Over-reaction to novelty, difficulty with transitions and change

—Difficulty with self-regulatory functions including problems with attention, anxiety, modulation of activity level, arousal states, and impulsivity

—Difficulty with motor planning (praxis) and sequencing of oral motor, gross motor, fine motor, and visual motor skills

—Problematic social skills: gaze avoidance, social anxiety

—Difficulty with social language skills including phrase, sentence, and topic perseveration, as well as tangential speech

—Speech production complicated by fast rate, disordered rhythm, and verbal dyspraxia resulting in unintelligible speech

—Cognitive deficits ranging from learning disabilities to severe mental retardation

—Limited adaptive skill and life role development

These cognitive, communicative, and sensory difficulties preclude learning through a traditional classroom model. For the individual with FXS, integrated services involving the occupational therapist, speech/language pathologist, and behavioral psychologist are often critical to a successful educational program. The cognitive and speech/language skills, as well as the sensorimotor skills addressed by occupational therapy, vary significantly in the population with FXS. What may benefit a severely affected individual with FXS is inappropriate for a child in the high-functioning range. Thus, the educational and therapeutic needs of each child with FXS must be assessed on an individual basis. Chapter 11 describes specific components to be addressed in developing an individualized education plan (IEP) or IFSP. Some programming goals have been outlined in exhibit 10.1 as a reference for both school staff and parents.

Evaluation of academic, cognitive, adaptive, social-emotional, speech/language, motor, and sensory processing skills of the child with FXS is challenging. Formal assessment is often limited because of attentional and behavioral problems, social anxiety, and/or sensory processing difficulties. However, with a little creativity and adaptability on the part of both the examiner and the child, much can be accomplished.

Initially, the physical testing environment should be assessed and adapted to

**Exhibit 10.1**

**Programming Goals for an Individualized Educational Plan**

1. Occupational therapy using a sensory-integrative approach to
   a. Manage sensory defensiveness to minimize effect on learning and behavior.
   b. Improve adaptability to changes in routine and environment.
   c. Establish an organized behavior state and facilitate sustained attention.
   d. Decrease ritualistic behaviors.
   e. Improve oral, fine, and gross motor skills.
   f. Improve postural control.
   g. Improve motor planning skills, specifically in areas of initiation, ideation, planning, sequencing, and execution. Utilize imitation skills to expand praxis.
   h. Expand repertoire of life roles.
2. Speech/language therapy to
   a. Normalize oral sensitivity and improve oral motor functioning for speech.
   b. Increase receptive and expressive vocabulary.
   c. Increase the use of vocabulary as it applies to life skill development.
   d. Decrease perseverative language.
   e. Increase social language skills: maintaining topics, taking turns, initiation of conversations, use of a variety of speech acts.
   f. Work on problem-solving skills as related to real-life situations.
   g. Reduce rate and normalize rhythm.
3. Combined occupational and speech therapies to use sensory integration strategies to develop speech, language, play, pragmatic skills, and life role development.
4. Education and behavior intervention to
   a. Identify level of cognitive and adaptive behavior function.
   b. Increase attending behaviors in all situations.
   c. Reinforce compliance to direct cues.
   d. Decrease maladaptive behaviors.
   e. Adapt curriculum to appropriate developmental level.
   f. Increase independence of daily living skills: dressing, eating, toileting.
   g. Increase positive coping skills in the school setting through consultation with family, occupational and speech therapists, and teachers.
   h. Increase opportunities for social interactions with same-age peers.
   i. Increase mainstreaming with normal age-appropriate peers.
   j. Manage anxiety.
5. Team education to develop a common knowledge base around FXS.

provide the most uncluttered and quiet atmosphere. (Exhibit 10.2 outlines specific modifications to be considered in the assessment environment.) Flexibility in terms of seating arrangements, eye contact, the establishment of meaningful reinforcers to be used during testing, and use of calming techniques are only some of the areas to be considered. Prior knowledge of sensory defensiveness in the child is essential, as this will dictate how the examiner physi-

**Exhibit 10.2**
**Modifications to Assessment Environment**

- Child to be well rested and on medication schedule.
- Schedule the evaluation at the time of day optimal for the child.
- Identify all environmental adaptations and reinforcers that may be helpful in maintaining attention.
- Specifically adapt the environment:
  Eliminate all distractions possible.
  Make the child comfortable by providing alternative seating (gym ball, seat wedge, sided chair).
  Modify lighting.
  Have calming materials available as needed.
  Allow the child movement breaks if needed.
  Allow avoidant eye gaze. Don't insist on eye contact.
  Allow increased response time to ensure that the child has had the opportunity to respond to the best of his or her ability. You may need to redirect perseverative and impulsive responses.

cally handles the child, proximity in seating, physical lighting of the evaluation room, as well as assessment.

Formal assessment is often easily accomplished provided the necessary adaptations have been made. However, with many children, information gathered from observation, parent interviews, review of records, or a trial period of diagnostic therapy will reveal more about the child's strengths and weaknesses than will formal testing. The examiner must remain open, flexible, and creative in the assessment process.

The decision for classroom placement must be based on individual needs and ability (Baroff 1986; Spiridigliozzi 1994). Although PL 94-142 sometimes has been misinterpreted as a mandate that all special education students should be mainstreamed into regular classrooms, the public law does not require mainstreaming. Instead, appropriate education must be provided with specific procedures defined to protect that right. Mainstreaming can be a positive educational practice if the regular classroom teacher has had special education training or experience (Walker et al. 1989). Modifications of the mainstreaming experience can also benefit the child. One example is reverse mainstreaming, in which a small number of typical peers attend the special education classroom. A variety of structured play and leisure activities can help the handicapped and non-handicapped children accept each other and learn together. A typical day describing activities for a child in a resource room and a child in a more inclusive setting is outlined in tables 10.1 and 10.2.

**Table 10.1**
**Typical Day: Resource Room**

| Day "A" | Monday | Tuesday |
|---|---|---|
| 8:15–9:00 | OT/Sensory integration and calming with aide in resource room | OT/Sensory integration and calming with aide in resource room |
| 9:00–10:00 | Reading, spelling, etc., in resource room | Reading, spelling, etc., in resource room |
| 10:00–11:00 | Computer, greet Julie, Edmark in resource room | Computer, greet Julie, Edmark in resource room |
| 11:00–11:45 | Lunch, physical activity, meds, OK in resource room | Lunch, physical activity, meds, OK in resource room |
| 11:45–12:15 | OT/Sensory activities, tactile and proprioceptive systems in resource room | OT/Sensory activities, tactile and proprioceptive systems in resource room |
| 12:15–12:40 | Heavy work jobs + schedule interruption tolerance in resource room | Heavy work jobs + schedule interruption tolerance in resource room |
| 12:40–1:00 | Speech | CD Rom in resource room |
| 1:00–1:25 | Music | Music |
| 1:25–3:20 | Spelling, community helpers, physical activity in resource room, dismissal | Spelling, community helpers, physical activity in resource room, dismissal |

Transitioning from one activity to another or one setting to another can be extremely disruptive for the child with FXS because of sensory modulation difficulties. These manifest most severely when "newness" or novelty occurs, as registered in the limbic system of the brain. Acting out, resistance, and tantruming may result from this difficulty in shifting cognitive sets. These behaviors should be recognized as a response to making transitions rather than as purposeful defiance. Teachers, aides, school staff, and volunteers should be aware of this and consistent in their responses to the child during times of transition. Specific strategies to aid in transitioning are the following:

| Wednesday | Thursday | Friday |
|---|---|---|
| OT/Sensory integration and calming with aide in resource room | OT/Sensory integration and calming with aide in resource room | OT/Sensory integration and calming with aide in resource room |
| Reading, spelling, etc., in resource room | Reading, spelling, etc., in resource room | Reading, spelling, etc., in resource room |
| Computer, greet Julie, Edmark in resource room | Computer, greet Julie, Edmark in resource room | Computer, greet Julie, Edmark in resource room |
| Lunch, physical activity, meds, OK in resource room | Lunch, physical activity, meds, OK in resource room | Lunch, physical activity, meds, OK in resource room |
| OT/Sensory activities, tactile and proprioceptive systems in resource room | OT/Sensory activities, tactile and proprioceptive systems in resource room | OT/Sensory activities, tactile and proprioceptive systems in resource room |
| Heavy work jobs + schedule interruption tolerance in resource room | Heavy work jobs + schedule interruption tolerance in resource room | Heavy work jobs + schedule interruption tolerance in resource room |
| Speech | CD Rom in resource room | Art |
| Music | Music | Music |
| Spelling, community helpers, physical activity in resource room, dismissal | Spelling, community helpers, physical activity in resource room, dismissal | Spelling, community helpers, physical activity in resource room, dismissal |

—Prepare the child for change on a level that he or she will understand. This may include using a picture schedule or verbally explaining what is to come. Reviewing the daily schedule through pictures at the beginning of the day may also be useful.

—Use a song describing upcoming changes ("It's time to line up for lunch now").

—Develop a routine using a signaling system to indicate that a change in activity is at hand (i.e., ring bell, use timer, show hand signal).

**Table 10.2**
**Typical Day: Inclusion Model**

| Day "B" | Monday | Tuesday |
|---|---|---|
| 8:15–9:00 | OT/Sensory integration and calming with aide in resource room | OT/Sensory integration and calming with aide in resource room |
| 9:00–10:00 | Classroom with Mrs. Brown | Classroom with Mrs. Brown |
| 10:00–11:00 | P.E. | P.E. |
| 11:00–11:45 | Lunch, meds, recess | Lunch, meds, recess |
| 11:45–12:15 | Calming in the classroom and quiet reading | Calming in the classroom and quiet reading |
| 12:15–12:40 | Heavy work + schedule interruption | Heavy work + schedule interruption |
| 12:40–1:00 | Speech | CD Rom in resource room |
| 1:00–1:25 | Music | Music |
| 1:25–3:20 | Spelling, community helpers, functional reading, physical activity in resource room, dismissal | Spelling, community helpers, functional reading, physical activity in resource room, dismissal |

*Source:* Marcia L. Braden, Ph.D.

—Utilize goal-directed, task-relevant responsibilities, such as taking keys to the next teacher, collecting and carrying assignments, and carrying a basket of lunch boxes to the lunch room.

—Consult with the occupational therapist about specific adaptive activities to help with transitions. Some of these activities may include the use of "heavy work," which may calm and organize the child. Examples are pushing in all the chairs before moving on; carrying heavy objects between classrooms/activities, such as books, a loaded backpack, or a basketful of supplies to be used in the next task; or carrying or moving an object with purposeful intent, which often can make a transition smoother.

There is no specific educational program, curriculum, or classroom placement for students with FXS. Each program must be individualized to meet the students' specific needs. Community-based programs may work best for some,

| Wednesday | Thursday | Friday |
|---|---|---|
| OT/Sensory integration and calming with aide in resource room | OT/Sensory integration and calming with aide in resource room | OT/Sensory integration and calming with aide in resource room |
| Classroom with Mrs. Brown | Classroom with Mrs. Brown | Classroom with Mrs. Brown |
| P.E. | P.E. | P.E. |
| Lunch, meds, recess | Lunch, meds, recess | Lunch, meds, recess |
| Calming in the classroom and quiet reading | Calming in the classroom and quiet reading | Calming in the classroom and quiet reading |
| Heavy work + schedule interruption | Heavy work + schedule interruption | Heavy work + schedule interruption |
| Speech | CD Rom in resource room | Art |
| Music | Music | Music |
| Spelling, community helpers, functional reading, physical activity in resource room, dismissal | Spelling, community helpers, functional reading, physical activity in resource room, dismissal | Spelling, community helpers, functional reading, physical activity in resource room, dismissal |

a regular education classroom may be best for another, and some time in special education integrated into a community-based or inclusion experience may work for others. All individuals should have the opportunity to spend time with same-age peers and be provided with adequate support and the adaptations necessary to be successful. Parents play a critical role in this decision-making process and offer the most valuable information regarding their child. The program planning and decision-making process regarding the focus of the education plan (i.e., functional vs. academic) should be made by the educational team, in which the parents play a critical part.

Higher-functioning children with FXS may do well in the regular classroom. Many children with FXS demonstrate strong verbal and behavioral imitation skills. Because of this, placement in a regular classroom, where development of normal socialization skills can be encouraged, is desirable. In deciding educational placement for a child, educators and parents need to consider many factors. Some questions to ask when determining placement include:

1. What is the placement objective for this student?
   - Social interaction
   - Behavioral modeling
   - Academic stimulation
   - Skill development
   - Extracurricular activities
2. What are the benefits/disadvantages of the inclusive model for this student?
3. What are the benefits/disadvantages of a noninclusive classroom?
4. Is it possible to develop a program or setting that incorporates the best of both philosophies?
5. Will the necessary educational and environmental adaptations for this student be implemented?

## Occupational Therapy and Fragile X

To understand and work effectively with individuals with FXS, one must recognize underlying deficits in sensory-processing and/or sensory-integrative functions. Modulation and discriminative difficulties, for example, are commonly seen in this population, although the degree of deficit in each individual may vary.

The central nervous system (CNS) has evolved with complex interrelationships of the sensory modalities (Nobak 1975; Marks 1978; Sarnat and Netsky 1981; Smith 1985; Kandel et al. 2000). Ayres (1965) recognized this principle and investigated its importance in the study and treatment of children with a variety of CNS disorders. This research indicated that dysfunction in the proprioceptive, vestibular, tactile, and visual systems could adversely affect the development of higher-level functions (Ayres 1972, 1978). Ayres postulated that treatment enhancing basic sensory integration would have a positive influence on motoric, tactile, emotional, and cognitive functions. She defined sensory integration as "the neurological process that organizes sensation from one's own body and from the environment and makes it possible to use the body effectively within the environment" (Ayres 1972, 1989).

The spatial and temporal aspects of inputs from different sensory modalities are interpreted, associated, and unified. Sensory integration is information processing: The brain must select, enhance, inhibit, compare, and associate the sensory information in a flexible, constantly changing pattern; in other words, the brain must integrate it.

Occupational therapy using a sensory integration approach has been an effective form of intervention for certain diagnostic groups. Importantly, some populations previously studied display behaviors similar to those seen in the population with FXS. Among these are children with autism, who may be hypersensitive to touch (Ayres and Tickle 1980) or preschoolers with autism who show a decrease in nonengaged social behavior and an increase in mastery play (Case-Smith and Bryan 1999), individuals with stereotypic rocking behavior (Bonadonna 1981), and children who display self-stimulatory or self-injurious behavior (Bright et al. 1981; Storey et al. 1984). There is also evidence that sensory integrative therapy can facilitate the development of language skills in children with mental retardation, developmental delay, learning disabilities, and autism (Kawar 1973; Meegrum et al. 1981; Kantner et al. 1982; Reilly et al. 1983; Densom et al. 1989). See Vargas and Camilli (1999) for a meta-analysis of sensory integration (SI) treatment studies. They demonstrate the specific motor gains made in SI treatment, as well as its benefits in comparison to non-SI approaches.

The quality of higher-level functioning in the CNS may depend on the integrity of more basic integration, with the individual's behavior often a clue as to this integrity (Ayres 1979). This basic level of integration is believed to occur at a neural level and function in a systems manner. These systems, or clusters, are categorized for ease of understanding into (1) sensory modulation disorders including self-regulatory functions, registration impairments, and sensory defensiveness and (2) sensory discrimination disorders influencing body scheme development and use, postural-ocular control, and the process of motor planning (praxis). As these basic sensory processing problems manifest, they affect higher-level skill development, ranging from problems with learning to social interaction to difficulty playing and motor planning. Disorganization in early-developing functions sets a pattern of disruption that makes higher-level communication and cognitive skills slow and disrupted (exhibit 10.3). For example, if there has been inadequate vestibular-proprioceptive integration, individuals may struggle with balance, awareness of where and how their bodies are moving through space and comfort with this movement, and postural-ocular control (Fisher et al. 1991). These are components of sensory discrimination processing difficulties. Vestibular-proprioceptive processing deficits are seen in sensory modulation disorders as well. These manifest as a spectrum disorder ranging from fearful or avoidant responses to movement/gravity challenges, including having the feet off the ground, to seeking behaviors toward intense movement or movement substitute experiences. Examples of this are an individual's visual fascination with spinning tops or toys, watching water twirling out of a faucet, repetitive toilet flushing, and rocking of the body or parts of the body. These may be used to satisfy a need for movement input. Ayres has postulated that this type of self-stimulatory behavior may be an attempt to stimulate the vestibular system (1979). Baranek and Berkson (1994) identified an association between sensory hypersensitivity and self-stimulatory behavior.

Another basic sensory system involves the sense of touch, known as the tac-

**Exhibit 10.3**
**Hierarchy of Attributes Related to Human Communication**

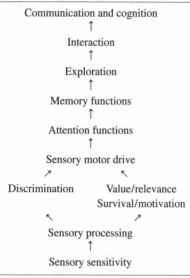

*Source:* After Pattie Oetter and Marci Laurel (1989).

tile system. Sensory modulation disorders in this system include tactile defensiveness (part of the larger syndrome of sensory defensiveness; Wilbarger 1988), which is manifested by hypersensitivity to touch (Ayres 1972; Baranek and Berkson 1994). Persons may prefer wearing long-sleeved clothing or avoiding light touch while seeking out deep pressure, craving hugs, or crashing into things. They may even bite or hit themselves when overly anxious in an attempt at self-modulation through pressure and proprioceptive receptors (Ayres 1979). Sensory defensiveness is typified as a lack of recovery to sensory input creating a tendency to react negatively or with alarm to sensory input that is generally considered nonharmful, and it can happen in any or all sensory systems (Wilbarger and Wilbarger 1991). Sensory defensiveness may lead to decreased interactions with care givers and other children, peers, and adults, resulting in a disruption of the natural development of social interaction and language (Short-de Graaff 1988). Poor discrimination of tactile perceptions makes it difficult to tell a quarter from a dime in your pocket and makes walking in the sand a "tripping" experience.

The visual system should help with navigation as well as accommodation to changes in the visual field, such as looking at a teacher pointing at a chalkboard and then referring to your tabletop notes and back to the overhead projection.

Modulation of visual input makes this typical classroom event possible. With disordered visual modulation, this same classroom event is an agonizing experience. Gaze avoidance is often the result of sensory modulation disorders.

Olfactory stimuli, which input at the cortical rather than the brain-stem level (Scott 1986) and which influence the limbic system and memory (Nobak 1975; Gustavson et al. 1987), may cause primitive defensive or nondiscriminatory behavior. One study demonstrated that children with FXS initially perceive nonaversive scents as either noxious or undifferentiated (Burns and Hickman 1989). This response to olfactory stimuli is yet another example of disorganized sensory processing.

Early learning occurs through the child's basic sensory experiences with people and with the environment. For meaningful interaction to occur, a child must be at a normal level of arousal (Windeck and Laurel 1989). Arousal difficulties are a large component of sensory modulation/self-regulatory problems. Most individuals with FXS report trouble tolerating typical amounts of sensory input. Miller et al. (1999) offer support for a basic disruption in the typical sensory responding and habituation mechanisms across sensory modalities. In their studies, individuals with FXS show unusual, marked over-responsiveness and poor habituation as measured by electrodermal reactivity (EDR) (see chap. 1). When sensory over-responsivity is coupled with unpredictable environments and the social demands of our culture, we see resultant characteristic fragile X behavior of unpredictable withdrawal, flight, fear, and fight behaviors. Social anxiety contributes to "overload" in the sensory systems, and sensory modulation problems make social situations very difficult to manage. These reciprocal deficits make developing and maintaining an appropriate level of arousal or alertness very difficult. People function at their optimum when they are in their range of balance between over- and under-responsivity to sensory input, interaction, and environmental and task demand. When this balance is not easily achieved or maintained, functioning in a socially driven context is nearly impossible. This is characteristic of individuals with FXS (Belser and Sudhalter 1995; Miller et al. 1999).

The end products of sensory integration with which we are ultimately concerned are the variety of life roles individuals occupy and the skills one acquires to competently fill these occupations, as student, son, mother, friend, or worker. Through the knowledge provided by the theories of sensory integration, the occupational therapist is able to shed light on complicated processes that are clearly impairing a person's ability to efficiently learn and develop the variety of roles that each person is entitled to richly explore. Because individuals with FXS have such marked sensory processing difficulties, they frequently are unable to achieve this roundedness in their life roles. Clinical experience has taught us that, without applied sensory integrative theory, this squelching of potential happens too frequently. Yet with intervention, new realms of developmental possibilities are discovered. Improvements in sensory processing at all levels may lead to improved sensory integration and subsequent output, both motor and vocal (de Quiros 1976; Luria 1976; de Quiros and Scharager 1978; Zivin 1979; Clark and Steingold 1982; Bellman and Goldberg 1984; Windeck and Laurel 1989).

The goal of therapy is to help the person develop more adaptive responses to the challenges life presents. At certain times, achieving an adaptive response may require the therapist to focus on the underlying basic sensory systems—vestibular, proprioception, and tactile—and how they underlie and contribute to later skills in auditory, visual, and language areas is at the crux of intervention. At other times, an adaptive response may best be facilitated by helping the individual to learn a specific skill, such as catching a ball or using a bus schedule. Because the treatment is all "OT," any of a range of goals and adaptive responses may be facilitated. Using classic sensory-integrative approaches has proven to be effective in treating sensory discrimination-based problems in particular. Treatment of sensory modulation problems uses sensory-integrative theory to help understand the complex issues of hypersensitivities to environmental stimuli and struggles with social anxiety. General principles that can be applied therapeutically to maintain a more normal level of arousal during therapy, school, or work or at home include the use of a "sensory diet," a concept formulated by Pat Wilbarger (1995) (exhibits 10.4 and 10.5). The use of the "Step-SI" treatment model (Stackhouse and Wilbarger 1998) as a means of structuring the sensation, task, environment, predictability, self-monitoring, and interactions in a treatment session, classroom, or home program is highly recommended.

Throughout testing and in therapy sessions, the therapist must understand basic sensory processing principles. The appropriate environment and activities should be provided. The therapist must also be sensitive to the complex, sometimes stereotypic needs and behaviors of the individual with FXS and respond with appropriate intervention. A reassuring firm touch, a quieter voice, or singing rather than speaking instructions may be indicated. Treatment may involve the use of particular aromas the person finds pleasant and calming. For example, midway through a testing session in which the response to a variety of nonnoxious smells had been assessed, a young man became very agitated. He demanded "I want that strawberry again" and reached for the olfactory vials. He also began biting his hand impulsively. The therapist recognized the importance of acknowledging the agitation this person felt and was able to help with verbalizing his emotional state. Once the reason for stereotypic, sometimes self-abusive behavior is expressed and the person's emotional state is acknowledged, alternative behaviors can be suggested and demonstrated. The therapist in this situation said, "It is uncomfortable to be tested. All your life, people have evaluated you. You get so upset sometimes that you have to bite

**Exhibit 10.4**
**Calming Activities**

This exhibit is intended for use as a guide for calming. The rationale and references supporting calming activities are complex and are briefly outlined in this chapter. Correct implementation of these activities should be done under the direction of a registered occupational therapist.

**Deep pressure input** through the muscles, joints, and skin is one of the safest and most effective calming inputs.
- swaddling or wrapping in blankets
- pillows to nestle, wrestle, and cuddle in; use a variety of sizes and textures
- weighted blankets, weighted or inflatable vests or cuffs at wrists/ankles
- wearing of Ace wraps on arms, legs, trunk; wearing of spandex under garments or neoprene gloves, shorts, headbands, etc.
- wedging into a "squeeze machine" (Grandin and Scariano 1988)
- wedging into a barrel with pillows
- use of a gymnastic ball to roll over a person with careful pressure

**Heavy work** is active pressure type input to the muscles and joints through pushing, pulling, lifting, carrying, "working"!
- kneading bread dough, stirring baking mixes, using a rolling pin
- vacuuming, carrying the laundry, carrying any load, mowing the lawn
- pushing the grocery cart, pulling a wagon, riding a bike
- stacking chairs, scrubbing tables
- doing push-ups or pushing against a wall
- climbing stairs; using stairstep or rowing machine; rowing a boat
- pushing feet on bungee cord at a desk
- carrying a backpack

**Heavy work in the hands** is an effective technique that can be used easily in multiple environments. This is characterized as "fidget and focus."
- using Play-Doh therapy/putty work
- having access to one or preferably more small manipulative toys with which to simply "fidget"
- using "worry stones" that are pleasant to hold and caress
- attaching rubber tubing to backpack strap to pull on as needed
- attaching a telephone cord type key chain to belt loop to pull on or "fidget"
- finger knitting, craft activities

**Oral motor inputs** have a "heavy work" component as well as effecting regulating mechanisms on more complex levels (Oetter et al. 1993).
- chewing on frozen grapes, fruit leather, licorice, pretzels, gum, rubber tubing, etc.
- sucking through resistive, long, or "silly" straws for liquids, to move game pieces, etc.
- using blow toys (some are even silent!), blowing cotton through a maze, blowing game pieces

*(continues)*

**Exhibit 10.4** (*Continued*)

---

- farm work: caring for animals, collecting eggs, shoveling, hoeing, the possibilities are endless
- rock climbing, back-packing
- sporting opportunities dependent on interest and tolerance levels
- commercial child playlands, especially at OFF PEAK hours
- make the most of local parks, museums, etc. Build in focus opportunities by doing scavenger hunts or slow and skilled movement experiences. Go at quiet rather than busy times.

These activities need to be individualized and usually are used in combination. The best recommendation is to utilize them in a "sensory diet" format (see exhibit 10.5). Accommodations for classroom/work and home need to incorporate these principles/ activities. See exhibit 10.6 for additional ideas.

---

*Source:* Compiled by Lois Hickman, MS OTR, and Tracy Murnan Stackhouse, OTR, from numerous sources, including our best teachers and the kids and families with whom we work.

your hand to calm down. Here's another way to feel better." This therapist demonstrated how the patient could rub his arms and press hard on the top of his head. The young man was able to relax and to complete the testing. Techniques such as this can be done independently or with the assistance of family, friends, or staff and are listed in exhibit 10.4.

Sensory integration is both a theory of brain-behavior relationships and an intervention approach (Fisher et al. 1991). It is used as a component of occupational therapy practice and incorporated into the intervention by many other professionals as well. At its foundation, SI treatment capitalizes on the plasticity of the nervous system (Parham and Mailloux 1996). As discussed in chapter 5, the work of Greenough and colleagues (1999, 2000) suggests that this is a critical aspect of understanding development and FXS. Critical to understanding the aim of SI treatment is the point that SI is not aimed at curing any particular disability. Rather, the aim of treatment is to facilitate efficient sensory processing, promote capabilities, and minimize dysfunction. This is true of both SI therapy and the field of occupational therapy.

It is critical for therapists and educators working with individuals with FXS to understand that many behavioral problems result from sensory-integrative deficits and are not intentional acts on the part of the child. The underlying cause of behavioral problems in this population must be examined, as it will have a significant effect on the type of therapy used to change undesirable behaviors. A strict behavior modification program may not be appropriate if behaviors are resulting from sensory-integrative deficits. However, working together the occupational therapist (OT) and psychologist will usually best manage difficult situations.

**Exhibit 10.5**
**Principles and Approaches of the Sensory Diet**

1. The sensory qualities of certain activities have a "modulating" influence on behavior. Deep pressure touch, proprioception, heavy work, and rhythmic movement, in general, promote organization. Other activities and sensory input such as using fidget toys, oral motor activities, or vibration can also be calming.
2. Sensorimotor activity must be available and repeated throughout the day to help the individual maintain an optimal level of organization. This is especially true during transitions, in highly stimulating environments, and at times when it is difficult to maintain attention or when activity is discouraged.

SCHEDULE:
It is sometimes helpful to make a schedule for deep pressure, tactile input, and joint compression (together sometimes referred to as the Wilbarger "brushing" protocol) and various activities for yourself.

| Time | Daily Activities and Accompanying Moderate Activity | "Brushing" and Joint Compression | Other Activity |
|---|---|---|---|
| 7:00 | | | |
| 8:00 | | | |
| 9:00 | | | |
| 10:00 | | | |
| 11:00 | | | |
| 12:00 | | | |
| 1:00 | | | |
| 2:00 | | | |
| 3:00 | | | |
| 4:00 | | | |
| 5:00 | | | |
| 6:00 | | | |
| 7:00 | | | |
| 8:00 | | | |
| 9:00 | | | |
| 10:00 | | | |

| Transitions | Time | Modulating Activity | Leisure | Time | Activity |
|---|---|---|---|---|---|
| 1. AM Routine: | | | 1. | | |
| 2. PM Routine: | | | 2. | | |
| 3. Other transitions: | | | 3. | | |

(Park time, sports, martial arts, coloring, etc.)

*(continues)*

**Exhibit 10.5** (*Continued*)

| Mealtime | Time | Modulating Activity |
|----------|------|---------------------|
| 1. Before: | | |
| 2. During: | | |
| 3. After: | | |

Notes on Adaptations

| To Environment: | To Interaction: | To Tasks: |
|-----------------|-----------------|-----------|
| (Provide quiet spaces, be aware of sensations present and adaptations) | (Use calm, rhythmic voice, pressure touch, and respect the sensory issues) | |

Components:

Deep pressure touch is firm touch like massage.

Proprioception is the sensation of joints and muscles. These joint senses give information about the movement, location, and force exerted on joints and muscles.

Heavy work is a kind of proprioception and includes anything that makes muscles work against resistance. This includes whole-body action and is best described as push, pull, lift, play, move! Use of hands, as in "fidgeting" with toys, is also heavy work.

Oral activity such as chewing, sucking, blowing helps to focus and organize. Use in meals, in snacks, and at play. This is like "heavy work" for the mouth.

Movement such as swinging, rocking, jumping, tumbling is particularly powerful, especially when done in specific positions. Rhythmic movement is also very calming in contrast to fast, changeable movement.

*Source:* Developed by Pat Wilbarger, Julie Wilbarger, and Tracy Stackhouse.

## Speech and Language Therapy and Fragile X

Minimal formal research on specific speech and language treatment regimes with individuals who have FXS has been reported. There are, however, many strategies that address the learning-disabled, mentally retarded, and autistic populations. Intervention strategies found useful with those populations can be used with individuals who have FXS.

Therapy goals for each child should be determined by his or her specific strengths, weaknesses, and skills in a variety of areas. Sensory-integrative dysfunction and cognitive and attentional deficits will significantly affect speech/language development and learning. Before speech and language therapy is initiated, these areas of difficulty must be addressed. Assessment and knowledge of the sensory integration and cognitive and attentional domains are vital to planning speech and language therapy. To establish a strong foundation for future learning, one must apply the therapeutic principles of each area.

General guidelines in program planning for speech and language therapy have been compiled in table 10.3. Many of the suggestions are based on clini-

**Table 10.3**
**Speech-Language Deficits and Intervention Strategies for the Child**
**with Fragile X Syndrome**

| Deficit Area | Intervention Strategies |
|---|---|
| Attention | Use child's interest areas. |
| | Supplement auditory with visual input, including photographs. |
| | Keep auditory and visual distractions at a minimum. |
| | Work in small, partitioned area. |
| | Use headphones to dampen sound if they'll be tolerated. |
| | Use calming activities provided by the occupational therapist, including brushing and joint compression. |
| | Work for several short periods of time. |
| | Adapt the environment as necessary. |
| Delayed onset of expressive speech | Use a total communication approach; fade out signs as verbalizations increase. |
| | Reinforce any attempts at speech; shape responses by modeling correct utterances. |
| | Encourage oral exploratory play; use suggestions to work with oral motor deficits that affect early sound production and language skills. |
| Rate, rhythm, "cluttering" | Model correct rate/rhythm. |
| | Melodic intonation therapy (Albert et al. 1973; Sparks and Holland 1976; Helfrich-Miller 1994). |
| | Be aware of the effect of low muscle tone on respiration and rate. |
| | Increase self-monitoring. |
| | Voice synthesizer for auditory and visual feedback. |
| | Model a rhythmic voice; use movement and activities to emphasize appropriate rhythm and rate. |
| | Use suggestions from occupational therapy to help calm and focus. |
| Oral and verbal dyspraxia | Music, singing, movement. |
| | Integrate therapy with occupational therapist. |
| | See suggestions for rate. |

*(continues)*

**Table 10.3** (*Continued*)

| *Deficit Area* | *Intervention Strategies* |
| --- | --- |
| Oral motor deficits<br>• Stuffing mouth | Understand that many of the oral problems may arise from poor awareness and proprioceptive feedback. |
| • Oral sensitivity to touch, textures, temperatures | Use appropriate deep pressure input, massage, and vibration. |
| • Chewing on toys, clothes<br>• Low tone | Work on normalizing sensitivity throughout the body under the guidance of an OT when working on sensitivity issues in the oral area. |
| | Be open to doing oral motor interventions in a group setting, which allows the fragile X child to see models and take turns. |
| | Use foods with a variety of tastes and textures as well as bubbles and other motivating toys. |
| | Have highly structured tasks; use cues as needed. |
| | Allow child to perform activities himself if tactile defensiveness interferes with performance. |
| | Cold or warm stimulation may be tolerated easily and may help with tolerance of touch to oral area you usually can't touch (ice, cold food, wet washcloth, warm water bottle, warm hand). |
| | Chew on gum, aquarium tubing, fruit leather, turkey jerky. |
| | Use straws for drinks, pudding, applesauce, yogurt. |
| | Mouth toys: kazoo, harmonica, blower, popsicle, slushy. |
| Auditory memory | Elicit attention before task.<br>Pair auditory information with visual cue.<br>Rhythm and music to cue recall.<br>Use short instructions intrinsic to the task. |
| Abstract reasoning, problem-solving skills | Use realistic, meaningful materials of interest to the child.<br>Begin at the concrete level and systematically increase the level of abstraction.<br>Teach skill sets for specific problem-solving activities.<br>Use games/activities on computer. |
| Verbal perseveration, tangential comments, topic maintenance | Allow increased processing time.<br>Model desired utterances. |

**Table 10.3** (*Continued*)

| Deficit Area | Intervention Strategies |
|---|---|
| | Reduce the complexity of utterances to child's level. |
| | Use dramatic play to encourage natural social interactions. |
| | Monitor anxiety level and adapt accordingly (calming and focusing activities). |
| | Provide opportunities to practice a variety of speech acts. |
| | Redirect the child verbally. |
| | Have the child reauditorize to help process. |
| | Emphasize "topic" through the use of high-interest materials. |
| | Use a motor activity (jumping, clapping, pushing on the wall) paired with a verbal activity to "break" the perseveration. |
| Responding to questions | Use fill-ins instead of direct questioning. |
| | Give choices. |
| | In the group setting, do not ask the fragile X child first. |
| | Minimize the need for eye contact. |
| | Use a visual response mode; let the child say the answer after selecting it from an array of pictures/words. |
| Eye contact | Often develops after familiarity with speaker. |
| | Don't train out of context. |
| | Recognize sensory limitations to eye contact. |
| | Don't give constant eye contact yourself. |
| | Position the child so eye contact is not always demanded (i.e., off to side). |
| | Focus on joint attention rather than eye contact. |
| | Use dark glasses. |

General Strategies
- Because imitative skills are often strong for fragile X individuals, use small groups consisting of higher-functioning children to augment individual therapy.
- Maintain close coordination of goals between all those working with the child. Use the parents to follow through on home programs.
- Evaluate the need for combined speech-language and occupational therapies.

*Source:* Scharfenaker and Shopmeyer 1994.
*Note:* These are only a few of the many strategies that have been successful. Be creative!

cal experience and our understanding of the specific learning style of individuals with FXS.

Individuals with FXS usually exhibit difficulties with topic maintenance, tangential comments, initiation of conversation, short-term memory, cluttering, verbal and motor dyspraxia, abstract reasoning, perseveration (repetition of words, phrases, sentences, or topics), and eye gaze (see chaps. 1 and 6). Many of these deficits relate to the disorder of pragmatics. Pragmatics is the study of the conversational act and its components. The purpose of conversation is to control or influence a listener's thoughts, beliefs, actions, and attitudes (Lucas 1980). Conversation may serve a variety of communicative functions: labeling, denying, requesting, or stating information, among others. For an individual to be proficient in pragmatic or conversational skills, he or she must have developed a repertoire of socially acceptable rules and strategies for influencing the listener. One must be able to use the correct linguistic structures as well as nonverbal cues (eye contact, gestures, body posture) to get a message across effectively. A child with pragmatic difficulties may not have developed the linguistic knowledge necessary to communicate effectively or may not use conversational rules and strategies appropriately. In addition, they may not be able to correctly interpret verbal and nonverbal messages from others. Sensory processing problems may also affect the child by disrupting the development of appropriate pragmatic skills. For example, a child with FXS may demonstrate sensory defensiveness to such a degree that he or she becomes easily overwhelmed by the children in the classroom bumping into or brushing up against him or her. The child may react by withdrawing from those social and classroom group experiences necessary to learn appropriate pragmatic skills. Difficulties with conversational rules and strategies are common within the population of FXS.

One of the more distinctive pragmatic features of the FXS population is the use of verbal perseveration. As with repetitive self-stimulatory behaviors (such as hand biting and rocking), verbal perseveration may reflect the individual's difficulty with inhibition of responses. Perseveration may also be an anxiety-based response to excessive language demands. For example, increased receptive and expressive as well as pragmatic demands may cause the individual with FXS to become anxious, resulting in increased use of perseveration (Sudhalter 1992, 2000). Anxiety is often experienced during formal assessments. As the assessment demands become more complex, perseveration is more frequent. Perseveration may also provide the individual with FXS a conversational time filler as well as increased time for processing information, as has been documented in aphasics without FXS (Travis 1971; Arwood 1984). By providing more time for processing, the therapist is more apt to elicit an appropriate response, and conversation may be facilitated. Additionally, use of specific hands-on techniques provided by the occupational therapist can help to diminish anticipatory anxiety and hyperarousal. These techniques can be used by the parent, occupational therapist, speech/language pathologist, and teacher or classroom aide to help reduce anxiety and subsequent related communication problems such as verbal perseverations.

Because there is such variability of speech and language deficits among individuals with FXS, a thorough assessment of pragmatic skills is necessary. Although formal assessment tools are available through publishers, many therapist-made tools are equally sensitive. Suggestions for developing specific pragmatic treatment programs for individuals with FXS can be drawn from the related fields of autism and developmental disabilities. Pragmatic skills programs that take advantage of naturally occurring events in the child's environment, provide functional use of skills, facilitate the spontaneous use of communication, and encourage a wide generalization of learning are most beneficial with this population (Stokes and Bauer 1977). Conversely, a dogmatic approach to teaching pragmatics may inhibit or disrupt social interaction and communication (Wetherby 1986) and is not desirable.

Individuals with FXS who demonstrate strong verbal and social imitative skills should have academic and therapeutic opportunities with others functioning at the same or a slightly higher language level. Many of the suggestions listed in table 10.3 are applicable in a group setting. These include using the group's interest areas, using visual cues, and allowing extra response time. Modeling of correct utterances (reducing the complexity of therapist verbalizations), expansion (expanding the child's utterance with one or two words), and parallel talk (verbalizing what the patient is doing or thinking) are useful in improving pragmatics (Koegel et al. 1987). Modeling and expansion are also used to target the growth of specific linguistic structures. These techniques have been used successfully with the autistic population (Schwartz and Leonard 1985; Scherer and Olswang 1989). A fast rate of speech, oral and verbal dyspraxia, and difficulties with auditory memory and abstract reasoning skills also require direct work. Although specific therapeutic techniques for these deficits can be found in the general speech and language literature, some adaptations should be made in structure and presentation when working with individuals with FXS. Suggestions for adaptations in the academic and therapy setting are found in exhibit 10.6.

The intelligibility of speech of individuals with FXS is affected by the degree to which dyspraxia, speech rate, and overall oral motor functioning work together. Dyspraxia is a disruption in motor planning skills. Motor planning comprises several steps: ideation, initiation, and execution. The ability to plan for the fine, precise, rapid movements for speech production is compromised in many children with dyspraxia. Motor planning for speech is often a concern with these individuals, as is decreased tone, tactile sensitivity issues, and stability within the jaw, tongue, lips, and upper body. Many children lack the over-

**Exhibit 10.6**
**Classroom Accommodations**

Children with fragile X syndrome have significant social anxiety, sensory processing, cognitive, and regulation problems that make living and learning in a school setting challenging for themselves and their teachers and peers.

The following recommendations are based on an integrated intervention style that incorporates the principles of sensory processing theory and specific behavior management methods focused on FXS. (See exhibit 10.5, Sensory diet.) Many are common-sense suggestions drawn from the learning disabilities literature. Not all will be applicable to every child with FXS.

1. Use the sensory diet as outlined in exhibit 10.5. Remember that this must be implemented under the guidance of the occupational therapist.
2. Children with FXS are often fidgety or motorically overactive in a school environment. Those working with the child need to determine the basis of this behavior. Some common causes of the behavior include
   - Poor postural control
   - Poor self-regulation
   - Sensory defensiveness
   - Task avoidance
   - Poor understanding of expectations
A. If problems are related to postural control:
   1. Adjust the chair so the child is given feedback about where he or she is in space (i.e., line edges with foam strips, have the child sit on a water-filled hemorrhoid cushion, etc.).
   2. Give frequent breaks from tabletop work, since the child has a difficult time maintaining sitting positions and fatigues more quickly than other children due to weakness in postural muscle control (i.e., activities done on floor or standing).
   3. Adjust the chair and table to a height suitable for the child to best perform tabletop work (feet touching the floor; table height just below the child's elbows).
   4. Allow the child to stand at the desk, to work on the floor in a prone-on-elbows position, or to move while working.
B. If problems are related to poor self-regulation:
   1. One approach is to allow some kind of movement of the body, hands, or mouth.
      - Consider a rocking chair, therapy ball, or bean bag chair for at least part of the day.
      - Allow seat breaks (be messenger, run errands, pass out materials).
      - Have the child hook a bungee cord to the front of his chair and place his or her feet on it so the child can move his or her legs while seated.
      - Give the child something to fidget with in the hands (a squishy ball, therapy tubing, any of a variety of held toys meant to keep kids' hands busy, not electronic).
      - Give opportunity for oral input if appropriate (gum to chew, food with strong texture, hard candy to suck).

**Exhibit 10.6** (*Continued*)

---

2. Another approach will be opportunities for muscles and joints to work or receive pressure.
   - Give joint compression or deep pressure exercise before requiring the child to sit for prolonged periods (push-ups on wall or chair, heavy lifting or carrying).
   - Have the child stack the chairs or rearrange furniture.
   - Have the child carry a basket of books to the library (use this at transition times as well).
3. An alternate approach focuses more on development of cognitive strategies than on sensory techniques.
   - Use of *Think Aloud* (Camp and Bush 1981)
   - Develop awareness strategies around self-regulation and modulation.

C. If problems are related to sensory defensiveness:
   1. Be sure the occupational therapist is overseeing the direct treatment of the defensiveness and that a sensory diet is in place and being used daily.
   2. Keep visual and auditory distractions to a minimum. Position the child near the teacher to help facilitate the child's attention to classroom instructions.
      - Be aware of the significant impact smells have on individuals with FXS. Decrease the use of perfume, be aware of cafeteria odors, etc.
      - For the child who experiences tactile hypersensitivity, allow the child to stand at the end of the line and arrange classroom seating to minimize the risk of the child's being jostled or bumped by classmates. Keep enough distance between desks to minimize problems.
      - Minimize the need for changing visual references ("Look at me," "Look at the blackboard," "Look at your paper," etc.).
      - Be aware of your interaction style: voice quality and how you touch and approach students. Make sure to use a calming manner in all respects.
      - Multiple light sources, especially fluorescent lighting, can be very overloading and may need to be changed. Halogen or natural lighting is recommended.

D. If problems are related to task avoidance:
   1. Use choices within structure. ("Would you like to work standing or sitting?").
   2. Follow through with consequences.

E. If problems are related to poor understanding of expectations:
   1. Use clear, concise directions, with visual backup as needed.
   2. Provide choices.
   3. Allow movement.
   4. Give physical or verbal redirection.

---

all tone in the trunk area to provide adequate support and stability for adequate respiratory patterns and volume. This affects the ability to use controlled and sustained vocalizations with sufficient volume. Poor oral motor and verbal planning skills in addition to low tone, as well as decreased jaw and upper body stability, may contribute to the development of other poor motor functioning for speech. Poor trunk and upper body stability, jaw and tongue instability and differentiation, low oral tone, and oral and verbal dyspraxia all contribute to problems in the oral motor functioning area. These difficulties are worsened by the arousal state of the child, requiring intervention through occupational therapy.

Sensitivity of the oral area is another area of concern in this population. Hyper-, hypo-, and mixed sensitivity may be observed. Normalizing sensitivity to tactile input is the goal in working in this area. Many children may have difficulty with production of specific sounds due to the way some phonemes "feel" in their mouths, at times heightening oral sensitivity (Marshalla 1994). In working on tactile sensitivity, it is important to start with normalizing sensitivity throughout the entire body first and not work on the oral area alone. If normalizing sensitivity is worked on in any area without the benefit of the whole body, the abnormal sensitivity in that area will most likely only be dissipated and soon return (Marshalla 1994). A prescribed program for normalizing sensitivity may include use of such equipment as washcloths, toothettes, toothbrushes, ice, and a variety of snack foods, such as crackers, pretzels, gum, and other snacks that provide "heavy work" in the mouth as well as a variety of textures. Increasing jaw stability, strength, and control gives the child the opportunity to practice increased and varied tongue and lip movements. A full oral motor assessment and understanding of the anatomy and physiology of this area are critical in developing a therapy plan to work on the oral motor area. Several excellent sources in the area of oral motor functioning are Morris (1977, 1982, 1988) and Marshalla (1992, 1996). Additionally, specific suggestions for working on oral motor skills in FXS are included in *The Fragile X Child* (Shopmeyer and Lowe 1992).

The nonverbal individual with FXS presents a particular challenge to the speech/language pathologist. The general speech/language literature reports that, if children do not acquire speech by the time they are seven years of age, the chance of them developing speech is quite small.

Taylor et al. (2001) found that only a very small percentage of children with FXS (1–2%) do not develop speech and must learn to rely on an augmentative/alternative system. Physical features, most clinical markers, and CGG repeat number of the full mutation do not predict severe language delay in fragile X syndrome. A total communication approach (the use of sign in combination with verbal output) has been useful in stimulating language growth. Therapists have noted that, as the child's spontaneous verbalizations increased, the use of sign language decreased and gradually faded out (Scharfenaker and Hickman 1989). General motor skills, including motor planning and sequencing skills, should be assessed before the use of sign language. The *Assessment, Behavior Management & Communication Training Program* by Krug et al. (1980) has been used successfully with several moderately handicapped, nonverbal children with FXS. Sign language and speech imitation are taught independently and then combined to form a total communication system when the student initiates vocalizations while signing. As speech production increases, the use of signs fades. The curriculum is centered on the child's interests and desires. Programming is presented through a hierarchical series of structured cues and responses, allowing quick and easy assessment of progress and areas of need.

The technology in the area of augmentative and alternative communication is rapidly expanding. If total communication or sign language is not helpful to a specific child, alternative communication systems can be evaluated. The Picture Exchange Communication System (PECS) is an alternative/augmentative program that teaches minimally verbal or nonverbal children to spontaneously initiate communication interactions (Frost and Bondy 1994). The child learns to exchange a single picture for a desired object, eventually moving into creating simple sentences. This program can be highly successful in teaching functional communication. Many clinicians report that this system is very useful for children with FXS who have severe verbal dyspraxia. The decision to use a specific communication device or computer is based on evaluation of the child's motor, cognitive, perceptual, social, and communicative skills and needs. Augmentative and alternative communication can be used by children at a wide variety of levels and for multiple purposes. Use of augmentative communication devices can help decrease frustration and build language skills while verbal language is being developed. Montgomery (1980), Schiefelbush (1980), Musselwhite and St. Louis (1982), Silverman (1982), and Yoder (1982) provide useful information in evaluating appropriate alternative communication choices for children.

## Integrating Occupational and Speech Therapies: A Rationale

The complexities of facilitating development in a child with FXS often necessitate the collaboration of multiple professionals. Specifically, the combining of OT and speech has been identified as a primary recommendation at different times throughout the child's life-span. A combined occupational–speech language therapy approach can facilitate the integration of sensory, language, and cognitive skills for the individual with FXS. Individuals with FXS have difficulty maintaining focus and attention, which interferes with the goals of speech therapy. However, with the support provided by the occupational therapist, using sensory integrative techniques, the person with FXS can benefit from more cognitive and language-related activities. Another common problem, that of oral and verbal dyspraxia, also lends itself well to the combined approach (Windeck and Laurel 1989). Use of movement, rhythm, music, singing, and limericks can facilitate and enhance motor planning and sequencing (Sparks et al. 1974; Sparks and Holland 1976).

**Table 10.4**

**Models of Combined Occupational (OT) and Speech/Language (SL) Therapy**

| Model Type | Description |
|---|---|
| Cotreatment | The OT and SL see the child together during a joint treatment session. This model is used when the hierarchy in exhibit 10.3 is marked by difficulties in the lower processing aspects that significantly hinder developmental change at the top of the chart. |
| Consultation | The OT and SL consult with each other (and with the parents or other team members) regarding treatment goals, techniques, and carry-over. Treatment or therapy may then be carried out by someone other than the consultant. |
| Group treatment | Several children are seen by one or more team members in a group setting, as the scaffolding and models provided by peers may provide important means of facilitating sensory-motor, language, or other skills needed at some particular time in development. |
| Individual treatment | Child or family is seen by one particular team member, who is also aware of and incorporating the goals of the other team members. |
| Ordering of therapy | Child's appointment times/class schedule is devised in such a way as to capitalize on one aspect of the intervention approach that may provide a means of supporting a later intervention (i.e., a child may be seen for OT ahead of speech to facilitate postural control and breath support for speech/language production). |

Table 10.4 illustrates the various ways in which occupational and speech/language therapies might work together. The therapists need to decide which model works best in their particular setting. Exhibit 10.3 illustrates how higher-level skills are built on more basic sensory modalities. This model should be referred to when devising individual intervention plans.

Children and adults diagnosed as having FXS have common behavioral characteristics, but they also have significant individual differences, strengths, and weaknesses. Even though a treatment session is planned to follow a certain sequence, the reciprocal therapeutic interactions between therapists and clients must reflect the client's and the group's immediate and evolving needs.

The educational challenge with this population is to adapt teaching materials that promote success through familiar contexts. The phenomenon of incidental learning is also important and is reflected in the high score usually obtained by boys with FXS on the Faces and Places subtest of the Kaufman Assessment Battery for Children (K-ABC) (Kemper et al. 1988). Abilities or skills may be acquired by patients in a subtle and informal way. Again, this seems to be related to interest area as well as associated contexts. The patient with FXS may produce information in a rather nonchalant manner, to the surprise of parents and educators. The acquired information is often unrelated to the designated curricular focus and seems to be acquired incidentally or without formal teaching. Many teachers remark that children with FXS learn best when observing situations and activities peripherally rather than through direct involvement.

When establishing an appropriate curriculum, integrating the child's incidentally acquired knowledge is important. For example, when teaching numbers, a clock, microwave touch plate, computer keyboard, or license plates may be used in preference to flashcards, workbooks, or number lines. Flags, cars, or product labels may be used when teaching reading or vocabulary. The identification and use of high-interest materials may also reduce student resistance and distractibility. An assessment of interests can be helpful when creating curricular content and strategies.

Educators recognize the influence of the environment on learning. Classroom noise, teacher-peer interactions, lighting, and curricular materials will significantly affect the learning environment of the individual with FXS. As these variables are identified, modifications can be made to facilitate learning. Exhibit 10.6 presents some useful suggestions for altering the environment and programs to fit the needs of children with FXS. Visual processing is a relative strength for many boys with FXS (Hodapp et al. 1992; Kemper et al. 1988). Using this strength (e.g., when giving instructions) is often more useful than limiting the presentation to auditorily presented instruction. Examples would be pairing verbal instructions with drawing or acting out stories and actions.

Often individuals with FXS experience motor deficits manifested in poor eye-hand coordination and motor dyspraxia (Levitas et al. 1983; Friefeld and MacGregor 1993). This has implications for academic expectations related to writing. Even though the individual demonstrates motivation to draw or write, the task becomes so difficult that inappropriate behavioral responses can emerge. Wide-margin paper or paper with nubbed lines to guide motor output through tactile input can be beneficial. Adaptive devices such as pencil grip, primary-sized pencils, or markers may provide more tactile input and promote better production. Templates or fine motor tracing devices are also useful in providing structure and boundaries when the individual is first learning to draw or write. Storytelling while the individual moves the pencil from left to right can provide motivation to comply. For example, a child might be given a picture of a car on the left margin, a copy of a logo from a favorite fast-food chain on the right margin, and a line between. A story could assist in completing the task of driving his car to McDonald's and staying on the road as he drives.

## Assistive Technology

Assistive technology (AT) covers an exceptionally broad range of devices and services that are able to meet the needs of diverse populations. Individuals with FXS can use AT to enhance learning opportunities, build independence, and improve communication across activities and environments. To appropriately apply AT, one must first determine the goal and then find the tool that will be used to accomplish the desired outcome.

Use of technology in the educational setting has become commonplace. AT encompasses any piece of equipment that aids a person's ability to complete tasks. These tasks may include educational, vocational, communicative, and recreational endeavors and activities of daily living. Recent federal regulations have focused the attention of students, educators, and parents on the use of assistive devices and services. AT is explicitly written into the language of the Individuals with Disabilities in Education Act (IDEA, PL 105-17). IDEA states that school systems must provide AT to children and youth with disabilities when these devices and services are necessary for the student to obtain a free and appropriate education.

An *assistive technology device* is any item, piece of equipment, or product system, whether acquired commercially off the shelf, modified, or customized, that is used to increase, maintain, or improve the functional capabilities of a child with a disability. An *assistive technology service* is any service that directly assists a child with a disability in the selection, acquisition, or use of an AT device. Services include:

—The evaluation of the needs of such a child, including a functional evaluation of the child in the child's customary environment;

—Purchasing, leasing, or otherwise providing for the acquisition of AT devices by such a child;

—Selecting, designing, fitting, customizing, adapting, applying, maintaining, repairing, or replacing of AT devices;

—Coordinating and using other therapies, interventions, or services with AT devices, such as those associated with existing education and rehabilitation plans and programs;

—Training or technical assistance for such a child or, where appropriate, the family of such a child; and

—Training or technical assistance for professionals (including individuals providing education and rehabilitation services), employers, or other individuals who provide services to, employ, or are otherwise substantially involved in the major life functions of such a child.

AT devices can be placed on a continuum by the amount of "technology" and general availability involved in their use and implementation. These categories range from high-tech to no-tech. The highest technological solution may not be the most practical for many situations. Examples of high-tech devices are synthesized voice output communication aides and laptop computers. Light-tech devices may include portable keyboards and software specifically developed to support a skill. Low-tech devices tend to be available in retail stores, are used by the general public, and include items such as watches that speak the time, recording devices, and educational software. No-tech, as the name implies, requires no electricity to operate. These devices range from picture schedules representing routines to pencil grips.

The means of representing language for the person who will be using the AT is very important. Additionally, the amount of information presented at any given time and the complexity of the information must be taken into account before AT device implementation. Graphic representation of language has been extensively studied to identify levels of complexity in pictures (Buekelman 1988). This research has helped to determine at what level an individual will be able to use a symbol to represent a linguistic concept. In addition to the actual symbol being used, the extent to which the person using the AT is able to learn and retain the assigned meaning for pictures is considered. For example, although the picture for "more" can be based on sign language (two hands together) and is abstract, it may be made meaningful through the modeling of its meaning in structured play situations.

AT encompasses many modes of learning, teaching, organizing, and demonstrating knowledge. Following are examples of areas of life functioning in which AT may benefit an individual with FXS.

—Graphic representations of schedules and routines can help an individual move through his or her day with greater independence, deal with unusual changes in routines, and have a sense of confidence in unfamiliar situations.

—Voice output communication aides can help individuals communicate with unfamiliar listeners, make needs known across environments, and demonstrate knowledge, frustration, and social closeness.

—Situation-specific communication boards can help an individual order a meal at a restaurant, engage in recreational pursuits, and learn language related to specific activities.

—Communication picture dictionaries can help an individual demonstrate knowledge by pointing to a picture of an item, write words for which the picture can be identified but the spelling is not known, and relate information that is not necessarily related to here and now.

—Software that is specific to functional tasks or specific skill sets (i.e., making change or reading environmental print) can help an individual learn a new skill, practice a task, and demonstrate mastery.

—A pager or personal timer with multiple settings can help an individual remember to take medication, arrive for work with reduced outside assistance, and complete a list of chores.

AT is put into place based on the information gathered from all other realms of related services. Therefore, a single piece of AT may be used to reach goals from an occupational therapist, speech/language pathologist, and the classroom teacher. Working as a team to determine the types of AT that will be most beneficial to a person with FXS is imperative. The team should include all parties with a vested interest, including the person who will be using the AT, family members, teachers, therapists, vocational rehabilitation specialists, educational assistants, social workers, and/or psychologists. One process for determining the type of AT that will meet an identified goal is a needs-based process (see table 10.5). The goal behavior is identified first. This is followed by a discussion of what is happening at the current time. Ideas are generated to help bridge the gap between what is happening and what will happen when the goal is accomplished. After this, the AT that can be used to assist in the accomplishment of the goal is identified, keeping in mind all levels of AT. Finally, the people who will be responsible for the availability, functioning, and implementation of the AT are identified.

## Computer Technology

The benefits of computers in regular and special education classrooms have been documented (Maddux 1984; Mokros and Russell 1986). Microcomputers have been used successfully with children with FXS in both the academic and therapy settings. The visual presentation of microcomputers capitalizes on the strong visual skills of children with FXS. A computer allows the child to learn independently of the teacher and also gives an important sense of control over learning (Ellis and Sabornie 1986). The colorful nature of many programs helps to focus a child's attention. However, many microcomputers lie idle in classrooms or are used primarily as reinforcing games for classwork finished early. Regular and special education teachers should be encouraged and instructed in how to use microcomputers effectively in the classroom.

In many situations, a computer allows a child to actively participate in his or her education and demonstrate abilities and potential. Additionally, it can be used as a tool to teach. Children do not have to have mastery of any skills to begin using a computer. For many children with FXS, the computer is a tool that can help to hold attention and allow for meaningful learning to take place. Additionally, computers provide the ability to produce written communication without the significant motor component that is required when writing with a paper and pencil. Computers can create a much more positive and productive environment for writing. Finally, having experience with computers can allow a child to be an expert in the class, providing peers with valuable information about how software works and helping others to solve problems.

Many types of software are available for a variety of topics in special education. Programs that teach the basic skill of cause-effect are available, as are programs in problem-solving skills for the higher-functioning child. Special concerns in evaluating software for the child with FXS include the auditory and visual distractibility of the program and its complexity. Placing the keyboard on the floor with the child lying in front of it or having the child sit in a bean bag chair with the keyboard in his or her lap may be more beneficial than using traditional seating. Similarly, special adaptations for keyboards are available. A child's cognitive level and visual-spatial, memory, motor, and language skills must be evaluated so that appropriate software can be matched to the student. The input of the occupational therapist in assessing perceptual-motor abilities, recommending optimal seating, and suggesting approaches to help the child focus attention is also beneficial.

When determining the specific computer for a child, several factors come into play. The decision must be based on the child's unique strengths and needs, as well as the type of equipment currently available on the market. In most situations, the equipment that is available at home and at school can be used. Frequently, what is required to make old hardware functional is new software or adaptive peripherals. Ultimately, a recommendation is based on a combination of the child's needs and what is available for use.

When determining how technology can be used in the school setting, it is important to consider how it is being used and the possibilities for other use. Within the language of the IEP, technology can fit into several categories. These include characteristic of service, annual goals, short-term goals, supplementary aides, and related services. The IEP should include information about why this technology is being used and how it is to be used (i.e., in a group, for written communication, to practice math concepts). It is important to remember that the "goal" is not increased computer use, but rather, increased opportunities to learn or be involved and that the computer is one tool to achieve this goal.

In determining the appropriateness of computer technology for a child, an important first step is to determine whether the computer is a meaningful object to a child. For many children who have poor attending abilities, the computer can be a tool to build attention. Does the child attend to the monitor when visual changes occur? Does the child seem to be taking more cues from the auditory feedback? Will the child attend to the action and attempt to reactivate it

**Table 10.5**
**Needs-based Process**

| What is the goal? | What is currently happening? | What needs to happen? | What technology will be used? | Who will implement? |
|---|---|---|---|---|
| JD will move from one kindergarten activity to another with minimal assistance. | JD requires 1-1 assistance to physically transition across all activities. Frequently, tantrums make it difficult for him to refocus on class activities. | Cueing to anticipate changes. Physical movement between activities | Give designated transition object 1 minute before change of activities. Use a picture schedule of the events of the day, including a picture for "something different." Use an individual picture schedule with removable pictures. | The educational assistant will hand JD the object and, initially, verbally tell student what will happen next. Teacher will move an arrow from picture to picture throughout the day. Initially, educational assistant takes JD to the schedule and assists to attend to the pictures, remove the just completed task, and place it in a box. |
| KP will indicate preference within structured activities. | KP takes what she wants by either grabbing from others or going to the cabinets to take things out until she finds what she wants. | KP needs a limited set of choices. KP needs a way to vocalize that she wants something. | During art activities, pictures of the necessary materials will be on KP's workspace. KP will sign or will touch a single-message voice output device to say, "I want," and then point | 2x2-inch pictures of art supplies will be created and placed in an envelope on the side of KP's desk. The teacher will pull the appropriate pictures before the activity. |

| Goal | Problem | Need | Solution | Action |
|---|---|---|---|---|
| | | | | of the process for requesting and reviewing the choices. |
| DL will arrive at work on time with the appropriate materials. | DL is frequently late to catch the bus. DL usually leaves his lunch or coat at home. | Needs a reminder to leave for the bus stop with enough time to catch the bus. Needs a form to check that he has all of his belongings. | A timed message will be sent to DL's pager 10 minutes and 5 minutes before he needs to leave. A checklist will be placed at the door including items that DL needs to take and do before leaving for the bus. | Voc-Rehab will set up paging schedule, and family will purchase pager. Family will determine the list of items to include and placement. If needed, an additional form for leaving work will be made. |
| SM will participate in a daily, open-ended creative writing task. | SM becomes frustrated with the activity. She disrupts other students. | Needs a prompt for writing. Needs an alternative to pencil and paper to accomplish writing. Needs help with spelling new words. | SM will have a word or picture on an index card to cue her into the day's topic. SM will have access to an electronic means of writing. SM will have a picture dictionary to look up new words. | SM and Dad will decide on topic and make a card as part of her nightly homework. Trials with a portable keyboard, auditory feedback word processing, and word prediction will take place. Teacher will find a selection of dictionaries. He and SM will determine which is most functional. |

when it stops? How big a change has to occur or how long in duration in order for the child to notice? For some children the change must be a combination of auditory and visual feedback to be meaningful.

Software content falls into four basic areas: pre-academic, academic, language, and recreation/leisure. Many times one piece of software can be used for multiple purposes. For example, the beginning graphics program, *Kid Pix,* by Broderbund can be used to build understanding of cause-effect relationships through the use of many of its tools. Object, color, and shape identification and letter and number recognition can be addressed. Sound-symbol correspondence can be practiced with the stamps and the letters. Math concepts ranging from counting to fractions to multiplication are all possible. A story can be written and sequenced together later. And a picture can be made to hang on the refrigerator.

Choosing software that is open-ended and interactive can go a long way toward finding quality software for a child. Software that does not require a specific response can be very beneficial for developing choice-making skills and confidence in learning. Another characteristic is multiple purposes or levels. Software that offers multiple levels of difficulty (i.e., exploration, basic, advanced information) can also help enliven the program. Some software programs, costs, and publishing companies are listed in appendix 2.

The Alliance for Technology Access has several member centers across the United States. These centers provide information and programs for children with disabilities, their families, and professionals working with them. The centers emphasize the use of specially adapted computers to reinforce learning and play skills and guide parents and professionals in choosing developmentally appropriate software for their children and students (appendix 2).

## Integrated Service Approach

The benefit of early education intervention programs has long been supported (Caldwell and Stedman 1977). One of the earlier surveys commissioned by Elliott Richardson, secretary of Health, Education and Welfare, indicated that educational programs for preschool handicapped children, whether infants or five-year-olds, could significantly improve the quality of the children's lives. Of particular interest was the finding that the effects of early intervention were most salient when they occurred during the period of rapid development. In addition, if access to the child could be gained in the early years (one to two years of age) when language was emerging, the programs were even more effective than if begun later. This intervention contributed to the child's social and intellectual development. Several preschool programs have been successful with autistic children with pervasive developmental delays. The approach is usually developmental, with an emphasis on language and affect development within an integrated setting (Strain 1987; Rogers and Lewis 1989).

Young children with FXS present with great variability in their acquisition of developmental milestones. Many children are identified to function within the average range on intellectual testing and demonstrate relative strengths in vocabulary development (chap. 6). Others are observed to present with global developmental delays, hypotonia, and significant behavioral problems. Findings from a longitudinal study at the University of North Carolina document great difficulties across five developmental domains: cognition, communication, adaptive, motor, and personal-social. Boys 24–72 months with FXS demonstrated significant delays in relation to agemates. At every age tested, scores for boys with FXS were higher on the motor and adaptive domains and lower on communication and cognitive (Bailey et al. 1998).

Many young children with FXS also present with a secondary diagnosis of autism (25%) or autistic-like features (Bailey et al. 1998). They may have significantly delayed and deviant communication patterns, be perseverative in actions or topics, and engage in self-stimulatory behaviors on a level that interferes with their ability to learn or engage in developmentally appropriate play and interaction.

Many young children with FXS are described to thrive in educational and therapy programs similar to those designed for children with autism or other significant communicative disorders. Many children do well in very structured programs with an organized, planned set of activities within an organized physical environment. Programs such as the TEACCH model (Schopler 1974) or the Denver model (Rogers et al. 2000) have been described by parents and therapists to be very successful models in promoting language and social skill development in young children with FXS. Structured teaching, visually cued instruction, and incidental teaching of social communication are the basic components of these programs. Important additions for the child with FXS would include the use of group instruction and sensory support strategies.

Clinical interviews with parents of young children with FXS support the benefit of intensive behavioral intervention such as applied behavior analysis (ABA). These programs consist of an intervention plan with structure and reinforcement provided at high intensity, using very precise teaching techniques. "Lovaas Therapy," a very specific type of behavior intervention, can only be provided by a practitioner directly affiliated with Lovaas. Many other intensive behavioral interventions have evolved from the Lovaas approach and model similar philosophy. Most often, services are intensive (30–40 hours per week) and are conducted one to one with a therapist trained in the specific technique. Goals are to maximize success by breaking down tasks into targets that are achievable and rewardable. These types of programs are helpful for many children to develop such skills as attention, cooperation, and imitation. The emphasis is placed on these skills, as they are necessary for higher-level learning.

ABA strategies can occur in one-to-one settings, special education classrooms, or full inclusion environments. An ABA curriculum may include the following (Maurice et al. 1996):

—Attending skills

—Imitation skills

—Receptive language skills

—Expressive language skills

—Preacademic skills

—Self-help skills

As children grow this type of program may continue to be appropriate. Many boys with FXS demonstrate a decrease in specific behavioral symptoms associated with a diagnosis of autism as they grow older (see chap. 1).

Research studies are necessary to document this change over time. Learning in a typical classroom is difficult for many school-aged individuals with FXS. Social anxiety, sensory processing, attention problems, and hyperactivity and cognitive delay affect the individual's tolerance and ability to learn. Individuals with FXS are relatively strong visual learners and have significant auditory processing problems. Relatively well-developed abilities of remembering and recognizing visual gestalts often lead to strengths in sight reading. Many benefit from a simultaneous approach to teaching. Individuals with FXS consistently demonstrate poor arithmetic skills. This finding is true of both sexes across all age and IQ levels.

Individuals with FXS do best when provided with materials of high interest in a typical, realistic setting and when developmental expectations are appropriate. Strong emphasis on visually based, simultaneous curriculums is encouraged (see chap. 11).

Social skills groups for skill development and support may be beneficial in this challenging area. While social skills are sometimes seen as a relative strength in FXS, the social anxiety and subtleties of pragmatics may be more difficult to manage. Specific programming aimed at alleviating anxiety and building skill may be helpful. Programs such as "Circle of Friends" (1979) or MAPS (McGill Action Planning System; Vandercook and York 1989) are successful for many students.

## Behavior Plan

Behavior plan continuums have been successful for many individuals with FXS. These types of thoughtful and preventive intervention strategies involve a plan that may begin with preventive environmental supports in place and may allow full participation of the student. It may progress to a more directed, supported method of management involving such strategies as leaving the room to calm down, talking with an adult, or redirection to a particular goal-directed activity (see chaps. 9 and 11). This midpoint in the continuum would involve the support of another. The end point in the continuum may involve suspension of the activity, removal from the room, or restraint if the behavior cannot be managed with the support of an adult.

The plan is developed to provide the student with the environmental supports necessary to be most successful in an inclusive setting. There is a documented description of behaviors that would signal escalating problems and specific methods of dealing with the behaviors. The goal would be to intervene at the earliest stage of escalation and also to have a responsible, well-designed, and well-communicated plan in place if the intervention did not work. A 1997 amendment to IDEA requires that, if a student with a disability has behavior problems, the IEP team should consider strategies like a proactive behavior intervention plan, based on a functional behavior assessment (see chaps. 9 and 11).

Keogh (1992) also discusses a neuropsychologic training program to increase attention, concentration, memory, and abilities to organize, plan, and sequence. She describes five exercises that are most appropriate for higher-functioning or older children: Ace to King, Attributes, Master Mind, Simon, and What's in the Square.

Understanding the impact of sensory integration difficulties in the child with FXS is important. For a non–special education classroom teacher to be effective with children with FXS in a mainstreaming experience, it is critical to understand possible interfering behaviors associated with the syndrome: strong reaction to change, overstimulation, poor verbal output on command, hypotonia, difficulty with fine motor tasks, and academic deficits. It is also important to be aware of the events that may exacerbate levels of anxiety, especially when in a large group with a variety of distractions. For instance, confrontation, loud yelling, and inflexibility often lead to further stimulation and eventual outbursts of behavior (exhibits 10.7 and 10.8). Please refer to chapter 11 for more information regarding curriculum development.

A plateau and then decline in IQ scores is typically seen in the majority of males with FXS (chap. 6; Dykens 1994). This seems to be related to deficits in abstract reasoning and higher linguistic abilities that are emphasized in cognitive testing during middle and later childhood. Consequently, the learning potential may be greatest during preschool and early school years (Paul et al. 1987). Early sensory integration and attentional deficits often contribute to difficulty in learning for the child with FXS. Hypersensitivity to sounds, sights, and touch makes normal interactions with one's environment difficult at best

**Exhibit 10.7**
**General Instructional Suggestions**

---

Provide:
- Responsibilities that are appropriate for the child's level of understanding
- Clear, consistent rules
- Instructions in very small, simple steps
- Consistent daily routines, especially around transitions
- Frequent positive reinforcement and recognition of effort
- Positive redirection (tell the child what he or she *can* do)
- Recognition of and reward for self-control

In addition:
- Recognize that many behaviors are not intentional and are the result of sensory overload.
- Supervise closely during transition times.
- Ignore minor inappropriate behavior.
- Use a calm, quiet voice when teaching.
- Using a rhythmic voice with exaggerated intonation is also useful in holding attention.
- Do not require eye contact; it will develop as the child becomes comfortable in the setting.
- If the child has difficulty with initiation of conversation, provide cues using the cloze technique. For example, in a discussion about a weekend activity the teacher may say, "Aaron, over the weekend you. . . ." Using comments rather than direct questioning is also recommended.

Other ideas to think about:
- Generalization is difficult. The child needs to be taught responses and reactions for a number of situations.
- Involve the child in activities to enhance memory skills (act as messenger, group leader, assistant).
- Use the child's interests and achievements outside of school to teach and redirect.
- Help the child get started by modeling and talking through the first couple of steps.
- Model appropriate behavior when too much is going on (ask for quiet time, headphones, or to move).
- Seat the child near a good role model (kids with FXS are great imitators).
- Acknowledge positive behavior of others nearby.
- Look for opportunities for the child to display strengths or leadership skills.
- Use private visual signals to cue the child to stay on task.

Encourage self-organization early on:
- When working at desk, make sure only necessary materials are available.
- Help the child organize; give the child a place for everything (label with pictures or words).
- Use visual checklists and schedules.
- Send home daily or weekly progress reports or a notebook for everyone to make comments in.
- Mark papers where to start and stop; mark borders with bright colors.

---

.**Exhibit 10.7** (*Continued*)

---

Maximize time in the general education classroom:
* Preventive behavior plan and sensory diet in place
* Small group instruction with positive reinforcement of effort
* Audiotaped instructions that can be reviewed repeatedly
* "Fact groups" on cards/pictures related to topic at hand
* Hands on opportunities or experiential activities
* Reference materials bookmarked on the computer

---

and interferes with social, motor, play, and emotional development (Scharfenaker and Schreiner 1989). Therefore, the need for a multidisciplinary and integrated approach at this age level is critical for the child with FXS.

Many children with FXS are extremely sensitive to environmental stimuli, especially to touch and movement. As a result, there may be difficulty modulating behavior, and they may exhibit hostility or aggressiveness or may simply withdraw to avoid being overwhelmed by the environment. For these children, individual occupational therapy may be preferred, with sensory-integrative treatment structured to reduce these hypersensitive responses. The therapist may work with the child in a dimly lit room and use only essential play equipment. Additional structure and calming may be provided by using taped environmental sounds or music with a strong underlying beat. Initially, transitions may be facilitated by holding the child firmly and carrying him in a prone position from one activity to the next. Additional techniques are suggested in exhibit 10.4.

## Speech and Language

The relationship between functional and symbolic play and language acquisition is well established (Bates 1979; McCune-Nicolich 1981; Ungerer and Sigman 1984). An early intervention program must be based on interactive play in a natural setting through which communication can evolve. Play provides children with an opportunity for observation and imitation of others, which are basic prerequisites for language and learning (Bloom and Lahey 1978).

The role of speech/language pathologists in early intervention is multidimensional. Therapists must provide direct or consultative services within the classroom as part of the multidisciplinary team. They must provide parents with ongoing suggestions on how they can apply speech/language intervention techniques at home. In addition, therapists must integrate intervention techniques from other disciplines into the therapy program.

For the infant and toddler, the therapy techniques of imitation, modeling, and

**Exhibit 10.8**
**Academics**

---

**Literacy**
- Use music to teach prereading and other academic skills by presenting new information in a song.
- Pair the child with FXS with a buddy when reading aloud. This will reduce the pressure to perform.
- Give the child an opportunity to read into a tape recorder or use a microphone.
- Encourage the child to listen to stories on audiotape and try to follow the text in the book.
- Look at magazines or the pictures in word books, as a way of building language and prereading skills.
- Use the sight word approach to reading, with a long-range goal of backing into phonics.
- Individual words can be taught by printing the word on one side of an index card and gluing a picture of the object or action on the back.
- Try a "word family" approach to reading.
- Video-tape reading a report and play it back to the classroom instead of doing it in person.
- Capitalize on the child's interests (sports, cooking, gardening, etc.).
- Read in the context of real experiences (when cooking, driving, vacationing, etc.).
- Use computer programs such as "living books" (see appendix).
- Read books with limited vocabulary and a high level of contextual cues (i.e., *Go Dog Go*).

**Prewriting skill development**
- Allow the child to use alternative means of communicating what he or she knows (e.g., using a rubber stamp to mark the answer rather than circling the response).
- Use oral tests where the teacher reads the question individually and grades the child's verbal response.
- Spell words for the child and tell him or her when you have reached the end of the word.
- Allow the child to use stencils to write letters and words.
- Use a simple word-processing program on a computer that has large letters.
- Consider computers for teaching; they are visually motivating and nonjudgmental.
- Frequent opportunities to write in meaningful contexts (phone messages, grocery lists, weekend activities)
- Access to a word-processing program and encouragement to use it
- Spelling words on audiotape
- Computer programs such as "Cowriter" and "Writeout Loud" (see appendix)
- Use of handwriting curriculum (Handwriting without Tears, by Jan Olsen, OTR)

**Numbers**
- Teach one-to-one correspondence using meaningful examples (e.g., setting the table for a certain number of people).
- Teach math concepts in the context of a practical activity when possible (e.g., learning which coins to use in a vending machine).
- Let the child use his or her own counters, especially objects that are of high interest to the child.

---

**Exhibit 10.8** (*Continued*)

---

- Try the Touch Math curriculum approach, where the positions of small dots on the numbers are memorized and used as counters.
- Use an area of interest to assist in learning to identify numbers (e.g., license plates, sports jerseys).
- Reduce the number of math problems on a single page to one or two.
- Repeated application of number concepts to daily activities (counting snack items, pencils, silverware)
- Application to areas of high interest (presidents to learning coin names)
- Use of dice, board games, and card games to teach concepts

---

*Source:* Many of these suggestions are reprinted with permission from Spiridigliozzi et al. 1994.

---

expansion are most beneficial. Facilitating imitation of environmental and animal sounds may be the starting point of therapy for very young children. Modeling and expansion can then be used as receptive and expressive vocabulary increases.

In development, every new skill is based on previously acquired skills that are then adapted to accommodate the next level. This adaptation process was theoretically presented by Gilfoyle et al. (1982) in their book, *Children Adapt*. Elementary and middle school–aged children with FXS usually have not developed the skills that would enable them to cope with the complicated adjustments involved in development through childhood. The physical, emotional, and intellectual changes common to early adolescent development intensify the problems. The ability to screen out environmental stimuli, a sense of competence and self-reliance, and tolerance for change may not develop. At a time when peer acceptance is gaining importance, children with FXS are apt to exhibit behaviors that alienate them from group interaction. A clinical study with a group of learning-disabled teenagers without FXS (Jones et al. 1986) demonstrated that learning style, communication, and pragmatic areas were affected by sensory integration difficulties. Underlying all of these dysfunctional areas was the complication of a poor self-image.

Emotional complications such as anxiety, depression, and angry outbursts may emerge and must be dealt with. Treatment in a group setting to address areas of need using occupational, speech, educational, and emotional support is critical. Exhibits 10.4 and 10.7 offer suggestions for this age group. Chapter 8 discusses the many beneficial medications useful in dealing with behavior and attentional problems.

In school-aged children with FXS, we begin to see the effects of early childhood struggles on life performance. This is just one of the reasons why early intervention is so critical. It is also one of the reasons why continued support from therapeutic specialists is often required to help manage the range of difficulties the kids are dealing with throughout their schooling and on into adulthood.

Occupational therapy intervention should use a sensory integration frame of reference to provide the basis of understanding for many of the problems experienced by school-aged children with FXS. These difficulties may include poor sensory modulation including sensory defensiveness and difficulty managing arousal levels, poor postural development, dyspraxia, immature fine motor skills and hand development, difficulty with visual motor skills, continued overdependence with daily living skills, and limited social and recreational pursuits.

These problem areas are best treated using sensory integration as a foundation and augmenting this with adaptations for fine motor and visual motor and life skill tasks, a comprehensive home program using a "sensory diet" approach (exhibit 10.5) (Wilbarger 1995), and facilitation of community and school inclusion.

For the school-aged child, a thorough assessment of speech/language, occupational therapy, and academic needs will help direct the focus of speech therapy and determine the frequency of intervention. In general, small-group speech/language therapy is beneficial, yet individual therapy offers one-on-one therapist-student interaction and decreased distractions. A combination of group and individual therapy therefore is optimal.

For optimal learning to occur, the school-aged child with FXS often needs some physical classroom accommodations. These are listed in exhibit 10.6. Most of these changes are easy to make and benefit many other children in the classroom as well. Either combined occupational therapy and speech therapy or consultation between occupational therapy, speech/language pathology, and classroom teacher is critical for carryover of services and to provide a common groundwork from a sensory processing perspective from which language, speech, and academics can develop.

During the school years, peer modeling should play an important role in speech/language therapy. Small groups are best in teaching pragmatic skills through role playing, modeling, and problem solving (Lucas 1980). Typical experiences and topical interests of the group can further be used to increase motivation and ultimately increase generalization of learned skills. The input of an occupational therapist is important in providing calming and focusing strategies for the group.

Peer tutoring is a useful strategy when working with individuals with FXS in a variety of educational therapeutic settings. Tutoring provides the student with more individualized teaching and with repetition and practice. Tutoring within the classroom, rather than having a child removed from the room, is preferable. In addition, this technique encourages and gives the student a chance to practice social and pragmatic skills (Jenkins and Jenkins 1981; Wilson et al. 1994).

## Late Adolescence through Adulthood

As the child with FXS progresses through junior high and high school, the emphasis often will shift to prevocational and vocational training. Much information can be drawn from the literature that describes vocational training for handicapped students in general (Mithaug and Hagmeier 1978; Wehman and Hill 1981, 1982; Levy 1983; Wehman et al. 1985). Many investigators think that vocational training begins too late in the school experience and that comprehensive training, including training in social and pragmatic competence, should occur at all levels of schooling (Brown et al. 1979; Wimmer 1981; Hamre-Nietupski et al. 1982; Hayes 1987). Academic skills, however, should not be abandoned at this time. Little opportunity is given for these young adults to explore personalized vocational options, let alone continue academic skill development. Although it is true that most of these individuals will need the focused effort of the team to learn and generalize the independent living skills necessary for adult life, this should not be at the expense of continuing academic skill development.

Preparation for employment must be individually determined. Transition plans may be included in the IEP by tenth grade to determine how this will happen. Some individuals require more time to learn a certain skill, and instruction should begin early on. Transition planning documents may include things such as long-range career goals, long-range living goals, independent living, vocational skills, academics, transportation, medical issues, and leisure time development.

Important information pertinent to job training and placement can be derived from the general behavioral and cognitive features of the population with FXS. For example, an adult who has difficulty screening out visual and auditory stimuli would not be a good candidate for sacking groceries at a supermarket. Because of the excellent imitative skills of most individuals with FXS, placement with more severely handicapped or emotionally/behaviorally disturbed adults would not be desirable, as maladaptive behaviors would most likely be imitated. Other general conditions when placing individuals with FXS in a vocational setting are listed in table 10.6.

Alterman et al. (1992) assessed the vocational abilities and work habits of a small group of adults with FXS. They identified well-developed psychomotor skills and work habits, relative to other mild to moderately retarded adults. An obstacle in vocational training, however, is the attentional deficits that continue through adulthood.

**Table 10.6**
**Considerations in Vocational Planning**

| Client Considerations | Employer Considerations |
| --- | --- |
| *Environment* | |
| Overall noise level | Understanding of employee's sensory needs, strengths, and deficits |
| Level of auditory, visual, olfactory, tactile distractions; degree of sensitivity to various stimuli | Willingness to modify work setting to encourage optimal performance by reducing distractibility and length of day |
| | Willingness to provide rest periods for needed calming or exercise; flexibility in providing time off for scheduled therapies |
| Physical proximity of other employees | Willingness to modify physical setting and work station |
| Number of other employees | Willingness to modify work setting |
| | Ability to provide independent work stations, carrels, or small area to work alone |
| *Basic Skills* | |
| Verbal and motor imitation | Willingness to assess environmental hazards and potential safety issues |
| | Understanding of possible emotional or physical outbursts and causes |
| Visual discrimination and memory | Ability to give clear expectations for appropriate social interaction |
| Auditory memory and sequencing | Willingness to provide charts, diagrams, and picture schedules to prompt appropriate sequence of work tasks |
| Complexity of receptive and expressive language | Ability to reduce verbal input and augment visually |
| Complexity of motor skills | Limited tasks that require fine motor planning |
| Difficulty with novel tasks | Willingness to encourage repetition and familiarity of tasks |
| Client's interests | Work tasks that include high interest |
| | Prompts and visual cues that include high-interest materials |
| *Social and Work Skills* | |
| Personal grooming | Ability to include grooming cues and additional programming during the work day |
| Impulsive social language | Ability to prepare other employees for SI deficits |
| | Discouragement of inappropriate verbalization |

**Table 10.6** (*Continued*)

| Client Considerations | Employer Considerations |
|---|---|
| Ability to interact appropriately with other employees and public | Availability to encourage social interaction while prompting appropriate social skills and training within the work setting |
| Degree of independence in using transportation | Willingness to prompt and encourage use of mass transit or alternative methods to transport |
| Physical strength and stamina | Limitation of job tasks requiring manual strength |

Melzer et al. (1992) described a vocational training program for males with FXS with the three major goals of

1. Development of social skills necessary for suitable behavior in society
2. Vocational rehabilitation according to individual capabilities and placement within a protective framework or within the productive and competitive work force
3. Placement within a special hostel to function with maximum independence according to capabilities

In developing the vocational experience for the individual with FXS, environmental limitations are as critical as cognitive and behavioral ones. The occupational therapist, then, plays an important part in vocational planning. Coping with the challenges of late adolescence and adulthood can be especially stressful for individuals with FXS and their families. All of the expected maturation issues common to a normal individual can be compounded by the sensory integrative problems and behavioral anomalies with which the person with FXS has dealt since infancy. Behavioral responses to sensory sensitivity or defensiveness are often maladaptive and may include ritualistic movements, self-abuse (i.e., biting the back of the hand), aggression, and withdrawal.

The beneficial effect of sensory integrative methods, including vibratory and vestibular stimulation, with adults with mental retardation has been documented (Ottenbacher and Altman 1984; Clark and Miller 1978). Vigorous physical activity, which would naturally include vestibular and proprioceptive input, has also been reported to have a calming influence (Autism Research Review 1989; Elliott et al. 1994). Exercise tapes may be used to augment a treatment program for individuals with FXS. The ability to mimic behaviors, love of imitation of movement, a fascination with visual stimuli, and interest in music could make this approach useful. Because of the importance of fostering social interaction, it is advisable to have this type of exercise program incorporated into a group setting. Leisure skills that can contribute to self-regulatory and praxis functions are very beneficial. A well-rounded sensory diet will include a rich leisure component.

Techniques to decrease auditory, visual, and tactile sensitivity should be incorporated into work and living situations, as well as into therapy sessions. The adult with FXS should be encouraged to assume increasing responsibility for making self-calming part of the daily routine. Individual psychotherapy may also be helpful in teaching calming techniques and controlling anger and frustration.

The speech/language pathologist can provide needed support in vocational planning. Specific vocabulary and social skills necessary for the job and a more independent lifestyle should be emphasized. These can be taught most effectively through the use of small groups in a real-life experiential setting. Social skills development is equally important, as it is necessary to understand and relate to others in the work environment. Social communication skills such as greetings, making requests, and turn taking should be incorporated into the communication and academic curriculum. Verbalization of emotions must be taught as an alternative to violent behavioral outbursts, which often occur when a patient is overwhelmed by stimuli. Problem-solving skills around conflict resolution are essential for the individual with FXS in any work setting.

Facilitating the transition from school to work is the ultimate goal of public education. To encourage the vocational training and placement process, one should address several areas in an academic setting. Dalrymple (1986) provided a model for transition that was suggested for the autistic population. Based on behavioral and language similarities, this model can also be used with the adolescent individual with FXS. Overall competency, self-care, and language, social, academic, and prevocational skill development are recommended. Dalrymple (1986) suggested that basic academic skill building will further assist in an effective transition. Within the population with FXS, basic attending and listening skills are critical. These skills can be trained by involving the adolescent in a listening program that will require attending for a sustained period and by having the individual follow oral directions of increasing length and difficulty. Pharmacologic intervention may also improve attention during the adolescent period, as in earlier childhood. Taking advantage of the visual strengths, one can provide a sequence of tasks in a visual format that will cue the adolescent/adult to the next step of the sequence in the workplace.

Academic emphasis in vocational training should be presented in a functional format (real coins vs. plastic coins, real job applications, actual work objects from the real work environment, etc.). Training in identifying coins, making the correct change, budgeting, endorsing paychecks, and making deposits should be a part of the instructional program. Functional sight vocabulary or comprehension of basic instruction should also be the focus of the reading curriculum at this level.

Success in the workplace is dependent on a developed ability to make transitions and adjust to new environments and routines. The importance of training these skills early in the academic environment cannot be overemphasized. If the strong reaction to change is gradually desensitized during school placement, it will not be a problem when the workplace is entered. Appropriate behavior in the work environment is essential for compliance and success. Hyperactivity in the population with FXS can interfere with maintaining a job station and properly caring for work-related materials, although hyperactivity is usually improved by adulthood (Fryns 1985). Appropriate behavior should be trained by beginning with short work periods and extending them, with more work materials and distractors gradually introduced. This will build tolerance and reduce the likelihood of overstimulation in the workplace.

## The Application of Integrated Services to Girls with FXS

Cognitive functioning in females with FXS ranges from normal to severely retarded. The majority of females with the full mutation have significant cognitive deficits (chaps. 1 and 6). Affected females may exhibit behavioral problems similar to those of males with FXS but usually less severe. Poor eye contact, impulsivity, and attending problems, as well as difficulties with shyness, anxiety, and depression, may be present. Counseling (chap. 9) and medication (chap. 8) in addition to special education support (chap. 11) may be helpful for females affected by FXS (see exhibit 10.9). Many girls affected with FXS demonstrate a neuropsychologic profile consistent with a nonverbal learning disability (NLD) (Miezejeski and Hinton 1992). This is characterized by arithmetic difficulties without reading and spelling disabilities (Mazzocco et al. 1992b).

Deficits in math, especially with math reasoning and conceptual skills, have been reported (Kemper et al. 1986; Mazzocco et al. 1992a; Miezejeski and Hinton 1992). Often females have difficulty generalizing math concepts into a variety of situations for future problem solving. Algebraic formulas, symbolic associations that include missing elements, and the computation of word problems often cause great difficulty in this population. A curriculum that uses concrete and manipulative materials to introduce basic mathematic operations should be considered. Teaching methods should include patterns and visual gestalt whenever possible to reinforce complex mathematic processes (see appendix 3).

In the language area, problems with distractibility, inattentiveness, abstract reasoning, pragmatic language, topic maintenance, and a run-on narrative style have been reported (Madison et al. 1986; Hagerman 1987; see chap. 1). The prag-

**Exhibit 10.9**
**Intervention Strategies Suggested for Affected Heterozygous Females**

---

**Math Deficits**
• Use concrete manipulative materials to teach concepts and mathematical operations.
• Use visual cues whenever possible to reinforce mathematical operations.
• Allow additional time to reduce the possibility of provoking performance anxiety.
• Minimize auditory distractions during time periods when concentration is required (computation, problem solving).
• Use diagrams, illustrations, and visual patterns whenever teaching a new concept.
• Use repetition and patterning whenever rote memory tasks are required.

**Auditory, Memory, and Attentional Problems**
• Give specific instruction in a slow, simple, and concrete manner.
• Place the student near the instructor to ensure attention and concentration.
• Structure the environment to be void of auditory distractions (earphones, carrels, or seating arrangements).
• Vary the presentation to include frequent breaks to avoid attentional difficulties and lack of concentration.

**Visual Disorganization**
• Limit the amount to be copied from printed or written materials.
• Simplify visually presented materials to eliminate a cluttered or excessively stimulating format.
• Provide visual cues, such as color coding, numbering, and arrows, to organize written tasks.
• Give specific concrete cues when giving oral directions that require an organized format.
• Additional time may be required for written assignments.

---

matic language deficits may be related to a "tangential" and impulsive thought process that affects reasoning and problem-solving skills. These problems should be the focus of language therapy. The anxiety seen within the females may lead to some cases of selective mutism (Hagerman et al. 1999). Support and treatment from a psychologist and a speech pathologist is often necessary.

Important findings document specific executive function difficulties for females with FXS. Women with FXS perform worse on tasks of executive function and spatial processing. Recent evidence from Cornish et al. (1998) suggests that the spatial difficulties are less specific than previously thought, as no deficits are found when the tasks do not have a motor component. Specific executive function deficits in females with FXS are described in more depth in chapter 6.

Therapists have noted various sensory integration problems within the female population. As in males, sensory defensiveness, low muscle tone, a lack of trunk rotation (which can result in an inability to cross the midline), and dyspraxia can be seen. The defensiveness to touch and the shy, withdrawn behavior may contribute to poor interpersonal skills and may result in decreased pragmatic skills. The awkward movement patterns secondary to low tone, poor postural skills, and dyspraxia may limit a person's developing sense of their body and subsequently affect self-esteem. Leisure choices may be limited, and a sense of living a well-rounded, balanced lifestyle hard to achieve. With the presence of biological predisposition to depression, these sensory motor factors can contribute to emotional difficulties.

## Conclusion

Many new and varied intervention strategies have been presented in this chapter. The success of these strategies is based on the commitment, creativity, and flexibility of the multidisciplinary team treating the child. Parents, educators, therapists, and doctors all play an equal and integral role in determining academic and therapeutic goals for each child. Children with FXS are first and foremost individuals, and intervention needs to meet each child's varied and individual needs. We hope the information presented in this chapter will help you meet those needs.

## References

Albert, M., R. Sparks, and N. Helm. 1973. Melodic intonation therapy for aphasia. *Arch. Neurol.* 29:130–131.

Alliance for Technology Access. 1994. *Computer resources for people with disabilities.* Alameda, Calif.: Hunter House.

Alterman, D., M. Ya'acoby, and M. Schurr. 1992. Towards differential rehabilitation strategies in employment of fragile X adults. In R. J. Hagerman and P. McKenzie (eds.), *1992 International Fragile X Conference proceedings.* Dillon, Colo.: Spectra Publishing, pp. 273–279.

American Association on Mental Retardation. 2000. What is mental retardation? Internet site www.aamr.org

Anonymous. 1989. Physical exercise: A simple prescription for behavior problems? *Autism Res. Rev.* 3:1–7.

Armstrong, J., and K. Jones. 1994. Assistive technology and young children: Getting off to a great start! *Closing the Gap,* Aug/Sept, pp. 131–132.

Arnold, L. E., D. I. Clark, L. A. Sachs, S. Jakim, and S. Smithies. 1985. Vestibular and visual rotational stimulation as treatment for attention deficit and hyperactivity. *Am. J. Occup. Ther.* 39:84–91.

Arwood, E. L. 1984. *Pragmaticism: Treatment for language disorders.* Rockville, Md.: National Student Speech, Language, Hearing Association.

Ayres, A. J. 1965. Patterns of perceptual motor dysfunction in children: A factor analytic study. *Percept. Mot. Skills* 20:335–368.

———. 1972. *Sensory integration and learning disabilities.* Los Angeles: Western Psychological Services.

———. 1978. Learning disabilities and the vestibular system. *J. Learn. Disabil.* 11:30–41.

———. 1979. *Sensory integration and the child.* Los Angeles: Western Psychological Services.

———. 1989. *Sensory integration and praxis test.* Los Angeles: Western Psychological Services.

Ayres, A. J., and Z. Mailloux. 1981. Influence of sensory integration procedures on language development. *Am. J. Occup. Ther.* 35:383–390.

Ayres, A. J., and L. S. Tickle. 1980. Hyper-responsivity to touch and vestibular stimuli as a predictor of positive response to sensory integration procedures by autistic children. *Am. J. Occup. Ther.* 34:375–381.

Bailey, D. B., Jr., D. Hutton, and M. Skinner. 1998. Early developmental trajectories of males with fragile X syndrome. *Am. J. Ment. Retard.* 103:29–39.

Baranek, G. T., and G. Berkson. 1994. Tactile defensiveness in children with developmental disabilities: Responsiveness and habituation. *J. Autism Dev. Disord.* 24:437.

Baroff, G. S. 1986. *Mental retardation: Nature, cause, and management.* New York: Hemisphere Publishing, pp. 337–340.

Bates, E. 1979. *The emergence of symbols: Cognition and communication in infancy.* New York: Academic Press.

Bellman, K., and L. Goldberg. 1984. Common origin of linguistic and movement abilities. *Am. J. Physiol.* 6:915–921.

Belser, R. C., and V. Sudhalter. 1995. Arousal difficulties in males with fragile X syndrome: A preliminary report. *Dev. Brain. Dysfunct.* 8:270–279.

Birren, F. 1979. *Color and human response.* New York: Van Nostrand Reinhold.

Bloom, L., and M. Lahey. 1978. *Language development and language disorders.* New York: Wiley.

Bonadonna, P. 1981. Effects of a vestibular stimulation program on stereotypic rocking behavior. *Am. J. Occup. Ther.* 35:775–781.

Braden, M. 1991. A screening instrument for FRA-X males. Ph.D. dissertation, University of Denver.

———. 1992. Behavioral assessments. In R. J. Hagerman and P. McKenzie (eds.), *1992 International Fragile X Conference proceedings.* Dillon, Colo.: Spectra Publishing, pp. 161–163.

———. 1989. *Logo reading system.* 219 E. St. Vrain, Colorado Springs, Colo. 80903.

———. 2000. Fragile: handle with care—more about fragile X syndrome including adolescents and adults (revised). Colorado Springs, Colo. 719-633-3773.

Bradley, M. 1994. Computers for the very young: From the ridiculous to the sublime. *Closing the Gap,* Jun/Jul, pp. 1–6.

Bright, T., K. Brittick, and B. Fleeman. 1981. Reduction of self-injurious behavior using sensory integrative techniques. *Am. J. Occup. Ther.* 35:167–172.

Brown, J., M. Braden, and W. Sobesky. 1991. *Fragile X syndrome: Diagnosis, treatment, and research.* Baltimore: Johns Hopkins Univ. Press, p. 321.

Brown, L., M. Branston, S. Hamre-Nietupski, F. Johnson, B. Wilcox, and L. Gruene-wald. 1979. A rationale for comprehensive longitudinal interactions between se-verely handicapped students and non-handicapped students and other citizens. *AAE-SPH Rev.* 4:3–14.

Brown, L., P. Schwarz, A. Udvari-Solner, E. F. Kampschroer, et al. 1991. How much time should students with severe intellectual disabilities spend in regular education classrooms and elsewhere? *J. Assoc. Persons Severe Handicaps* 16(1):39–47.

Brown, W. H., S. L. Odom, and M. A. Conroy. 2001. An intervention hierarchy for pro-moting preschool childrens' peer interactions innaturalistic environment. *Topics Early Childhood Special Educ.* In press.

Buekelman, D. R., and P. Mirenda. 1988. *Augmentative and alternative communication: Management of severe communication disorders in children and adults,* 2d ed. Bal-timore: Brookes Publishing.

Burns, E., and L. Hickman. 1989. Integrated therapy in a summer camping experience for children with fragile X syndrome. *S.I. Int. News* 17:1–3.

Caldwell, B., and D. Stedman. 1977. *Infant education: A guide for helping handicapped children in the first three years.* Durham, N.C.: Walker Publishing.

Camp, B. W., and M. S. Bush. 1981. *Think aloud: Increasing social and cognitive skills—a problem solving program for children.* Champaign, Ill.: Research Press.

Campbell, P. H., W. F. McInerney, and M. A. Cooper. 1984. Therapeutic programming for students with severe handicaps. *Am. J. Occup. Ther.* 38:594–602.

Case-Smith, J., and T. Bryan. 1999. The effects of occupational therapy with sensory in-tergration emphasis on preschool-age children with autism. *Am. J. Occup. Ther.* 53:489–497.

Clark, S., and L. Miller. 1978. A comparison of apparent and sensory integrative meth-ods on developmental parameters in profoundly retarded adults. *Am. J. Occup. Ther.* 32:86–92.

Clark, F., and L. Steingold. 1982. A potential relationship between occupational therapy and language acquisition. *Am. J. Occup. Ther.* 36:42–44.

Cohen, I. L. 1992. The behavioral phenotype of fragile X syndrome. In R. J. Hagerman and P. McKenzie (eds.), *1992 International Fragile X Conference Proceedings.* Dil-lon, Colo.: Spectra Publishing, pp. 121–145.

Commerce Clearing House Editorial Staff. Americans with Disabilities Act of 1990: Law and explanation. Chicago: CCH. 1990 [the law itself, presented in as readable a form as possible].

Cornish, K., F. Muner, and J. Wilding. 1998. A unique pattern of working memory deficits in fragile X males. Presented to the Sixth International Fragile X Conference, Asheville, N.C., July.

Cronister, A., R. Schreiner, M. Wittenberger, K. Amiri, K. Harris, and R. J. Hagerman. 1991. The heterozygous fragile X female: Historical, physical, cognitive and cyto-genetic features. *Am. J. Med. Genet.* 38:269–274.

Dalrymple, N. 1986. *Transitional autism program.* Bloomington, Ind.: Indiana Univ. Press.

Densom, J. F., G. A. Nuthall, J. Bushnell, and J. Horn. 1989. Effectiveness of a sensory integrative treatment program for children with perceptual motor difficulties. *J. Learn. Disabil.* 22:221–229.

de Quiros, J. 1976. Diagnosis of vestibular disorders in the learning disabilities. *J. Learn. Disabil.* 9:51–58.

de Quiros, J., and O. Schrager. 1978. *Neuropsychological fundamentals in learning disabilities.* San Rafael, Calif.: Academic Therapy Publications.

Dykens, E. M., R. M. Hodapp, and J. F. Leckman. 1994. *Behavior and development in fragile X syndrome.* Thousand Oaks, Calif.: Sage Publications.

Ellis, E. S., and E. J. Sabornie. 1986. Effective instruction with microcomputers: Promises, practices and preliminary finding. *Focus Except. Child.* 19:1–16.

Farber, S. 1982. *Neurorehabilitation: A multisensory approach.* Philadelphia: W. B. Saunders.

Fisher, A. G., E. Murray, and A. Bundy, eds. 1991. *Sensory integration theory and practice.* Philadelphia: F. A. Davis.

Freund, L., and A. L. Reiss. 1991. Cognitive profiles associated with the fragile X syndrome in males and females. *Am. J. Med. Genet.* 38:542–547.

Friefeld, S., and D. MacGregor. 1993. Sensory motor coordination in boys with fragile X syndrome. In J. A. Holden and B. Cameron (eds.), *Proceedings of the First Canadian Fragile X Conference, Ongwanda Resource Center, Kingston, Ontario,* pp. 59–65.

Frost, L., and A. Bondy. 1994. *The Picture Exchange Communication System.* Cherry Hill, N.J.: Pyramid Educational Consultations.

Fryns, J. P. 1985. X-linked mental retardation. In *Medical genetics: Past, present and future.* New York: Alan R. Liss, pp. 309–319.

Giangreco, M. 1986. Delivery of therapeutic services in special education programs for learners with severe handicaps. *Phys. Occup. Ther. Pediatr.* 6:5–15.

Gilfoyle, E., A. Grady, and J. Moore. 1982. *Children Adapt.* Thorofare, N.J.: Charles B. Slack.

Goosens, C., S. Crain, and P. Elder. 1992. *Engineering the preschool environment for interactive, symbolic communication.* Communication Publications. Chapel Hill, N.C.: Univ. of North Carolina Press.

Grandin, T., and M. Scariano. 1988. *Emergence labeled autistic.* Nova, Calif.: Arena Press.

Greenough, W. 1999. Experience, brain development and links to mental retardation. Presented to the Biennial Meeting of the Society for Research in Child Development, Albuquerque, N.M., April.

Greenough, W. T. 2000. FMRP and synaptic protein synthesis. Presented to the Seventh International Fragile X Conference, Los Angeles, July 19–21.

Gustavson, A., M. Dawson, and D. Bonett. 1987. Androstenal, a putative human phoneme, affects human (*Homo sapiens*) male choice preference. *J. Comp. Psychol.* 101:210–212.

Hagerman, R. J., and A. Smith. 1983. The heterozygous female. In R. J. Hagerman and P. McBogg (eds.), *The fragile X syndrome: Diagnosis, biochemistry, and intervention.* Dillon, Colo.: Spectra Publishing, pp. 83–94.

Hagerman, R. J., and W. Sobesky. 1989. Psychopathology in fragile X syndrome. *Am. J. Orthopsychiatry* 59:142–152.

Hagerman, R., Hills, J., Scharfenaker, S., and H. Lewis. 1999. Fragile X syndrome and selective mutism. *J. Med. Genet.* 83:313–317.

Hamre-Nietupski, S., J. Nietupski, P. Bates, and S. Maurer. 1982. Implementing a community-based educational model for moderately/severely handicapped students: Common problems and suggested solutions. *J. Assoc. Severely Handicap.* 7:38–43.

Hatten, D., D. Bailey, J. Roberts, M. Skinner, L. Mayhew, R. Duffee Clark, E. Waring, and J. Roberts. 2000. Early intervention services for young boys with fragile X syndrome. *J. Early Interv.* 23:235–251.

Hayes, R. 1987. Training for work. In P. Cohen and A. Donnellan (eds.), *Handbook of autism and pervasive developmental disorders.* New York: Wiley, pp. 360–370.

Helfrich-Miller, K. 1994. Melodic intonation therapy and developmentally apraxic children. *Clin. Communication Disord.* 4:175–182.

Hodapp, R., J. Leckman, E. Dykens, S. Sparrow, D. Zelinsky, and S. Ort. 1992. K-ABC profiles in children with fragile X syndrome, Down syndrome, and nonspecific mental retardation. *Am. J. Ment. Retard.* 97:39–46.

Holder, E. 1995. Inclusion for children with fragile X syndrome. *Natl. Fra. X Adv.* 1(1):5–7.

Huss, A. 1976. Touch with care or a caring touch. *Am. J. Occup. Ther.* 31:11–18.

Hutchinson, D. J. 1983. The transdisciplinary approach. In J. B. Curry (ed.), *Mental retardation: Nursing approaches to care.* St. Louis: C. V. Mosby, pp. 65–74.

Jenkins, J. R., and L. Jenkins. 1981. *Cross age and peer tutoring: Help for children with learning problems.* Reston, Va.: Council for Exceptional Children.

Jones, A., P. Currier, and L. Hickman. 1986. Pragmatics camp and offshoot programs for the adolescent language-learning disabled population. Presented to the Colorado Speech and Hearing Association, Breckenridge, Colo.

Kandel, E., J. Schwartz, and T. Jessell, eds. 2000. *Principles of neuroscience,* 4th ed. New York: McGraw-Hill.

Kantner, R., B. Kantner, and D. Clark. 1982. Vestibular stimulation effect on language development in mentally retarded children. *Am. J. Occup. Ther.* 36:36–41.

Kawar, M. 1973. The effects of sensorimotor therapy on dichotic listening in children with learning disabilities. *Am. J. Occup. Ther.* 27:226–231.

Kemper, M. B., R. J. Hagerman, R. S. Ahmad, and R. Mariner. 1986. Cognitive profiles and the spectrum of clinical manifestations in heterozygous fra(X) females. *Am. J. Med. Genet.* 23:139–156.

Kemper, M. B., R. J. Hagerman, and D. Altshul-Stark. 1988. Cognitive profiles of boys with the fragile X syndrome. *Am. J. Med. Genet.* 30:191–200.

Keogh, M. 1992. Intervention to enhance attention skills in children with attention deficit hyperactivity disorder. In R. J. Hagerman and P. McKenzie (eds.), *1992 International Fragile X Conference proceedings.* Dillon, Colo.: Spectra Publishing, pp. 251–259.

Koegel, R., M. O'Dell, and L. Koegel. 1987. A natural language teaching paradigm for nonverbal autistic children. *J. Autism Dev. Disord.* 17:187–200.

Krug, D. A., J. R. Arick, and P. J. Almond. 1980; 1993. *ASIEP Examiner's Manual* (Autism Screen Instrument for Educational Planning): An assessment and educational planning system for autistic, severely handicapped, and developmentally disabled persons. Texas: Pro-Ed.

Krug, D., J. Rosenblum, P. Almond, and J. Arick. 1980. *Assessment, behavior management, and communication training program.* Portland, Oreg.: ASIEP Education.

Leckman, J. F., R. M. Hodapp, E. M. Dykens, S. S. Sparrow, D. Zylinsky, and S. I. Ort. 1989. Evidence for a specific profile of cognitive processing among fragile X males. Presented at the Fourth International Workshop on Fragile X Syndrome and X-linked Mental Retardation, New York, September.

Levitas, A., R. Hagerman, M. Braden, B. Rimland, P. McBogg, and I. Matus. 1983. Autism and the fragile X syndrome. *J. Dev. Behav. Pediatr.* 4:151–158.

Levy, S. 1983. School doesn't last forever: Then what? Some vocational alternatives. In E. Shoper and G. Mesibov (eds.), *Autism in adolescents and adults.* New York: Plenum, pp. 133–148.

Lowe, F., L. Jacob, and S. Kaye. 1995. Models and techniques for combined treatment. *Natl. Fra. X Adv.* 1(1):5–6.

Lucas, E. V. 1980. *Semantic and pragmatic language disorders: Assessment and remediation.* Rockville, Md.: Aspen.

Luria, A. 1976. *Cognitive development: Its cultural and social foundation.* Cambridge: Harvard Univ. Press.

Madison, L., C. George, and J. Moeschler. 1986. Cognitive functioning in the fragile X syndrome: A study of intellectual memory and communication skills. *J. Ment. Defic. Res.* 30:129–148.

Maes, B., M. Van Walleghem, and J. Fryns. 1992. Social-emotional characteristics of adult mentally retarded men. In R. J. Hagerman and P. McKenzie (eds.), *1992 International Fragile X Conference proceedings.* Dillon, Colo.: Spectra Publishing, pp. 147–160.

Magun, W. M., K. Ottenbacher, S. McCue, and R. Keefe. 1981. Effects of vestibular stimulation on spontaneous use of verbal language in developmentally delayed children. *Am. J. Occup. Ther.* 35:101–104.

Marks, L. 1978. *The unity of the senses.* New York: Academic Press.

Marshalla, P. 1992. *Oral-motor techniques in articulation therapy.* Seattle: Innovative Concepts.

———. 1994. *Oral-motor techniques in articulation therapy.* Presented at the meeting Oral-Motor Techniques in Articulation Therapy, Denver, March, pp. 25–26.

———. 1996. Oral-Motor Training Kit. Temecula, Calif.: Speech Dynamics.

Mazzocco, M. M., R. J. Hagerman, and B. F. Pennington. 1992a. Problem-solving limitations among cytogenetically expressing fragile X women. *Am. J. Med. Genet.* 43: 78–86.

Mazzocco, M. M., R. J. Hagerman, A. Cronister-Silverman, and B. F. Pennington. 1992b. Specific frontal lobe deficits among women with the fragile X gene. *J. Am. Acad. Child Adolesc. Psychiatry* 31:1141–1148.

McCune-Nicolich, L. 1981. Toward symbolic functioning: Structure of early pretend games and potential parallels with language. *Child Dev.* 52:785–797.

McKibben, E. H. 1973. The effect of additional tactile stimulation in a perceptual-motor treatment program for school children. *Am. J. Occup. Ther.* 27:191–197.

Meegrum, W., K. Ottenbacher, S. McCue, and R. Keefe. 1981. Effects of vestibular stimulation on spontaneous use of verbal language in developmentally delayed children. *Am. J. Occup. Ther.* 35:101–104.

Melzer, Y., A. McGhee, M. Feigenbaum, and D. Schurr. 1992. Stages in vocational training for fragile X clients. In R. J. Hagerman and P. McKenzie (eds.), *1992 International Fragile X Conference proceedings.* Dillon, Colo.: Spectra Publishing, pp. 281–282.

Miezejeski, C., E. Jenkins, A. Hill, K. Wisniewski, J. French, and W. Brown. 1986. A profile of cognitive deficit in females from fragile X families. *Neuropsychologia* 24: 405–409.

Miller, L. J., D. N. McIntosh, J. McGrath, V. Shyu, M. Lampe, A. K. Taylor, F. Tassone, K. Neitzel, T. Stackhouse, and R. J. Hagerman. 1999. Electrodermal responses to sensory stimuli in individuals with fragile X syndrome: A preliminary report. *Am. J. Med. Genet.* 83:268–279.

Minskoff, E. H. 1980. Teaching approach for developing non-verbal communication skills in students with social perception deficits. Part I: The basic approach and body language clues. *J. Learn. Disabil.* 13:9–15.

Mithaug, D., and L. Hagmeier. 1978. The development of procedures to assess prevocational competencies of severely handicapped young adults. *AAESPH Rev.* 3:94–115.

Mokros, R. J., and S. J. Russell. 1986. Learner-centered software: A survey of microcomputer use with special needs students. *J. Learn. Disabil.* 19:185–190.

Montgomery, J. 1980. *Non-oral communication: A training guide for the child without speech.* Exemplary/Incentive Dissemination Project, ESEA, Title IV-C, Plavan School, Fountain Valley, Calif.

Morris, S. E. 1977. *Program guidelines for children with feeding problems.* Edison, N.J.: Childcraft Education Corp.

———. 1982. *The normal acquisition of oral feeding skills: Implications for assessment and treatment.* Central Islip, N.Y.: Therapeutic Media.

Morris, S. E., and M. D. Klein. 1988. *Pre-feeding skills.* Tucson: Communication Skill Builders.

Musselwhite, C., and K. St. Louis. 1982. *Communication programming for the severely handicapped: Vocal and non-vocal strategies.* San Diego: College Hill Press.

Nobak, C. 1975. *The human nervous system.* New York: McGraw-Hill.

O'Connor, R. 1995. *Boys with fragile X syndrome: The fragile X awareness series for children.* Denver: National Fragile X Foundation.

Odom, S. L., and W. H. Brown. 1993. Social interaction skills interventions for young children with disabilities. In C. Peck, S. Odom, and D. Bricker (eds.), *Integrating young children with disabilities into community programs: Ecological perspectives on research and implementation.* Baltimore: Paul H. Brooks, pp. 39–64.

Oetter, P., E. Richter, and S. Frick. 1993. M.O.R.E.: Integrating the mouth with sensory and postural functions. Hugo, Minn.: PDP Press.

Ottenbacher, K. 1982. The effect of a controlled program of vestibular stimulation on the incidence of seizures in children with severe developmental delay. *Phys. Occup. Ther. Pediatr.* 2:25–33.

Ottenbacher, K., and R. Altman. 1984. Effects of vibratory, edible and social reinforcement on performance of institutionalized mentally retarded adults. *Am. J. Ment. Defic.* 89:201–204.

Parham, D., and Z. Mailloux. 1996. Sensory integration. In J. Case-Smith, A. Allen, and P. Pratt (eds), *Occupational therapy for children.* St. Louis: Mosby, pp. 307–352.

Paul, R., P. Dykens, J. Leckman, M. Watson, W. Breg, and D. Cohen. 1987. A comparison of language characteristics of mentally retarded adults with fragile X syndrome and those with nonspecific mental retardation and autism. *J. Autism Dev. Disord.* 17: 457–468.

Reilly, C., D. Nelson, and A. Bundy. 1983. Sensorimotor versus fine motor activities in eliciting vocalizations in autistic children. *Occup. Ther. J. Res.* 3:199–212.

Richter, E., and P. Oetter. 1990. Environmental matrices for sensory integrative treatment. In S. Merrill, ed. *Environmental Implications for Occupational Therapy Practice.* Rockville, MD.: American Occupational Therapy Association.

Rogers, S., and D. DiLalla. 1991. A comparative study of the effect of a development based preschool curriculum on young children with autism and young children with other disorders of behavior and development. *Topics Early Childhood Special Educ.* 11:29–47.

Rogers, S., and B. F. Pennington. 1991. A theoretical approach to the deficits in infantile autism. *Dev. Psychopathol.* 3:137–162.

Rogers, S. J., J. M. Herbision, H. C. Lewis, J. Pantone, and K. Reis. 1986. An approach for enhancing symbolic communicative interpersonal functioning of young children with autism or severe emotional handicaps. *J. Dis. Early Child.* 10:135–148.

Rogers, S. J., and H. Lewis. 1989. An effective day treatment model for young children with pervasive developmental disorders. *JAACAP* 28:207–214.

Sarnat, H., and M. Netsky. 1981. *Evaluation of the nervous system.* New York: Oxford Univ. Press.

Scharfenaker, S., and L. Hickman. 1989. Combined speech-language and occupational therapy and the fragile X child. *Fragile X Assoc. Mich. Newslett.* 2:4–5.

Scharfenaker, S., and R. Schreiner. 1989. Cognitive and speech-language characteristics of the fragile X syndrome. *Rocky Mount. J. Commun. Disord.* 5:25–35.

Scharfenaker, S., and B. Shopmeyer. 1994. Speech-language deficits and intervention strategies for the fragile X child. Handout presented at the Fourth Annual International Fragile X Conference, Albuquerque, June 9–14.

Scharfenaker, S., and T. Stackhouse. 1995. Speech-language and occupational therapy: A combined approach. *Natl. Fra X Adv.* 1:4–5.

Scherer, N., and L. Olswang. 1989. Using structured discourse as a language intervention technique with autistic children. *J. Speech Hear. Disord.* 54:383–394.

Schiefelbush, R., ed. 1980. *Nonspeech language and communication.* Baltimore: Univ. Park Press.

Schwartz, R., and L. Leonard. 1985. Lexical imitation and acquisition in language impaired children. *J. Speech Hear. Disord.* 50:31–39.

Scott, J. 1986. *The olfactory bulb and central pathways.* Basel: Birkhauser Verlag.

Shopler, E. 1974. *Division Teacch.* Chapel Hill: Univ. of North Carolina.

Shopmeyer, B., and F. Lowe. 1992. *The fragile X child.* San Diego: Singular Publ. Co.

Short-de Graaff, M. 1988. *Human development for occupational and physical therapists*. Baltimore: Williams & Wilkins.

Silverman, F. 1982. *Communication for the speechless*. Englewood Cliffs, N.J.: Prentice-Hall.

Smith, C. 1985. *Ancestral voices and evolution of human consciousness*. Englewood Cliffs, N.J.: Prentice-Hall, pp. 5–93.

Sparks, R., and A. Holland. 1976. Method: Melodic intonation therapy for aphasia. *J. Speech Hear. Disord.* 41:287–297.

Sparks, R., N. Helm, and R. Albert. 1974. Aphasia rehabilitation resulting from melodic intonation therapy. *Cortex* 10:303–316.

Spiridigliozzi, G., A. Lachiewicz, C. MacMordo, A. Vizoso, C. O'Donnell, A. McConkie-Rosell, and D. Burgess. 1994. *Educating boys with fragile X syndrome: A guide for parents and professionals*. Durham, N.C.: Duke Univ. Medical Center.

Stackhouse, T. 1994. Sensory integration concepts and fragile X syndrome. *Am. Occup. Ther. Assoc. S.I.* (special interest section newsletter) 17:2–6.

Stackhouse, T. M., and J. Wilbarger. 1998. Step SI: A clinical reasoning model for sensory modulation. Presented at the AOTA National Conference, Baltimore, March.

Sternat, J., R. Messina, J. Nietupski, S. Lyons, and L. Brown. 1977. Occupational and physical therapy services for severely handicapped students: Toward a naturalized public school service delivery model. In E. Sontag, J. Smith, and N. Certo (eds.), *Educational programming for the severely and profoundly handicapped*. Reston, Va.: Council for Exceptional Children, pp. 263–277.

Stokes, T., and D. Bauer. 1977. An implicit technology of generalization. *J. Appl. Behav. Anal.* 10:349–367.

Storey, K., P. Bates, N. McGhee, and S. Dycus. 1984. Reducing the self-stimulatory behavior of a profoundly retarded female through sensory awareness training. *Am. J. Occup. Ther.* 38:510–516.

Strain, P. S. 1987. Comprehensive evaluation of intervention for young autistic children. *Top. Early Child. Spec. Ed.* 7:97–110.

Sudhalter, V. 1992. The language system of males with fragile X syndrome. In R. J. Hagerman and P. McKenzie (eds.), *1992 International Fragile X Conference proceedings*. Dillon, Colo.: Spectra Publishing, pp. 165–166.

———. 2000. Language dysfunction in fragile X syndrome. Presented to the Seventh International Fragile X Conference, Los Angeles, July.

Taylor, R., R. O'Connor, S. Scharfenaker, and R. Hagerman. 2001. Severe language impairment in fragile X syndrome: Clinical and molecular correlates and treatment approaches. *J. Dev. Behav. Pediatr.* (submitted).

Theobald, T., D. Hay, and C. Judge. 1987. Individual variation and specific cognitive deficits in the fra(X) syndrome. *Am. J. Med. Genet.* 28:1–11.

Travis, L., ed. 1971. *Handbook of speech pathology and audiology*. Englewood Cliffs, N.J.: Prentice-Hall.

Turk, J. 1992. Behavioral assessments. In R. J. Hagerman and P. McKenzie (eds.), *1992 International Fragile X Conference proceedings*. Dillon, Colo.: Spectra Publishing, pp. 165–166.

Uma, K., H. R. Nagendra, R. Nagarathna, S. Vaidehi, and R. Seethalakshmi. 1989. The integrated tool for mentally retarded children: A one-year controlled study. *J. Ment. Defic. Res.* 33:415–421.

Ungerer, J. A., and M. Sigman. 1984. The relation of play and sensorimotor behavior to language in the second year. Child Dev. 55:1448–1455.

U.S. Congress. 1975. Public Law 94-142, Education for All Handicapped Children Act of 1975. Washington, D.C.

U.S. Congress. 1986. Public Law 99-457, Individualized Family Service Plan. Washington, D.C.

Vandercook, T., and J. York. 1989. The McGill Action Planning System (MAPS): A strategy for building the vision. *Assoc. Persons Severe Handicaps* 14:205–215.

Vargas, S., and G. Camilli. 1999. A meta-analysis of research on sensory integration treatment. *Am. J. Occup. Ther.* 53:189–198.

Walker, D., J. Palfrey, M. Handley-Derry, and J. Singer. 1989. Mainstreaming children with handicaps: Implications for pediatricians. *J. Dev. Behav. Pediatr.* 10:151–156.

Webb, G., J. Halliday, D. Pitt, C. Judge, and M. Leversha. 1982. Fragile (X)(q27) sites in a pedigree with female carriers showing mild to severe mental retardation. *J. Med. Genet.* 19:44–48.

Weber, J. D. 1994. *Transitioning "special" children into elementary school.* Boulder, Colo.: Books beyond Borders.

Wehman, P., and J. Hill. 1981. Competitive employment for moderately and severely handicapped individuals. *Except. Child.* 47:338–345.

———. 1982. Preparing severely handicapped youth for less restrictive environments. *J. Assoc. Sev. Handicap.* 7:33–39.

Wehman, P., J. Kregel, and J. M. Barus. 1985. From school to work: A vocational transition model for handicapped students. *Except. Child.* 52:25–37.

Wetherby, A. 1986. Ontogeny of communicative functions in autism. *J. Autism Dev. Disord.* 16:295–316.

Wilbarger, P. 1995. The sensory diet: Activity programs based on sensory processing theory. *Am. Occup. Ther. Assoc. S.I.* (special interest section newsletter) 18(2):1–4.

Wilbarger, P., and J. L. Wilbarger. 1988. Sensory affective disorders: Beyond tactile defensiveness. Presented at the Sensory Integration Workshop, Denver, Colo.

———. 1991. Sensory defensiveness in children aged 2–12. Santa Barbara, Calif.: Avanti Educational Programs.

Wilson, P., T. Stackhouse, R. O'Connor, S. Scharfenaker, and R. J. Hagerman. 1994. *Issues and strategies for educating children with fragile X syndrome: A monograph.* Dillon, Colo.: Spectra Publishing Co.

Wimmer, D. 1981. Functional learning curricula in the secondary schools. *Except. Child.* 47:610–616.

Windeck, S., and M. Laurel. 1989. A theoretical framework combining speech language therapy with sensory integrative treatment. *Am. Occup. Ther. Assoc. S.I.* (special interest section newsletter) 12(1).

Yoder, D., ed. 1982. Communication interaction strategies for the severely communicatively impaired. *Top. Lang. Disord.* 2.

Zivin, D., ed. 1979. *The development of self-regulation through private speech.* New York: Wiley.

## Recommended Reading

Ayres, A. 1979. *Sensory integration and the child.* Los Angeles: Western Psychological Services.

Braden, M. 2000. *Fragile: Handle with care. Understanding fragile X syndrome,* 2d ed.

Dykens, E. M., R. M. Hodapp, and J. F. Leckman. 1994. *Behavior and development in fragile X syndrome.* Thousand Oaks, Calif.: Sage Publications.

O'Connor, R. 1995. *Boys with fragile X syndrome: The fragile X awareness series for children.* Denver: Dakali Corp.

Russell, L., A. Grant, S. Joseph, and R. Fee. 1994. *Planning for the future: Providing a meaningful life for a child with disability.* Evanston, Ill.: American Publ. Co.

Schopmeyer, B. B., and F. Lowe. 1992. *The fragile X child.* San Diego: Singular Publishing Group.

Smith, R. 1993. *Children with mental retardation.* Rockville, Md.: Woodbine House.

Spiridigliozzi, G., A. Lachiewicz, C. MacMurdo, A. Vizoso, C. O'Donnell, A. McConkie-Rosell, and D. Burgess. 1994. *Educating boys with fragile X syndrome: A guide for parents and professionals.* Durham, N.C.: Duke Univ. Medical Center.

Weber, J. 1994. *Transitioning "special" children into elementary school.* Boulder, Colo.: Books beyond Borders.

Weber, J. D., ed. 2000. *Children with FXS: A parent's guide.* Bethesda, Md.: Woodbine House.

Wilson, P., T. Stackhouse, R. O'Connor, S. Scharfenaker, and R. Hagerman. *Issues and strategies for educating children with fragile X syndrome.* Dillon, Colo.: Spectra Publ. Co.

Wright-Talamante, C., A. Cheema, J. E. Riddle, D. W. Luckey., A. K. Taylor, and R. J. Hagerman. 1996. A controlled study of longitudinal IQ changes in females and males with fragile X syndrome. *Am. J. Med. Genet.* 64:350–355.

## Web Sites

www.fragileX.org
www.fraxa.org
www.SLnetwork.org
www.aavap.org
www.aota.org
www.asha.org
www.thearc.org
www.autism-society.org
www.ataccess.org
www.nichcy.org
www.ataccess.org
www.ed.gov/offices/OSERS/
www.ldresources.com
http://janweb.icdi.wvu.edu/kinder/index.htm

# CHAPTER 11
# Academic Interventions

## Marcia L. Braden, Ph.D.

Just as our understanding of the FMR-1 protein has increased, so has our knowledge of successful academic interventions for persons with fragile X syndrome (FXS). The academic research laboratory has been confined to clinics and classrooms. Very little scientific data have been generated because of the arduous task of matching subjects and teaching strategies within a group large enough to yield statistical significance. Most intervention strategies have been developed through clinical trial and error and, when successful, applied to others who carry the FXS diagnosis. Some strategies have been adapted from those used with other populations, such as persons with autism, learning disability, or Down syndrome.

Learning can be difficult for individuals with FXS, especially when the level of affliction is significant. Exactly how the FMR-1 protein affects brain functioning is still being investigated (chaps. 1, 4, and 5). The lack of scientific data that test specific educational methods makes formulating well-designed strategies more difficult. Several studies, however, have been reported and replicated and have given rise to the identification of a cognitive phenotype (chap. 6) and a subsequent characterization of relative strengths and weaknesses in males affected by FXS. More is known about the cognitive processing style of females affected with FXS, in part because of a higher prevalence and better mental functioning. It is much easier to evaluate groups of females and extract evidence to formulate a particular theory than it is to study groups of males.

Although this chapter will discuss academic intervention with both males and females affected with FXS, the greatest challenge is with the males. Many strategies already defined in the literature have proven helpful in remedial work with females with FXS. Those interventions will be cited as they relate to specific areas of academic development and the application to males affected by the syndrome.

*Fragile X Syndrome: Diagnosis, Treatment, and Research,* third edition, ed. Randi Jenssen Hagerman and Paul J. Hagerman (Baltimore: Johns Hopkins University Press, 2002), © The Johns Hopkins University Press.

## Cognitive Foundations for Academic Strategies

Because individuals with FXS are being diagnosed at an earlier age, there is a greater overall awareness of presenting behaviors, speech/language deficits, and delayed motor development. These deficits form the cornerstone of a cognitive phenotype that includes significant processing deficits. The cognitive style of those with FXS is linked to physical, behavioral, and processing deficits. It is clear from clinical experience that the deficit areas defined in the phenotype interfere with cognitive development and learning overall because cognitive development requires the ability to pay attention, problem solve, and recall information (Sobesky et al. 1994; Sudhalter 1992; Scharfenaker et al. 1996).

Perhaps the most salient piece of research regarding learning presented early in the literature was that of Kemper et al. in 1988. The Kemper study was replicated by Hodapp et al. in 1992 and has evolved as the standard by which we define learning. The study and those that followed identified a particular processing style for males with FXS that has formed the foundation from which intervention strategies have been developed. Many suggest that defining the processing style may also provide answers to questions about problem behaviors, speech and language deficits, and poor motor planning.

The profile indicates a specific style of cognitive processing (table 11.1; exhibit 11.1). The studies suggest that males with FXS perform better on tasks that require a simultaneous approach to understanding information. The conceptual framework for simultaneous processing lies within a neuropsychologic context.

Kaufman (1983) asserts that simultaneous processing is a holistic approach to problem solving, accomplished by processing many stimuli at once instead of one stimulus at a time, as is the case with sequential processing. Kaufman believes that the ability to form gestalt perceptions develops early. The formation of gestalt comprehension initially relies on lower-level intellectual functions such as configurations and deriving meaning from pictures and visual pat-

**Table 11.1**
**Cognitive Profile: Studies of IQ in Males with Fragile X Syndrome**

| Study | IQ Test | n | Age (yr) | Cognitive Profile |
|---|---|---|---|---|
| Dykens et al. 1987 | K-ABC | 14 | 7–28 | Sequential < Simultaneous/Achievement |
| Kemper et al. 1988 | K-ABC | 20 | 4–12 | Sequential < Simultaneous/Achievement |
| Hodapp et al. 1992 | K-ABC | 10 | 6–10 | Sequential < Simultaneous/Achievement |

**Exhibit 11.1**
**Cognitive Features in Males with Fragile X Syndrome (K-ABC)**

---

Fragile X IQ < DD controls' IQ
Fragile X Achievement score > DD controls' Achievement score
Fragile X has more variation across subtests than do DD controls.
Fragile X Simultaneous (mean 71) IQ > Sequential (mean 62) IQ

---

*Source:* Kemper et al. 1988.
*Note:* Fragile X = 20 (experimental); children with developmental delays (DD) = 20 (control).

terns (Kaufman 1983). Young children with FXS often perform well and even better than those in normed age groups on tasks relying heavily on simultaneous processing. This is due in part to artifacts in the test design but also to a preferred processing style that very often emerges early in development and, in this population, compensates for deficient language and sequential processing deficits.

The cognitive profile initially defined by Kemper et al. (1988) describes a learning style that is unique. Although individuals with FXS demonstrate a continuum of affectedness, there are certain similarities in how they process information (chap. 6). As tasks become more abstract, simultaneous processing is more closely related to creative problem solving. If individuals with FXS are unable to develop higher-level processing, they may be unable to grasp more complicated concepts.

Information presented using a simultaneous approach resembles a "visual whole." Clinical experience has proven that individuals with FXS best understand information that is presented in that format (Braden 2000a, 2000b). The use of pictures, diagrams, and visual associations supplies the glue to solidify long-term memory of novel tasks. Long-term memory has been noted by several investigators as a relative strength (Dykens et al. 1987; Kemper et al. 1988; Hodapp et al. 1992).

As more clinical studies have emerged, the significance of this cognitive profile has become more important in the development of academic strategies and curricular adaptations (Gibb 1992; Mazzocco et al. 1993; Spiridigliozzi et al. 1994). We also know from earlier studies that sequential tasks, short-term memory, and visual motor planning tend to be more difficult for males with FXS (Dykens et al. 1987; Kemper et al. 1988; Hodapp et al. 1992). In the second edition of this book, Bennetto and Pennington posited a connection between these deficit areas and impairment of executive functioning (Bennetto et al. 1996). An expansion of their theory with application to academic strategies will be provided later in this chapter.

## Matching of Processing Style with Teaching Methods

The Kemper study further implicated academic treatment methods. As discussed earlier, simultaneous processing involves a specific style of information processing that has a theoretical foundation in both neuropsychology and cognitive psychology. Simultaneous processing requires spatial integration of stimuli in order to solve problems. Individuals with FXS can process the sum of parts to a problem but not the individual parts themselves without a context. This style of acquiring information is counter to most traditional teaching methods.

Traditional curricular structure most often includes a scope and sequence of skills. One skill is presented and learned to provide the prerequisite for the next skill to be learned. In addition to the overall curricular structure, teaching methods often include a sequential presentation. For example, to teach reading involves the acquisition of phonemes, which are then blended together in a sequential manner from left to right, which ultimately results in the reading of a word. This phonetic process requires the learner to use cognitive processes that are commonly deficient in males with FXS. When the reading method uses a phonetic approach, the child is required to

1. attend to the stimuli
2. recall the symbol
3. pair the symbol with a sound
4. recall the sound with the symbol
5. hold the sound/symbol while moving on to the next symbol
6. attend to the next symbol
7. repeat the earlier steps and blend the sound-symbols to form a word

In addition to the cognitive components, the Kemper study provided the impetus to espouse learning theory that several clinicians have subsequently included in their work (Schopmeyer et al. 1992; Scharfenaker et al. 1996). Individuals with FXS seem to better perform those tasks that are familiar and repetitive. When a group of males with FXS was compared to a control group, their achievement scores were significantly higher than the scores of the intelligence tests (Kemper et al. 1988). This suggests that novel and unrelated tasks are more difficult for individuals with FXS. The obvious fallout affects performance on intelligence testing because the material presented in intelligence testing is intended to be novel to preserve the integrity of the test.

There are several reasons why individuals with FXS perform better on achievement testing, one being the comfort of familiarity. Familiarity reduces anxiety because the outcome is predictable. In direct contrast, the performance of novel tasks requires flexible thinking, impulse control, and reduced performance anxiety.

Males with FXS seem to struggle with working memory (holding information while solving problems), and it follows that the performance of novel tasks would be affected (Freund and Reiss 1991). Flexibility of thought is also required when solving a novel problem. Individuals with FXS often habituate a certain approach, which results in frustration if the approach is applied without success to a novel task.

## Students with FXS in the Classroom

Because a child spends much of the day at school, it is incumbent on those who educate children to understand what they need. The classroom environment is typically busy, fast-paced, and noisy and includes a variety of transitions. Often adults and peers interface daily with sophisticated social interaction. A child with FXS may find this environment particularly frustrating because of the cognitive and behavioral profile defined earlier in this chapter.

During the elementary school years, individuals with FXS often experience significant academic growth, especially if early intervention programs were provided on an intensive basis. At this point, it is common for school districts to explore inclusive educational opportunities. Although some early education placements include individuals with FXS with typical preschool peers, it is generally more productive to employ intensive therapies (occupational therapy [OT], speech/language therapy, cognitive training, and behavioral intervention) at an early age and transition the young child into an included environment later. This model provides a stronger foundation for successful academic achievement and social development in the elementary school environment (chap. 10).

Problems with attention will obviously interact with the learning acquisition rate. Although attending behaviors usually increase through early intervention training, it is still important to include attending as a basic component in the educational process. Many learning activities within an elementary environment require attention. Frequently, classroom management rules require basic attending behaviors from children. Behaviors such as waiting in line, raising a hand, and waiting until called upon are prerequisites to becoming a viable classroom member. Cooperation through turn taking may also be important to success in an integrated environment. If the child with FXS is able to comply with these basic requirements, there will be less need for reprimand and redirection from the teacher, thus promoting acceptance from typical peers.

Even children who exhibit minimal cognitive deficits experience speech/language deficits (Hagerman et al. 1985; Sudhalter et al. 1990; Sobesky et al.

1994). Language deficits are often due to auditory processing difficulties. Language becomes the keystone to social acceptance and social reciprocity. Speech intelligibility may be affected by anxiety, causing verbal interaction to be problematic. Even though the youngster wants very much to communicate with his peers, his organization of thought and ability to maintain a topic in conversation may be impaired (chap. 6). Typical peers may become impatient or may begin to speak for the one with FXS in an attempt to continue the conversational exchange.

Research tells us that individuals with FXS perform better on tasks that are repetitive and familiar. Novel tasks promote anxiety, creating fear and an obsession to avoid the unfamiliar. During the elementary school years, it is important to foster problem solving by introducing novel tasks and observing the outcome. If the child consistently avoids the novel task, note the ways in which he avoids the task (diverting attention, acting out, becoming confused or disinterested, perseverating, or becoming aggressive). These avoidance behaviors provide evidence that he is resisting. To desensitize the child, one must reinforce solution finding without creating additional stress. Anticipating sustained perseverance while supporting the outcome is important. As the number of attempted tasks increases, the process will help decrease the negative reaction to anything new.

## Environment

The environment in which one learns can be as important as *what* is learned, especially with this population. Because individuals with FXS exhibit a variety of behaviors that seem to be reactionary, it is good educational practice to control the environment as often as possible in order to foster learning.

Variables have been observed to affect an academic outcome. For example, Braden's dissertation results (1991) identified routine changes to be more difficult for individuals with FXS than for the control group, negative for FXS. As would be expected, the normal classroom setting includes numerous transitions throughout the day, from subject area changes to physical transitions and classroom movement. Reassuring the student with FXS requires a consistent and predictable learning environment. It is often necessary to provide a visual schedule to reduce the anxiety often associated with routine change (fig. 11.1).

Specific placement in the classroom may also be warranted. Often the student with FXS demonstrates higher vigilance that competes with focus and concentration. If the student is positioned in the front of the class with clear access to a door or exit, attending behaviors improve and the need for hypervigilance decreases.

The size of the classroom is also an important factor. A smaller group set-

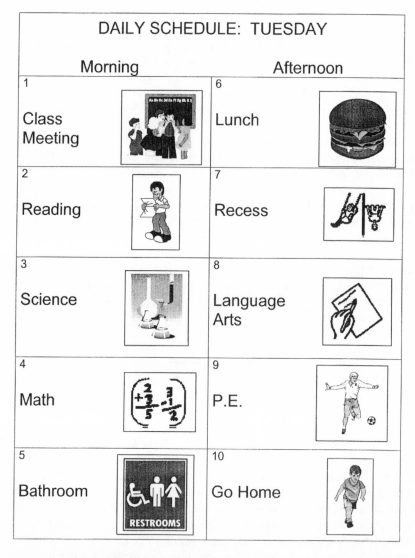

**Fig. 11.1.** A visual schedule may reduce the anxiety associated with transitions.

ting is more conducive to learning, especially when novel tasks are presented. The size of the classroom often correlates with the noise level, and individuals with FXS are very sensitive to noise (chap. 10). It is not uncommon to see a boy with FXS cover his ears if the noise level is too loud or becomes overwhelming. Motor excesses such as hand flapping, moving, and rocking may increase if the environment is particularly noisy. Every attempt to reduce the noise level in the classroom should be made, especially for children at younger ages when coping skills are not as developed. If several classroom placements are available, it is best to choose a classroom with structure and a low noise level. This is usually promoted by the teacher and is reflective of a particular teaching style.

Individuals with FXS may also avoid noisy environments such as cafeterias, gymnasiums, and theaters. The student's attendance at a portion of a presentation, game, or lunchtime will provide an opportunity to become desensitized and gradually reduce the anxiety associated with larger and more crowded environments. Some individuals with FXS never acclimate to noisy environments and require special accommodations under those conditions.

Recent school law has encouraged the inclusion of children with disabilities among those who are typically developing (Individuals with Disabilities Education Act of 1997). Often in an inclusive setting, a teacher assistant is assigned to the student with FXS to facilitate participation and learning. The model shown in exhibit 11.2 has been used in several included environments where accommodations are necessary.

**Exhibit 11.2**
**Model for Adaptation of Curriculum and Classroom Accommodations**

1. The case manager (special educator) solicits study units from the regular education teachers at least a week ahead of the actual presentation.
2. The case manager adapts the curriculum to accommodate the student's level of functioning and processing style to incorporate the student's strengths into the presentation.
3. The case manager trains the teaching assistant to facilitate the adaptations in the regular education classroom.
4. The teaching assistant preteaches skills whenever possible as appropriate in the included environment.
5. The teaching assistant's role is multifaceted and includes
   • teaching an alternative activity in or out of the regular education classroom based on the individual's ability to access the curriculum.
   • providing cues and instructional support in the regular education classroom.
   • teaching in a small group (2–3 adolescents) using indirect instruction and side dialog. This can be done in the special education or regular education classroom, depending on need.
   • teaching social skills in a small group and in vivo experiences.
6. The team meets weekly to make adjustments to the curriculum and develop accommodations. The team includes a case manager, a regular education teacher when appropriate, and a teaching assistant.

## How to Teach

Because an individual with FXS is more comfortable with familiarity, the tenets of a traditional educational process can become problematic. It is obvious that learning requires the acquisition of new information. Because learning constantly integrates new into familiar information, it is prudent to include teaching techniques that use incidentally acquired knowledge. This can be accomplished by using acquired information and integrating that information into a more structured teaching format. Typically, incidentally acquired information has been learned in a natural environment without instructional constraints. This kind of teaching reduces performance anxiety and fosters long-term memory.

There are, however, times when it is impossible to avoid novel tasks in an educational setting. Several strategies have been effective in overriding the anxiety created by learning novel tasks (Braden 2000b). For example, when novel tasks are presented in familiar formats, the familiarity is more likely to override the anxiety created by the unfamiliarity. Interspersing high-interest material within an unfamiliar learning format is another viable method. The interest overrides the anxiety, allowing the learner to focus and concentrate.

The following learning characteristics are present in many persons with FXS. These traits may require certain academic and environmental accommodations, as offered.

### Executive Functioning

Children with FXS show a deficit in executive function (Pennington et al. 1998). This neuropsychologic term includes the ability to formulate a plan, sum up intention, and execute it (chap. 6). Executive function also requires flexibility in problem solving. It is not unusual to watch a child with FXS struggle attempting to begin a task. This is particularly apparent before beginning a written exercise. The child may be stymied, turning his pencil over and over, erasing excessively or staring off, waiting for assistance. This may be perceived as a stalling technique but is more likely due to an inability to execute a response. If the therapist begins the trial or task and asks the child to finish or complete it, the rate of success will increase. Another technique, backward chaining, begins an exercise by providing the beginning but leaving the end segments unfinished in greater and greater increments until the child is able to complete the entire answer without prompting.

### Closure

Experience has demonstrated that children with FXS prefer completion or closure of information. It is not uncommon to observe a child finishing a puzzle before moving on or filling in a blank before leaving a task. This need for completion can become a compulsion that may interfere with daily functioning. Rather than focus on the negative aspects of the behavior, educators have begun to use it as a means to stimulate oral and written responses. For example, if a child is disturbed about an experience at school and is unable to verbalize the sequence of the infraction, a parent may use this closure technique to gain information. For example, instead of asking, "Who hit you?" or "Where did this happen?" the parent may say something like, "Today on the playground you got ———." "When you were hit, Susie said ———." As the incident is pieced together by the parent and more information is gradually added to the story line, the incident can be better understood from the child's perspective.

Another example includes presenting an unfinished sample to promote task completion. Using a hangman format (_ _ t) to teach the spelling of c-a-t forces completion of the whole word, which will often override any sequential deficits ordinarily associated with spelling.

## Indirect Instruction

It is not uncommon for children with FXS to become stymied by a direct question. A direct question, in isolation, may force a response without the benefit of contextual information. The same question asked in a more relaxed format will result in spontaneous recall. Clinicians have found that using peers as teaching models can facilitate learning in an indirect fashion. Instructing several children in a group enables the teacher to teach a lesson without worry from the child with FXS that he will be called upon for a response. Teaching a group of peers provides a filter through which an interaction can occur, which ultimately promotes more participation from the student with FXS. This strategy is similar to peer mediation (Myles and Simpson 1998), where peers are used to promote initiation in social interactions. The advantage of this model, according to Myles, is that the challenged peer is more naturally integrated into a social and school community.

## Associative Learning

As a result of their simultaneous learning style, it is easier for children with FXS to recall information if it is related to or associated with a bigger whole. For example, a child may learn a jingle or song before he is able to identify different letters or numbers. Individuals with FXS often demonstrate attention deficits and hyperactivity. Information presented in isolation without association may become distorted or forgotten. It is important to include high-interest materials in the school curriculum. An interest inventory, completed by parents, teachers, and caretakers, provides educators with ideas from which to create teaching materials. For example, one student interested in television weather maps used the maps to learn geographic locations, states, and capitals.

## Long-term Memory

Generally, children with FXS have good long-term memory (Kemper et al. 1988; Hodapp et al. 1992). Simultaneous processing generates good long-term memory. When the learner is given multiple stimuli within a context, the information is more likely to be retained. For example, long-term memory can be triggered by an association that is often the by-product of the simultaneous processing style. A child may be shown a map that will conjure up a memory about a road map his family used when traveling from California to Texas. This association then activates a memory that may include a fact or general information pertinent to the conversation.

## Focus and Concentration

Focus and concentration are mentioned by researchers as distinct features of a behavioral phenotype (Hagerman 1996; Braden 2000a; Sobesky 1996). Teachers often describe a child with FXS as distractible and unable to concentrate, even for short periods. It is important, when assessing these behavioral characteristics, to identify times when the behavior occurs. It is not unusual, for example, to watch a student with FXS go from concentrating on a task to being completely distractible. Sometimes, the change or shift to another task can contribute to distractibility. As mentioned earlier in this chapter, lack of focus and concentration can be a direct result of environmental conditions, low-interest material, or anxiety.

Before teaching a lesson, it is important to consider the factors that may affect concentration. Several strategies can assist in promoting better focus and concentration. Exhibit 11.3 lists strategies that can be used to increase attention during instructional periods.

## What to Teach

In general, most parents of children with FXS want the educational process to support their child, to maximize the child's full potential. As mentioned in the introduction, academic acquisition varies and is generally tied to the level of affectedness. Thus, a specific standard of what should be taught and at what age is difficult to determine. Based on clinical experience, a general sense of educational objectives can be beneficial.

As the child develops, a better sense of his strengths and weaknesses can

**Exhibit 11.3**
**Proactive Behavioral Strategies**

Provide small group instruction.
Allow seating in the back section of a room.
Allow seating near an exit.
Provide structure and predictability.
Reduce the level of environmental noise/sound.
Allow additional processing time.
Use natural lighting whenever possible.
Avoid crowded areas.
Predict transitions and signal with visual cues.
Provide nonverbal cues and feedback.
Role play behavioral consequences.
Provide calming activities (SI intervention).
Encourage physical activity.
Allow removal from stressful events.
Encourage breaks and "down time."

help one formulate a learning rate. As this process continues, finding the right balance between teaching academic skills and teaching those that are more functional (self-help and skills of independent functioning) becomes a significant issue. Some level of academic knowledge is necessary to learn functional skills. For example, to follow a recipe, one must be able to read and follow a sequence of directions. To measure ingredients, one must be able to recognize numerals and decipher size.

At an early age the child must be provided with knowledge that will foster independent functioning without restrictive supports. It is far more natural for the individual with FXS to live independent of family within a multilevel support system that can be accessed based on need. This issue should be addressed early and supported throughout the academic experience. As the child develops into a preadolescent, the programming emphasis may shift from one weighted more heavily with academics to one with a more vocational bias with community-based instruction.

The formulation of a curricular structure requires examination of those learning traits unique to this population and of the corresponding adaptations necessary to access as much of the typical curriculum as possible. Emphasis on modifying certain behavioral traits that may compete with the natural acquisition of skills must be considered.

Braden (2000a) developed a Suggested Curriculum Guide appropriate for use with this population, presenting systematically the skills necessary for mastery. The sequence is projected through four levels of academic development: preschool, elementary school, middle school, and high school. The targeted skill areas include attending behaviors, language, problem solving, social/sexual development, and academics.

Most children with FXS experience learning problems due to a variety of reasons (Sudhalter 1992; Dykens et al. 1987; Braden 2000a). Cognitive deficits along with difficulties with attentional processing contribute to academic weaknesses. The Kemper study concluded that individuals with FXS achieved higher scores in reading and spelling than in math. This research finding has been reinforced through clinical experience.

## Math

The math difficulties indigenous to the females affected by FXS are also present in the males. Providing cognitive restructuring about the execution of math may have strong implications for remediation. Teaching models should include a component to address faulty cognition, which may contribute to phobic reactions and anxiety. If these kinds of strategies are included, higher cognitive ability is required. This might exclude the majority of males affected by FXS.

The ability to learn and apply mathematics has a strong effect on functional life skills. Effective teaching is essential and occurs only if strategies are multimodal and systematic. Introducing concepts using concrete, hands-on materials will set the stage for higher-order learning. Mercer and Miller (1992) described a teaching generalization strategy that moves from concrete to representational and then to abstraction. Although this intervention has been proposed for students with learning disabilities (Maccini and Hughes 1997), there may be application to those with FXS.

Various causal factors have been identified as contributing to poor math performance. As mentioned earlier, the sequential processing deficits commonly observed in the FXS group make difficult the conceptualization of mathematical abstracts. Because these deficits are so significant and far reaching, lack of confidence and perseverance becomes a secondary disability in the acquisition of math skills. In addition, difficulty with attention, working memory, and visual-spatial relationships factor into poor math performance.

Because math is sequential and requires the learner to build systematically from one step to the next, the curriculum used in regular education classrooms will probably need to be adapted. Instruction must include demonstration, practice, and positive reinforcement. It may be necessary to review the skills expected and systematically focus on those that are functional, discarding those that are extraordinary. This method of curricular adaptation is called *skill streaming*. If this method becomes necessary, the child's ability should be consistent with curricular expectations. Adapting the curriculum requires assistance from a special educator familiar with FXS and the child, along with the parent and classroom teacher.

Math as a functional skill should be carefully considered whenever an educational plan is developed. Basic skills to include are number identification, value, money, time telling, and reading tables/recipes. The more proficient the child becomes, the more independent he will be.

Deficits in math, especially in math reasoning and conceptual skills, have been reported (Kemper et al. 1986; Mazzocco et al. 1992a; Miezejeski and Hinton 1992). Often females have difficulty generalizing math concepts to a variety of situations for future problem solving. Algebraic formulas, symbolic associations that include missing elements, and the computation of word problems often cause great difficulty in this population. A curriculum that uses concrete and manipulative materials to introduce basic mathematic operations should be considered. Teaching methods should include patterns and visual gestalt whenever possible to reinforce complex mathematic processes. Suggested materials are listed in appendix 3.

## Reading

Reading, unlike math, is less contingent on sequential processing. Reading success can be acquired using a variety of methods. Learning to read can be accomplished using a simultaneous approach. The configuration of a word and the contextual meaning can provide enough information for the learner to read successfully.

Generally, clinicians and teachers have had more success teaching reading to children with FXS using a high-interest, whole language–based approach. When a phonetic or sequential approach is used, children with FXS lose interest and often experience failure (Braden 2000b).

Reading for various purposes should be noted as an instructional plan is developed. The pragmatics of reading has functional impact. For example, teaching the specific vocabulary necessary to read a grocery list, follow directions, cook from a recipe, or read a daily planner is essential for independence.

If the student's ability level is higher, simple word recognition and recall become the foundation for general information such as reading forms for content, perusing a newspaper, or reading a TV schedule. As the reading program progresses, the understanding of factual information transcends into more abstract verbal reasoning, and the student begins to understand inferences, predicting outcomes and drawing conclusions.

The sequential deficits noted throughout this chapter may interfere most with comprehension of complex and abstract concepts. Using a cloze technique often works well to help the reader increase general comprehension. This technique is similar to that described earlier regarding the remediation of executive functioning deficits. In the cloze technique one presents a paragraph with intact beginning and ending sentences. Words are then systematically omitted throughout the passage. The reader is expected to fill in the blanks based on the content. The content provides the information necessary to formulate an understanding of the passage.

Individuals with FXS can and do learn to read, some quite successfully. Generally, reading for pleasure is rarely observed in males with FXS. Females, on the other hand, often read for enjoyment. Reading proficiency is determined by early intervention strategy instruction and level of affectedness.

Clinical experience has identified commercial reading programs appropriate for use with this population (Braden 2000a). The most successful programs use a visual approach with pictures to aid in comprehension and conceptual orientation. The Edmark Reading program is an example. This program progresses from level I to level II and can accommodate readers through a third- to fourth-grade reading level. A computerized counterpart can augment the printed material. The Logo Reading System (Braden 1989) uses well-known fast-food logos as a vehicle through which to teach word recognition. The words are generalized into word families and ultimately sentence strips. This program readies the reader to move on to a more traditional reading curriculum.

## Written Language

Individuals with FXS vary in their language ability. Usually, we write what we can say. Males with FXS are often tangential in their initiation of spontaneous oral language, and written language may reflect the same differential. Often, a picture can be used to stimulate language. As the story is expressed, a scribe can convert the oral language into written form.

Fine motor and motor planning deficits have been noted by several clinicians (chap. 1). Motor planning deficits affect writing (chap. 10). Individuals with FXS may become frustrated trying to copy from or write down information. The help of a scribe decreases the level of frustration associated with written language. Keyboarding may provide another alternative to written language, reducing the frustration created by poor motor planning and fine motor control.

## Curricular Adaptations

At different times during the school experience, it may be necessary to decide what is most important to teach. Clearly, a common goal is to use the educational process to advance the learner to the greatest possible level of independence.

At various junctures, one may need to discuss placement options as well. For example, it may be more prudent to include the child in a special education

**Exhibit 11.4**
**Decision Tree for Curricular Adaptations**

---

Can the student with FXS understand and interact with the curriculum used in regular education placement?

| No | Yes |
|---|---|
| ↓ | ↓ |
| If the functioning level is minimally delayed, curricular expectations are adapted based on functioning level; for example, the reading level is lower, but understanding of content is within normal limits. | No adaptations are necessary. May require time adjustments or other accommodations, such as skill streaming existing curricula to include only those skills that are important to maintaining competency in the classroom/course. |

↓

If the functioning level is moderately delayed, curricular adaptations include a parallel curriculum in which the same content is taught but with less volume and complexity of content.

↓

If the functioning level is significantly delayed and curricular adaptations cannot be provided because of the level of cognitive functioning and delayed academic skills, a differentiated curriculum is used. This curriculum is different from the one presented in the regular education placement.

---

placement at an early age so that intensive individual therapies and instruction may occur without interference with classroom routine. As the learning process continues and the child has the skills necessary to be a viable classmate, it may be more appropriate to include him with typically developing peers with special education support to help with academic accruement. If individuals with FXS are included, it may be necessary to evaluate the curriculum to determine the application and/or need for adaptations. Exhibit 11.4 illustrates curriculum design variables.

Later on, the same dilemma arises when decisions regarding the focus of future instruction are made. By the time the child reaches the age of 14, schools are required to begin to make plans for the transition from school to an adult life and into the community. The transition plan is set by the requirements of the Individuals with Disabilities Education Act (IDEA).

As this transition plan develops, it may be necessary to access a technical or vocational instructional track. It may be possible at that point for the adolescent with FXS to benefit from a vocational curriculum without major modifications. On the other hand, instruction of specific skills that are somewhat technical but critical to the final task outcome may require individualized instruction in the special education classroom. The school may provide work-study experiences within the school environment to teach entry-level work skills or to test certain work behaviors. In addition to work-related skills, other social and behavioral domains are explored to determine any needs related to accessing community resources to foster independent functioning.

At times during the school experience, it may be too difficult to adapt the curriculum enough to be meaningful. For example, if the student with FXS does not demonstrate reading skills necessary to benefit from an existing civics lesson, the special education staff may need to develop an adapted curriculum that parallels the existing curriculum but is different in instructional complexity.

## Prevocational/Vocational Training

During the middle school years, vocational interests are explored within a variety of environments. The term *prevocational* is often used in middle school to define training for the work experience. Part of the instructional time is spent assessing prerequisite work behaviors such as attending, asking for help, indicating when a job has been completed, and working under supervision. Environmental work conditions, job content, skill requirements, staff ratio, acceptable behavior, and production rates are explored during middle school. Results from this process, which is ongoing, are shared with the high school staff and used to match student to job placements in and out of the school.

A variety of vocational experiences have proven successful for those with

**Exhibit 11.5**
**Preferred Vocational Components**

Predictable routine with a consistent schedule
Limited transitions, consistent staff, flexibility of work stations
Open-ended, nonconstrained work environment
Nonsequential tasks without excessive time constraints
Quiet environment, especially void of loud noises
Enclave work settings and supportive coworkers
Job coaches to give gentle reminders and prompt at task behaviors
Verbal task direction augmented by visual systems/pictures, diagrams, or symbols
Opportunities to access space to employ self-calming techniques (break time, cafeteria, taking walks, etc.)

FXS. Whenever possible, school programs should provide a rotation of job placements early so that interest and competence can be assessed. As the student progresses through high school, work experience studies (WES) can provide academic credit and, at the same time, provide environments in which appropriate work behaviors can be practiced. This kind of program allows flexibility so that the individual with FXS can move from one job to another and experience a variety of work settings and work types before entering the world of work after graduation. Exhibit 11.5, generated from clinical experience with individuals with FXS, delineates the necessary components for successful vocational experiences.

## Social Development

Even though individuals with FXS demonstrate social behaviors, they often lack the skills necessary to effectively interact with others. It is extremely important to provide the vehicle through which their obvious interest can develop into a meaningful exchange of ideas.

Social skills are correlated with speech/language development but are not mutually exclusive. Waiting to teach social skills until speech fully develops is a mistake. The interaction develops by using turn taking to teach social reciprocity, the give and take of interaction. This can be expanded into lengthy verbal exchanges and ultimately the cultivation of good family and personal relationships.

During the elementary school years, the child with FXS is usually included within his typical peer group through most of the day. Even if the student with FXS is significantly affected, there are valuable units of time in the classroom when academic instruction is not the entire focus and social experiences may be of benefit. These periods can include group work, experiential centers, and cooperative learning. The elementary classroom environment is more conducive to accepting individual differences. Elementary school teachers typically receive more training in developmental models, learning style, and individualized instruction, making inclusion more effective at this age.

If a paraprofessional (teacher's aide) is assigned to provide one-to-one support to the student with FXS, it is important to define that role in a way that does not interfere with the posits of inclusion. For example, giving the child with FXS options to access supports is best. During times of high stress, the paraprofessional can be available to encourage calming activities and direct sensory integration support. At other times when a social component is emphasized, the paraprofessional can facilitate social interaction within a group of children.

Children at this age tend to accept individual differences across the board and are usually unaware of academic deficits. A general feeling of equality is shared. The individual with FXS is usually well liked because he is socially engaging, fun to be with, and easily integrated.

It is important to encourage the child with FXS to participate in social activities such as scouts, music lessons, sports, or church groups as much as possible during this developmental period. Imitating typical peers and learning socially appropriate behaviors through repeated exposure will promote skill development that will pay off for many years to come (Sobesky 1996; Braden 2000a).

The social skills training model included in exhibit 11.6 can be facilitated by a paraprofessional, teacher, school counselor, or social worker. This model can be used to provide the foundation for the acquisition of interactive skills within a natural environment at school and in social activities.

The social behavior typically manifested during the middle school years is immature, even though the physical development of those with FXS is perfectly normal. This paradox presents a difficult dilemma because our society expects normal social behavior from those who look normal. Teaching age-appropriate behavior at this point becomes the focus. Because individuals with FXS respond well to rules, it is effective to note immature social behaviors with comments such as the following: "That is what your little sister would do." "Now that you are 14 and wearing a Bronco jersey, you don't chew with your mouth open anymore."

Social/sexual behaviors also require a fair amount of program planning. Commonly, the prerequisite social behaviors are reinforced during preschool and elementary school. When the preadolescent moves to the middle school environment, new challenges present. A normal interest in heterosexual relationships is intensified at this stage of development. The adolescent with FXS may become obsessed with male/female relationships. Looking at magazine ads and television surfing for romantic and intimate interaction are common ways to satisfy a need to gain vicarious access to the experience.

Sex education at this point of development should include open discussion about curiosity. If sexual curiosity is not discussed, the adolescent feels that it is shameful and tries to hide his interest. If voyeurlike behavior is not addressed openly, it takes on a repressed quality that feeds obsessive-compulsive behavior and could result in misunderstood motivation with legal ramifications (Braden 2000a).

Developing social behaviors is imperative because individuals with FXS need to be accepted in order to build competence and credibility in the world of work. Issues involving typical peers present during the middle and high school years. Heterosexual relationships will be modeled, and individuals with FXS will be exposed to those behaviors at school. Dating, school dances, and extracurricular activities are all part of the middle and high school experience. Appropriate participation can be successful if adequate social behaviors have been learned.

**Exhibit 11.6**
**Social Skills Training Model**

---

*Level 1*

---

Turn Taking with an Adult

- Parent/teacher chooses a toy or activity of high interest.
- Adult verbally models "my turn" or, if the individual is nonverbal, points to self and takes a turn.
- Adult gives the individual a game piece, toy, etc., and says "your turn," pointing to him and shaping the pointing to self.

- Individual indicates desired object, toy, or activity.
- Individual waits his turn and imitates the role model.
- Individual points to himself, picks up game piece, toy, etc., and takes a turn.

This process continues for at least five exchanges.

Variations: Pegs, Lego building, drawing a person (hangman), drawing cards from a deck, passing objects back and forth, etc.

Turn Taking with Another Child

- Adult acts as facilitator and prompts whenever necessary.

- Individuals wait and take turns, pointing or verbalizing when it is their turn.

---

*Level 2*

---

Verbal Exchange with an Adult while Developing
Spontaneously Initiated Verbal Interaction

- Adult gives individual a compliment: "I like your shirt."
- Individual repeats, "I like your shirt."

- Individual responds with "Thank you."
- Adult responds with "Thank you."

As the interaction becomes spontaneous and the individual initiates the compliment without prompts from the facilitator, the adult begins the generalization step.

Generalization Step: This step can be facilitated by a visual cue such as pecs, photograph, icon, rebus symbol, or sentence strip. Trainer holds up visual cue to prompt a broader array of complimentary statements. For example, picture of a face to prompt facial features or a sentence strip to cue, "I like your Lego space ship," "I like your drawing," etc.

---

*Level 3*

---

Verbal Exchange Using Facts of Personal Information
Already Mastered in Isolation

- Adult asks (from a list of personal information questions):
  "Do you have a brother?"
  "What is his name?"
  "Do you have a pet?"
  "Where do you live?"

- Individual answers the question and asks the same question.

Generalization Step: Adult facilitates this interaction between two students and prompts whenever necessary.

---

*(continues)*

**Exhibit 11.6** (*Continued*)

---

### *Level 4*

---

#### Taking Turns Talking to an Adult

This level is facilitated by a traveling notebook provided by parents to teacher/therapist. The parent includes information related to an experience, event, book read, movie, trip taken, etc. This information forms the basis for discussion. It is later replaced by a chart that the child fills in and uses in place of a sentence strip.

| | |
|---|---|
| • Adult says, "Talk to me," and passes talking stick to the individual. If necessary, prompts discussion about an event discussed in the notebook. | • Individual responds with information about a specific event, movie, or experience. |
| • Adult asks questions related to the information shared and begins to count the number of reciprocal exchanges, dealing out cards. | • Individual responds to the question and offers a reciprocal response. A card is given after each appropriate exchange. |

At the end of the discussion, cards are counted and tallied on personal interaction sheets.

#### Taking Turns Talking to Another Group Member

| | |
|---|---|
| • Adult facilitates interaction between two individuals within a group milieu. | • Members pass the talking stick back and forth. The stick cues the turn and reinforces waiting a turn. |
| • Adult begins the discussion with, "Talk to (other group member) about your trip to the zoo (or any other event noted in the traveling notebook)." | • Individual responds to other group member but waits his turn. |

---

### *Level 5*

---

#### Taking Turns Talking and Listening

This level is to reinforce the importance of sharing talking time and listening. Questioning after listening is prompted verbally or with a visual icon or symbol. Formulating questions appropriate to the discussion is also reinforced. Cards and the talking stick can also be used to signal the speaker.

| | |
|---|---|
| • Adult holds up visual icon or a current event from a newspaper or presents an idea to be discussed. | • Group member responds with appropriate verbal exchange. |
| | • Group member passes talking stick to group member of his choice and listens. |
| • Group member formulates a question about the subject discussed. | • Group member answers the question and listens. |

Variation: Discussions can be based on newspaper events (can use Weekly Readers or kids' sections of the newspaper), sports events (males with fragile X syndrome usually love sports), or contrived scenarios about taking a trip to Disney World, a local amusement park, a TV game show, etc.

---

**Exhibit 11.7**
**Sex Education**

---

*Changes in You: An Introduction to Sexual Education through an Understanding of Puberty,* Peggy Sigel (James Stanfield Publishing Co.)

*Circles: A Multi-media Package to Aid in the Development of Appropriate Social/Sexual Behavior in the Developmentally Disabled Individual,* Marilyn Champagne and Leslie Walder-Hirsch (James Stanfield Publishing Co.)

*Life Horizons: "Sexuality and the Mentally Handicapped,"* Winifred Kempton (James Stanfield Publishing Co.)

*The Family Education Program Manual,* Katherine Simpson (Planned Parenthood: Shasta-Diablo, 1291 Oakland Boulevard, Walnut Creek, CA 94596; 510-935-4066)

*Human Sexuality: A Portfolio for Persons with Developmental Disabilities,* 2d ed., Victoria Livingston and Mary E. Knapp (Planned Parenthood of Seattle–King Co., 2211 E. Madison Street, Seattle, WA 98112-5397; 206-328-7716)

*Positive Approaches: A Sexuality Guide for Teaching Developmentally Disabled Persons,* Lisa Maurer (Planned Parenthood of Delaware, 625 Shipley Street, Wilmington, DE 19801; 302-655-7293)

*Safe and Okay: Elementary Level. A NO-GO-TELL! Curriculum for Disabled Children* (grades 3–6), Shella Brener and Elizabeth J. Krents (Child Abuse and Disabled Children Prog., Lexington Center, Inc., 30th Avenue and 75th Street, Jackson Heights, NY 11370; 718-899-8800)

*Special Education: Secondary F.L.A.S.H. (Family Life and Sexual Health). A Curriculum for 5th through 10th Grades,* Jane Stangle (Seattle–King County Dept. of Health, Family Planning Publication, 110 Prefontaine Avenue South, Suite 300, Seattle, WA 98104; 206-296-4672)

---

*Source: New Hampshire Challenge,* fall 1999.

## Sex Education

This area is very important but one of the most difficult to discuss. Religious and ethical considerations may preclude honest and open communication about sexual issues. Many typical peers are sexually active at this stage of development, regardless of parental influence. The problem can be extremely complex and far reaching. It is not easy to teach others how to respond as you wish, but it is possible to educate the individual with FXS about ways to respond to issues of privacy, exploitation, voyeurism, and sexual conduct (Krumm 1999). Exhibit 11.7 lists sexual education programs suggested for use with the FXS population.

## Behavioral Characteristics

Children with FXS sometimes have behavior problems that can interfere with learning (chap. 1). Teachers and therapists should be aware of these behaviors

**Exhibit 11.8**
**Common Behaviors in Children with Fragile X Syndrome**

| | |
|---|---|
| Hyperactivity (ADHD) | Excessive motion, darting about, rushing, difficulty staying still |
| Impulsivity | Difficulty waiting until needs can be met; requiring immediate attention; making decisions quickly without forethought |
| Limited attention span and concentration (ADD) | Difficulty sustaining attention, easily distracted, unable to focus and attend |
| Difficulty tolerating changes in routine | Easily upset by changes in schedule, routine, people, or expectations |
| Ritualistic and repetitive behavior | Compulsive repetition of hand movements, behavioral rituals such as turning lights off and on, closing doors and drawers, and verbal repetition or perseveration |
| Social anxiety or shyness | Difficulty interacting with others on request; avoiding eye contact, handshakes, or other forms of social interaction |
| Aggression | Hitting or striking out at others, often directed toward the primary care giver |

*Source:* Braden 2000a.

when developing behavior-management strategies, making classroom accommodations, and developing individual programming. Exhibit 11.8 lists behaviors often seen in children with FXS. Not all children will exhibit the behaviors listed. It is common, however, to observe these behaviors in children as they pass through certain developmental levels. Research shows that, as children with FXS mature into adulthood, many of the behavioral symptoms manifested subside (Braden 1991), resulting in a decrease in behavioral excesses, often including aggression.

## Anxiety and Behavior

The effects of anxiety on behavior have been described in the normal population and in females affected with FXS (Bourne 1995; Sobesky 1996; Braden 2000a). Anxiety may manifest in panic attacks so debilitating that daily functioning is affected. Females with FXS report fluctuating between a flight or fight response when they become anxious. Simply put, when they feel that they are losing control, they become anxious and want to leave, or escape the environment that is causing the anxiety (chap. 1). On the other hand, the response may be more consistent with a fight reaction, which may result in verbal or physical abuse. The anxiety overrides impulse control and may result in atypical behavioral patterns (Scharfenaker et al. 1996; Braden 2000a, 2000c; Sobesky 1996). Similar behavioral manifestations have been noted in males with FXS. Physicians may recommend the use of medications to help manage the behavioral problems while reducing the anxiety (chap. 8). Although this can be an effective treatment for males and females with FXS (Tranfaglia 1995; Hagerman 2000; chap. 8), it should be cautioned that medication, without adjunct programming, may fall short (chap. 9).

Educational and clinical staff, as well as care givers, must understand the effects of anxiety on behavior. Although it is important to address behaviors and provide boundaries, it is equally important to understand the causes of the behavior before implementing or designing a behavioral program (chap. 9). In other words, treating the symptom (the behavioral outbursts), rather than the cause, may result in an ineffectual behavior program.

Some behaviors seem to come and go without apparent antecedents or causes. These behaviors can increase when the individual with FXS becomes nervous, anxious, or aroused. For example, complimenting an individual with FXS may bring out feelings of anxiety due to insecurity about how to respond when put on the spot (Braden 2000a, 2000c; Sobesky 1996). The attention given to the individual with FXS may create perceived inadequacies and embarrassment. The anxiety may interfere with attempts to cope, resulting in fear or a need to avoid any subsequent experience that is similar.

## Behavior Intervention Plans

Because children with FXS can exhibit behavior that interferes with learning, it is important to develop and include a behavior intervention plan (BIP) in the individualized education plan (IEP). Under IDEA, children cannot be denied a free and appropriate public education because they have behavior problems (Braden 2000a). If the behavior interferes with learning, they are required to have a BIP. This plan encourages educators to carefully address behavior by understanding its function before developing an intervention (see also chap. 9).

Most behaviors, even disruptive behaviors, persist only while serving a purpose. For example, infants learn that, when they cry, they get attention: being fed, changed, or played with. That behavior persists as long as it gets the desired attention. When children learn to communicate their needs using gestures or verbal language, it is no longer necessary to cry or scream. If the verbal attempts to get the necessary attention fail, the child reverts back to disruptive and noisy behavior to get the desired response. Children learn over time that their behavior leads to something called a *consequence*. The consequence can be positive or negative.

Educational researchers and educators working with children with FXS have also learned that at times a behavior results from something that has just happened. For example, a child who begins to flap his hands may have just experienced excessive noises or a large crowd of people that caused arousal and overstimulation. When this happens, the event before the behavior is the *antecedent*. After extensive study and clinical experience of both the causes and the function of behavior for children with FXS (and other children with disabilities) (Maurice et al. 1996; Sobesky 1996; Braden 2000a; Hagerman 2000), educators and therapists have learned effective methods to help change negative or disruptive behavior.

It is important to analyze the antecedents when identifying the target behavior to be reduced or increased. In addition, there are ways to observe and analyze the function of a behavior as well (Maurice et al. 1996; Braden 2000; Myles et al. 1998). A behavior may serve as an avoidance or escape mechanism. Children may prefer punishment (time out, loss of privilege) to continuing a task they dislike. Because numerous factors can play into behavioral episodes, it is important to observe the child over several days and in various settings. This gives the observer a better idea of what function the behavior serves and under what conditions.

Myles and Simpson developed a functional assessment tool that qualifies the behavior. This approach notes not only when the behavior occurs but also under what conditions (structured activities, group, playing with others or alone, during times of transitions, in the morning or evening, and within certain environments (such as the classroom, gym, or library).

The following are examples of behavior plans taken from actual cases.

### Functional Behavior Analysis and Behavior Intervention Plan

Presenting Problem: Jan is an eighth grader at Saint Mary's Middle School. Jan has fragile X syndrome with a full mutation. Jan is very shy and tends to avoid social interaction. She has recently developed excessive picking behaviors. She began picking scabs from insect bites, scrapes, and cuts this summer. Now that school has begun, she is picking more often and seems to engage in the picking behavior in times of stress. She is picking scabs at night and puts Band-Aids over bleeding scabs when she goes to school because she becomes embarrassed.

Frequency: Jan picks at herself approximately 15 times a day.

Function of Behavior: It seems that Jan is inept at coping with high stress created by social interaction at school, as outlined in exhibit 11.9.

Discussion of Function and Conditions: Because the target behavior has increased since school began, the school environment may provoke anxi-

**Exhibit 11.9**
**Jan's Behavior Intervention Plan**

| Antecedent | Behavior | Consequence |
|---|---|---|
| Jan becomes anxious about a social interaction. | Jan picks at a wound. | Jan puts a Band-Aid over her wound. |
| Jan engages in deep relaxation exercises when anxious. | Jan becomes relaxed. Jan practices deep relaxation exercises when she's in speech class or before going to lunch each day at school. | Jan does not pick at her skin. |

Baseline: 15X a day.

**Exhibit 11.10**
**Functional Behavior Assessment**

Name _____

Behavior to Target_____ Staff Member_____

Date of Assessment_____ Location_____

Function of the Behavior_____

| Time | Antecedent | Behavior | Consequence |
|---|---|---|---|
|  |  |  |  |
|  |  |  |  |
|  |  |  |  |
|  |  |  |  |
|  |  |  |  |
|  |  |  |  |
|  |  |  |  |
|  |  |  |  |
|  |  |  |  |

ety. The analysis revealed that Jan's behavior escalated during speech class, most likely because Jan anticipated speaking in front of the class. The behavior also escalated during lunchtime and unstructured situations when Jan may become stressed about social expectations. Exhibit 11.10 provides a template for a functional behavioral assessment.

## Example of Behavioral Intervention Plan I

Target Behavior: Cursing at school

Baseline: Multiple days, averages 10× a day

Functional Behavior Assessment: David was observed in his school placement from 9:00 A.M. until 3:00 P.M. He was observed in his regular education classroom, playground, lunchroom, special education classroom,
auditorium, and gym class, as outlined in exhibit 11.11.

The assessment clearly implicates transition and anticipation of large-group
activities in either the gym or the auditorium. The cursing seems to be a function of his anxiety and decreases when the pressure to go into a crowded and
noisy environment is removed. The behavior intervention plan (exhibit 11.12)
should incorporate that knowledge into managing David's behavior.

The most important element to any plan is data collection. If a plan is working, it can be substantiated through the test of frequency and change from the

**Exhibit 11.11**

**Functional Behavior Assessment for David**

| Time | Antecedent | Behavior | Consequence |
|---|---|---|---|
| 9:35 | Lining up in regular education classroom to go to PE class. | Curses | Teacher redirects to sit down and wait. |
| 9:40 | David is sitting and class has left. | Cursing decreases | Teacher walks David to the gym for PE. |
| 9:45 | David is walking to PE with teacher. | Cursing increases | David is removed from PE and returns to classroom. |
| 9:55 | David is in the classroom. | Cursing stops | Teacher gives David positive reinforcement. |
| 12:00 | David lines up to go to the cafeteria for lunch. | Curses | David stays in the classroom to eat and isn't allowed to join his class in the lunchroom. |
| 12:15 | David eats his lunch alone in the classroom with teaching assistant. | Cursing stops | David goes out to recess. |
| 12:30 | Teacher discusses procedure to leave classroom and go into the auditorium for a presentation. | Curses | David is ignored. |
| 12:35 | Cursing is ignored and the classmates line up. | Cursing increases | David is asked to take a note to the office instead of following his class to the auditorium. |

**Exhibit 11.12**
**Behavior Intervention Plan for David**

---

Targeted Behavior: Cursing at school
Frequency: Averages 10X day
Consequences/Interventions Attempted:
  Time out, peer buddy escort, loss of privileges, extinction
Functional Behavior Assessment:
  Antecedent is transition into loud, crowded environment. Function of behavior is to
  avoid an experience that creates anxiety.
Level 1
  1. David anticipates transition to loud, crowded environment.
  2. Teacher presents him with three forced choice picture cards:
    • Stay in classroom
    • Go to PE or any other environment that is loud and crowded
    • Help with a school job
    Teacher ignores cursing and reinforces adaptive behavior.
Level 2
  1. David anticipates the transition and tells teacher he cannot go to the auditorium, gym,
    etc. (he refrains from cursing).
  2. David is given forced choice cards to desensitize reaction.
    • Go to auditorium, gym, etc., for 2 minutes in the beginning of the class.
    • Go to auditorium, gym, etc., for 2 minutes at the end of the class.
  3. Teacher reinforces his choice and success without cursing.

---

*Source:* Braden 2000a.

baseline. The baseline data are always gathered before a behavior program en-
sues, and data gathering continues throughout the intervention phase. When a
predetermined pass criterion is met, the program can be faded and data taken
once a week.

## Example of Behavioral Intervention Plan II

Target Behavior: Bites index finger (school only)
Baseline: Averages 20X a day (school only)
Functional Behavior Assessment: Tim was observed at his school placement
  from 9:00 to 2:00 on Monday and from 12:00 to 3:00 on Wednesday. He
  was observed in all included and special education classes (exhibit 11.13).
Discussion of Function: An analysis indicates that Tim bites his finger or
  pushes against his finger whenever he is excited or amused. Consequences
  have not effectively reduced the behavior. The behavior seems to be used
  as a way to calm down an autonomic reaction to a pleasurable or excitable

**Exhibit 11.13**
**Functional Behavior Assessment for Tim**

| Time | Antecedent | Behavior | Consequence |
|------|-----------|----------|-------------|
| 9:20 | Watching cartoon video in home room | Bites and pushes with teeth against index finger | Ignored |
| 10:15 | Waiting to take a turn playing bongo drum in music | Bites index finger | Told he couldn't have a turn |
| 11:45 | Waiting in line for turn on relay team in PE | Pushes against index finger with teeth | Peers on team tell him to stop |

**Exhibit 11.14**
**Behavioral Intervention Plan for Tim**

Targeted Behavior: Bites index finger (school only)
Frequency: Averages 20X a day (school only)
Consequences/Interventions Attempted:
   Verbal reminders, wearing gloves, keeping hands busy, redirection
Functional Behavior Assessment:
   Antecedent is anticipation of an exciting or humorous event. Function of behavior is to calm himself in some way, bringing deep pressure to his sensory system.

| Antecedent | Behavior | Consequence |
|-----------|----------|-------------|
| Tim becomes overstimulated (watches video, becomes excited or amused) | Bites finger, pushes finger against teeth | When Tim begins to bring his finger to his mouth, immediately hand him a squeeze ball, nerf ball, or other apparatus to push on instead of his finger. The trainer reinforces the use of the replacement behavior and ignores the biting or pushing on finger. |

condition. Because it is a nonvoluntary reaction, completely eliminating the behavior by punishing Tim would prove nonproductive. An important component of this behavior program is to provide Tim with an alternative behavior to replace his finger biting. For example, he may be conditioned to push his hands together, squeeze his hands together, or fold his hands when he becomes excited. Exhibit 11.14 outlines Tim's behavior plan.

## Teaching Girls

As mentioned earlier in this chapter, girls with FXS are generally affected to a lesser degree than are boys. Many girls with FXS do have learning disabilities and emotional difficulties. Girls often function so "normally" that early identification is unusual. Girls may have difficulties with depression and mood disorders. A large number of girls are shy and socially phobic. They may worry excessively about what others may be thinking (chap. 1). Exhibit 11.15 lists characteristics that are often seen in girls with FXS.

Even though much has been written about girls with FXS (Sobesky et al. 1996; Kemper et al. 1988; Freund and Reiss 1991; chap. 1), very little has been written about teaching girls. Girls are often recognized for their creative writing ability and enjoy written language and English classes. As is the case with the males affected with FXS, the girls, too, experience difficulty in math, auditory memory, and visual organization. Bennetto and Pennington (1996) and chapter 6 outline a neurocognitive profile in females with a full mutation. Exhibit 11.16 lists areas of deficit and provides strategies that have proven successful in the intervention process. It is believed that memory improves with associations and external structure (Grigsby et al. 1992).

When it comes to social interaction, girls become intimidated and anxious. Even though a girl may experience anxiety at school, parents will often find themselves frustrated by the lack of assertion their daughter demonstrates at school while exhibiting a controlling nature at home. Parents may hear constant complaints about school, while teachers hear few. Girls with FXS can often benefit from social language groups or friendship groups at school and in private therapy. Social skills can be taught in much the same way as academic skills. The school staff should be consulted about social behavior at school. They may have a very different view of the girl's social functioning, peer interaction, and class participation. The school social worker or counselor may be of assistance and a good resource for the child and family.

There are several studies related to the emotional functioning of girls with FXS. Sobesky (1996) notes findings suggesting that girls with a full mutation have problems with shyness, social anxiety, attentional problems, and poor eye contact. As the girls mature, there are a myriad of difficulties relating to both emotional and cognitive difficulties. Although adult females with a full mutation seem to experience these deficits more extensively, some females with a premutation also experience anxiety disorders, panic disorders, and social phobias (Franke et al. 1996, 1998).

**Exhibit 11.15**
**Symptom Checklist for Females**

Name: _____

Date of Birth: _____

Age: _____

Full mutation _____     Premutation_____

No. of CGG repeats _____     Year DNA Tested _____

Current medications_____     Dosages_____

|  | mild | moderate | severe |
|---|---|---|---|
| Aggressive/behavioral outbursts | | | |
| Anxious | | | |
| Cognitive delays | | | |
| Closes eyes while talking | | | |
| Clumsiness, poor motor planning | | | |
| Diagnosed bipolar disorder | | | |
| Hyperactivity | | | |
| Impulsive | | | |
| Interpersonal problems | | | |
| Lack of initiation | | | |
| Language delays (odd communication patterns) | | | |
| Math difficulties | | | |
| Mood instability | | | |
| Outgoing, gregarious | | | |
| Panic attacks | | | |
| Premature puberty | | | |
| Sensitivity | | | |
| Shy | | | |
| Social anxiety | | | |
| Visual/spatial difficulties (gets lost, directions difficult) | | | |

Please add any additional symptoms not included above:

**Exhibit 11.16**
**Suggested Strategies for Girls**

---

Suggested Strategies for Math
  Use concrete manipulative materials to teach concepts and mathematical operations.
  Use visual cues whenever possible to reinforce mathematical operations.
  Allow additional time to reduce the possibility of provoking performance anxiety.
  Minimize auditory distractions during time periods when concentration is required
    (computation, problem solving).
  Use diagrams, illustrations, and visual patterns whenever teaching a new concept.
  Use repetition and patterning whenever rote memory tasks are required.
Suggested Strategies for Auditory Memory
  Give specific instructions in a slow, simple, and concrete manner.
  Place the student close to the instructor to ensure attention and concentration.
  Structure the environment to eliminate auditory distractions—use earphones, carrels, or
    seating arrangements.
  Vary presentation to include frequent breaks to avoid attention difficulties and lack of
    concentration.
Suggested Strategies for Visual Organization
  Limit amount to be copied from printed or written materials.
  Simplify visually presented materials to eliminate a cluttered or excessively stimulating
    format.
  Provide visual cues—such as color coding, numbering, and arrows—to organize written
    tasks.
  Give specific concrete cues when giving oral directions that require an organized format.
  Give additional time for written assignments, when needed.

---

Clinical observations indicate that young girls with a full mutation are often referred to clinic because of symptoms of attention deficit hyperactivity disorder (ADHD). Poor impulse control, a related feature of ADHD, may interact with cognitive deficits, fueling negative experiences with decision making and behavior conducive to independence (chap. 1).

Adult females with FXS report diagnoses when reflecting on their medical and school histories during intake. There is diagnostic confusion in their childhood history. It is unclear whether many of the symptoms often observed in earlier development (anxiety, obsessive-compulsive disorder, and ADHD) are comorbid with psychiatric disorders diagnosed at adulthood or are precursors to a later expression of a psychiatric disorder (Papolos and Papolos 1999).

Bipolar disorder has been seen in some adult females with FXS. They have also reported early learning disabilities with problems focusing and concentrating. There may be a connection between earlier symptoms of poor attention span and obsessive behaviors and a subsequent psychiatric diagnosis as an adult (chap. 1). At any rate, if the girl affected by FXS does not meet the qualifications to access special education services through IDEA, it may be appropriate to access services under a section 504 plan. This 504 plan mandates that *individuals with impairments that substantially limit a major life activity, such as learning, are entitled to academic adjustments and auxiliary aids and services, so that courses, examinations, and services will be accessible to them.* The following information is taken from a 504 plan written for a girl with FXS.

## CASE STUDY: RATIONALE FOR ACCOMMODATIONS

Even though Sara has had a difficult ninth-grade year, it is incumbent on all providers to support Sara and provide her with the necessary skills to access her true potential and foster independence. Her academic challenges and emotional status are clearly correlated. It is critical to address her school failures while carefully considering the merit of her current school placement. Simply repeating her ninth-grade experience will not remediate her learning deficits. Additionally, she is not learning compensatory strategies to improve her performance. She is in need of alternative teaching methods to help her succeed. The following accommodations and curricular adaptations are offered.

Because Sara is easily distracted and needs access to a low-distraction environment, the following accommodations are warranted:

—Preferential seating away from distraction with access to a private study area (study carrel) and a place to work 1:1 or in a small group

—Preferential seating near the instruction so the teacher can summon her attention without humiliating or ostracizing her

Because Sara may demonstrate poor impulse control, she may require the following behavioral strategies:

—Firm boundaries with consequences she understands

—Scheduled and frequent breaks

—Systematic procedural remedy to slow down her immediate reaction (e.g., stop, count back from 10 to 0, count by twos to 50, recite months of the year, etc.)

Because Sara may engage in off-task behavior, she may require the following modifications:

—Redirect her behavior.

—Query her need for a break to refocus.

—Give her a preferred task to substitute for the task she is having trouble pursuing and then reintroduce the original task.

—Offer Sara choices of breaks, tasks, and schedules.

Because Sara becomes anxious and subconsciously may fear failure, she may need help with the following:

—Exempt her from timed tasks and tests.

—Substitute some written tests with oral tests.

—Decrease the length of her assignments.

—Initially limit the amount of homework, gradually adding more as she is able to tolerate the increase.

—Positively reinforce her successes.

Because Sara has difficulty with concentration and working memory, to include executive functioning deficits (formulating a plan of action and initiating), the following accommodations may be necessary:

—Allow additional time to complete work and for tests.

—Allow frequent breaks.

—Skill stream those academic areas that are particularly difficult; include only skills that will enhance her functionality.

Because Sara demonstrates symptoms similar to those of a nonverbal learning disorder (right-hemisphere learning disorder), she may require the following accommodations:

—Special considerations can be made for disorganization, tardiness, navigation difficulty, and understanding of spatial relationships.

—Novel situations may be very difficult and force anxiety. Sara is adept at hiding her discontent and fear. She has begun to avoid dealing with her academic disappointments.

—All instruction needs to be direct and concrete. Sara will not understand ambiguous cues. Write out specific expectations for any situation Sara may misconstrue.

—Begin a task and ask Sara to complete it. Use backward chaining as a method to assist with her executive functioning issues.

Because Sara demonstrates difficulty reading social ambiguity and initiating social interactions, the following accommodations will be necessary:

—Enroll her in a social skills group to practice social risk taking and reciprocity.

—Give her feedback related to social behavior that is always positive and constructive.

—Implement case management using mentors and role playing to build social strategies.

—Implement a concrete social skills training curriculum to assist Sara in expanding her social interaction.

## Premutation Carriers

Most individuals with the premutation are unaffected cognitively, although exceptions to this rule are outlined in chapter 1. If a child with the premutation demonstrates significant learning or emotional problems, the academic interventions outlined above can be tailored to the child's specific problems. Most premutation carriers whom the teacher encounters will be the mothers of the children affected by FXS. These mothers are remarkable for their insight and strength in finding interventions that can help their children.

They are called *carriers* because they carry a specific gene they pass on to their children. I call them carriers because they carry all the hopes and dreams possible for their children. They carry their fears, anxiety, struggles, defeat, and pain. They are capable of carrying the joy of success and the disappointment of developmental delays all at the same time. They carry a favorite toy, an old picture or a funny cap to bring comfort and security wherever they go. They carry mental ammunition to their school placement staffings and strategies for treatment. They carry the strength to defy all odds and march on with fortified courage and unconditional love. These are the carriers I know.

## References

Bennetto, L., and B. F. Pennington. 1996. The neuropsychology of fragile X syndrome. In R. J. Hagerman and A. Cronister (eds.), *Fragile X syndrome: Diagnosis, treatment, and research,* 2d ed. Baltimore: Johns Hopkins Univ. Press, pp. 210–248.

Bourne, E. J. 1995. *The anxiety and phobias workbook.* Oakland, Calif.: New Harbinger Publications.

Braden, M. 1989. The Logo Reading System, 100 E. St. Vrain #200, Colorado Springs, CO 80903.

———. 1991. A Screening Instrument for FRA-X Males. Ph.D. dissertation, University of Denver.

———. 1999. Sex education for children with disabilities: A beginning conversation. *New Hampshire Challenge,* PO Box 579, Dover, NH 03821-0579.

———. 2000a. *Fragile: Handle with care; more about fragile X syndrome—adolescents and adults.* Dillon, Colo.: Spectra Publishing Co.

———. 2000b. Education. In J. D. Weber (ed.), *Children with fragile X syndrome: A parent's guide.* Bethesda, Md.: Woodbine House, pp. 243–305.

———. 2000c. Treatment of aggression in children and adults with fragile X syndrome. *Foundation Quarterly,* spring 2000.

Brown, J., M. Braden, and W. E. Sobesky. 1991. The treatment of emotional and behavioral problems. In R. J. Hagerman and A. C. Silverman (eds.), *Fragile X syndrome: Diagnosis, treatment, and intervention.* Baltimore: Johns Hopkins Univ. Press.

Dykens, E. M., R. M. Hodapp, and J. F. Leckman. 1987. Strengths and weaknesses in the intellectual functioning of males with fragile X syndrome. *Am. J. Med. Genet.* 28:13–15.

Edmark Reading Program, Edmark, PO Box 9702, Redmond, WA 98073-9721.

Franke, P., W. Maier, M. Hautzinger, O. Weiffenbach, M. Gansicke, B. Iwers, F. Poustka, S. G. Schwab, and U. Froster. 1996. Fragile-X carrier females: Evidence for a distinct psychopathological phenotype? *Am. J. Med. Genet.* 64:334–339.

Franke, P., M. Leboyer, M. Gansicke, O. Weiffenbach, V. Biancalana, P. Cornillet-Lefebre, M. F. Croquette, U. Froster, S. G. Schwab, F. Poustka, M. Hautzinger, and W. Maier. 1998. Genotype-phenotype relationship in female carriers of the premutation and full mutation of *FMR-1. Psychiatry Res.* 80:113–127.

Freund, L., and A. L. Reiss. 1991. Cognitive profiles associated with the FraX syndrome in males and females. *Am. J. Med. Genet.* 38:542–547.

Gibb, C. 1992. The most common cause of learning difficulties: A profile of fragile X syndrome and its implications for education. *Educ. Res.* 34(3).

Graham, P. J., J. Turk, and F. Verhulst. 1999. Behavioural and cognitive psychotherapies. In *Child psychiatry: A developmental approach.* Oxford: Oxford Univ. Press, pp. 401–420.

Grigsby, J., M. B. Kemper, and R. J. Hagerman. 1992. Verbal learning and memory among heterozygous fragile X females. *Am. J. Med. Genet.* 43:111–115.

Hagerman, R. J. 1996. Physical and behavioral phenotype. In R. J. Hagerman and A. Cronister (eds.), *Fragile X syndrome: Diagnosis, treatment, and research,* 2d ed. Baltimore: Johns Hopkins Univ. Press, pp. 3–87.

———. 2000. Treatment of aggression in children and adults with fragile X syndrome. *Foundation Q,* winter 2000.

Hagerman, R. J., M. Kemper, and M. Hudson. 1985. Learning disabilities and attentional problems in boys with the fragile X syndrome. *Am. J. Dis. Child.* 139:674–678.

Hodapp, R. M., J. F. Leckman, E. M. Dykens, S. Sparrow, D. Zelinsky, and S. Ort. 1992. K-ABC profiles in children with fragile X syndrome, Down syndrome, and nonspecific mental retardation. *Am. J. Ment. Retard.* 97:39–46.

Individuals with Disabilities Education Act of 1997, 20 U.S.C. 1400 et seq.

Kaufman, A. S., and N. P. Kaufman. 1983. *Kaufman Assessment Battery for Children: Administration and scoring manual.* Circle Pines, Minn.: American Guidance Services.

Kemper, M. B., R. J. Hagerman, R. S. Ahmad, and R. Mariner. 1986. Cognitive profiles and the spectrum of clinical manifestations in heterozygous fragile (X) females. *Am. J. Med. Genet.* 23:139–156.

Kemper, M. B., R. J. Hagerman, and D. Altshul-Stark. 1988. Cognitive profiles of boys with the fragile X syndrome. *Am. J. Med. Genet.* 30:191–200.

Krumm, J. 1999. Sex education for children with disabilities. *New Hampshire Challenge* 12(1):12–19.

Maccini, P., and C. A. Hughes. 1997. Mathematics interventions for adolescents with learning disabilities. *Learn. Disabil. Res. Pract.* 12(3):168–176.

Maurice, C., G. Green, and S. C. Luce. 1996. *Behavioral intervention for young children with autism.* Austin, Tex.: PRO-ED.

Mazzocco, M. M. M., and R. O'Connor. 1993. Fragile X syndrome: A guide for teachers of young children. *Young Children,* Nov, pp. 73–77.

Mercer, D. D., and S. P. Miller. 1992. Teaching students with learning problems in math to acquire, understand, and apply basic math facts. *Remedial Special Educ.* 13(3): 19–35.

Miezejeski, C. M., and V. J. Hinton. 1992. Fragile X learning disability: Neurobehavioral research, diagnostic models and treatment options. In R. J. Hagerman and P. McKenzie (eds.), *International Fragile X Conference proceedings.* Dillon, Colo.: Spectra Publishing, pp. 165–166.

Myles, B. S., and R. L. Simpson. 1998. *Asperger syndrome: A guide for educators and parents.* Austin, Tex.: PRO-ED.

Papolos, D. F., and J. Papolos. 1999. *The bipolar child.* New York: Random House.

Pennington, B. F., and L. Bennetto. 1998. Toward a neuropsychology of mental retardation. In J. A. Burack, R. M. Hodapp, and E. Zigler (eds.), *Handbook of mental retardation and development.* Cambridge: Cambridge Univ. Press, pp. 80–114.

PL 94-142, Education for All Handicapped Children Act of 1975 (23 August 1977), 20 U.S.C. 140 et seq; *Federal Register* 42(163), 42474–42518.

PL 99-457, Education of the Handicapped Act Amendments of 1986 (22 September 1986), *Congressional Record* 132(125), H 7893–7912.

Scharfenaker, S., R. O'Connor, T. Stackhouse, M. Braden, L. Hickman, and K. Gray. 1996. An integrated approach to intervention. In R. J. Hagerman and A. Cronister (eds.), *Fragile X syndrome: Diagnosis, treatment, and research,* 2d ed. Baltimore: Johns Hopkins Univ. Press, pp. 349–411.

Schopmeyer, B. B., and F. Lowe. 1992. *The fragile X child.* San Diego: Singular Publishing Co.

Sobesky, W. E. 1996. The treatment of emotional and behavioral problems in fragile X. In R. J. Hagerman and A. Cronister (eds.), *Fragile X syndrome: Diagnosis, treatment, and research,* 2d ed. Baltimore: Johns Hopkins Univ. Press, pp. 332–348.

Sobesky, W. E., B. F. Pennington, C. Porter, C. E. Hull, and R. J. Hagerman. 1994. Emotional and neurocognitive deficits in fragile X. *Am. J. Med. Genet.* 51:378–385.

Sobesky, W. E., A. K. Taylor, B. F. Pennington, L. Bennetto, D. Porter, J. Riddle, and R. J. Hagerman. 1996. Molecular/clinical correlations in females with fragile X. *Am. J. Med. Genet.* 64:340–345.

Spiridigliozzi, G., A. Lachiewicz, C. MacMordo, A. Vizoso, C. O'Donnell, A. McConkie-Rosell, and D. Burgess. 1994. *Educating boys with fragile X syndrome: A guide for parents and professionals.* Durham, N.C.: Duke Univ. Medical Center.

Sudhalter, V. 1992. The language system of males with fragile X syndrome. In R. J. Hagerman and P. McKenzie (eds.), *International Fragile X Conference proceedings.* Dillon, Colo.: Spectra Publishing, pp. 107–120.

Sudhalter, V., I. L. Cohen, W. Silverman, and E. G. Wolf-Schein. 1990. Conversational analyses of males with fragile X, Down syndrome, and autism: Comparison of the emergence of deviant language. *Am. J. Ment. Retard.* 94:431–441.

Tranfaglia, M. R. 1995. A parent's guide to drug treatment of fragile X syndrome. West Newbury, Mass.: FRAXA Research Foundation.

# CHAPTER 12

## *FMR1* Gene Expression and Prospects for Gene Therapy

Paul J. Hagerman, M.D., Ph.D.

This chapter is divided into two parts, related to one another but with distinct focus and purpose. The first part describes very recent work regarding the expression of the *FMR1* gene. This field has changed radically since the second edition of this book was published in 1996, as has the view of possible molecular approaches to the treatment or cure of fragile X syndrome (FXS). Thus, the first part of this chapter sets the stage for a discussion of how one might approach molecular genetic therapies for FXS—the second part of this chapter.

### Expression of the *FMR1* Gene

### The Conventional Model

FXS usually arises as a consequence of an expanded CGG repeat in the promoter region of the fragile X mental retardation 1 (*FMR1*) gene (Oberlé et al. 1991; Pieretti et al. 1991; Sutcliffe et al. 1992; Yu et al. 1992; Devys et al. 1993). In the general population, a wide range of repeat numbers (5–50 CGG repeats) is tolerated without clinical involvement or significant loss of repeat stability (Pieretti et al. 1991; Fu et al. 1991; Brown et al. 1993; Snow et al. 1993). For women with moderately expanded CGG elements in the premutation range (55–200 repeats), the propensity for transmission of full mutation alleles (>200 repeats) increases with higher repeat number (Fu et al. 1991; Heitz et al. 1992; Snow et al. 1993; Nolin et al. 1996; chaps. 2 and 3). Although carriers of CGG expansions in the premutation range are often stated to be clinically normal (Reiss et al. 1993; Mazzocco et al. 1993), a subset of premutation carriers

*Fragile X Syndrome: Diagnosis, Treatment, and Research,* third edition, ed. Randi Jenssen Hagerman and Paul J. Hagerman (Baltimore: Johns Hopkins University Press, 2002), © The Johns Hopkins University Press.

do manifest clinical features, including mood lability, anxiety, prominent ears, and/or mild developmental delays (Loesch et al. 1987, 1994; Rousseau et al. 1994; Smits et al. 1994; Dorn et al. 1994; Hagerman et al. 1996; Riddle et al. 1998; Franke et al. 1998; Tassone et al. 2000d; chap. 1). For individuals in the full mutation range (>200 repeats), the *FMR1* promoter region and CGG element are usually methylated at positions of CpG dinucleotides, which often leads to silencing of the *FMR1* gene (Oberlé et al. 1991; Pieretti et al. 1991; Bell et al. 1991; Sutcliffe et al. 1992; Devys et al. 1993). In the absence of transcriptional activity, no *FMR1* protein (FMRP) is produced, resulting in FXS (Pieretti et al. 1991).

The conventional model for FXS can thus be summarized as follows: Clinical involvement in FXS is due to reductions in or absence of FMRP *as a direct consequence of* methylation-coupled silencing of the *FMR1* gene.

However, this model does not explain why some premutation carriers are clinically involved. In particular, whereas silencing of the *FMR1* gene is generally believed to be a consequence of methylation of the promoter region and CGG repeat, this process does not normally occur in the premutation range. Thus, it is often supposed that all clinically involved individuals with premutation alleles in blood are actually mosaic for repeat size, with full mutation alleles in the central nervous system (CNS); this "mosaicism" conjecture can be referred to as the "blood versus brain" dichotomy. Moreover, unless one accepts the mosaicism argument (namely, that all clinically involved individuals with premutation alleles in blood actually have full mutation alleles in brain), it remains unclear why many premutation carriers are unaffected. One possibility is that the spectrum of clinical involvement in premutation individuals is due to "second-gene" effects.

In the absence of a direct measure of repeat size in CNS tissues, it is not possible to rule out cryptic mosaicism in every case where individuals with premutation alleles (in blood) are clinically affected. Nevertheless, it is now clear that premutation alleles themselves *can* give rise to clinical involvement in some cases. This conclusion draws on three developing lines of evidence. First, there are now reports of mild involvement in daughters of transmitting males (Tassone et al. 2000d). Since no male has ever been observed to pass a full mutation on to his daughters, it is highly unlikely that full mutation alleles exist within the CNS of these daughters. Second, premature ovarian failure (POF) is present in approximately 16% of carriers of premutation alleles but is no higher than in the general population in females with the full mutation (Vianna-Morgante et al. 1996; Allingham-Hawkins et al. 1999). Thus, POF is considered to be a form of clinical involvement in FXS that is unique to premutation alleles. What makes this argument compelling is not so much the existence of POF in the premutation range as its absence in the full mutation range. Third, nine males have now been observed with premutation alleles in the 78–

100 repeat range who have progressive cerebellar tremor associated with executive function defects as well as a generalized neurodegenerative process (Hagerman et al. 2001; chap. 1). Although this last set of observations is highly suggestive of a process involving premutation alleles, a similar process in the full mutation range or comorbidity with other genes leading to neurodegeneration have not been ruled out.

## *FMR1* Gene Expression in Carriers of Premutation CGG Expansions

The basis for the variable clinical picture among individuals with premutation alleles is not known at present. However, clinical involvement in premutation carriers predicts that FMRP levels would be at least moderately diminished within the premutation range and that any observed reductions would be secondary to reduced gene activity.

### FMRP Levels

FMRP levels have generally been thought to be normal for alleles in the premutation range (Devys et al. 1993; Verheij et al. 1993; Feng et al. 1995a; Kaufmann et al. 1999; Tassone et al. 1999), although most individuals studied had repeat sizes in the lower portion of the premutation range (<100 repeats). Using the immunocytochemical staining method of Willemsen et al. (1995, 1997), FMRP levels were determined for an additional group of premutation males (Tassone et al. 2000c). In agreement with the first prediction of the model, protein levels (percentage of lymphocytes staining positively) were moderately diminished in the upper portion of the premutation range. Thus, at the level of FMRP production, the model and the clinical picture are qualitatively consistent.

### *FMR1* Messenger RNA Levels

The second prediction of the model requires that transcriptional activity (*FMR1* mRNA levels) also be reduced in the upper portion of the premutation range; that is, protein levels would be reduced as a direct result of decreased gene activity. However, against expectations, mRNA levels are actually substantially increased in the upper premutation range, with an average fivefold elevation over normal levels for males with CGG repeats in the 100–200 repeat range, and are slightly but significantly elevated (mean 2.1-fold elevation; $p = 0.0039$) in the 55–100 repeat range (Tassone et al. 2000a, 2000c; fig. 12.1). For females with alleles in the premutation range, the mean mRNA elevations are not as pronounced; however, the variation in mRNA levels is greater than for males (Tassone et al. 2000a). Both of these findings are consistent with the variation in activation ratio, defined as the fraction of normal, active X chromosomes, in females with premutation alleles.

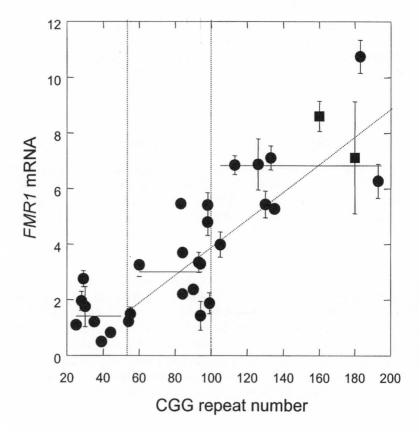

**Fig. 12.1.** Plot of *FMR1* mRNA levels as a function of CGG repeat number in the premutation range. *Source:* Adapted from Tassone et al. 2000a.

Two elements of the foregoing studies were critical for establishing that *FMR1* mRNA levels are elevated in the premutation range. First, mRNA levels were determined using the method of quantitative *f*RT-PCR (fluorescence reverse transcription-polymerase chain reaction) (Livak et al. 1995; Gibson et al. 1996; Heid et al. 1996). Methodologic details can be found in Tassone et al. (2000c) and references cited therein. The fluorescence method permits measurements of DNA levels at each cycle of the PCR amplification process. This continuous assay allows measurements to be made at much lower DNA concentrations, in a region of log-linear DNA amplification, where the ratios of fluorescent signals between sample and control are directly and quantitatively proportional to the concentrations of the original mRNA samples. In addition, the automated format permits multiple PCR measurements to be made for each sample. The protocol used by Tassone et al. (2000c) involves 24 separate reactions (concentration profiles, primary and secondary controls) for each mRNA determination (e.g., fig. 12.1), thus eliminating problems due to contaminated PCR reactions. To date, quantitative ƒRT-PCR measurements have been performed on nearly three hundred patients (Tassone et al. 2000a, 2000b, 2000c, 2000d, 2001, unpublished work).

The second and perhaps more important element for establishing elevated mRNA levels was that ƒRT-PCR measurements were performed initially on males with alleles in the upper premutation range (100–200 CGG repeats) (Tassone et al. 2000c). Such measurements were performed in an effort to understand the basis for clinical involvement in premutation males. Since premutation alleles are rarely methylated, elevated mRNA levels were observed for every male carrier of a high-premutation allele, thus providing substantial statistical weight to the observations.

The observation of elevated *FMR1* mRNA levels in premutation males establishes unequivocally that premutation alleles give rise to dysregulation of gene expression. Thus, although no direct, causal link has been established between the levels of *FMR1* mRNA in peripheral blood leukocytes and clinical involvement in premutation individuals, there now exists a biochemical correlate that supports such a mechanistic linkage in brain. However, such a causal relationship raises another problem: why do some male carriers of premutation alleles seem to escape any clinical involvement? Indeed, why do the vast majority of female carriers not suffer from POF, and why do many carrier males in their fifties and sixties seem to avoid the development of an action tremor (see chap. 1)? These questions are at the forefront of current research and must be addressed by better population data, particularly for the prevalence of tremor, and a better understanding of the neurochemical consequences of premutation alleles. It is likely that the spectrum of involvement in carriers of premutation alleles may reflect the interplay of *FMR1* and additional genetic loci.

The observation of mildly reduced FMRP levels in spite of elevated mRNA poses two related questions: why are the protein levels reduced, particularly in the presence of elevated message, and why are message levels elevated? With regard to the first question, Feng et al. (1995b) observed with cell lines that translation of the *FMR1* mRNA is impaired for alleles in the full mutation range, presumably due to the presence of the expanded CGG repeat in the 5′UTR (untranslated region) of the *FMR1* mRNA. It is possible that such an impediment to translation, albeit in a milder form, extends into the premutation range. The translation defect has profound implications for therapies for FXS, since it is not sufficient to reactivate the gene itself without also developing methods for circumventing the block to translation.

With regard to the second question, Tassone et al. (2000c) proposed that the elevated mRNA levels represent a response to the translation defect. In essence, the cell would attempt to compensate for reduced FMRP levels by stimulating production of mRNA. Thus, clinical manifestations would be mild in the upper premutation range *because* elevated mRNA levels can partially overcome the translation deficit. An alternative explanation for the elevated mRNA levels, namely, that the expanded CGG repeats increase *FMR1* mRNA stability, is unlikely because *FMR1* mRNA from premutation alleles decays in vivo with essentially the same lifetime as mRNA from normal alleles (Tassone et al. 2000c).

Although the observations of Feng et al. (1995b) and of Tassone et al. (2000c) provide support for a feedback mechanism, direct proof of this hypothesis is lacking. Specifically, a translational defect has not been demonstrated in the premutation range, and its nature has not been characterized in detail in the full mutation range. Moreover, increased transcriptional activity, as an explanation for the elevated mRNA levels, has not been demonstrated by direct means. Even if elevated mRNA levels are due to increased gene activity, one must show that such elevations in activity are due to feedback induction; that is, increased activity is a response to lowered protein concentration and/or function. Finally, it is also possible that the expanded CGG repeat could be acting in *cis* to increase transcription (i.e., independently of protein levels). These issues constitute an important research front in the study of *FMR1* gene expression. With regard to the issue of feedback induction, Tassone et al. (2000a) have observed normal mRNA levels for a mutant (I304N) *FMR1* gene from a severely affected male (De Boulle et al. 1993). This result implies that feedback upregulation, if operable, does not simply respond to altered FMRP *function.*

## Males with Allele Size Mosaicism

Mosaicism in FXS is commonly used to refer to individuals who harbor both premutation and full mutation (CGG expansion) alleles. With a more rigorous definition of mosaicism, namely, two or more alleles for the same gene locus (maternal or paternal) within an individual, essentially all individuals with expanded alleles are mosaic, since size heterogeneity, particularly in the full mutation range, is observed in nearly all carriers of expanded alleles. *FMR1* mRNA levels have been determined for a group of six males who possess both premutation and full mutation (methylated) alleles (Tassone et al. 2000a). The mRNA levels were broadly distributed, threefold reduced (mosaic with 14% premutation alleles) to sixfold elevated (56% premutation alleles) relative to normal controls, with an average elevation of approximately twofold. If one corrects for the fraction of premutation alleles, assuming that only those alleles are active, then the resulting average (6.5-fold elevation) is in good agreement with the observations for premutation carriers (Tassone et al. 2000c). Moreover, the range is considerably narrowed, suggesting that variations in the fraction of premutation alleles are responsible for the broad variation in message level. However, one important caveat with this interpretation is that hypermethylated, full mutation alleles are not always silent, as will be discussed in a subsequent section.

## Males with Full Mutations with Methylation Mosaicism

For CGG elements that exceed 200 repeats (full mutation alleles), the CG-rich promoter region (including the CGG element itself) generally becomes methylated, with consequent loss of activity of the gene (transcriptional silencing) (Oberlé et al. 1991; Pieretti et al. 1991). However, unmethylated alleles have been described in the full mutation range, and males with unmethylated, full mutation alleles are usually associated with a less severe phenotype (Loesch et al. 1993; McConkie-Rosell et al. 1993; Hagerman et al. 1994; Merenstein et al. 1994, 1996; Rousseau et al. 1994; Smeets et al. 1995; de Vries et al. 1996; Lachiewicz et al. 1996; Wang et al. 1996; Wöhrle et al. 1998; Burman et al. 1999; Taylor et al. 1999). This general observation of a less severe phenotype in the absence of methylation implies that transcription of full mutation alleles can take place with reasonable efficiency. Consistent with the relatively mild phenotypes for males with unmethylated, full mutation alleles, such "high-functioning" males have FMRP levels that are only moderately reduced (Hagerman et al. 1994; Smeets et al. 1995; de Vries et al. 1996; Tassone et al. 1999).

A priori, reduced FMRP levels could be due either to the aforementioned deficit in translation, or to a reduction in the efficiency of transcription of unmethylated, full mutation alleles. To address this issue, mRNA levels were determined for a group of fifteen full mutation males whose alleles possess varying levels of methylation (0 to 95%) (Tassone et al. 2000a, 2000b). The observed range of expression was nearly 30-fold, with a strong association between mRNA levels and the fraction of unmethylated alleles. Correcting for percent methylation (assuming that methylated alleles are silent; but see below), nearly all mRNA levels are substantially above normal (mean 5.6-fold elevation). Even in the absence of any correction, the highest levels are comparable to the highest levels in the premutation range. Thus, unmethylated full mutation alleles in the 200–400 repeat range are capable of being transcribed with efficiencies that are similar to those for alleles in the premutation range. This observation provides added support for the model in which silencing is due to methylation and postmethylation events (see below). Furthermore, the elevated mRNA levels support the argument that lowered FMRP levels are a consequence of an impediment to translation (fig. 12.2). Finally, the results underscore the need to target translation, not simply gene (transcriptional) activation, in therapeutic approaches for FXS.

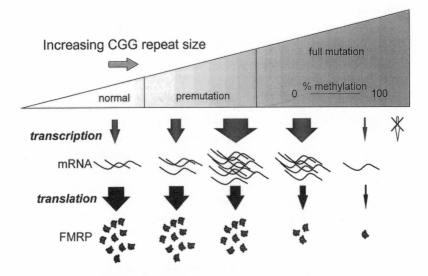

**Fig. 12.2.** Diagram of the influence of CGG repeat size and methylation status on transcription and translation of the *FMR1* gene.

## Males with Highly Methylated Full Mutation Alleles

For CGG repeats in the full mutation range, the CG-rich region of the *FMR1* gene is usually hypermethylated with loss of gene activity (gene silencing) (Oberlé et al. 1991; Pieretti et al. 1991); the attendant lack of FMRP results in FXS. Because hypermethylation is closely associated with silencing in FXS, hypermethylation per se, as usually defined by resistance to promoter cleavage by methyl-sensitive enzymes, is often taken as evidence that the *FMR1* gene is transcriptionally silent, particularly in the absence of FMRP. As a consequence, expression of FMRP in patients with hypermethylated (enzyme-resistant), full mutation alleles is usually interpreted as being due to occult premutation alleles within the cell population. However, recent observations suggest that more than half of the males with enzyme-resistant, FMRP-negative, full mutation alleles nevertheless produce some *FMR1* mRNA, with some individuals producing near-normal levels of mRNA (Tassone et al. 2001).

Tassone et al. (2001) demonstrated that for at least a subset of the males, the observed mRNA was unlikely to have been produced by occult premutation alleles. Their conclusion was based on a series of control experiments in which it was demonstrated that premutation alleles, if present, could have been detected at the 1% level. Since the highest *FMR1* mRNA levels found to date are no more than about 10-fold elevated over normal levels (Tassone et al. 2000a,

2000b, 2000c), occult premutation alleles (<1%) could not account for *FMR1* mRNA levels that are above 10% of normal levels—roughly one-third of the males in the study. Thus, it is not generally valid to assume that enzyme resistance and/or absence of FMRP are indicative of a transcriptionally silent *FMR1* gene.

It is not known why some males with hypermethylated, full mutation alleles produce *FMR1* mRNA while others do not, although it is possible that methylation of a specific subset of CpG elements is critical for silencing (de Graaff et al. 1995; Stöger et al. 1997; Kumari and Usdin 2000). This is an area of active research, since identification of critical methylation events for silencing may lead to therapies specifically directed toward those sites. It is also interesting that none of the males studied by Tassone et al. (2001) had more than 10% FMRP-positive lymphocytes, as measured by immunocytochemical staining (Willemsen et al. 1995, 1997). This lack of protein is likely to be due to a defect in translation, as discussed above.

### *FMR1* mRNA Levels in Females with Premutation and Full-Mutation Alleles

Most studies of *FMR1* expression have been performed in males, since the expression data are not confounded by the effects of varying activation ratio (AR). Not surprisingly, in a study of 43 females, 35 with premutation alleles and 8 with full mutation alleles, there was much greater variation in expression levels compared to males with comparable repeat expansions (Tassone et al. 2000a). In the premutation range, the dispersion of mRNA levels was much greater than for the males and the mean levels were less elevated. Similar effects were observed in the full mutation range, with mean levels being less elevated than for males. However, when a simple (approximate) correction to account for AR was applied to the data, the estimated mRNA levels of active, expanded alleles were consistent with the levels observed for males (Tassone et al. 2000a). Thus, mRNA expression data are consistent with two basic clinical observations for females, namely, broader variation in clinical involvement, and generally less severe clinical involvement (see chap. 1).

### Prospects for Gene Therapy

In the most general sense, *gene therapy* can be defined as any manipulation of the cells of an individual that alters the expression of a particular gene of interest. This might involve replacement of a missing or partially deleted gene (e.g., dystrophin gene of Duchenne muscular dystrophy) or elimination *and* replacement (or modification) of a gene whose mutated form is toxic (e.g., huntingtin gene of Huntington disease). For some disorders, gene-therapy approaches may involve isolation of cells from the patient, followed by alteration or replacement of an abnormal gene and return of the modified cells to the patient. Such "ex vivo" approaches hold particular promise for diseases that involve circulating cells (e.g., leukemias, thalassemias). However, for neurodevelopmental disorders, including FXS, genetic "correction" of the abnormal gene must be accomplished within the individual (in vivo). Gene therapy in vivo presents several daunting challenges, including efficient delivery of the genetic agent to the appropriate cells (e.g., neurons) and the appropriate regulation of the agent within the target cells. These hurdles have yet to be overcome for any neurologic disorder; however, for FXS, there are reasons for optimism, as will be discussed at the end of this section.

In the following discussion, potential avenues to gene therapy of FXS will be divided into four categories: reactivation of transcriptionally "silent" genes (including the *FMR1* gene) using drugs that are not gene-specific; introduction of copies of the normal *FMR1* gene into the cells of fragile X patients; delivery of FMRP directly to patient cells through the use of a short, specialized peptide, termed a transducing "tag," attached to the FMRP molecules; enhancement of the expression of the endogenous *FMR1* gene in ways that capitalize on an understanding of its specific mechanisms of expression. Although all four categories will be addressed, the following discussion reflects a clear bias in favor of the last two categories, for reasons that should become clear.

## General Reactivation of Transcriptionally "Silent" Genes

For fully expanded alleles (>200 CGG repeats), transcriptional silencing is not caused by the repeat expansion per se, since full mutation alleles that remain unmethylated continue to produce relatively high levels of mRNA (Sutcliffe et al. 1992; Tassone et al. 2000b). Rather, silencing is initiated by methylation of the cytosine (C) base of CG dinucleotides within the CG-rich regulatory region, including the repeat region (Oberlé et al. 1991; Pieretti et al. 1991; Bell et al. 1991; Sutcliffe et al. 1992; see also Bestor 2000). It is not known how the cell recognizes and specifically methylates *FMR1* genes with expanded repeats (see Hsieh and Fire 2000 for a general review of recognition and silencing) or why some full mutation repeats remain unmethylated. However, it is clear that this process likely takes place during early development (Monk et al. 1987; Kafri et al. 1992). The methylated C residues act as signals for the recruitment of other proteins that direct the silencing process, in part through deacetylation of histones that are associated with methylated DNA (Coffee et al. 1999; reviews by Wu and Grunstein 2000 and by El-Osta and Wolffe 2000).

The process of methylation-coupled silencing is a very general (normal) mechanism for gene regulation in humans (Holliday et al. 1975; Riggs et al.

1975; Sager et al. 1975) and is responsible for ensuring expression of a single copy of X-linked genes and for "imprinting" of autosomal genes (Lyon 1994; Goto and Monk 1998; Falls et al. 1999; Laan et al. 1999; Cheung et al. 2000; Saitoh and Wada 2000). However, in FXS, this imprinting process is abnormal, resulting in the silencing of a gene that would otherwise be active (Oberlè et al. 1991; Bell et al. 1991; Wöhrle and Steinbach 1991; Hornstra et al. 1993). Although DNA methylation correlates with the transcriptional silencing of genes, the specific mechanisms by which DNA methylation influences transcription are only beginning to be elucidated. Methyl-C residues appear to act as signals for the recruitment of methyl-C binding proteins (e.g., MECP2; Amir et al. 1999; van den Veyver and Zoghbi 2000; Ballestar et al. 2000), which in turn recruit histone deacetylases. The latter enzymes remove acetyl groups from the N-terminal regions of histones, a process that is closely linked to silencing.

Therapies directed toward *general* gene reactivation (i.e., reactivation of many or all genes with similar silencing mechanisms) could, in principle, operate at two levels, namely, through demethylation of the C residues or through inhibition of the subsequent process of histone deacetylation. No method for direct demethylation has been demonstrated; however, 5-azadeoxycitidine (5-azadC), a nucleotide analog that inhibits methylation of C residues, can reduce the net number of methylated C residues in actively dividing cells after several rounds of cell division (Jones 1985; Haaf 1995). Using this approach, Chiurazzi et al. (1998) demonstrated that *FMR1* gene activity could be partially restored (15%) in a cell line derived from an individual with a methylated, full mutation allele.

The observations of Chiurazzi et al (1998) represent an important "proof-of principle" for the role of methylation in silencing of the *FMR1* gene. However, 5-azadC is not likely to play any therapeutic role for fragile X patients, for at least three reasons. First, the therapeutic targets (neurons) in fragile X patients are generally nondividing; thus, agents such as 5-azadC, which require dividing cells, will have no effect. Second, any process involving *general* gene reactivation (i.e., capable of reactivation of thousands of genes) is very high risk, since other normally suppressed genes, including cellular oncogenes and transposable elements, may also be reactivated (Jensen et al. 1999). Third, 5-azadC is associated with significant toxicity.

With regard to the second approach for general gene reactivation, use of histone deacetylase inhibitors, several studies have demonstrated that inhibitors such as sodium butyrate (or phenylbutyrate), trichostatin A (TSA), trapoxin, and depudecin, can also *partially* relieve transcriptional silencing of methylated DNA (Yoshida et al. 1990, 1995; Selker et al. 1998; Bunn 1999). Those results imply that histone acetylation/deacetylation does regulate transcription, with acetylated histones being associated with actively transcribing genes. Using this approach, Chiurazzi et al. (1999) did see a small degree of reactivation (1–

2%) of the *FMR1* gene after treatment with either TSA or phenylbutyrate. However, Coffee et al. (1999) failed to see any *FMR1* gene activity when fragile X cells were treated with TSA.

The results of these two investigations are not necessarily inconsistent, since the degree of reactivation is likely to depend on the specific cell line being used. However, the low levels of reactivation reported by Chiurazzi et al. (1999) would not be expected to yield any therapeutic result, since protein levels would remain undetectable. Furthermore, as with 5-azadC, any general reactivation poses the risk of reactivating genes whose gain of function may be deleterious to the patient, and agents such as TSA are also toxic. Thus, methods involving general gene reactivation do not appear to represent viable approaches for the treatment of FXS.

## Gene-Transfer Methods

For many disorders of genetic origin, particularly where the coding portion of the involved gene is mutated or deleted, the greatest prospect for genetic correction lies with the therapeutic introduction of a normal copy of the gene (transgene). The field of gene transfer is evolving rapidly and, as of 2000, more than three hundred clinical trials have been initiated with various disease targets and gene-transfer protocols. An excellent review of recent developments in this area has been presented by Mountain (2000). As of the first part of 2000, all clinical trials have involved either ex vivo approaches, in which genes are introduced into isolated cell populations (e.g., cells collected from blood) before their return to the body, or by regional introduction into the target tissues. The latter approaches include direct injection of transgenes into tissues such as muscle to treat limb ischemia (Baumgartner et al. 1998) or their installation into the airway to treat cystic fibrosis (Wagner 1998). It is unlikely that gene-transfer methods will be used in the short term for introduction of transgenes (including *FMR1*) into the CNS, except for direct injection into otherwise-lethal CNS tumors. However, given the rapidly developing strategies for viral-mediated transfer, the situation may soon change.

### Viral Carriers

Approximately two-thirds of gene-transfer protocols have used viral carriers, with most protocols employing adenovirus, retroviruses, and adeno-associated virus. In all instances, the original viruses have been "gutted," a process whereby genes conferring viral pathology have been removed, to be replaced by the gene of interest. Advantages and disadvantages of each of these viruses are summarized in the review by Mountain (2000). For FXS, retrovirus-mediated gene transfer is unlikely, since transfer and integration of retroviral agents generally requires proliferating cell populations (e.g., immune cells, tumors); neuronal cell populations are predominantly nondividing after birth. Furthermore, retroviruses are rapidly inactivated by various mechanisms, thus limiting their use for in vivo gene therapy. Among the retroviruses, modified lentiviruses can deliver genes to nondividing cells, although they appear to target cells mainly within the blood lineage. A recent review of retroviral vectors has been presented by Buchschacher and Wong-Staal (2000). Adeno-associated viruses (AAVs) do have the potential for in vivo delivery of transgenes to a range of target tissues, and such viruses can deliver transgenes to nondividing cells (Schwarz 2000; Peel and Klein 2000; Smith-Arica and Bartlett 2001). Current limitations of the AAVs include the prospect of insertional mutagenesis. For all of the viruses employed thus far for gene therapy trials, several obstacles remain, including low transfer efficiency, viral immunogenicity, and unpredictable duration and extent of expression of the transgene. However, with the rapid development of second- and third-generation viral vectors, these obstacles are gradually being overcome.

### Nonviral Methods for Gene Transfer

DNA is rapidly degraded in blood; thus, delivery of naked DNA (or RNA) is not a viable option for the treatment of neurodevelopmental disorders such as FXS. Formation of complexes of DNA with cationic lipids affords improved protection from degradation and has allowed the delivery of genes to target tissues in human trials (Alton et al. 1999). One drawback of lipid-mediated delivery is that transfection efficiency is generally quite low, possibly due to poor cellular uptake or sequestration of the complexes in cytoplasmic organelles, although this situation is improving through the use of newer lipid formulations (Stein 1999; Maurer et al. 1999; Katsel and Greenstein 2000).

As an alternative approach, branched polycations (polyethyleneimine, PEI) hold promise as general gene-delivery vehicles, due in part to the greater stability and transformation efficiency of the DNA-polycation complexes (10–100-fold greater than cationic lipids; Densmore et al. 2000). DNA complexed with PEI is remarkably resistant to DNases—nearly a millionfold protection over naked DNA—and the complex appears to escape the lysosomal fate of the DNA-cationic lipid complexes (Godbey et al. 2000). PEI-p53 tumor suppressor gene, delivered by aerosol to mouse lung, was able to significantly reduce the number of metastatic tumors in the lung, demonstrating both efficient delivery of the p53 gene to tumor cells and efficient cellular expression of the transgene (Gautam et al. 2000). One additional advantage of PEI over various viral delivery vehicles is its ability to transfer extremely large transgenes (over 2 Mb) to target cells (Marschall et al. 1999), whereas viral delivery is limited to 4–8 kb.

For either viral or nonviral carriers, the potential exists for delivery of the protein-coding portion of the *FMR1* gene without the expanded CGG repeat, thus avoiding the associated problems of CGG-mediated gene silencing and reduced translation from *FMR1* mRNA with the expanded CGG repeat. However, problems associated with inefficient gene delivery remain daunting. Furthermore, unless delivery of the active *FMR1* transgene is cell-type-specific, the transgene itself may introduce neuropathology. For example, whereas the *FMR1* gene is normally active in neurons, FMRP is not detected in neighboring glial cells (Feng et al. 1997; chaps. 4 and 5), and the consequences of expressing *FMR1* in the latter cell type are not known. In addition, overexpression of an *FMR1* transgene may create its own, additional pathology: in transgenic mice, overexpression of *FMR1* leads to behavioral problems in heterozygous animals (Peier et al. 2000), and the inability to produce mammalian cells that overproduce FMRP (Ceman et al. 1999) presages possible lethality in homozygous animals and toxicity in humans. Thus, both appropriately targeted expression and proper regulation of the *level* of expression are likely to be of critical importance in the design of any gene-transfer therapy for FXS. The use of large transgenes with all of the native regulatory elements associated with the *FMR1* gene may yield both proper cell-specific expression and appropriate levels of expression, although none of the current viral vectors would support such large transgenes (>40 kbp).

### The Delivery of FMRP Directly to Cells Using a Transducing Peptide "Tag" Attached to the FMRP Molecules

In principle, one might envision correcting the clinical abnormalities associated with FXS by therapeutic administration of the protein (FMRP) itself, as is done with injections of insulin for the treatment of type I (insulin-dependent) diabetes, or even the oral administration of the enzyme, lactase, for lactose intolerance. However, the latter two examples are specialized cases: insulin normally operates as a circulatory factor in blood, regulating glucose uptake into cells through its interactions with receptors on the outer surface of cells; lactase is normally found in the GI tract, where it functions to break down dietary lactose. By contrast, FMRP is found only inside cells; thus, any effective therapy using FMRP per se must involve not only its efficient delivery to the appropriate target tissues (e.g., brain), but also its transport into cells (e.g., neurons).

In general, injected proteins can neither cross the blood-brain barrier to reach brain tissues nor enter cells. However, in 1988 two groups (Green and Lowenstein 1988; Frankel and Pabo 1988) independently observed that the trans-activator protein (Tat) of human immunodeficiency virus (HIV) was capable of being taken up by cells. This ability to move across cell membranes is conferred by a small, basic region of the Tat protein, termed a *protein transduction domain* (PTD),

$$\text{Tyr}_{47}\text{-Gly-Arg-Lys-Lys-Arg-Arg-Gln-Arg-Arg-Arg}_{57}$$

which spans amino acid residues 47 to 57 of Tat (Green and Lowenstein 1988; Mann and Frankel 1991; Ezhevsky et al. 1997; Vives et al. 1997).

A remarkable feature of the Tat PTD is its ability to confer transducing capability on many other proteins when coupled to those proteins (Anderson et al. 1993; Fawell et al. 1994; Nagahara et al. 1998; Schwarze et al. 1999; Vocero-Akbani et al. 2000; Barka et al. 2000; Mi et al. 2000; Schwarze and Dowdy 2000). Moreover, transducing capability has been demonstrated in nearly all cell types, and in whole organs and animals (Schwarze et al. 1999; Mi et al. 2000; Barka et al. 2000). It is not known how the PTD carries proteins across cell membranes; however, PTD-mediated transduction does not appear to involve any specific cell receptors, nor does it appear to involve endocytosis (Vives et al. 1997; Derossi et al. 1996). Dowdy and coworkers have demonstrated that protocols involving denaturation of the Tat PTD-protein fusions markedly improve transducing efficiency (Schwarze et al. 1999; Vocero-Akbani et al. 2000), although this procedure is not an absolute requirement for PTD function.

The Tat PTD holds obvious potential as a means for delivering FMRP to neurons and other involved cell types in fragile X patients, and at least four research groups have been working on this approach for at least two years as of this writing (no results to report thus far). At this point it is worth considering both the (potential) advantages of this mode of therapy and the possible pitfalls. There are at least two significant advantages of Tat PTD-FMRP-based therapy over various gene-delivery methods. First, Tat PTD-mediated delivery is reported to be highly efficient, with rapid delivery of Tat PTD-coupled proteins to most, if not all tissues (including brain) of whole animals. Second, because intracellular Tat PTD-protein levels decay over a period of several hours to one day, adverse consequences of overdelivery are likely to be reversible (as in many forms of conventional drug therapy).

Despite the potential utility of a Tat-PTD-FMRP fusion protein for therapeutic intervention in FXS, there are several potential problems with this approach that must be borne in mind. First, FMRP protein levels normally vary widely in different cell types, even within brain. For example, as noted in the previous section, FMRP levels are high in neurons, but there is little or no FMRP expression in neighboring glial cells (Feng et al. 1997). Thus, the delivery of uniform levels of the Tat-PTD-FMRP fusion protein to all cell types may be toxic at FMRP levels that are too low to be therapeutically effective. Second, repeated (e.g., daily) injections may lead to an immunological reaction to the fusion protein, particularly if delivered in denatured form; such a response is likely to be more pronounced in individuals who are producing no endogenous FMRP. Third, as a practical matter, the fusion protein may not be sufficiently stable in blood to deliver the necessary levels to brain tissues. Fourth, the fusion protein may not be active in the intended target cells, either as a consequence of improper refolding or due to the fused PTD itself.

The above caveats notwithstanding, the PTD fusion protein approach holds promise for treatment of FXS. Moreover, even if Tat PTD-FMRP fusion proteins do not turn out to be useful, there are other ways in which the Tat PTD might be exploited. For example, the Tat PTD might be used to carry other peptides into cells such that the interaction of neuron-specific proteins (or RNAs) with the Tat PTD fusion peptides is required for some function, such as *FMR1* reactivation (see following section). Thus, the *general* transducing function of the Tat PTD could be effectively converted to a neuron-*specific* function by other neuron-specific factors that are already present in the cell. An additional variation on the PTD-based scheme might involve the use of the Tat PTD to deliver oligonucleotides (modified DNA or RNA species) into cells (see following section). This capability has already been demonstrated by Allinquant et al. (1995), who used a related PTD from the fruitfly (*Drosophila*) (the ANTP PTD from the *Drosophila antennapedia* gene) to carry an antisense DNA into cells.

## Enhancement of the Expression of the Endogenous *FMR1* Gene

All of the potential therapeutic approaches discussed thus far rely on relatively general mechanisms—general gene reactivation; introduction of exogenous genes; delivery of FMRP via Tat PTD—that do not take into account the specific mechanisms of expression of the *FMR1* gene. However, as detailed in the first section of this chapter, several aspects of the patterns of *FMR1* gene expression, encompassing both gene transcription and protein synthesis (translation) may afford more specific approaches to treatment. Moreover, if elevated *FMR1* mRNA levels directly cause clinical involvement in individuals with expanded CGG repeats (e.g., premature ovarian failure; cerebellar tremor and cognitive decline; see chaps. 1 and 3), efforts directed solely toward increasing gene activity or protein levels may not relieve certain features of the disorder.

In the following paragraphs, several potential approaches are outlined that would exploit specific features of *FMR1* expression. These approaches would include targeted gene reactivation in those individuals with full mutations whose *FMR1* gene is truly silenced, and more efficient use of existing *FMR1* mRNA for those premutation and full mutation individuals whose *FMR1* gene retains at least partial activity. It should be appreciated that this section is necessarily speculative; however, it is presented in the spirit of stimulating a more general discussion of the ways in which FMRP production can be increased using the endogenous gene, since the native *FMR1* gene, even with the expanded CGG repeat, holds the greatest promise for correct tissue-specific regulation.

## Targeted Reactivation of the *FMR1* Gene Based on Sequence-specific Disruption of Silencing Factors

A significant fraction of males with full mutation alleles that are completely methylated at one or more sites of (methyl-sensitive) enzyme cleavage nevertheless continue to produce some mRNA, demonstrating that the *FMR1* gene in those individuals retains at least partial activity. This observation has a direct bearing on approaches to targeted reactivation of the *FMR1* gene, since it implies that only a small part of the promoter region of the *FMR1* gene, perhaps no more than a few dozen base pairs, may need to be targeted for reactivation. It is known that some transcription factors (e.g., α-PAL) that interact with the *FMR1* promoter are sensitive to the methylation status of their binding sites (Stöger et al. 1997; Kumari and Usdin 2000), and these sites (or adjacent elements) may prove to be productive targets for reactivation.

Identification of specific targets for reactivation within the *FMR1* promoter may also benefit from the completion of an ongoing effort to map the positions of methylated C residues for various levels of endogenous gene activity (Tassone and Hagerman, unpublished). It is hoped that a better understanding of the relationship between gene activity and specific positions of methylation will lead to more focused approaches for targeted reactivation of the *FMR1* gene. Such approaches would include targeted disruption of chromatin proteins within specific regions of the promoter.

## Targeted Disruption of Chromatin Proteins

The general reactivation approaches discussed above (e.g., using inhibitors of methylation) are not likely to be used for treatment of FXS. Nevertheless, those approaches (Chiurazzi et al. 1998, 1999; Coffee et al. 1999) have demonstrated that silencing of the *FMR1* gene involves, at least in part, methyl-coupled recruitment of histone deacetylases, whose action leads to an inactive form of chromatin. Since methylation of the promoter does not, by itself, cause silencing—modified protein-DNA interactions are required (Wu and Grunstein 2000; El-Osta and Wolffe 2000)—methods that disrupt such interactions, even locally, may lead to reactivation.

Over the past several years, a number of strategies have been developed for targeted disruption of protein-DNA interactions; such approaches include triple-helix forming oligonucleotides (Giovannangeli and Hélène 1997, 2000), peptide nucleic acids (PNA; DNA bases linked with a peptidelike backbone) (Nielsen et al. 1991; Good and Nielsen 1997), and complex polyamide minor groove binding drugs (Gottesfeld et al. 1997; White et al. 1998). Although these reagents are able to disrupt even strong protein-DNA interactions, and can do so in a relatively sequence-specific fashion, they are restricted to a relatively small number of possible targets; thus, additional work is required to further tailor these molecules to sequences within the *FMR1* promoter.

More recently, Lohse et al. (1999) demonstrated that "pseudocomplementary" PNA duplexes, in which each PNA strand pairs more tightly with the target DNA than it does with its oligomeric complement, are capable of efficient double strand invasion of 80% of all possible DNA (decamer) targets. While such pseudocomplementary PNA duplexes are capable of disruption of protein-DNA interactions in vitro under low salt conditions, in their present form they are not useful under the salt conditions normally found in the cell. Moreover, the highly CG-rich *FMR1* promoter region is not expected to lend itself to the pseudocomplement strategy, which requires 40–50% AT base pairs (Nielsen 2000). However, given the rapid pace of development of these targeting reagents, it is hoped that a new generation of oligonucleotides will be useful for reactivating the *FMR1* promoter.

## Targeted Enhancement of Translation of the *FMR1* mRNA

FMRP levels begin to decrease in the upper portion of the premutation range, despite increasingly elevated mRNA levels, with reductions in FMRP becoming much more pronounced in the full mutation range (for active, full mutation alleles). These data, combined with the earlier observations of impaired translation in the full mutation range (Feng et al. 1995b), suggest that the CGG expansion within the 5'UTR of the message acts—directly or indirectly—to impede translation of *FMR1* mRNA. Thus, irrespective of the intrinsic activity of the *FMR1* gene or of efforts to reactivate silenced genes, the translation defect must be circumvented.

It is not known how the CGG element might reduce translational efficiency. The most straightforward possibility is that a highly structured CGG region (in the RNA) blocks the normal process of scanning from the 5' cap to the start codon (Kosak 1989, 1991a, 1991b, 1999). Estimates of the free energy of folding of the CGG repeat and surrounding regions of the 5'UTR, suggest that such elements would be far more stable than needed to block scanning. However, it seems unlikely that the translation defect arises solely as a consequence of a failure to scan from the 5'cap through a highly structured CGG region to the start codon. Indeed, one difficulty with the scanning model is that it predicts that translation would be blocked for CGG repeats in the upper end of the normal range, whereas people with more than 50 repeats are clinically normal, with essentially normal FMRP levels. It is therefore more likely that the CGG repeat acts in concert with other elements, perhaps regulatory proteins, to control translation, and that expanded CGG repeats act in some fashion to disrupt this interaction.

Observations by Chiang et al. (2001) suggest that translation of the *FMR1* mRNA partially circumvents the problem of scanning by using a second mechanism, namely, initiation via an internal ribosome entry site (IRES; Pelletier and Sonenberg 1988; Jang et al. 1988; Sachs 2000). Originally identified as a mechanism used by picornaviruses (e.g., poliovirus) to circumvent virally induced suppression of host translation, IRESs have now been identified in the 5'UTRs of several key regulatory proteins, including platelet-derived growth factor (Bernstein et al. 1997), the c-myc proto-oncogene (Nanbru et al. 1997), apoptotic protease activating factor (Coldwell et al. 2000), and ornithine decarboxylase (Pyronnet et al. 2000), among others.

IRESs work by providing a second target for initiation factor binding to the 5'UTR that is independent of the normal requirement for binding to the 5' end (cap) of the mRNA. From the perspective of the current discussion of possible approaches to therapy, an *FMR1* IRES presents a target for trans-acting factors that could induce (or enhance) translation from existing message. It is now well known that IRESs display remarkable cell type specificity as well as developmental specificity (e.g., Pilipenko et al. 2000; Coldwell et al. 2000; Pyronnet et al. 2000; Créancier et al. 2000), due in part to interactions of tissue-specific, *trans*-acting proteins with the IRES element (Johannes and Sarnow 1998; Pilipenko et al. 2000). To circumvent the normal scanning mechanism for an mRNA that does not possess an IRES, De Gregorio et al. (1999) engineered a protein that could, in effect, convert a non-IRES sequence element in the 5'UTR into an IRES, thus allowing that message to avoid the need for cap-dependent initiation. This general approach holds potential for addressing the translation block in FXS.

A second, more speculative approach to circumventing the translation block is suggested by a mechanism used in plants, termed *shunting* (Fütterer et al. 1993; Donzé et al. 1995; Schmidt-Puchta et al. 1997; Schärer-Hernández and Hohn 1998; Hemmings-Mieszczak and Hohn 1999; Ryabova and Hohn 2000; Pooggin et al. 2000). For some genes in plants, the mRNA has a built-in bypass mechanism that allows the scanning ribosome to "hop" around a region of stable structure. This physical structure in the 5'UTR is termed a *shunt*. Of course, shunts in plant mRNAs are not of direct help for the translation block in *FMR1* mRNA; however, it has been demonstrated that shunts can be used *in trans* with different mRNAs (Fütterer et al. 1993), opening up the possibility of using *trans* shunts in FXS. These latter possibilities are currently being investigated in the Hagerman laboratory.

## Conclusions

Research over the past few years has dramatically changed the level of understanding of *FMR1* gene expression. Emerging models of gene expression, including reduced protein production in the face of elevated mRNA levels, strongly implicate a second block to protein expression at the level of translation initiation. This observation has important ramifications for treatment of FXS, since it is now understood that gene reactivation—without circumventing the block to translation—will not fully correct the protein deficit. Therefore, a two-pronged approach must be taken to molecular therapies for FXS if the endogenous gene is to be used. Methods that use protein delivery or exogenous genes would circumvent the translation and gene reactivation problems, but these latter methods must overcome a different set of hurdles, including delivery of the proper amounts of therapeutic agents to the correct target tissues and cell types. However, given the rapid development of therapeutic tools and greater understanding of mechanism, there is reason for genuine optimism that enduring molecular therapies will be developed in the short term. This optimism stems not only from the pace of research, but also from the fact that FMRP is apparently needed for brain function throughout life—that is, correct delivery of the protein is likely to have some benefit for current, not just future generations.

Finally, in support of a common theme of this chapter, the coding portion of the *FMR1* gene is normal in the vast majority of cases. Thus, use of the endogenous gene is a real possibility. Indeed, the bias of this review is toward the use of non–gene replacement approaches, so that alterations in expression are titratable and reversible—more like classical drug therapy.

## Acknowledgments

This work was supported by the Boory Family fund and the Cooper/Kraff/Fishman Family fund. The author also thanks Dr. Flora Tassone for many fruitful discussions and for her outstanding contributions to the field of fragile X research.

## References

Allingham-Hawkins, D. J., R. Babul-Hirji, D. Chitayat, J. J. Holden, K. T. Yang, C. Lee, R. Hudson, H. Gorwill, S. L. Nolin, A. Glicksman, E. C. Jenkins, W. T. Brown, P. N. Howard-Peebles, C. Becchi, E. Cummings, L. Fallon, S. Seitz, S. H. Black, A. M. Vianna-Morgante, S. S. Costa, P. A. Otto, R. C. Mingroni-Netto, A. Murray, J. Webb, and F. Vieri. 1999. Fragile X premutation is a significant risk factor for premature ovarian failure: The international collaborative POF in fragile X study—preliminary data. *Am. J. Med. Genet.* 83:322–325.

Allinquant, B., P. Hantraye, P. Mailleux, K. Moya, C. Bouillot, and A. Prochiantz. 1995. Downregulation of amyloid precursor protein inhibits neurite outgrowth in vitro. *J. Cell Biol.* 128:919–927.

Alton, E. W., M. Stern, R. Farley, A. Jaffe, S. L. Chadwick, J. Phillips, J. Davies, S. N. Smith, J. Browning, M. G. Davies, M. E. Hodson, S. R. Durham, D. Li, P. K. Jeffrey, M. Scallan, R. Balfour, S. J. Eastman, S. H. Cheng, A. E. Smith, D. Meeker, and D. M. Geddes. 1999. Cationic lipid-mediated *CFTR* gene transfer to the lungs and nose of patients with cystic fibrosis: A double-blind placebo-controlled trial. *Lancet* 353: 947–954.

Amir, R. E., I. B. van den Veyver, M. Wan, C. Q. Tran, U. Francke, and H. Y. Zoghbi. 1999. Rett syndrome is caused by mutations in X-linked MECP2, encoding methyl-CpG-binding protein 2. *Nat. Genet.* 23:185–188.

Anderson, D. C., E. Nichols, R. Manger, D. Woodle, M. Barry, and A. R. Fritzberg. 1993. Tumor cell retention of antibody Fab fragments is enhanced by an attached HIV TAT protein-derived peptide. *Biochem. Biophys. Res. Commun.* 194:876–884.

Ballestar, E., T. M. Yusufzai, and A. P. Wolffe. 2000. Effects of Rett syndrome mutations of the methyl-CpG binding domain of the transcriptional repressor MeCP2 on selectivity for association with methylated DNA. *Biochemistry* 39:7100–7106.

Barka, T., E. W. Gresik, and H. van der Noen. 2000. Transduction of TAT-HA-(-galactosidase fusion protein into salivary gland-derived cells and organ cultures of the developing gland, and into rat submandibular gland in vivo. *J. Histochem. Cytochem.* 48:1453–1460.

Baumgartner, I., A. Pieczek, O. Manor, R. Blair, M. Kearney, K. Walsh, and J. M. Isner. 1998. Constitutive expression of phVEGF165 after intramuscular gene transfer promotes collateral vessel development in patients with critical limb ischemia. *Circulation* 97:1114–1123.

Bell, M. V., M. C. Hirst, Y. Nakahori, R. N. MacKinnon, A. Roche, T. J. Flint, P. A. Jacobs, N. Tommerup, L. Tranebjaerg, U. Froster-Iskenius, B. Kerr, G. Turner, R. H. Lindenbaum, R. Winter, M. Pembrey, S. Thibodeau, and K. E. Davies. 1991. Physical mapping across the fragile X: Hypermethylation and clinical expression of the fragile X syndrome. *Cell* 64:861–866.

Bernstein, J., O. Sella, S-Y. Le, and O. Elroy-Stein. 1997. PDGF2/*c-sis* mRNA leader contains a differentiation-linked internal ribosomal entry site (D-IRES). *J. Biol. Chem.* 272:9356–9362.

Bestor, T. H. 2000. The DNA methyltransferases of mammals. *Hum. Mol. Genet.* 9: 2395–2402.

Brown, W. T., G. E. Houck, Jr., A. Jeziorowska, F. N. Levinson, X. Ding, C. Dobkin, N. Zhong, J. Henderson, S. S. Brooks, and E. C. Jenkins. 1993. Rapid fragile X carrier screening and prenatal diagnosis using a nonradioactive PCR test. *JAMA* 270:1569–1575.

Buchschacher, G. L., and F. Wong-Staal. 2000. Development of lentiviral vectors for gene therapy for human disorders. *Blood* 95:2499–2504.

Bunn, H. F. 1999. Induction of fetal hemoglobin in sickle cell disease. *Blood* 93:1787–1789.

Burman, R. W., P. A. Yates, L. D. Green, P. B. Jackey, M. S. Turker, and B. W. Popovich.

1999. Hypomethylation of an expanded *FMR1* allele is not associated with a global DNA methylation defect. *Am. J. Hum. Genet.* 65:1375–1386.

Ceman, S., V. Brown, and S. T. Warren. 1999. Isolation of an FMRP-associated messenger ribonucleoprotein particle and identification of nucleolin and the fragile X-related proteins as components of the complex. *Mol. Cell Biol.* 19:7925–7932.

Cheung, W. L., S. D. Briggs, and C. D. Allis. 2000. Acetylation and chromosomal functions. *Curr. Opin. Cell Biol.* 12:326–333.

Chiang, P-W., L. Carpenter, and P. J. Hagerman. 2001. Identification of an IRES element in the 5'UTR of the *FMR1* mRNA. *J. Biol. Chem.* In press. Published online 08/06/01.

Chiurazzi, P., M. G. Pomponi, R. Willemsen, B. A. Oostra, and G. Neri. 1998. In vitro reactivation of the *FMR1* gene involved in fragile X syndrome. *Hum. Mol. Genet.* 7: 109–113.

Chiurazzi, P., M. G. Pomponi, R. Pietrobono, C. E. Bakker, G. Neri, and B. A. Oostra. 1999. Synergistic effect of histone hyperacetylation and DNA demethylation in the reactivation of the *FMR1* gene. *Hum. Mol. Genet.* 8:2317–2323.

Coffee, B., F. Zhang, S. T. Warren, and D. Reines. 1999. Acetylated histones are associated with *FMR1* in normal but not fragile X-syndrome cells. *Nat. Genet.* 22:98–101.

Coldwell, M. J., S. A. Mitchell, M. Stoneley, M. MacFarlane, and A. E. Willis. 2000. Initiation of Apaf-1 translation by internal ribosome entry. *Oncogene* 19:899–905.

Créancier, L., D. Morello, P. Mercier, and A-C. Prats. 2000. Fibroblast growth factor 2 internal ribosome entry site (IRES) activity ex vivo and in transgenic mice reveals a stringent tissue-specific regulation. *J. Cell Biol.* 150:275–281.

De Boulle, K., A. J. M. H. Verkerk, E. Reyniers, L. Vits, J. Hendrickx, B. Van Roy, F. van den Bos, E. de Graaff, B. A. Oostra, and P. J. Willems. 1993. A point mutation in the *FMR-1* gene associated with fragile X mental retardation. *Nat. Genet.* 3:31–35.

de Graaff, E., P. Rouillard, P. J. Willems, J. Smits, A. P. Rousseau, and B. A. Oostra. 1995. Hotspot for deletions in the CGG repeat region of *FMR1* in fragile X patients. *Hum. Mol. Genet.* 4:45–49.

De Gregorio, E., T. Preiss, and M. W. Hentze. 1999. Translation driven by an eIF4G core domain *in vivo*. *EMBO J.* 18:4865–4874.

Densmore, C. L., F. M. Orson, B. Xu, B. M. Kinsey, J. C. Waldrep, P. Hua, B. Bhogal, and V. Knight. 2000. Aerosol delivery of robust polyethyleneimine-DNA complexes for gene therapy and genetic immunization. *Mol. Ther.* 1:180–188.

Derossi, D., S. Calvet, A. Trembleau, A. Brunissen, G. Chassaing, and A. Prochiantz. 1996. Cell internalization of the third helix of the Antennapedia homeodomain is receptor-independent. *J. Biol. Chem.* 271:18188–18193.

de Vries, B. B., C. C. Jansen, A. A. Duits, C. Verheij, R. Willemsen, J. O. van Hemel, A. M. van den Ouweland, M. F. Niermeijer, B. A. Oostra, and D. J. Halley. 1996. Variable *FMR1* gene methylation of large expansions leads to variable phenotype in three males from one fragile X family. *J. Med. Genet.* 33:1007–1010.

Devys, D., Y. Lutz, N. Rouyer, J. P. Bellocq, and J. L. Mandel. 1993. The *FMR-1* protein is cytoplasmic, most abundant in neurons and appears normal in carriers of a fragile X premutation. *Nat. Genet.* 4:335–340.

Donzé, O., P. Damay, and P-F. Spahr. 1995. The first and third uORFs in RSV leader RNA are efficiently translated: Implications for translational regulation and viral RNA packaging. *Nucl. Acids Res.* 23:861–868.

Dorn, M. B., M. M. Mazzocco, and R. J. Hagerman. 1994. Behavioral and psychiatric disorders in adult male carriers of fragile X. *J. Am. Acad. Child Adolesc. Psychiatry* 33:256–264.

El-Osta, A., and A. Wolffe. 2000. DNA methylation and histone deacetylation in the control of gene expression: Basic biochemistry to human development and disease. *Gene Expr.* 9:63–75.

Ezhevsky, S. A., H. Nagahara, A. M. Vocero-Akbani, D. R. Gius, M. C. Wei, and S. F. Dowdy. 1997. Hypophosphorylation of the retinoblastoma protein (pRb) by cyclin D:Cdk4/6 complexes results in active pRb. *Proc. Natl. Acad. Sci. USA* 94:10699–10704.

Falls, J. G., D. J. Pulford, A. A. Wylie, and R. L. Jirtle. 1999. Genomic imprinting: Implications for human disease. *Am. J. Pathol.* 154:635–647.

Fawell, S., J. Seery, Y. Daikh, C. Moore, L. L. Chen, B. Pepinsky, and J. Barsoum. 1994. Tat-mediated delivery of heterologous proteins into cells. *Proc. Natl. Acad. Sci. USA* 91:664–668.

Feng, Y., L. Lakkis, D. Devys, and S. T. Warren. 1995a. Quantitative comparison of *FMR1* gene expression in normal and premutation alleles. *Am. J. Hum. Genet.* 56: 106–113.

Feng, Y., F. Zhang, L. K. Lokey, J. L. Chastain, L. Lakkis, D. Eberhart, and S. T. Warren. 1995b. Translational suppression by trinucleotide repeat expansion at *FMR1*. *Science* 268:731–734.

Feng, Y., C. A. Gutekunst, D. E. Eberhart, H. Yi, S. T. Warren, and S. M. Hersch. 1997. Fragile X mental retardation protein: Nucleocytoplasmic shuttling and association with somatodendritic ribosomes. *J. Neurosci.* 17:1539–1547.

Franke, P., M. Leboyer, M. Gansicke, O. Weiffenbach, V. Biancalana, P. Cornillet-Lefebre, M. F. Croquette, U. Froster, S. G. Schwab, F. Poustka, M. Hautzinger, and W. Maier. 1998. Genotype-phenotype relationship in female carriers of the premutation and full mutation of *FMR-1*. *Psychiatr. Res.* 80:113–127.

Frankel, A. D., and C. O. Pabo. 1988. Cellular uptake of the Tat protein from human immunodeficiency virus. *Cell* 55:1189–1193.

Fu, Y. H., D. P. Kuhl, A. Pizzuti, M. Pieretti, J. S. Sutcliffe, S. Richards, A. J. Verkerk, J. J. Holden, R. G. Fenwick, S. T. Warren, B. A. Oostra, D. L. Nelson, and C. T. Caskey. 1991. Variation of the CGG repeat at the fragile X site results in genetic instability: Resolution of the Sherman paradox. *Cell* 67:1047–1058.

Fütterer, J., Z. Kiss-László, and T. Hohn. 1993. Nonlinear ribosome migration on cauliflower mosaic virus 35S RNA. *Cell* 73:789–802.

Gautam, A., C. L. Densmore, and J. C. Waldrep. 2000. Inhibition of experimental lung metastasis by aerosol delivery of PEI-p53 complexes. *Mol. Ther.* 2:318–323.

Gibson, U. E., C. A. Heid, and P. M. Williams. 1996. A novel method for real time quantitative RT-PCR. *Genome Res.* 6:995–1001.

Giovannangeli, C., and C. Helene. 1997. Progress in developments of triplex-based strategies. *Antisense Nucleic Acid Drug Dev.* 7:413–421.

————. 2000. Triplex technology takes off. *Nat. Biotech* 18:1245–1246.

Godbey, W. T., M. A. Barry, P. Saggau, K. K. Wu, and A. G. Mikos. 2000. Poly(ethyleneimine)-mediated transfection: A new paradigm for gene delivery. *J. Biomed. Mater. Res.* 51:321–328.

Good, L., and P. E. Nielsen. 1997. Progress in developing PNA as a gene-targeted drug. *Antisense Nucleic Acid Drug Dev.* 7:431–437.

Goto, T., and M. Monk. 1998. Regulation of X-chromosome inactivation in development in mice and humans. *Microbiol. Mol. Biol. Rev.* 62:362–378.

Gottesfeld, J. M., L. Neely, J. W. Trauger, E. E. Baird, and P. B. Dervan. 1997. Regulation of gene expression by small molecules. *Nature* 387:202–205.

Green, M., and P. M. Lowenstein. 1988. Autonomous functional domains of chemically synthesized human immunodeficiency virus Tat Trans-activator protein. *Cell* 55: 1179–1188.

Haaf, T. 1995. The effects of 5-azacytidine and 5-azadeoxycytidine on chromosome structure and function: Implications for methylation-associated cellular processes. *Pharmacol. Ther.* 65:19–46.

Hagerman, R. J., C. E. Hull, J. F. Safanda, I. Carpenter, L. W. Staley, R. O'Connor, C. Seydel, M. M. Mazzocco, K. Snow, S. N. Thibodeau, et al. 1994. High functioning fragile X males: Demonstration of an unmethylated fully expanded *FMR-1* mutation associated with protein expression. *Am. J. Med. Genet.* 51:298–308.

Hagerman, R. J., L. W. Staley, R. O'Conner, K. Lugenbeel, D. Nelson, S. D. McLean, and A. K. Taylor. 1996. Learning-disabled males with a fragile X CGG expansion in the upper premutation size range. *Pediatrics* 97:122–126.

Hagerman, R. J., M. Leehey, W. Heinrichs, F. Tassone, R. Wilson, J. Hills, J. Grigsby, B. Gag, and P. J. Hagerman. 2001. Action tremor and generalized brain atrophy in older males with the fragile X premutation. Submitted.

Heid, C. A., J. Stevens, K. J. Livak, and P. M. Williams. 1996. Real time quantitative PCR. *Genome Methods* 6:986–994.

Heitz, D., D. Devys, G. Imbert, C. Kretz, and J. L. Mandel. 1992. Inheritance of the fragile X syndrome: Size of the fragile X premutation is a major determinant of the transition to full mutation. *J. Med. Genet.* 29:794–801.

Hemmings-Mieszczak, M., and T. Hohn. 1999. A stable hairpin preceded by a short open reading frame promotes nonlinear ribosome migration on a synthetic mRNA leader. *RNA* 5:1149–1157.

Holliday, R., and J. E. Pugh. 1975. DNA modification mechanisms and gene activity during development. *Science* 187:226–232.

Hornstra, I. K., D. L. Nelson, S. T. Warren, and T. P. Yang. 1993. High resolution methylation analysis of the *FMR1* gene trinucleotide repeat region in fragile X syndrome. *Hum. Mol. Genet.* 2:1659–1665.

Hsieh, J., and A. Fire. 2000. Recognition and silencing of repeated RNA. *Annu. Rev. Genet.* 34:187–204.

Jang, S. K., H-G. Kräusslich, M. J. H. Nicklin, G. M. Duke, A. C. Palmenberg, and E. Wimmer. 1988. A segment of the 5′ nontranslated region of encephalomyocarditis virus RNA directs internal entry of ribosomes during in vitro translation. *J. Virol.* 62:2636–2643.

Jensen, S., M-P. Gassama, and T. Heidmann. 1999. Taming of transposable elements by homology-dependent gene silencing. *Nat. Genet.* 21:209–212.

Johannes, G., and P. Sarnow. 1998. Cap-independent polysomal association of natural mRNAs encoding c-myc, BiP, and eIF4G conferred by internal ribosome entry sites. *RNA* 4:1500–1513.

Jones, P. A. 1985. Altering gene expression with 5-azacytidine. *Cell* 40:485–486.

Kafri, T., M. Ariel, M. Brandeis, R. Shemer, L. Urven, J. McCarrey, H. Cedar, and A. Razin. 1992. Developmental pattern of gene-specific DNA methylation in the mouse embryo and germ line. *Genes Devel.* 6:705–714.

Katsel, P. L., and R. J. Greenstein. 2000. Eukaryotic gene transfer with liposomes: Effect of differences in lipid structure. *Biotechnol. Annu. Rev.* 5:197–220.

Kaufmann, W. E., M. T. Abrams, W. Chen, and A. L. Reiss. 1999. Genotype, molecular phenotype, and cognitive phenotype: Correlations in fragile X syndrome. *Am. J. Med. Genet.* 83:286–295.

Kozak, M. 1989. Circumstances and mechanisms of inhibition of translation by secondary structure in eucaryotic mRNAs. *Mol. Cell Biol.* 9:5134–5142.

———. 1991a. Effects of long 5′ leader sequences on initiation by eukaryotic ribosomes in vitro. *Gene Expr.* 1:117–125.

———. 1991b. An analysis of vertebrate mRNA sequences: Intimations of translational control. *J. Cell Biol.* 115:887–903.

———. 1999. Initiation of translation in prokaryotes and eukaryotes. *Gene* 234:187–208.

Kumari, D., and K. Usdin. 2000. Interactions of the transcription factors USF1, USF2 and alpha-Pal/Nrf-1 at the *FMR1* promoter: Implications for Fragile X mental retardation syndrome. *J. Biol. Chem.* 276:4357–4364.

Laan, L. A., A. v Haeringen, and O. F. Brouwer. 1999. Angelman syndrome: A review of clinical and genetic aspects. *Clin. Neurol. Neurosurg.* 101:161–170.

Lachiewicz, A. M., G. A. Spiridigliozzi, A. McConkie-Rosell, D. Burgess, Y. Feng, S. T. Warren, and J. Tarleton. 1996. A fragile X male with a broad smear on Southern blot analysis representing 100–500 CGG repeats and no methylation at the EagI site of the *FMR-1* gene. *Am. J. Med. Genet.* 64:278–282.

Livak, K. J., S. J. Flood, J. Marmaro, W. Giusti, and K. Deetz. 1995. Oligonucleotides with fluorescent dyes at opposite ends provide a quenched probe system useful for detecting PCR product and nucleic acid hybridization. *PCR Methods Appl.* 4:357–362.

Loesch, D. Z., D. A. Hay, G. R. Sutherland, and P. N. Howard-Peebles. 1987. Phenotypic variation in male-transmitted fragile X: Genetic inferences. *Am. J. Med. Genet.* 27:401–417.

Loesch, D. Z., R. Huggins, D. A. Hay, A. K. Gedeon, J. C. Mulley, and G. R. Sutherland. 1993. Genotype-phenotype relationships in fragile X syndrome: A family study. *Am. J. Hum. Genet.* 53:1064–1073.

Loesch, D. Z., D. A. Hay, and J. Mulley. 1994. Transmitting males and carrier females in fragile X—revisited. *Am. J. Med. Genet.* 51:392–399.

Lohse, J., O. Dahl, and P. E. Nielsen. 1999. Double duplex invasion by peptide nucleic acid: A general principle for sequence specific targeting of double stranded DNA. *Proc. Natl. Acad. Sci. USA* 96:11804–11808.

Lyon, M. F. 1994. The inactivation center and X chromosome imprinting. *Eur. J. Hum. Genet.* 2:255–261.

Mann, D. A., and A. D. Frankel. 1991. Endocytosis and targeting of exogenous HIV-1 Tat protein. *EMBO J.* 10:1733–1739.

Marschall, P., N. Malik, and Z. Larin. 1999. Transfer of YACs up to 2.3 Mb intact into human cells with polyethyleneimine. *Gene Ther.* 6:1634–1637.

Maurer, N., A. Mori, L. Palmer, M. A. Monk, K. W. Mok, B. Mui, Q. F. Akhong, and P. R. Cullis. 1999. Lipid-based systems for the intracellular delivery of genetic drugs. *Mol. Membr. Biol.* 16:129–140.

Mazzocco, M. M., F. Pennington, and R. J. Hagerman. 1993. The neurocognitive phenotype of female carriers of fragile X: Additional evidence for specificity. *J. Dev. Behav. Pediatr.* 14:328–335.

McConkie-Rosell, A., A. M. Lachiewicz, G. A. Spiridigliozzi, J. Tarleton, S. Schoenwald, M. C. Phelan, P. Goonewardena, X. Ding, and W. T. Brown. 1993. *Am. J. Hum. Genet.* 53:800–809.

Merenstein, S. A., V. Shyu, W. E. Sobesky, L. Staley, E. Berry Kravis, D. L. Nelson, K. A. Lugenbeel, A. K. Taylor, B. F. Pennington, and R. J. Hagerman. 1994. Fragile X syndrome in a normal IQ male with learning and emotional problems. *J. Am. Acad. Child Adolesc. Psychiatry* 33:1316–1321.

Merenstein, S. A., W. E. Sobesky, A. K. Taylor, J. E. Riddle, H. X. Tran, and R. J. Hagerman. 1996. Molecular-clinical correlations in males with an expanded *FMR1* mutation. *Am. J. Med. Genet.* 64:388–394.

Mi, Z., J. Mai, X. Lu, and P. D. Robbins. 2000. Characterization of a class of cationic peptides able to facilitate efficient protein transduction in vitro and in vivo. *Mol. Ther.* 2:339–347.

Monk, M., M. Boubelik, and S. Lehnert. 1987. Temporal and regional changes in DNA methylation in the embryonic, extraembryonic and germ cell lineages during mouse embryo development. *Development* 99:371–382.

Mountain, A. 2000. Gene therapy: The first decade. *TIBTECH* 18:119–128.

Nagahara, H., A. Vocero-Akbani, E. L. Snyder, A. Ho, D. G. Latham, N. A. Lissy, M. Becker-Hapak, S. A. Ezhevsky, and S. F. Dowdy. 1998. Transduction of full-length TAT fusion proteins into mammalian cells: TAT-p27Kip1 induces cell migration. *Nat. Med.* 4:1449–1452.

Nanbru, C., I. Lafon, S. Audigier, M-C. Gensac, S. Vagner, G. Huez, and A-C. Prats. 1997. Alternative translation of the proto-oncogene *c-myc* by an internal ribosome entry site. *J. Biol. Chem.* 272:32061–32066.

Nielsen, P. E.. 2000. Peptide nucleic acids: On the road to new gene therapeutic drugs. *Pharmacol. Toxicol.* 86:3–7.

Nielsen, P. E., M. Egholm, R. H. Berg, and O. Buchardt. 1991. Sequence selective recognition of DNA by strand displacement with a thymine-substituted polyamide. *Science* 254:1497–1500.

Nolin, S. L., F. A. Lewis, 3rd, L. L. Ye, G. E. Houck, Jr., A. E. Glicksman, P. Limprasert, S. Y. Li, N. Zhong, A. E. Ashley, E. Feingold, S. L. Sherman, and W. T. Brown. 1996. Familial transmission of the *FMR1* CGG repeat. *Am. J. Hum. Genet.* 59:1252–1261.

Oberlé, L., F. Rousseau, D. Heitz, C. Kretz, D. Devys, A. Hanauer, J. Boue, M. F. Bertheas, and J. L. Mandel. 1991. Instability of a 550-base pair DNA segment and abnormal methylation in fragile X syndrome. *Science* 252:1097–1102.

Peel, A. L., and R. L. Klein. 2000. Adeno-associated virus vectors: Activity and applications in the CNS. *J. Neurosci. Meth.* 98:95–104.

Peier, A. M., K. L. McIlwain, A. Kenneson, S. T. Warren, R. Paylor, and D. L. Nelson. 2000. (Over)correction of *FMR1* deficiency with YAC transgenics: Behavioral and physical features. *Hum. Mol. Genet.* 9:1145–1159.

Pelletier, J., and N. Sonenberg. 1988. Internal initiation of translation of eukaryotic mRNA directed by a sequence derived from poliovirus RNA. *Nature* 334:320–325.

Pieretti, M., F. P. Zhang, Y. H. Fu, S. T. Warren, B. A. Oostra, C. T. Caskey, and D. L. Nelson. 1991. Absence of expression of the *FMR-1* gene in fragile X syndrome. *Cell* 66:817–822.

Pilipenko, E. V., V. P. Pestova, V. G. Kolupaeva, E. V. Khitrina, A. N. Poperechnaya, V. I. Agol, and C. U. T. Hellen. 2000. A cell cycle-dependent protein serves as a template-specific translation initiation factor. *Genes Dev.* 14:2028–2045.

Pooggin, M. M., T. Hohn, and J. Futterer. 2000. Role of a short ORF in ribosome shunt on the CaMV RNA leader. *J. Biol. Chem.* 275:17288–17296.

Pyronnet S., L., L. Pradayrol, and N. Sonenberg. 2000. A cell cycle-dependent internal ribosome entry site. *Mol. Cell* 5:607–616.

Reiss, A. L., L. Freund, M. T. Abrams, C. Boehm, and H. Kazazian. 1993. Neurobehavioral effects of the fragile X premutation in adult women: A controlled study. *Am. J. Hum. Genet.* 52:884–894.

Riddle, J. E., A. Cheema, W. E. Sobesky, S. C. Gardner, A. K. Taylor, B. F. Pennington, and R. J. Hagerman. 1998. Phenotypic involvement in females with the *FMR1* gene mutation *Am. J. Ment. Retard.* 102:590–601.

Riggs, A. D. 1975. X inactivation, differentiation, and DNA methylation. *Cytogenet. Cell Genet.* 14:9–25.

Rousseau, F., D. Heitz, J. Tarleton, J. MacPherson, H. Malmgren, N. Dahl, A. Barnicoat, C. Mathew, E. Mornet, and I. Tejada. 1994. A multicenter study on genotype-phenotype correlations in the fragile X syndrome, using direct diagnosis with probe StB12. 3: The first 2,253 cases. *Am. J. Hum. Genet.* 55:225–237.

Ryabova, L. A., and T. Hohn. 2000. Ribosome shunting in the cauliflower mosaic virus 35S RNA leader is a special case of reinitiation of translation functioning in plant and animal systems. *Genes Dev.* 14:817–829.

Sachs, A. B. 2000. Cell cycle-dependent translation initiation: IRES elements prevail. *Cell* 101:243–245.

Sager, R., and R. Kitchen. 1975. Selective silencing of eukaryotic DNA. *Science* 189:426–433.

Saitoh, S., and T. Wada. 2000. Parent-of-origin specific histone acetylation and reactivation of a key imprinted gene locus in Prader-Willi syndrome. *Am. J. Hum. Genet.* 66:1958–1962.

Schärer-Hernández, N., and T. Hohn. 1998. Nonlinear ribosome migration on cauliflower mosaic virus 35S RNA in transgenic tobacco plants. *Virology* 242:403–413.

Schmidt-Puchta, W., D. Dominguez, D. Lewetag, and T. Hohn. 1997. Plant ribosome shunting in vitro. *Nucleic Acids Res.* 25:2854–2860.

Schwarz, E. M. 2000. The adeno-associated virus vector for orthopaedic gene therapy. *Clin. Orthop.* (379 Suppl): S31–39.

Schwarze, S. R., and S. F. Dowdy. 2000. In vivo protein transduction: Intracellular delivery of biologically active proteins, compounds and DNA. *Trends Pharmacol. Sci.* 21:45–48.

Schwarze, S. R., A. Ho, A. Vocero-Akbani, and S. F. Dowdy. 1999. In vivo protein transduction: Delivery of a biologically active protein into the mouse. *Science* 285:1569–1572.

Selker, E. U. 1998. Trichostatin A causes selective loss of DNA methylation in *Neurospora. Proc. Nat. Acad. Sci. USA* 95:9430–9435.

Smeets, H. J., A. P. Smits, C. E. Verheij, J. P. Theelen, R. Willemsen, I. Van de Burgt, A. T. Hoogeveen, J. C. Oosterwijk, and B. A. Oostra. 1995. Normal phenotype in two brothers with a full *FMR1* mutation. *Hum. Mol. Genet.* 4:2103–2108.

Smith-Arica, J. R., and J. S. Bartlett. 2001. Gene therapy: Recombinant adeno-associated virus vectors. *Curr. Cardiol. Rep.* 2001 3:43–49.

Smits, A., D. Smeets, B. Hamel, J. Dreesen, A. de Haan, and B. van Oost. 1994. Prediction of mental status in carriers of the fragile X mutation using CGG repeat length. *Am. J. Med. Genet.* 51:497–500.

Snow, K., L. K. Doud, R. Hagerman, R. G. Pergolizzi, S. H. Erster, and S. N. Thibodeau. 1993. Analysis of a CGG sequence at the *FMR-1* locus in fragile X families and in the general population. *Am. J. Hum. Genet.* 53:1217–1228.

Stein, C. A. 1999. Two problems in antisense biotechnology: In vitro delivery and the design of antisense experiments. *Biochim. Biophys. Acta* 1489:45–52.

Stöger, R., T. M. Kajimura, W. T. Brown, and C. D. Laird. 1997. Epigenetic variation illustrated by DNA methylation patterns of the fragile-X gene *FMR1. Hum. Mol. Genet.* 6(11):1791–1801.

Sutcliffe, J. S., D. L. Nelson, F. Zhang, M. Pieretti, C. T. Caskey, D. Saxe, and S. T. Warren. 1992. DNA methylation represses *FMR-1* transcription in fragile X syndrome. *Hum. Mol. Genet.* 6:397–400.

Tassone, F., R. J. Hagerman, D. Ikle, P. N. Dyer, M. Lampe, R. Willemsen, B. A. Oostra, and A. K. Taylor. 1999. FMRP expression as a potential prognostic indicator in fragile X syndrome. *Am. J. Med. Genet.* 84:250–261.

Tassone, F., R. J. Hagerman, W. D. Chamberlain, and P. J. Hagerman. 2000a. Transcription of the *FMR1* gene in individuals with fragile X syndrome. *Am. J. Med. Genet.* 97:195–203.

Tassone, F., R. J. Hagerman, D. Z. Loesch, A. Lachiewicz, A. K. Taylor, and P. J. Hagerman. 2000b. Fragile X males with unmethylated, full mutation trinucleotides repeat expansions and elevated levels of *FMR1* messenger. *Am. J. Med. Genet.* 94:232–236.

Tassone, F., R. J. Hagerman, A. K. Taylor, L. W. Gane, T. E. Godfrey, and P. J. Hagerman. 2000c. Elevated levels of *FMR1* messenger RNA in carriers males: A new mechanism of involvement in the fragile X syndrome. *Am. J. Hum. Genet.* 66:6–15.

Tassone, F., R. J. Hagerman, A. K. Taylor, J. B. Mills, S. B. Harris, L. W. Gane, and P. J. Hagerman. 2000d. Clinical involvement and protein expression in individuals with the *FMR1* premutation. *Am. J. Med. Genet.* 91:144–152.

Tassone, F., R. J. Hagerman, A. K. Taylor, and P. J. Hagerman. 2001. A majority of fragile X males with methylated, full mutation alleles have significant levels of *FMR1* messenger RNA. *J. Med. Genet.* 38:453–456.

Taylor, A. K., J. F. Safanda, M. Z. Fall, C. Quince, K. A. Lang, C. E. Hull, I. Carpenter, L. W. Staley, and R. J. Hagerman. 1994. Molecular predictors of cognitive involvement in female carriers of fragile X syndrome. *JAMA* 271:507–514.

Taylor, A. K., F. Tassone, P. N. Dyer, S. M. Hersch, J. B. Harris, W. T. Greenough, and R. J. Hagerman. 1999. Tissue heterogeneity of the *FMR1* mutation in a high-functioning male with fragile X syndrome. *Am. J. Med. Genet.* 84:233–239.

van den Veyver, I. B., and H. Y. Zoghbi. 2000. Methyl-CpG binding protein 2 mutations in Rett syndrome. *Curr. Opin. Genet. Dev.* 10:275–279.

Verheij, C., C. E. Bakker, E. de Graaff, J. Keulemans, R. Willemsen, A. J. Verkerk, H. Galjaard, A. J. J. Reuser, A. T. Hoogeveen, and B. A. Oostra. 1993. Characterization and localization of the *FMR-1* gene product associated with fragile X syndrome. *Nature* 363:722–724.

Vianna-Morgante, A. M., S. S. Costa, A. S. Pares, and I. T. Verreschi. 1996. FRAXA premutation associated with premature ovarian failure. *Am. J. Med. Genet.* 64:373–375.

Vives, E., P. Brodin, and B. Leblus. 1997. A truncated HIV-1 Tat protein basic domain rapidly translocates through the plasma membrane and accumulates in the cell nucleus. *J. Biol. Chem.* 272:16010–10617.

Vocero-Akbani, A., N. A. Lissy, and S. F. Dowdy. 2000. Transduction of full-length Tat fusion proteins directly into mammalian cells: Analysis of T cell receptor activation-induced cell death. *Meth. Enzymol.* 322:508–521.

Wagner, J. A., T. Reynolds, M. L. Moran, R. B. Moss, J. J. Wine, T. R. Flotte, and P. Gardner. 1998. Efficient and persistent gene transfer of AAV-CTFR in maxillary sinus. *Lancet* 351:1702–1703.

Wang, Z., A. K. Taylor, and J. A. Bridge. 1996. *FMR1* fully expanded mutation with minimal methylation in a high functioning fragile X male. *J. Med. Genet.* 33:376–378.

White, S., J. W. Szewzyk, J. M. Turner, E. E. Baird, and P. B. Dervan. 1998. Recognition of the four Watson-Crick base pairs in the DNA minor groove by synthetic ligands. *Nature* 391:468–471.

Willemsen, R., S. Mohkamsing, B. de Vries, D. Devys, A. van den Ouweland, J. L. Mandel, H. Galjaard, and B. Oostra. 1995. Rapid antibody test for fragile X syndrome. *Lancet* 345:1147–1148.

Willemsen, R., A. Smits, S. Mohkamsing, H. van Beerendonk, A. de Haan, B. de Vries, A. van den Ouweland, E. Sistermans, H. Galjaard, and B. A. Oostra. 1997. Rapid antibody test for diagnosing fragile X syndrome: A validation of the technique. *Hum. Genet.* 99:308–311.

Wöhrle, D., and P. Steinbach. 1991. Fragile X expression and X inactivation. II. The fragile site at Xq27. 3 has a basic function in the pathogenesis of fragile X-linked mental retardation. *Hum. Genet.* 87:421–424.

Wöhrle, D., U. Salat, D. Glaser, J. Mucke, M. Meisel-Stosiek, D. Schindler, W. Vogel, and P. Steinbach. 1998. Unusual mutations in high functioning fragile X males: Apparent instability of expanded unmethylated CGG repeats. *J. Med. Genet.* 35:103–111.

Wu, J., and M. Grunstein. 2000. 25 years after the nucleosome model: Chromatin modifications. *Trends Biochem. Sci.* 25:619–623.

Yoshida, M., S. Horinouchi, and T. Beppu. 1990. Trichostatin A and trapoxin: Novel chemical probes for the role of histone acetylation in chromatin structure and function. *BioEssay* 17:423–424.

Yu, S., J. Mulley, D. Loesch, G. Turner, A. Donnelly, A. Gedeon, D. Hillen, E. Kremer, M. Lynch, M. Pritchard, G. R. Sutherland, and R. I. Richards. 1992. Fragile X syndrome: Unique genetics of the heritable unstable element. *Am. J. Med. Genet.* 50: 968–980.

# APPENDIX 1

# General Information about Fragile X Syndrome

Susan Harris

## Foundations

National Fragile X Foundation
P.O. Box 190488
San Francisco, CA 94119
Phone: 1-800-688-8765 or 925-938-9300
Fax: 925-687-9315
Email: natlfx@fragilex.org
Web Page: http://www.fragilex.org

FRAXA Research Foundation
P.O. Box 935
West Newbury, MA 01985-0935
Phone: 978-462-1866
Fax: 978-463-9985
Email: info@fraxa.org
Web Page: http://www.fraxa.org
Fragile X listserve: to subscribe, send email to listserv@listserv.cc.emory.edu
with, "SUBSCRIBE FRAGILEX-L" in the message body.

Fragile X Research Foundation of Canada
167 Queen Street West
Brampton, Ontario, Canada L6Y 1M5
Phone: 905-453-9366
Email: FXRFC@attglobal.net
Web Page: http://dante.med.utoronto.ca/Fragile-X/linksto.htm

The Fragile X Society (England)
53 Winchelsea Lane
Hastings, East Sussex TN35 4LG
Phone: 011-424-813147
Email: lesleywalker@fragilex.k-web.co.uk
Web Page: http://www.fragilex.org.uk

The International Fragile X Alliance (Australia)
263 Glen Elra Road
Nth Caulfield 3161
Melbourne, Australia
Phone: 03-9528-1910
Fax: 03-9532-9555
Email: jcohen@netspace.net.au

Fragile X Association of Australia, Inc.
15 Bowen Close
Cherrybrook, NSW, Australia
Phone: 019-987012
Email: fragilex@ozemail.com.au

## Reading for Families

*Fragile: Handle with Care; More about Fragile X Syndrome, Adolescents and Adults.* Braden, M. (2000) Dillon, Colo.: Spectra Publishing.

*Children with Fragile X Syndrome: A Parent's Guide.* Weber, J. (2000) Bethesda, Md.: Woodbine House.

*Behavior and Development in Fragile X Syndrome.* Dykens, E. M., Hodapp, R. M., and Leckman, J. F. (1994) Thousand Oaks, Calif.: Sage Publication.

*Educating Children with Fragile X Syndrome: A Guide for Parents and Professionals.* Copies can be obtained by calling Gail Spiridigliozzi at 919-684-5513.

*Fragile X Syndrome: Diagnosis, Treatment, and Research,* 3d edition. Hagerman, R. J., and Hagerman, P. J. (eds.) (2002) Baltimore: Johns Hopkins University Press.

*The Fragile X Child.* Schopmeyer, B. B., and Lowe, F. (1992) San Diego: Singular Publishing Co.

*The Fragile X Syndrome: A Handbook for Parents and Professionals.* Finucane, B., McConkie-Rosell, A., and Cronister-Silverman, A. (2002) National Fragile X Foundation.

*A Parent's Guide to Drug Treatment of Fragile X Syndrome.* Tranfaglia, M. R. (2000) West Newbury, Mass.: FRAXA Research Foundation.

*Seventh International Fragile X Conference Proceedings, July 19–23, 2000.* Miller, R. (ed.) (2001) San Francisco: National Fragile X Foundation.

*Straight Talk about Psychiatric Medications for Kids.* Wilens, T. E. (1999) New York: Guilford Press.

*Transitioning "Special" Children into Elementary School.* Weber, J. D. Books beyond Borders, 1881 Fourth Street, #108, Boulder, Colo. 80302 (1-800-347-6440).

*Issues and Strategies for Educating Children with Fragile X Syndrome: A Monograph.* Wilson, P., Stackhouse, T., O'Connor, R., Scharfenaker, S., and Hagerman, R. (1994) National Fragile X Foundation.

## Newsletters

*National Fragile X Foundation Newsletter.* Call the National Fragile X Foundation at 1-800-688-8765.

*FRAXA Research Foundation Newsletter.* Subscriptions through FRAXA, P.O. Box 935, West Newbury, MA 01985.

*The Fragile X Society Newsletter.* Subscriptions through the Fragile X Society (London), 237 Lyndhurst Avenue, Twickenham, Middlesex, England TW2 6BW.

## Reading for Children

*Boys with Fragile X Syndrome.* O'Connor, R. (1995) Can be obtained from the National Fragile X Foundation at 1-800-688-8765.

*I Feel Angry.* Moses, B. (1995) Wayland Publishers Ltd., 61 Western Road, Hove, East Sussex, England BN3 LJD.

*My Brother Has Fragile X Syndrome.* Steiger, C. (1998) Chapel Hill, N.C.: National Fragile X Foundation at 1-800-688-8765.

## General Family Support—Internet

The Family Village
http://www.familyvillage.wisc.edu
This site was organized by the Waisman Center of the University of Wisconsin–Madison.

The Family Village integrates resources and communication opportunities on the Internet for people with disabilities, their families, and those who support and serve them. Selections include: Library (information re: disabilities), Coffee Shop (connections with other families), Hospital (links re: health care concerns), Shopping Mall (assistive technology suppliers), and others.

Family Voices
http://www.ichp.edu/mchb/fv
Family Voices is a national grassroots network of families and friends speaking on behalf of children with special health care needs. Selections include:

About Family Voices, ACCESS-MCH/Family Voices, PIC Project, To Join Family Voices, Voices Newsletter, Español, Search.

National Parent Network on Disabilities (NPND)
http://www.npnd.org
NPND was established to provide a presence and national voice for parents of children, youth, and adults with special needs. NPND shares information and resources in order to promote and support the power of parents to influence and affect policy issues concerning the needs of people with disabilities and their families. The selections include news releases, the Friday Fax (weekly newsletter from the Department of Health and Human Services), conferences, federal issues, links to federal government sites, and information on IDEA.

PACER Center
http://www.pacer.org
PACER stands for Parent Advocacy Coalition for Educational Rights. Selections include: Publications (including order forms), Who We Are, PACER Center Articles, Events, Legislative Information (including alerts), Frequently Asked Questions, Projects, National Information (links to other organizations).

PEP: Parents, Educators, and Publishers
http://www.microweb.com/pepsite/index.html
The PEP site is intended as an informational resource for parents, educators, and children's software publishers. The creators of this site have developed its content in response to the interests and needs of these three audiences. Selections include: Children's Software Revue, Educational Software Publishers, Computer Camps, Shopper Resources, and Cool School Sites.

## Readings for Parents, Patients, and Teachers Regarding ADHD

### Books on ADHD

Barkley, R. A. 1995. *Taking Charge of ADHD: The Complete, Authoritative Guide for Parents.* New York: Guilford Press.
———. 1997. *ADHD and the Nature of Self Control.* New York: Guilford Press.
———. 1997. *Defiant Children: A Clinician's Manual for Assessment and Parent Training,* 2d edition. New York: Guilford Press.
Clark, L. 1989. *The Time-out Solution: A Parent's Guide for Handling Everyday Behavior Problems.* Chicago: Contempory Books.
Fowler, M. C. 1990. *Maybe You Know My Kid: A Parent's Guide to Identifying, Understanding, and Helping Your Child with Attention Deficit Hyperactive Disorder.* New York: Carol Publishing Group.

Garber, S. W., Garber, M. D., and Spizman, R. F. 1990. *If Your Child Is Hyperactive, Inattentive, Impulsive, Distractible . . . Helping the ADD (Attention Deficit Disorder) Hyperactive Child.* New York: Villard Books.

Hallowell, E., and Ratey, J. 1994. *Driven to Distraction: Recognizing and Coping with Attention Deficit Disorder from Childhood through Adulthood.* New York: Pantheon Books.

———. 1994. *Answers to Distraction.* New York: Pantheon Books.

Ingersoll, B. 1988. *Your Hyperactive Child: A Parent's Guide to Coping with Attention Deficit Disorder.* New York: Doubleday.

Ingersoll, B., and Goldstein, S. 1993. *Attention Deficit Disorder and Learning Disabilities: Realities, Myths, and Controversial Treatments.* New York: Doubleday Main Street Books.

Kelly, K., and Ramundo, P. 1996. *You Mean I'm Not Lazy, Stupid, or Crazy?!* New York: Fireside Books.

Nadeau, K. 1994. *Survival Guide for College Students with ADD or LD.* New York: Magination Press.

Nadeau, K. G. 1995. *A Comprehensive Guide to Attention Deficit Disorder in Adults: Research, Diagnosis, and Treatment.* New York: Brunner/Mazel.

Wilens, T. E. 1999. *Straight Talk about Psychiatric Medications for Kids.* New York: Guilford Press.

## Newsletters for ADHD

*Attention! The Magazine of Children and Adults with Attention Deficit Disorders* (449 N.W. 70th Avenue, Suite 208, Plantation, FL 33317).

*The ADHD Report.* New York: Guilford (72 Spring Street, New York, NY 10012).

*Challenge: The First National Newsletter on Attention Deficit (Hyperactivity) Disorder* (P.O. Box 2001, West Newbury, MA 01985).

## Readings for Pharmacotherapy in Children and Adolescents

Aman, M. G, and K. S. Langworthy. 2000. Pharmacotherapy for hyperactivity in children with autism and other pervasive developmental disorders. *Journal of Autism and Developmental Disorders* 30:451–459.

Biederman, J., and T. Spencer. 2000. Nonstimulant treatments for ADHD. *European Child and Adolescent Psychiatry* 9:51–59.

Green, W. H. 1995. *Child and Adolescent Clinical Psychopharmacology.* Baltimore: Williams & Wilkins.

Greenhill, L. L., J. M. Halperin, and H. Abikoff. 1999. Stimulant medications. *Journal of the American Academy of Child and Adolescent Psychiatry* 38:503–512.

Kutcher, S. P. 1997. *Child and Adolescent Psychopharmacology.* Philadelphia: Saunders.

McFee, R. B., and L. I. Weinstein. 2001. ADHD and adolescent psychopharmacology. *Journal of Adolescent Health* 28:255–256.

Popper, C. W. 2000. Pharmacologic alternatives to psychostimulants for the treatment of attention-deficit/hyperactivity disorder. *Child and Adolescent Psychiatric Clinics of North America* 9:605–646.

Riddle, M. A. 1995. Pediatric Psychopharmacology I. *Child Adolescent Psychiatry Clinics of North America* 4:1–260.

———. 1995. Pediatric Psychopharmacology II. *Child Adolescent Psychiatry Clinics of North America* 4:261–520.

Rosenberg, D. R., Holttum, J., and Gershon, S. I. 1994. *Textbook of Pharmacotherapy for Child and Adolescent Psychiatric Disorders.* New York: Brunner/Mazel.

Werry, J. S., and Aman, M. G. 1993. *Practitioner's Guide to Psychoactive Drugs for Children and Adolescents.* New York: Plenum.

Wiener, J. M. 1996. *Diagnosis and Psychopharmacology of Childhood and Adolescent Disorders.* New York: Wiley.

# APPENDIX 2

# Computer Software Information

Andrew Halpern, M.D., Lisa Nobel, M.S.,
and Kristen Gray, M.S.

## Recommended Software

Berta Max Educational Software Center
P.O. Box 31849
Seattle, WA 98103

*Berta Max Read Alongs* ($25)
A series of emergent and early reading books on the computer. Text is predictable with rhyme and repetition. Graphics are good and text is underlined as it is read by the speech synthesizer. Stories include ABC, counting, and Feet (Apple)

Big Top Productions
1-800-900-PLAY

*Hello Kitty Big Fun Deluxe* ($40)
Coloring book, piano, animal sounds, story book, and counting. CD-ROM

Bright Star
P.O. Box 485
Coarsegold, CA 93614
1-800-743-7725

*Dream Team Series* ($15–25)
Combination of visual and auditory feedback in interactive programs designed to teach early learning through middle elementary concepts. Some available in CD-ROM format. (Mac/IBM)
Alphabet Blocks, Beginning Reading, Early Math, Kid's Typing, Basic Spelling, Advanced Spelling

Brøderbund
17 Paul Drive
San Rafael, CA 94903
1-800-521-6263

*Playworld BUNDLE* ($90)
The Backyard, Playroom, The Tree House

*Living Books Series* ($35–$45)
The Living Books series combines sound and animation to bring children's literature to life. The story can be read aloud and virtually every object on the page can be manipulated in some way. CD-ROM
    Arthur's Teacher Trouble; Arthur's Birthday; Berenstein Bears Get in a Fight; Dr. Seuss ABC; Green Eggs and Ham; Harry and the Haunted House; Just Grandma and Me; Little Monster at School; The New Kid on the Block; Ruff's Bone; Sheila Rae, the Brave; The Tortoise and The Hare

*Amazing Writing Machine* ($40)
Journals, poetry, essays, stories and more. Includes feature to support building stories from a template. CD-ROM

*Kid Pix Studio* ($30–$40)
This is an excellent graphics and drawing program. Children can write by stamping letters, select stamps to put in their pictures, and draw in color. The alphabet talks, and sound effects can be added to pictures. Also integrates features of Kid Pix Companion. (Mac, IBM)

*Math Workshop* ($30–$40)
Highly interactive problem-solving software. Arithmetic and visual perceptual skills are addressed through seven different activities. Multiple skill levels are available (Mac, IBM)

*Print Shop or Deluxe* ($36)
This easy-to-use program allows the user to make signs, banners, and letters. It is an excellent tool for motivational writing and creation activities. (Apple, Mac, IBM)

*Where in —— Is Carmen San Diego Series* ($35)
Reading, attention to detail, discrimination between significant and insignificant facts, note taking, and a variety of other skills are used to catch a crook who flees to different parts of the world.

Creative Wonders
1-800-KID-XPRT

> *Early Learning* ($35)
> Sesame Street: Get Set to Learn, Elmo's Preschool, Sesame Street: Let's Make a Word
>
> *School House Rock Series* ($35–$40)
> Grammar Rock, Science Rock, America Rock, Math Rock

Davidson
1-800-567-4321

> *Kids Can Read—5 titles in a bundle* ($40)
> A collection of popular books converted to CD-ROM technology. The program will read the story, pronounce words individually, and even give definitions of words. It also creates a list of words that the reader needs to practice. Can read in Spanish or English. CD-ROM
>
> *Kid Phonics 1* ($40)
>
> *Kid Phonics 2* ($40)
>
> *Kid Keys* ($35)
> Talking animated typing program. Three activities to familiarize young children with keyboard functions. (IBM/Mac)
>
> *Math Blaster Series* ($35)
> Addition, subtraction, multiplication and division concepts are taught in a fun arcade game format. On disks further into the series concepts in the areas of geometry and algebra are explored. (Apple, Mac, IBM)
> > Math Blaster Mystery, Math Blaster: In Search of Spot, What's My Angle?
> > Alge-Blaster 3

Don Johnston Developmental Equipment, Inc.
P.O. Box 1000 N. Rand Road, Bldg. 115
Wauconda, IL 60084
1-800-999-4660

> *Big Calc* ($29)
> Large calculator program that has many features for manipulating numbers as well as the layout of the keypad. Has auditory feedback capabilities. (Mac)

*Blocks in Motion* ($79 starter kit)
Building blocks for the computer. New sets of bricks can be purchased for $25 each.

*Co:Writer* ($350)
A word prediction program that "guesses" the word to be typed based on the first few letters. It collects new words as you use them, and adds them to the lists of possibilities. This program makes writing much faster.

*Gateway Stories I and II* ($125)

*Gateway Authoring System* ($90)
Allows the reader to independently select, hear, and turn pages with a switch or mouse click. The authoring program allows you to insert graphics and text onto blank pages.

*Eensy and Friends* ($65)
Characters involved in cause/effect games that involve counting, dressing and prepositions.

*Write: Outloud* ($99)
All of the power of a fully functional word processor including a spell checker, with the added feature of speech. The speech output options are flexible enough to meet every user's needs. There is visual ribbon, which makes changing settings as easy as pointing and clicking.


Edmark Corporation
P.O. Box 3218
Redmond, WA 98073-3218

*Imagination Express Series* ($30 each)
Castle; Time Trip, USA; Pyramids; Ocean; Neighborhood; Rain Forest; Creative Writing programs. CD-ROM

*Kid's Desk* ($59)
A program which allows for single click access to individual applications. The system and other parts of the computer can be locked to avoid inadvertent loss. (IBM/Mac)

*Learning House Programs* ($30–$40)
Learn about a variety of concepts through interactive games and exploration. (IBM/Mac)
Bailey's Book House, Millie's Math House, Sammy's Science House, Stanley's Sticker Stories, Trudy's Time and Place House

*Mighty Math Series* ($60)
Interactive math programs in different levels. CD-ROM
Carnival Countdown, Zoo Zillions, Number Heroes, Calculating Crew, Cosmic Geometry, Astro Algebra

*Thinkin' Things 1* ($40)

*Thinkin' Things 2* ($40)

*Thinkin' Things 3* ($40)
Builds critical thinking skills and creativity. Musical patterns, logical comparison, and deductive reasoning addressed. (Mac/IBM) CD-ROM

*Strategy Games of the World* ($45)
Includes Mancala, Nine Men's Morris, and GO. Can play against computer or another person. CD-ROM

Information Services, Inc.
28 Green Street
Newbury, MA 01951
1-800-659-3399

*WriteAway* ($199)
This word prediction program "guesses" the next word being typed based on the first few letters. It has the ability to collect new words and add them to its dictionary. This program may greatly increase typing speed. This program is not transparent and must be used only with the accompanying word processor. (DOS/Windows)

IntelliTools
55 Leveroni Court, Suite 9
Novato, CA 94949
1-800-899-6687

*Click It!* ($99.95)
Software allows programming of any computer input. Allows for more than one switch to be used differentially within any software program.

*IntelliTalk* ($50)
A talking word processor which can speak letters, words, sentences, or any combination (Mac, IBM, Apple).

*IntelliPics* ($40)
This software allows the user to design software simply and creatively to be used with a mouse or the IntelliKeys, when an overlay is created using Overlay Maker. Specific concepts can be addressed in a fun, interactive way. (Mac)

*Overlay Maker* ($80)
This is a program which allows for the IntelliKeys to be programmed to meet an individual's needs.

Knowledge Adventure, Inc.
1311 Grand Central Avenue
Glendale, CA 91201
1-800-542-4240

*Jump\*start Learning System* ($20–$40 each)
A grade-based software series that targets various skills at each grade level.
Toddlers: computer mouse skills, letters and numbers, vocabulary, and music
Preschool: comprehension, phonics, mouse skills, letters and numbers, vocabulary, and music
Pre-K: letter order, quantities, problem solving, decision making, social roles, phonics, counting, vocabulary, and music
Kindergarten: letter combinations, reading & sentences, similarities & differences, sequencing, counting, art, time concepts, comprehension, listening skills, vocabulary, and music
1st Grade: spelling, literature, math, science, geography, phonics, reading, similarities & differences, sequencing, art, vocabulary, and music
2nd Grade: basic grammar, math, social studies, science, geography, vocabulary, writing, spelling, literature, reading, art, sequencing, comprehension, and phonics review
3rd Grade: history, science, geography, spelling, grammar, sentence structure, math, art, music, and astronomy
4th Grade: history, science, geography, parts of speech, spelling, grammar, story creation, math, art history, and music
5th Grade: history, logic, problem solving, deductive reasoning, map skills, science, geography, grammar, math skills (including geometry), and art history

Laureate Learning Systems, Inc.
110 E. Spring Street
Winooski, VT 05404-1837
1-800-562-6801
The purpose of this software series is to introduce the concepts of cause and effect, switch use, visual tracking, discrete pointing, and turn-taking. ($75)

*Creature Antics*

*Creature Capers*

*Creature Features*

*Creature Chorus*

*First Words Series* ($200 each)
This series is part of an entire language development program. It can be accessed in a variety of ways, including touch window and single switch. There is a Lesson Editor, which allows for customization of the software. Most pieces of software from this company can be run on a Macintosh with an Apple IIe emulator, and they are currently developing more Macintosh specific software.

Lawrence Productions
1800 S. 35th Street
Galesburg, MI 49053-9687
1-800-421-4157

These programs allow children to explore different environments on the computer. Children decide what McGee will play with and explore (Apple II available individually, Mac, IBM) ($32)

*McGee Series*

*McGee*

*McGee at Fun Fair*

*McGee Visits Katie's Farm*

The Learning Company
6493 Kaiser Dr.
Freemont, CA 94555
1-800-852-2255

*Ancient Empires!*

*Treasure Mountain!*

*Time Riders in American History*

*Gizmos and Gadgets*

*Operation Neptune*

*Midnight Rescue*

*Spell Bound*
Adventure games that use reading, math, science, comprehension, and critical thinking skills. (IBM, Macintosh)

*Reader/Writer Rabbit Series* ($40–$50 each)
Each piece of software works on different reading and writing skills, from letter recognition to word attack strategies. (IBM, Apple, Mac)

*Interactive Reading Journey* ($100)
Combines open-ended reading exploration with structured practice. Wide variety of concepts addressed. CD-ROM

*Math Rabbit Series* ($40)
Each piece of software works on different math skills, from number recognition to problem solving and arithmetic. (IBM, Apple, Mac)

*Interactive Math Journey* ($90)
Combines open-ended math exploration with structured practice. Wide variety of concepts addressed. CD-ROM

*The Writing Center (Mac)* ($55)

*The Bilingual Writing Center (Mac)*

*The Student's Writing Center (IBM)*

*The Children's Writing and Publishing Center (Apple)*

*The Children's Writing and Publishing Center Spanish Edition (Apple)*
All of the features of The Children's Writing and Publishing Center and much more. It includes a spell checker, thesaurus, and graphics. You can also import graphics from other programs. It will print in color or black and white. This is an easy-to-use and versatile word-processing program.

MacWarehouse
P.O. Box 3013
1720 Oak Street
Lakewood, NJ
08701-3013
1-800-255-6227

*OmniPage 3.0* ($459)
Optical Character Recognition software allows for scanned data to be treated as text files. Imperative if the goal is to work with the information scanned in a word-processing format.

Madenta Communications
Box 25 Advanced Technology Centre
9650 20 Avenue
Edmonton, Alberta, Canada
1-800-661-8406

*Screen Doors* ($365)
This is a word prediction, on-screen keyboard, and telephone program. The word prediction portion "guesses" the next word being typed based on the first few letters. It has the ability to collect new words and add them to its dictionary. This program greatly increases typing speed. The on-screen keyboard allows for typing using only a mouse or mouse emulator. The telephone feature allows for environmental control of the telephone through the computer and a modem. This program is "transparent" in that it can be used with any word processing program. Pieces of the program can be purchased as needed. (Mac)

*Telepathic* ($250)
This word prediction program "guesses" the next word being typed based on the first few letters. It has the ability to collect new words and add them to its dictionary. This program may greatly increase typing speed. This program is "transparent" in that it can be used with any word processing program. (Mac)

MECC
3490 Lexington Ave. N.
Saint Paul, MN 55126
1-800-228-3504
MECC produces numerous pieces of academic software, with subjects ranging from science, to problem solving, to telling time. These programs can often be used to integrate with classroom curriculum goals.

*Storybook Weaver Deluxe* ($55)
Create a storybook with a picture library, and fun fonts.

*Trail Programs* ($60)
Trail games incorporate multiple skills, including planning and problem solving. CD-ROM
Oregon Trail, Amazon Trail, Africa Trail, Maya Quest

Microsystems Software, Inc.
600 Worcester Road
Framingham, MA 01701-5342
1-800-828-2600

*HandiWORD* ($290)
This word prediction program "guesses" the next word being typed based on the first few letters. It has the ability to collect new words and add them to its dictionary. This program may greatly increase typing speed. This program is "transparent" in that it can be used with any word processing program. (DOS/Windows)

Orange Cherry Talking Schoolhouse
P.O. Box 390
Pound Ridge, NY 10576-0390

Many of the programs in this series are available bundled together on a CD-ROM for Macintosh.

*Talking Alpha Chimp* ($40)
Alphabet skills and early numbers are taught by Harry the Chimp. Three programs are included: Alphabet board, Number Tree, and alphabet Story. (IIgs/IBM)

*Jungle Safari* ($40)
Take a safari and learn about animals and their habitats. Prereaders can explore the animals by passing the reading sections. Motivating text for beginning and advanced readers. (IIgs)

*Talking First Words* ($40)
Introduction to word classes, such as nouns, verbs, and word families. Children complete sentences, solve riddles, and fill in missing letters. (IIgs/IBM)

*Talking Addition and Subtraction* ($40)
Beginning math problems are introduced, including number sets, picture problems, and a number line. Immediate feedback is provided for all input. (IIgs/IBM)

*Talking Clock* ($40)
Time telling skills are taught in hours, minutes, and seconds. (IIgs/IBM)

Tom Snyder Productions
90 Sherman Street
Cambridge, MA 02140
617-876-4433

*Flodd the Bad Guy* ($40–$50)

*Jack in the Beanstalk*
These programs are interactive storybooks. Children read the story, turn the page, and choose where the story goes. (IBM, Mac, Apple)

Toucan Software
21000 Nordhoff Street
Chatsworth, CA 91311
1-800-247-4641

Children create their own stories following familiar story lines and formats. Each program includes graphics and text generation. (Apple, IBM, Mac)

*Creative Writing Series* ($50–60 each)
Big Book Maker: Fairy Tales and Nursery Rhymes
Big Book Maker: Tall Tales and American Folk Heroes
Monsters and Make Believe
Comic Book Maker
Story Starters: Social Studies, Science
Dinosaur Days Plus
Robot Writer

Walt Disney Computer Software Inc.
500 S. Buena Vista Street
Burbank, CA 91521

*Mickey's ABC's, A Day at the Fair* ($27.95)

*Mickey's 123's, The Big Surprise Party* ($27.95)

*Mickey's Colors and Shapes, The Dazzling Magic Show* ($27.95)

*Mickey's Jigsaw* ($34.95)

*Beauty and the Beast Print Kit* ($13.95)

*Aladdin Print Kit* ($13.95)
Variety of programs which work on different skill areas. They all have popular Disney characters, high quality graphics, and auditory feedback. (IBM)

Weekly Reader Software
Optimum Resources, Inc.
10 Station Place
Norfolk, CT 06058

This is a fun series of software programs introducing a variety of concepts to children. These include ABC's, Numbers, Shapes, and Opposites, among others. (Apple/IBM/Mac)

*Talking Sticky Bear Series* ($25–$35 each)
Numbers, Math, Word Problems, ABC's, Typing, Reading, Opposites

William K. Bradford Publishing
310 School Street
Acton, MA 01720

These programs are classic and familiar stories (e.g., Princess and the Pea, The Three Little Pigs, Lima Bean Dream, etc.) that allow the children to read the story, create their own stories and a variety of other activities related to the story. The graphics on the screen move with a mouse, so children can interact with the story as they read it. (Apple)

*Explore-a-Classic* ($40–$50 each)

*Explore-a-Folktale*

*Explore-a-Science*

*Explore-a-Story*

## Other CD-ROM Disks

*MacMillan Dictionary for Children* ($30)
Includes almost 12,000 word entries, 1,000 illustrations, and 40 sound effects. You can hear a spoken version of any word by clicking on its pronunciation.

*Grolier's or Compton's Encyclopedia* ($240)
More than 33,000 articles featuring audio capabilities, hundreds of maps and thousands of pictures.

## Games

*Shanghai* (visual/perceptual)

*Tetris* (visual/perceptual)

*Lemmings (Psygnosis)* (problem solving)

*Columns* (visual/perceptual)

*Jeopardy* (knowledge base)

*Wheel of Fortune* (decoding skills/knowledge base)

*Mr. Potato Head* (Playskool)

*Candy Land Adventure* (Playskool)

## Technology Resource Centers

Nebraska Assistive Technology Project
Phone: (402) 471-0735
This organization can provide families with information regarding technology outreach centers, such as computer labs that may be available in various areas of the state.

Children's Charity Fund
7061 S. Tamiami Trail
Sarasota, FL 34238
Phone: 1-800-6HELPUS
This organization may fund assistive technology, including computers. Families may call for an application. After all information is submitted, applications are considered on a individual basis, and the process takes a few days.

Educational Resources
1550 Executive Dr.
Elgin, Illinois 60123
1-800-624-2926
They have a catalog through which software can be purchased.

American Printing House for the Blind
1839 Frankfort Avenue
P.O. Box 6085
Louisville, KY 40206-0085
Phone: 1-800-223-1839
This company has many books available on tape, including literature for all age levels.

# APPENDIX 3
# Learning Materials and Equipment

Andrew Halpern, M.D., Sarah Scharfenaker, M.A., C.C.C.,
Rebecca O'Connor, M.A., Tracy Stackhouse, O.T.R.,
Marcia L. Braden, Ph.D., and Kristen Gray, M.S.

Special Education Materials

Educational Resources
1550 Executive Dr.
Elgin, Illinois 60123
1-800-624-2926
    They have a catalog through which software can be purchased.

American Printing House for the Blind
1839 Frankfort Avenue
P.O. Box 6085
Louisville, KY 40206-0085
Phone: 1-800-223-1839
    This company has many books available on tape, including literature for all age levels.

Books On Tape Inc.
P.O. Box 7900
Newport Beach, CA 92658
Phone: 1-800-88-BOOKS
email: botcs@booksontape.com
web page: http://www.booksontape.com

Library for the Blind and Dyslexic
Princeton, NJ
Phone: (609) 452-0606

Pro Ed Publishers
8700 Shoal Creek Blvd.
Austin, TX 78757
Phone: 1-800-897-3202
   Lindamood Phoneme Sequencing Program for Reading, Spelling and Speech (LIPS)


Gander Publishing Company
553 Thain Way
Palo Alto, CA 94306
Phone: (415) 858-0971
Fax: (415) 858-0971
   Lindamood-Bell, "Visualizing & Verbalizing"


Educator's Publishing Service
31 Smith Place
Cambridge, MA 02138-1089
1-800-225-5750
   Orton Gillingham for reading and spelling


Innovative Learning Concepts, Inc.
6760 Corporate Drive
Colorado Springs, CO 80919
Phone: 1-800-888-9191
   Touch Math: Multisensory program for basic arithmetic and computation


Handwriting Without Tears, Janice Z. Olsen, OTR
Distributed by:
Fred Sammons, Inc.
Box 32
Brookfield, IL 60513
Phone: (800)-323-7305 or (312) 971-0610


Slantboard & Raised Line Paper
K&L Resources, Inc.
P.O. Box 2612
Springfield, VA 22152
Phone: (703) 455-1503
   Paper: Flaghouse catalog 250 sheets: $42 (800) 793-7900

Testing and Evaluation Strategies for Children with Williams Syndrome
(Early Intervention to Vocational Options)
Published by the William Syndrome Association
P.O. Box 297
Clawson, MI 48017-0297
Phone: (248) 541-3630

How to Participate in Your Child's IEP
Published by:
The Coordinating Council for Handicapped Children
20E Jackson Blvd. Room 900
Chicago, IL
    Publication #312-939-3513

*Reading (sight/visually based)*

Logo Reading System, by Marcia L. Braden, Ph.D.
219 E. Saint Vrain
Colorado Springs, CO 80903
    The Logo reading system uses well-known logos, traditional flash cards, sort
cards with placements, phrase cards, and matching/fine-motor worksheets.

Edmark Corporation
P.O. Box 3903
Bellevue, WA 98009-3903
    The Edmark Reading Program, Level 1, is a beginning reading and language
development program recommended for use with any individual who is considered a nonreader. The program contains 227 lessons presented in five formats: prereading, word recognition, direction book, picture/phrase matching,
and storybook lessons.

SRA (Science Research Associates, Inc.)
155 N. Wacker Drive
Chicago, IL 60606
    Corrective Reading comprehension develops the reasoning processes (ana-
logs, deductions, inductions, classification), vocabulary, and writing skills students need. Reasoning is taught, not just practiced, in carefully written lessons
that foster an experience of success and self-worth.

Merrill Reading Series
Merrill Publishing Co.
P.O. Box 508
Columbus, OH 43216-0508

The Merrill Linguistic Reading Program motivates students to become independent readers and encourages them to learn, to know, to think and to discover. The program offers reading in important areas such as science, health, history, mathematics, and literature.

Appletree-Dormac, Inc.
P.O. Box 270459
San Diego, CA 92128-0983
Appletree is an acronym for "A Patterned Program of Linguistic Expansion Through Reinforced Experiences and Evaluations." It is a language system that provides sequential procedures for construction and development of the basic sentence structures that are the foundation of verbal language. The program has six workbooks, a teacher's manual, and a pre-post test booklet.

Cloze Stories for Reading
Walker Education Book Corporation
720 Fifth Avenue
New York, NY 10019
This reading program uses a cloze technique that has proven successful with students who are affected with FXS. The progression of lessons presents words and then phrases with deletions. The learner is expected to fill in the spaces, which matches well their learning style.

Developing Every Day Reading Skills
Educational Design Inc.
47 West St.
New York, NY 10011
This series is an excellent presentation of tasks related to everyday functional skills such as reading maps, schedules, and recipes to figuring a budget and predicting costs of purchases.

First Sight Word Lotto
Lakeshore Learning Materials
2695 E. Dominguez St.
P.O. Box 6261
Carson, CA 90749
This game allows the learner to practice reading skills without the anxiety often created by a structured, formal reading format.

High Hat
American Guidance Services
Circle Pines, MN 55014-1796

This program includes a story line about a character that travels through a reading series. It is augmented by puppets and characters that allow for associations, as well as a contextual framework to comprehension.

The Master Blender
Walker Education Book Corporation
720 Fifth Ave.
New York, NY 10019

Although phonetic in its approach, this series provides visual patterns that make the reading process more viable.

Reading Milestones
Edmark Corporation
P. O. Box 3903
Bellevue, WA 98009-3903

Reading milestones is a comprehensive reading program for students who struggle with phonics-based instruction. It is a systematic, language-based approach that presents an attractive alternative to traditional reading programs.

Capture the Meaning
CC Publications
P.O. Box 23699
Tigard, OR 97223-0108

Here is an exciting new program that really teaches comprehension. Effective and easy to use, "Capture the Meaning: Strategies for Reading Comprehension" focuses on strategies for building comprehension. This 10-unit, 35-lesson program consists of teacher-guided instruction and practice, independent practice that includes individual and group activities, and tests—all designed to reinforce and build reading comprehension skills.

Reading Attainment System, 1987
Educational Design, Inc.
47 W. 13th Street
New York, NY 10011

This program is specially designed to supply practice for students who fail when basal texts reach the 3d-5th-grade reading level. Ease in reading comes only with practice at low reading levels. This system supplies that practice and produces fluency and confidence in students for whom ordinary methods of remediation have failed. Reading skills, vocabulary skills, and thinking skills are offered in three different sets of multiquestion exercises.

## Spelling

"I Can Print"
PRO-ED
5341 Industrial Oaks Boulevard
Austin, TX 78735

Designed to help students develop the necessary skills to form letters, begin writing sentences, and build handwriting fluency, "I Can Print" can be used as a developmental program in kindergarten, first grade, and special education. Also designed to be used as a remedial program for older children who have already learned to write but consistently have trouble with letter formation and spacing.

Spell Master
Chieftain Products Inc.
265 Champagne Dr.
Downsview, Ontario, Canada M3J 2C6

This game resembles Scrabble in that letter blocks are provided to match a visual configuration, which is augmented by a picture of the word. It is especially appropriate to test spelling because it can be used in lieu of written tests.

Right Line Paper
Pro Ed
8700 Shoal Creek Blvd.
Austin, TX 78757-6897

This paper provides raised lines to give tactile input to the writer. It is especially helpful to the learner with spatial deficits.

## Mathematics

"I Can Plus and Minus"
PRO-ED
5341 Industrial Oaks Boulevard
Austin, TX 78735

A complete arithmetic program based on learning theory and practical experience, this is a beginning series that moves from an assumption of no skill by the student through 116 ordered skills, culminating in regrouping two-place subtraction.

Good Apple Math Book
Grimm & Mitchell
6 Apple, Box 299
Carthage, IL 62321

Math can be fun when students discover how to apply basic skills in practical ways. Activities are based on nature, mail order catalogs, popular foods, calendars, etc. Complete instructions for a math center with 28 idea cards and four gameboards are included.

Big Money Market
Budget Town
Classroom Cash
Edmark Time Telling
Edmark Touch Money
Look'n Cook
Edmark
P. O. Box 9702
Redmond, WA 98073-9721

These programs all provide learning experiences in the application of mathematics.

Dino Math Tracks Game
Learning Resources
380 N. Fairway Dr.
Vernon Hills, IL 60061

This game includes three levels of challenge for children aged six and above. It teaches addition, subtraction, and place value.

Money Skills Package
Attainment Company
P. O. Box 930160
Verona, WI 53593-0160

This program provides real-life teaching application of money skills. It is particularly appropriate for older children.

Racko Game
Parker Brothers
CPG Products Corp.
Beverly, MA 01915

This game is appropriate for ages eight and higher. It uses cards and a rack to teach number sequence using increments of five through fifty.

Touch Math
Innovative Learning Concepts
6760 Corporate Dr.
Colorado Springs, CO 80919-1999

This series provides a visual overlay of dots configuring the numerals. It can be used to facilitate computation of all math operations.

## Social

"I Can Behave"
PRO-ED
5341 Industrial Oaks Boulevard
Austin, TX 78735

"I Can Behave" revolves around an illustrated storybook comprising 10 stories and 125 full-page drawings. Each of the 10 stories focuses on a specific classroom dilemma ("My Turn, Your Turn"—letting others talk; "Marvin and His Mouth"—using a quiet voice). Lessons include working independently, waiting for help, doing careful work, handling classroom frustrations, and sitting still.

"Social Skills for Daily Living"
American Guidance Services
Publisher's Building, P.O. Box 99
Circle Pines, MN 55014-1796

A proven, effective method for enhancing the social skills of mildly learning-disabled, mildly emotionally disturbed, and mildly mentally retarded adolescents and young adults aged 12 to 21.

All Feelings Are OK
Face Your Feelings
Center for Applied Psychology, Inc.
P. O. Box 1587
King of Prussia, PA 19406

This unique workbook includes four different Feelings Faces stamps and stamp pad. Opposite each picture children are asked to express their feelings about what is depicted in the picture and to answer follow-up questions about the feeling.

Social Skills Lessons & Activities—Pre-K through High School
The Center for Applied Research in Education
West Nyack, NY 10994

This is a ready-to-use curriculum based on real-life situations to help you build children's self-esteem, self-control, respect for the rights of others, and sense of responsibility for their own actions.

The Social Skills Game
Jessica Kingley Publishers
116 Pentonville Rd.
London, N19JB, England

This lively and exciting therapeutic board game helps children and adolescents who experience difficulties with relationships.

Ups & Downs with Feelings
Carole Gesma
4036 Kerry Court
Minnetonka, MN 55345
(612) 938-9163

This series explores feeling and mood changes in children and adolescents.

### Community Life/Functional Skills

Stepping Out Cues
Attainment Company
P. O. Box 930160
Verona, WI 53593-0160

This series takes instruction out of the classroom and into the community. Thirteen different cues make it possible to learn community skills without requiring academic ability. Users can catch a bus, pay for shoes, and use the telephone directory.

Life Skills Game Series
Cooking Class Game
You Tell Me Game
Community Skills Game
All About You Game
Looking Good Game
Eating Skills Game
Workplace Skills Game
Behavior Skills Game
Life Skill Game
Attainment Copany
P. O. Box 930160
Verona, WI 53593-0160

Eight popular games add to your life skill curriculum and make instruction fun; ideal for school or home.

## Training Institutes

All Kinds of Minds
P.O. Box 3580
Chapel Hill, NC 27515
Phone: (919) 933-8082
Fax: (919) 967-3590
email: AKOMinds@aol.com
web page: http://www.allkindsofminds.org/

## Books

D. F. Brackley, M. E. King-Sears, and D. Tessier-Switlick (1997). *Teaching Students in Inclusive Settings: From Theory to Practice.* Allyn & Bacon, Longwood Division

L. J. Meltzer, et al. *Strategies for Success, Classroom Teaching Techniques for Students with Learning Problems.* Austin, Tex.: Pro Ed publishers

## Product Information for Pragmatic Language Training

Academic Communication Associates
Publications Division, Dept. 83-C
4149 Avenida de la Plata
P.O. Box 586249
Oceanside, CA 92058
    Knowing What to Say!
    Talking on Purpose!
    Conversation Express
    Situation Communication (SITCOM)
    Pragmatic Language Intervention Resource


Communication Skills Builders
3830 E. Bellevue/P.O. Box 42050-E93
Tucson, AZ 85733
    Building Functional Social Skills, Group Activities for Adults
    INTERACT, A Social Skills Game
    A Sourcebook of Pragmatic Activities (Revised)
    A Sourcebook of Adolescent Pragmatic Activities
    Pragmatic Activities for Language Intervention
    Tackling Teen Topics
    Pragmatic-Language Trivia Junior

DLM
1 DLM Park
Allen, TX 75002
    CONVERSATIONS; Language Intervention for Adolescents
    Talk about It
    STARTLINE, Social Education/Communication


LinguiSystems
3100 4th Avenue
P.O. Box 747
East Moline, IL 61244
    Life Skills Workshop
    On My Own with Language
    Communication Workshop
    RAPP (Resource of Activities for Peer Pragmatics)
    Room 14, A Social Language Program
    FriendZee, A Social Skills Game


PRO-ED
8700 Shoal Creek Boulevard
Austin, TX 78758
    PALS: Pragmatic Activities in Language and Speech
    BEING ME: A Social/Sexual Training Program
    Teaching the Moderately and Severely Handicapped, Vol II: Communica-
        tion & Socialization (2d Ed)
    The Walker Social Skills Curriculum
    The ACCEPTS Program: A Curriculum for Children's Effective Peer and
        Teacher Skills
    The ACCESS Program: Adolescent Curriculum for Communication and Ef-
        fective Social Skills
    Peer Interaction Skills
    Talking, Listening, Communicating


The Psychological Corporation
555 Academic Ct.
San Antonio, IX 78204
    Conversation Connections: A Whole Language Preschool Program
    Let's Talk: for Children (LTC)
    Let's Talk: for Intermediate Level
    Let's Talk: for Developing Prosocial Communication Skills

The Reverside Publishing Co.
8420 Bryn Mawr Ave.
Chicago, IL 60631
SMALL TALK: Creating Conversation with Young Children

Thinking Publications
1713 Westgate Rd
P.O. Box 163
Eau Claire, WI 54702
Scripting: Social Communication for Adolescents
Skillstreaming the Adolescent
Skillstreaming the Elementary School Child
Skillstreaming in Early Childhood
Daily Communication
Communicate (game)
Communicate Junior (game)
Social Skill Strategies
SOCIAL STAR, General Interaction Skills

## Resources on the World Wide Web

Point your world wide web browser to the addresses below to discover many helpful educational tools and products offered via the Internet.

### *Assistive Technology*

| | |
|---|---|
| http://www.amdi.net/default.htm | AMDi Home Page |
| http://www.sentient-sys.com/ | DynaVox |
| http://www.greattalkingbox.com/ | Great Talking Box |
| http://www.independentliving.com/ | Independent Living Aids |
| http://www.maxiaids.com/ | Maxi-Aids |
| http://www.prentrom.com/index.html | PRC |
| http://www.sammonspreston.com/ | Sammons Preston |
| http://www.saltillo.com/ | Saltillo |
| http://www.words-plus.com/ | Words+ |

### *Computer Software and Peripherals*

| | |
|---|---|
| http://www.ablenetinc.com/ | AbleNet |
| http://attainment-inc.com/ | Attainment, Inc |
| http://www.donjohnston.com/ | Don Johnston |
| http://www.dkonlinestore.co.uk/us/ | Dorling Kindersley |
| http://www.dragonsys.com/ | Dragon |
| http://www.edmark.com/ | Edmark |

| | |
|---|---|
| http://www.hminet.com/ | Houghton Mifflin Interactive |
| http://www.intellitools.com/ | IntelliTools |
| http://www.kensington.com/ | Kensington |
| http://www.madenta.com/ | Madentec |
| http://www.mayer-johnson.com/ | Mayer-Johnson |
| http://www.tiac.net/users/poorrich/ | Poor Richards |
| http://www.slatersoftware.com/ | Slater |

### General Information and References

| | |
|---|---|
| http://www.abledata.com/ | ABLEDATA |
| http://www.iltech.org/catalog.htm | AT Catalog List |
| http://www.ataccess.org/ | ATA |
| http://www.atia.org/members.html | ATIA |
| http://www.cast.org/ | CAST |
| http://www.c-cad.org/ | C-CAD |
| http://www.itpolicy.gsa.gov/cita/ | CITA |
| http://www.csun.edu/cod/ | CSUN |
| http://www.closingthegap.com/ | CTG |
| http://www.dooronline.org/ | dooronline |
| http://www.fragilex.com/home.html | Fragile X |
| http://www.thegateway.org/ | Gateway |
| http://jg.cso.uiuc.edu/PG/welcome.html | Project Gutenberg |
| http://www.ideapractices.org/ | IDEA |
| http://yuri.org/isaac/isaac/index.html | ISAAC |
| http://www.ldresources.com/ | LD Resources |
| http://mindinstitute.ucdmc.ucdavis.edu/ | MIND |
| http://www.ed.gov/offices/OSERS/ | OSERS |
| http://www2.edc.org/NCIP/ | NCIP |
| http://www.nichcy.org/ | NICHY |
| http://www.sonic.net/nilp/ | NILP |
| http://www.resna.org/ | RESNA |
| http://www.stw.ed.gov/ | School to Work Council |
| http://trace.wisc.edu/ | Trace |

# APPENDIX 4

# Toilet Training the Child with Fragile X Syndrome

Franci Crepeau-Hobson and Rebecca O'Connor, M.A.

Clinical interviews with hundreds of parents of children with fragile X syndrome report that it takes longer than usual to toilet train the child with fragile X syndrome. The majority of families report that the process used is generally the same as that used with their other children. More support, reminders, practice, and patience are required. Few families report the need to engage in more formal or aversive techniques for training. The length of time it takes a child to learn generally depends on the child's developmental level or understanding, awareness of their body and sensations, and the degree of motoric or muscular difficulties.

Toilet training a child with fragile X syndrome requires a number of behaviors and abilities to be in place. The child needs to be able to physically perceive that he is wet and to communicate this. He needs to have significant periods of dryness (about two hours) and have a fairly regular time for voiding or bowel movements. He also needs the motor skills and muscle tone to get to the bathroom and to sit on the toilet unassisted. Eventually he needs to be able to coordinate the entire process of feeling the need to go, getting to the bathroom, sitting down (or standing up for some boys), and actually going. All of this requires appropriate timing as well.

If your child is lacking in one or more of these areas, toilet training will be even more challenging. It may require focus on training the child to go rather than on training him to *not* go. It will therefore be important for your child to be on a frequent toileting schedule, where he will have many opportunities to go.

The following should be considered as only guidelines and suggestions for toilet training your child. It is not intended to be a cookbook recipe that can be expected to be successful with all children. Every child is unique, including every child with fragile X syndrome. There is a wide range of variability when children with fragile X will be toilet trained. Not starting prematurely and being consistent can help cut down on frustration. In general, a relaxed approach works best.

Toilet training the child with fragile X syndrome often, though not always, takes the same form as it does with other children and involves teaching about the potty and what it's for. You may also need to teach your child about "wet" and "dry." When you check your child's diaper, let him know what you find. For example, if he's dry, say, "Good. Your pants are dry." You may also want to place his hand inside the diaper to feel that it is dry. If the child is wet, let him know this as well, and again allow him to feel what wet is. The "pretraining" can begin around age two and may also include allowing your child to watch other family members use the toilet so that he can see firsthand how it is supposed to work. This is also a good time to read books about toilet training and diapers to your child or watch potty training videos together. (Learning through Entertainment released a good video entitled "PottyTime." 1-800-23-POTTY). Once your child has an understanding of the potty, toilet training then shifts to establishing a baseline of your child's toileting behaviors.

It is generally easiest to start with bowel training. Keep a schedule of your child's elimination pattern to determine appropriate toileting times. Once you have a good idea of your child's pattern, begin placing your child on the toilet around the time he usually has a bowel movement. If your child has low muscle tone, a footstool or a small potty chair may help your child feel more secure. Encourage your child to move his bowels and leave him there for about 10 minutes. After this time period, help him off the toilet and praise him for trying and/ or succeeding. Continue this as a consistent pattern until bowel continence is achieved.

Urinary training can be started after bowel training is established. Use another record of elimination to determine when to place your child on the potty. At this point, you may want to put your child in training pants during the day. Using the elimination schedule, place your child periodically on the potty, being sure that enough time has elapsed so that he can feel the sensation of a full bladder. After 5 to 10 minutes, remove the child and praise him, regardless of whether or not he actually went in the toilet. Sometimes water-prompting can help relax the child's external sphincter muscle, which initiates urination. This involves slowly pouring a small amount of lukewarm water over the child's genitalia immediately after sitting the child on the toilet. Parents can begin to tell their children to go to the bathroom rather than actually placing them there. With increasing success, parents can begin to wait for the child to signal that he wants to go to the potty.

Nighttime toilet training should not begin until day training has been established. It is often helpful to reduce the child's fluid intake before bedtime to help him have more control. Begin by waking the child one or two times a night (depending on the child's nighttime elimination pattern) and have him sit for five minutes on the toilet each time. Remember to praise and encourage your child each time. Eventually, many children begin awakening by themselves when they need to go and begin to take care of nighttime toileting themselves.

Keep in mind that it is normal for any child, including those with fragile X syndrome, to regress or seem to lose toileting skills at times. Treat accidents lightly and remember that this is a process that cannot be rushed. Pushing a child who is not developmentally ready for toilet training may actually slow or completely disrupt the process. Forcing, scolding, or punishing a child into toilet training may only frighten the child and reduce the likelihood of toilet training success. Remember, patience, praise, and consistency are the keys to reaching this goal.

## Toilet Training Resources for Parents

### Books

Azrin, N. H., and R. M. Foxx. 1974. *Toilet training in less than one day.* New York: Pocketbook.

Baker, B. L., A. J. Brightman, J. B. Blacher, L. J. Heifetz, S. P. Hinshaw, and D. M. Murphy. 1989. *Steps to independence: A skills training guide for parents and teachers of children with special needs.* 2d ed. Baltimore: H. Brookes.

Clark, L. 1985. *SOS! Help for parents.* Bowling Green: Parents Press.

Foxx, R. M., and N. H. Azrin. 1973. *Toilet training persons with developmental disabilities: A rapid program for day and nighttime independent toileting.* Champagne: Research Press.

Linde, T. F., and T. Kopp. 1973. *Training retarded babies and preschoolers.* Springfield: Charles C. Thompson Publishing.

Mack, A. 1978. *Toilet learning: The picture book technique for children and parents.* Boston: Little, Brown & Company.

Smith, R. 1993. *Children with mental retardation: A parent's guide.* Rockville: Woodbine House.

Wilson, R. 1995. Generic habit-training program. *Autistic Behav.* 10:1–8.

### Video

Learning through Entertainment. 1990. *PottyTime.* Distributed by Video Distributors. (For information, call 1-800-23POTTY.)

# INDEX

504 plan, 462

L-Acetylcarnitine 303
Activation ratio 3, 6, 10, 118, 206, 210,
  226, 227, 234, 254, 467, 473
Adaptive functioning 217, 364–365
Adderall 55, 74, 301–303
Adenoviruses 476, 477
Adolescence 293–296
Adoption 268
AGG interruptions 236; influence on
  repeat stability 124; polarity 124
Aggression 68, 69, 294–296, 305,
  309–315, 343, 349, 350, 413, 450
Agoraphobia 341, 359
Alcoholism 39
Alleles: amplification of expanded 119;
  full mutation 465
Amantidine (Symmetrel) 303–304, 314
Amblyopia 18–19
Ampakines 318–319
Amyotrophic lateral sclerosis (ALS) 43
Antibody test, FMRP 178
Anticipation 115, 128, 152
Anticonvulsants: carbamazepine 40–
  43, 296–298, 309, 313; phenytoin
  (Dilantin) 40–41, 299–300, 308;
  valproic acid (Depakote) 68, 298–
  299, 309, 312–313
Anxiety 50, 54–57, 63–64, 72, 73,
  259, 260, 271, 290, 305, 309–313,
  316, 339, 341, 342, 350, 351, 355–
  359, 369, 370, 380, 388, 404, 413,
  431, 433, 436, 450–451, 453, 457–
  460, 466
Anxiolytic medications: buspirone
  (Buspar) 305, 358; clonazepam 314
Apnea 20, 35, 288

Applied behavioral analysis (ABA)
  403–404
Arthrodesis 21
Articulation 219, 290
Artificial yeast. *See* Yeast artificial
  chromosome
Ascertainment bias 209, 211
Asperger syndrome 5, 73, 76
Assistive technology 396–402
Ataxia 4, 35–40
Atkin syndrome 76
Attention deficit hyperactivity disorder
  (ADHD) 20, 55–57, 65, 71, 74, 210,
  224, 239, 260, 291–294, 300–309,
  311, 317, 341, 459–460; hyperactiv-
  ity 3, 27, 53–57, 68, 73, 76, 77, 236,
  260, 292–293, 300–309, 415, 450;
  pharmacotherapy 296–319
Atypical antipsychotics 313–316;
  olanzepine 314, 358; quetiapine 68,
  314–315; risperidone 68, 313–314
Augmentative and assistive communication (AAC) 392–393
Autism 3–4, 20, 49, 51, 57–63, 64, 66,
  68, 76, 207, 210, 214, 220, 221, 239,
  290, 291, 298, 305, 313, 342, 368,
  377, 402–404, 414; ADI-R 61;
  ADOS-G 61; CARS 60, 63; females
  63
Autonomic system 55–56
Autopsy 23–24
azadC (5-aza) 474

Bacterial endocarditis, subacute (SBE)
  293
Bedwetting (enuresis) 293
Behavior management 292, 344–351,
  357, 439, 451–457